Essentials of Neuropsychiatry and Clinical Neurosciences

Essentials of Neuropsychiatry and Clinical Neurosciences

Edited by

Stuart C. Yudofsky, M.D.

D.C. and Irene Ellwood Professor and Chairman,
Menninger Department of Psychiatry and Behavioral Sciences,
Baylor College of Medicine; Chief, Psychiatry Service,
The Methodist Hospital, Houston, Texas

Robert E. Hales, M.D., M.B.A.

Joe P. Tupin Professor and Chair,
Department of Psychiatry and Behavioral Sciences,
University of California, Davis School of Medicine;
Medical Director, Sacramento County Mental Health Services,
Sacramento, California

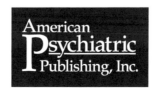

American Psychiatric Publishing, Inc.
Washington, DC
London, England

Copyright © 2004 American Psychiatric Publishing, Inc.
ALL RIGHTS RESERVED

Manufactured in the United States of America on acid-free paper

07 06 05 04 03   5 4 3 2 1

Typeset in Adobe's Revival and Formata

About the cover image:

The brain image on the front cover is from the SPL/NSL Brain Browser, a project developed by members of the Surgical Planning Laboratory (SPL), MRI Division, Department of Radiology, Brigham and Women's Hospital, Harvard Medical School; by members of the Clinical Neuroscience Division, Laboratory of Neuroscience, Department of Psychiatry, VAMC-Brockton, Harvard Medical School; and by collaborators from the Artificial Intelligence Laboratory of MIT. The Brain Browser and the expanded Anatomy Browser allow highly detailed, hierarchical representations of human anatomy to be viewed on ordinary computers. More information about the SPL/NSL Anatomy Browser can be found at http://www.spl.harvard.edu:8000/pages/papers/Anatomy Browser/current/index.html.

The work was supported in part by grants from the National Institutes of Health and National Institute of Mental Health to M.E. Shenton, R.W. McCarley, R. Kikinis, and F.A. Jolesz. The image is used with permission from Harvard University.

Special thanks to Katherine Taber, Ph.D., and Robin A. Hurley, M.D., for their help selecting the image.

American Psychiatric Publishing, Inc.
1000 Wilson Boulevard
Arlington, VA 22209-3901
www.appi.org

Library of Congress Cataloging-in-Publication Data
Essentials of neuropsychiatry and clincial neurosciences / edited by Stuart C. Yudofsky, Robert E. Hales.
   p. ; cm.
Includes bibliographical references and index.
ISBN 158562005X (alk. paper)
  1. Neuropsychiatry. I. Yudofsky, Stuart C. II. Hales, Robert E. III. American Psychiatric Publishing textbook of neuropsychiatry and clinical neurosciences. 4th ed.
  [DNLM: 1. Mental Disorders. 2. Nervous System Diseases. 3. Neuropsychology. WM 140 E785 2004]
RC341.E84 2004
616.8–dc21

2002043672

British Library Cataloguing in Publication Data
A CIP record is available from the British Library.

Dedicated to

Ethel Spector Person, M.D.

masterful clinician,

inspiring educator,

and

gifted theoretician and author

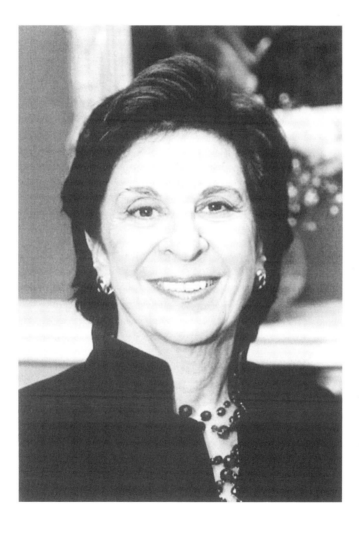

Modern-day pioneer

of the

integration of psychoanalytic theory and psychodynamic treatments

into contemporary medicine and neuropsychiatry

Contents

PART I

Neuropsychiatric Assessment

PART II

Neuropsychiatric Symptomatologies

PART III

Neuropsychiatric Disorders

PART IV

Neuropsychiatric Treatments

Contributors

Susan L. Andersen, Ph.D.
Assistant Professor, Department of Psychiatry, Harvard Medical School, Developmental Biopsychiatry Research Program and Laboratory of Developmental Psychopharmacology, McLean Hospital, Belmont, Massachusetts

Sylvia Askin-Edgar, M.D, Ph.D.
Instructor, Department of Neurology, University of California at Los Angeles School of Medicine, Los Angeles, California

Stephen K. Brannan, M.D.
Medical Director, Clinical and Medical Affairs, Cyberonics, Inc., Houston, Texas

Jeffrey L. Cummings, M.D.
Professor, Departments of Neurology and Psychiatry and Biobehavioral Sciences; Director, UCLA Alzheimer's Disease Center, University of California at Los Angeles School of Medicine, Los Angeles, California

Michael D. Franzen, Ph.D.
Associate Professor of Psychiatry (Psychology), Medical College of Pennsylvania Hahnemann University; Chief, Section of Psychology and Neuropsychology, Allegheny General Hospital, Pittsburgh, Pennsylvania

Kenneth L. Goetz, M.D.
Associate Professor of Psychiatry, Department of Psychiatry, Drexel University College of Medicine, Philadelphia, Pennsylvania

Robert E. Hales, M.D., M.B.A.
Joe P. Tupin Professor and Chair, Department of Psychiatry and Behavioral Sciences, University of California, Davis School of Medicine; Medical Director, Sacramento County Mental Health Services, Sacramento, California

L. Anne Hayman, M.D.
Research Fellow, Visual Explanations Laboratory, School of Health Information Sciences, University of Texas Health Science Center, Houston, Texas

Max Hirshkowitz, Ph.D., A.B.S.M.
Associate Professor, Menninger Department of Psychiatry and Department of Medicine, Baylor College of Medicine; Director, Houston VAMC Sleep Research Center, Houston, Texas

Diane B. Howieson, Ph.D.
Associate Professor of Neurology and Psychiatry, Oregon Health & Science University, Portland, Oregon

Frans J. Hugo, M.B.Ch.B., M.Med.(Psych.)
Neuropsychiatry Unit, Department of Psychiatry, University of Stellenbosch, Cape Town, South Africa

Robin A. Hurley, M.D.
Associate Chief of Mental Health, Salisbury Veterans Affairs Medical Center, Salisbury, North Carolina; Associate Professor, Menninger Department of Psychiatry and Behavioral Sciences, Department of Radiology, Baylor College of Medicine, Houston, Texas

Michelle Keightley, M.A.
Ph.D. candidate, Department of Psychology, University of Toronto, Toronto, Ontario, Canada

Dennis Kim, M.D.
Instructor, Department of Psychiatry, Harvard Medical School, Developmental Biopsychiatry Research Program and Clinical Evaluation Center, McLean Hospital, Belmont, Massachusetts

Kathryn J. Kotrla, M.D.
Associate Professor and Chair, Department of Psychiatry and Behavioral Sciences, Texas A&M University Health Science Center, College of Medicine; Medical Director, Mental Health & Behavioral Medicine, Central Texas Veterans Health Care System, Temple, Texas

Muriel D. Lezak, Ph.D.
Professor of Neurology and Psychiatry, Oregon Health & Science University, Portland, Oregon

Mark R. Lovell, Ph.D.
Assistant Professor of Orthopedics and Director, UPMC Sports Medicine Concussion Program, University of Pittsburgh School of Medicine, Pittsburgh, Pennsylvania

Roderick K. Mahurin, Ph.D.
Clinical Associate Professor, Department of Psychiatry and Behavioral Sciences; Research Scientist, Department of Neurology, University of Washington, Seattle, Washington

Helen S. Mayberg, M.D.
Professor of Psychiatry and Medicine (Neurology), Sandra Rotman Chair in Neuropsychiatry, Rotman Research Institute, University of Toronto, Toronto, Ontario, Canada

David J. Meagher, M.D., M.R.C.Psych., M.Sc. (Neuroscience)
Consultant Psychiatrist and Clinical Research Tutor, Midwestern Health Board, Limerick, Ireland

Deborah R. Medoff, Ph.D.
Assistant Professor, Schizophrenia-Related Disorders Program, Maryland Psychiatric Research Center, University of Maryland School of Medicine, Baltimore, Maryland

Mario F. Mendez, M.D., Ph.D.
Professor of Neurology and Psychiatry and Biobehavioral Sciences, University of California at Los Angeles School of Medicine; Director, Neurobehavior Unit, West Los Angeles Veterans Affairs Medical Center, Los Angeles, California

Carryl P. Navalta, Ph.D.
Instructor, Department of Psychiatry, Harvard Medical School, Developmental Biopsychiatry Research Program and Child Outpatient Services, McLean Hospital, Belmont, Massachusetts

Eric J. Nestler, M.D., Ph.D.
Lou and Ellen McGinley Distinguished Professor and Chair, Department of Psychiatry, The University of Texas Southwestern Medical Center, Dallas, Texas

Fred Ovsiew, M.D.
Associate Professor of Psychiatry; Chief, Clinical Neuropsychiatry; Medical Director, Adult Inpatient Psychiatry, University of Chicago Hospitals, Chicago, Illinois

James C. Patterson II, M.D., Ph.D.
Assistant Professor, Department of Psychiatry; Director, PET Neuroimaging Research, Biomedical Research Institute PET Imaging Center, Louisiana State University Health Sciences Center, Shreveport, Louisiana

Ann Polcari, Ph.D., R.N.
Research Associate, Developmental Biopsychiatry Research Program, McLean Hospital, Belmont, Massachusetts

Trevor R.P. Price, M.D.
Private practice of neuropsychiatry, geriatric psychiatry, and general adult psychiatry, Bryn Mawr, Pennsylvania

Robert G. Robinson, M.D.
Professor and Head, Department of Psychiatry, University of Iowa, Roy J. and Lucille A. Carver College of Medicine, Iowa City, Iowa

Peter P. Roy-Byrne, M.D.
Professor and Vice Chair, Department of Psychiatry and Behavioral Sciences, University of Washington School of Medicine; Chief of Psychiatry, Harborview Medical Center, Seattle, Washington

Harold A. Sackeim, Ph.D.
Professor of Clinical Psychology in Psychiatry and Radiology, College of Physicians and Surgeons of Columbia University; Chief, Department of Biological Psychiatry, New York State Psychiatric Institute, New York, New York

David W. Self, Ph.D.
Lydia Bryant Test Associate Professor, Department of Psychiatry, The University of Texas Southwestern Medical Center, Dallas, Texas

Jonathan M. Silver, M.D.
Clinical Professor of Psychiatry, New York University School of Medicine; Assistant Chair for Clinical Services and Research, Department of Psychiatry, Lenox Hill Hospital, New York, New York

Sergio E. Starkstein, M.D., Ph.D.
Associate Professor, Department of Psychiatry and Clinical Neurosciences, University of Western Australia, Fremantle Hospital, Fremantle, Australia

Dan J. Stein, M.D., Ph.D.
Director, Medical Research Council Unit on Anxiety Disorders, Department of Psychiatry, University of Stellenbosch, Cape Town, South Africa, and University of Florida, Gainesville, Florida

Yaakov Stern, Ph.D.
Professor of Clinical Neuropsychology in Neurology, Psychiatry, and Sergievsky Center, College of Physicians and Surgeons of Columbia University; Director of Neuropsychology, Memory Disorders Clinic, Department of Biological Psychiatry, New York State Psychiatric Institute, New York, New York

Katherine H. Taber, Ph.D.
Research Fellow, Visual Explanations Laboratory, School of Health Information Sciences, University of Texas Health Science Center, Houston, Texas

Carol A. Tamminga, M.D.
Professor of Psychiatry and Communities Foundation of Texas Chair in Brain Science, The University of Texas Southwestern Medical Center, Dallas, Texas

Martin H. Teicher, M.D., Ph.D.
Associate Professor, Department of Psychiatry, Harvard Medical School, Developmental Biopsychiatry Research Program and Laboratory of Developmental Psychopharmacology, McLean Hospital, Belmont, Massachusetts

Gunvant K. Thaker, M.D.
Professor of Psychiatry, University of Maryland School of Medicine; Chief, Functional Neuroimaging Laboratory, Maryland Psychiatric Research Center, Baltimore, Maryland

Paula T. Trzepacz, M.D.
Clinical Professor of Psychiatry and Neurology, University of Mississippi Medical School, Jackson, Mississippi; Adjunct Professor of Psychiatry, Tufts University Medical School, Boston, Massachusetts; and Lilly Research Laboratories, Indianapolis, Indiana

Gary J. Tucker, M.D.
Professor Emeritus, Department of Psychiatry and Behavioral Sciences, University of Washington, Seattle, Washington

Mahendra Upadhyaya, M.D.
Director of Geriatric Psychiatry Services, Covenant Health System, Lubbock, Texas

Katherine E. White, M.D.
Assistant Clinical Professor, Departments of Neurology and Psychiatry and Biobehavioral Sciences, University of California at Los Angeles School of Medicine, Los Angeles, California

Michael G. Wise, M.D.
Clinical Professor of Psychiatry, University of California, Davis; Adjunct Professor of Psychiatry, Uniformed Services University of the Health Sciences, F. Edward Hebert School of Medicine, Bethesda, Maryland

Stuart C. Yudofsky, M.D.
D.C. and Irene Ellwood Professor and Chairman, Menninger Department of Psychiatry and Behavioral Sciences, Baylor College of Medicine; Chief, Psychiatry Service, The Methodist Hospital, Houston, Texas

Neuropsychiatric Assessment

CHAPTER 1

Bedside Neuropsychiatry

Eliciting the Clinical Phenomena of Neuropsychiatric Illness

Fred Ovsiew, M.D.

> Unless we take pains to be accurate in our examinations as to the question propounded, our observations will be of little value. The investigator who simply asks leading questions…is not accumulating "facts," but is "organising confusion." He will make errors enough without adopting a clumsy plan of investigating which renders blundering certain.
>
> —*John Hughlings-Jackson (1880/1881)*

In this chapter, I aim to provide the neuropsychiatric clinician with a method for data gathering at the bedside. To this end, I review the tools offered by history taking and examination for discovering the contribution of cerebral dysfunction to psychological abnormality and behavioral disturbance.

In neuropsychiatry, attention to cerebral organization must not be matched by neglect of psychosocial variables, for these may have substantial impact on symptom expression, impairment, and disability. Thus, the naturalistic clinical examination cannot lose its relevance, even in the era of brain imaging and cognitive neuropsychology. Ideally, the clinical approach will be guided by the best available understanding of the fundamental principles of brain organization, but the rubrics provided below cannot be claimed as such elementary modules of cognition and behavior.

Taking the History

Obtaining a history is an active process on the part of the interviewer, who must have in mind a matrix to be filled in with information. The excuse "the patient is a poor historian" has no place in neuropsychiatry. The examiner must realize that it is he or she, and not the patient, who is the "historian," responsible for gathering information from all necessary sources and forming a coherent narrative. Discovering that the patient is unable to give an adequate account of his or her life and illness should prompt, first, a search for other informants and, second, a search for an explanation of the incapacity.

Birth

Maternal illness in pregnancy and the process of labor and delivery must be reviewed for untoward events associated with fetal maldevelopment, including bleeding and substance abuse during pregnancy, the course of labor, and fetal distress at birth and in the immediate postnatal period. Obstetric complications are associated with schizophrenia (Cannon et al. 2000; McNeil et al. 2000; Rosso et al. 2000b) and perhaps with mood disorder (Kinney et al. 1993a; Preti et al. 2000) and other psychiatric conditions (Capstick and Seldrup 1977; Raine et al. 1994; Schachar 1991).

Development

At times, the historian can gather information from the first minutes of extrauterine life, for example, when Apgar scores are available in hospital records. More commonly, parental recollection of milestones must be relied on. The ages at which the child crawled, walked, spoke words, spoke sentences, went to school, and so on can often be elicited from parents. Parents may be able to compare the patient with a "control" sibling. The infant's temperament—shy, active, cuddly, fussy, and so on—may give clues to persisting traits. School performance is an important marker of both the intellectual and the social competence of the child and often is the only information available about premorbid intellectual level. Childhood illness, including febrile convulsions, head injury, and central nervous system infection, is sometimes the precursor of adult neuropsychiatric disorder.

Handedness

The simplest and most obvious indicator of cerebral dominance is handedness. A few inquiries—asking the patient which hand he or she uses to write, throw, draw, and use a scissors or toothbrush—serve well to establish handedness (Bryden 1977). With some nonverbal patients (e.g., the severely mentally retarded), watching the patient catch a thrown ball or crumpled piece of paper is a simple examination for handedness.

Ictal Events

The clinician must be concerned with the phases of the paroxysm, starting with the prodrome, then the aura, then the remainder of the ictus (the aura being the onset or core of the ictus), then the aftermath. For any attack disorder, how frequent and how stereotyped the events are must be determined. Rapidity of onset and cessation; disturbance of consciousness or of language; occurrence of autochthonous sensations, ideas, and emotions and of lateralized motor or cognitive dysfunction; purposefulness and coordination of actions; memory for the spell; and duration of the recovery period must be ascertained. Beginning an inquiry about seizures by asking if the patient has just one sort of spell or more than one reduces confusion as history taking proceeds with a patient who has both partial and generalized seizures. Some patients with pseudoseizures will say that they have epileptic spells and then another sort that happens when they are upset.

Some of the abnormal experiences well known in temporal lobe epilepsy—the "elaborate" mental state described by Hughlings-Jackson (Bancaud et al. 1994; Gloor et al. 1982)—occur in mood disorders and in other psychiatric states as a putative marker of limbic dysfunction (Ardila et al. 1993; Atre-Vaidya et al. 1994; Persinger and Makarec 1993; Roberts et al. 1990; Silberman et al. 1985, 1994; Teicher et al. 1993). The phenomena can be elicited by questions about déjà vu and *jamais vu*, episodic sensory experiences such as visual illusions, paranormal experiences such as clairvoyance, and other paroxysmal experiences.

Head Injury

The length of the anterograde amnesia, from the moment of trauma to the recovery of the capacity for consecutive memory, can be learned either from the patient or from hospital records. The patient can say what the last memories before the accident are; from last memory to injury is the period of retrograde amnesia. The lengths of these intervals and the duration of coma are correlated with the severity of brain damage (Lishman 1998). Usually, posttraumatic amnesia is the best indicator.

Mild Cognitive Impairment

One commonly encounters patients with mild, chronic, stable, global cognitive disturbance not meeting the criteria for a diagnosis of dementia; the most frequent condition giving rise to this state is traumatic brain injury (Alexander 1995; Gutierrez et al. 1993, 1994). Lezak (1978) emphasized the patient's experience of perplexity, distractibility, and fatigue in mild and severe brain injury. In my experience, some cognitive symptoms reported by patients are so characteristic that they are nearly diagnostic of organic illness. Other features, such as emotional lability and irritability, are characteristic of, but less specific to, organic states.

The loss of the capacity for divided attention is highly characteristic of mild cerebral disease. Distractibility is heightened, and automatic tasks require attention and effort.

Appetitive Functions

Appetitive functions include sleep, eating, and sexual interest and performance. Disturbed sleep is common in patients with psychiatric disorders of any origin and in the general population as well. In a search for clues to organic factors in psychiatric illness, the clinician inquires about the pattern of disturbance: early waking in depressive illness, nighttime wakings related to pain or nocturnal myoclonus, excessive daytime sleepiness in narcolepsy and sleep apnea, sleep attacks in narcolepsy, and periodic excessive somnolence in Kleine-Levin syndrome and related disorders. Simple observation of a hospitalized patient by night nursing staff, or at home by family members, can reveal apneas or abnormal movements. Patterns of abnormal eating behavior can be recognized beyond the anorexia of depressive illness and food-avoidance in anorexia nervosa: the hyperphagia of hypothalamic disease, in which food exerts an irresistible attraction; the mouthing and eating of nonfood objects in bilateral amygdalar disease (part of the Klüver-Bucy syndrome); and the impulsive stuffing of food into the mouth irrespective of hunger in frontal disease (Mendez et al. 1995; G. Smith et al. 1998).

Sexual interest and performance are commonly disturbed in brain disease. Helping a patient discuss these matters can be a great relief to the patient. Hyposexuality seems to be a feature of epilepsy, although its mechanism is controversial (Morrell et al. 1994; Toone et al. 1989). A change in a person's habitual sexual interests, either quantitative or qualitative, occurring de novo in adult life, suggests organic disease (Cummings 1999).

Aggression

Features of aggressive behavior such as its onset and cessation; the patient's mental state and especially clarity of consciousness during the violent period; the patient's capacity for planned, coordinated, and well-organized action as displayed in the act; the patient's regret, or otherwise, afterward; and any associated symptoms may yield clues about the contribution of cerebral dysfunction to the behavior.

Personality Change

Persisting alterations in or exaggerations of personality traits, if not related to an abnormal mood state or psychosis, may be important indicators of the development of cerebral disease. Lability and shallowness of emotion, irritability, aggressiveness, loss of sense of humor, and coarsening of the sensibilities are often mentioned.

A particular set of personality traits is said to be distinctive in temporal lobe epilepsy, including mystical or religious interests, "humorless sobriety," tendency toward rage, interpersonal stickiness or "viscosity," and hyposexuality. Whether these traits are related to epilepsy, to the temporal lobe injury underlying epilepsy, or merely to psychopathology remains controversial (Bear et al. 1989).

Occupation

Exposures to heavy metals or volatile hydrocarbons and repeated blows to the head in boxers are examples of occupational causes of neuropsychiatric illness. Apart from etiological information, the clinician needs to know about the patient's work in order to gauge premorbid capacities and to assess disability.

Family History

Inquiring about the family history of neuropsychiatric illness relative by relative, even constructing a family tree with the assistance of collateral informants, is more revealing than asking questions such as "Is there any mental illness in the family?"

Examining the Patient

Asymmetry and Minor Physical Anomalies

Abnormal development of a hemisphere may be betrayed by slight differences in the size of the thumbs or thumbnails. A postcentral location of cortical lesions causing asymmetry is characteristic (Penfield and Robertson 1943). A small hemiface or hemicranium is usually ipsilateral to an epileptic focus (Tinuper et al. 1992).

Other physical anomalies are stable through childhood and give clues to abnormal neurodevelopment even in adulthood. The Waldrop scale is in common use (Table 1–1), but minor anomalies not included in that scale may be relevant (Ismail et al. 1998a). They may occur in healthy individuals, and no individual anomaly, except perhaps abnormal head circumference (Lainhart et al. 1997; Steg and Rapoport 1975), has a correlation with psychopathology. The deviant development can be traced to the first four months of fetal life, and either genetic or environmental factors can give rise to the disturbance of gestation (McNeil et al. 2000). Presumably, the relationship of the anomalies to the brain disorder lies in a disturbance of contemporaneous cerebral development.

Such anomalies are associated with schizophrenia (McNeil et al. 2000), even late-onset schizophrenia (Lohr et al. 1997). They may also be associated with mood disorder (Lohr et al. 1997), as well

TABLE 1–1. Waldrop scale of minor physical anomalies

Head
  Head circumference outside the normal range[a]
  Fine, "electric" hair that will not comb down
  More than one hair whorl
  Abnormal epicanthal folds of the eyes
  Hypertelorism or hypotelorism
  Low-set ears (entirely below the plane of the pupils)
  Malformed or asymmetrical ears
  High palate
  Furrowed tongue
Hands and feet
  Curved fifth finger (clinodactyly)
  Single palmar crease
  Wide gap between first and second toes
  Partial syndactyly of the toes
  Third toe longer than second

[a]The normal range of head circumference in adults is governed by a complex relation to height, weight, and sex. Roughly, for males the range is 54–60 cm (21.25–23.5 inches) and for females, 52–58 cm (20.5–22.75 inches) (Bushby et al. 1992).

as tardive dyskinesia (Waddington et al. 1995), autism (Gualtieri et al. 1982; Steg and Rapoport 1975), schizotypal personality disorder (Weinstein et al. 1999), violent delinquency in boys (Arseneault et al. 2000) and perhaps inhibited behavior in girls (Fogel et al. 1985), and violent behavior in criminals (Kandel et al. 1989). Thus they are best regarded as a nonspecific indicator of abnormal neurodevelopment (Ismail et al. 2000; Tarrant and Jones 1999), maldevelopment that may interact with psychosocial factors in the genesis of psychopathology (Pine et al. 1997). Dysmorphic features in a mentally retarded patient should lead to investigations to identify the cause of the retardation (Ryan and Sunada 1997).

Olfaction

Hyposmia or anosmia can be detected in Alzheimer's disease, Parkinson's disease, normal aging, schizophrenia, multiple sclerosis, subfrontal tumor, human immunodeficiency virus (HIV) infection, migraine, and traumatic brain injury (Brody et al. 1991; Eslinger et al. 1982; Harrison and Pearson 1989; Hirsch 1992; Kopala et al. 1994; Pinching 1977). The most common cause of hyposmia, however, is local disease of the nasal mucosa, and the examiner must exclude local disease before regarding the finding as having neuropsychiatric significance.

Stimuli that cause trigeminal irritation (e.g., ammonia) are not suitable. Floral and musk odors provide the greatest sensitivity. I use raspberry and cherry scented lip balm to test for olfactory defects.

Eyes

Dilated pupils associated with anticholinergic toxicity may be a clue to the cause of delirium, and small pupils associated with opiate intoxication may be a clue to substance abuse. Argyll Robertson pupils—bilaterally small, irregular, and reactive to accommodation but not to light—characteristically accompany neurosyphilis (Burke and Schaberg 1985; Luxon et al. 1979), but they also occur in sarcoidosis and other conditions (Dasco and Bortz 1989). Pupillary abnormalities other than Argyll Robertson pupils, such as bilateral tonic pupils, also may occur in neurosyphilis (Fletcher and Sharpe 1986).

A Kayser-Fleischer ring is nearly always present when Wilson's disease affects the brain (Demirkiran et al. 1996). This brownish-green discoloration of the cornea begins at the limbus, at 12 o'clock then 6 o'clock, spreading from each location medially and laterally until a complete ring is formed. It can be difficult to discern in patients with dark irises, so slit-lamp examination should supplement bedside inspection (Marsden 1987; Walshe 1986).

Visual Fields

When lesions disrupt the white matter of the temporal lobe, a congruent homonymous upper quadrantanopsia or even a full homonymous hemianopsia can result from involvement of Meyer's loop, the portion of the optic radiation that dips into the temporal lobe (Falconer and Wilson 1958; Tecoma et al. 1993). Such an abnormality can be seen in some patients with temporal lobe epilepsy. In cases of delirium from posterior cerebral or right middle cerebral artery infarction, hemianopsia may be the only pointer to a structural cause rather than a toxic-metabolic encephalopathy (Caplan et al. 1986; Devinsky et al. 1988).

Blinking

The normal response to regular one-per-second taps on the glabella (with the examiner behind the patient so that the striking finger is not within the patient's visual field and the patient is not responding to visual threat) is blinking to the first few taps, followed by habituation and no blinking. The normal spontaneous blink rate increases through childhood but is stable in adulthood at a rate of about 16 ± 8 (Zametkin et al. 1979).

Stevens (1978a) drew attention to abnormalities of blinking in schizophrenic patients and reminded us that Kraepelin, among other early investigators, had already commented on them. She found high rates of spontaneous blinking, paroxysms of rapid rhythmic blinking during episodes of abnormal behavior, and abnormal responses to glabellar tap. On glabellar tap, Stevens's patients either failed to blink, produced a shower of blinks, or failed to habituate. Although Stevens's patients were drug free, few were neuroleptic-naïve, so she could not distinguish between an abnormality intrinsic to schizophrenia and tardive dyskinesia (Stevens 1978b).

The rate of spontaneous blinking is quite insensitive to peripheral stimuli (ambient light, humidity, even deafferentation of the fifth nerve) but is under dopaminergic control (Ellsworth et al. 1991; Freed et al. 1980). Clinically, this process is manifested by a low blink rate in parkinsonism and the increase of blink rate with effective levodopa treatment (Karson et al. 1984). Thus, blink rate provides a simple, quantitative index of central dopamine activity. Failure to habituate to glabellar tap also is seen in parkinsonism and is called Myerson's sign.

Eye Movements

Stevens (1978a) also called attention to early observations by Kraepelin and others of a number of abnormal eye movements seen in psychotic patients. She noted gaze abnormalities, abnormality in eye contact with the examiner (e.g., fixed staring or no eye contact), impaired convergence movements, and irregular smooth pursuit movements.

However, jerky smooth pursuit movements are a common and nonspecific finding on bedside examination and do not reliably distinguish schizophrenic patients from healthy control subjects (E. Y. H. Chen et al. 1995).

Elucidating abnormalities of eye movement in neuropsychiatric patients requires separate examination of voluntary eye movements without fixation ("look to the left"), generation of saccades to a target ("look at my finger, now at my fist," with one hand on each side of the patient), and smooth pursuit ("follow my finger"). Failure of voluntary downgaze is a hallmark of progressive supranuclear palsy but is not always present early in the course (Collins et al. 1995). Limitation of voluntary upgaze is common in the healthy elderly. Inability to inhibit reflexive saccades to a target is characteristic of frontal disease and is seen in schizophrenia (Kennard et al. 1994); in its extreme, when any moving object captures the patient's gaze, this phenomenon is visual grasping (Ghika et al. 1995b). Milder manifestations can be elicited by instructing the patient to look at the examiner's finger when the fist moves, and vice versa, with one hand on each side of the patient (Shaunak et al. 1995). Slowed saccades, inability to make a saccade without moving the head or blinking, and other eye movement abnormalities are common in Huntington's disease (Leigh et al. 1983). Head-eye synkinesia occurs in schizophrenia (E.Y.H. Chen et al. 1995; Kolada and Pitman 1983) and in dementia. Abnormalities of eye movement (nystagmus, a VI [sixth nerve] palsy, or a gaze palsy) in a confused patient may indicate Wernicke's encephalopathy (Victor et al. 1989).

Apraxia of gaze (also called psychic paralysis of gaze and ocular apraxia) is, like other apraxias, a failure of voluntary movement with the preserved capacity for spontaneous movement (Rizzo 1993). Congenital ocular motor apraxia can be associated with other neurodevelopmental abnormalities (PeBenito and Cracco 1988). Patients with gaze apraxia may have difficulty with searching or scanning arrays or scenes. Gaze apraxia is a feature of Balint's syndrome (see the discussion in "Visuospatial Function," Disordered Reaching and Simultanagnosia, later in this chapter). In so-called apraxia of eyelid opening, patients have difficulty in initiating lid elevation. This disorder occurs in extrapyramidal disease, notably progressive supranuclear palsy (Grandas and Esteban 1994); with frontal lesions, especially right hemisphere infarction (Algoed et al. 1992); and as an isolated finding (Defazio et al. 1998). Ptosis is absent, and eye closure and reflex eye opening are normal. In apraxia of lid opening, as distinct from blepharospasm, the orbicularis oculi are not excessively contracted; in blepharospasm, the brows are lowered below the superior orbital margins (Grandas and Esteban 1994). Sensory tricks may be effective in initiating eye opening (Defazio et al. 1998), probably an indicator of extrapyramidal dysfunction in the disorder (thus making the term *apraxia* incorrect). Supranuclear disorders of eyelid closure may occur with bilateral frontal lesions, either structural (Ghika et al. 1988) or functional, as in the case of progressive supranuclear palsy (Grandas and Esteban 1994). Spontaneous blinking is intact. Often, other bulbar musculature is involved (Ross Russell 1980).

Facial Movement

A double dissociation in the realm of facial movement demonstrates that emotional movements and volitional movements are separately organized (Monrad-Krohn 1924; Wilson 1924). A paresis seen in movements in response to a command ("show me your teeth") is sometimes overcome in spontaneous smiling; this indicates disease in pyramidal pathways (Hopf et al. 1992). A severe impairment of voluntary control of the bulbar musculature with preservation of automatic movements is seen in bilateral opercular lesions, the anterior opercular or Foix-Chavany-Marie syndrome (Mao et al. 1989; Weller 1993). The inverse phenomenon—normal movement in response to a command but asymmetry of spontaneous emotional movements—is seen with disease in the supplementary motor area (Laplane et al. 1976), thalamus (Bogousslavsky et al. 1988; Graff-Radford et al. 1984; Hopf et al. 1992), temporal lobe (Remillard et al. 1977), and striatum and internal capsule (Trosch et al. 1990).

Speech

Dysarthria

Disorders of articulation are difficult to describe, although they often are easily recognized when heard. In pyramidal disorders, the speech output is slow, strained, and slurred. Often accompanying the speech disorder are other features of pseudobulbar palsy, including dysphagia, drooling, and disturbance of the expression of emotions. Usually, the causative lesions are bilateral. Bulbar, or flaccid, dysarthria is marked by breathiness and nasality, as well as impaired articulation. Signs of lower motor neuron involvement can be found in the bulbar musculature. The lesion is in the lower brain stem. Scanning speech is a characteristic sign of disease of the cerebellum and its connections; the rate of speech output is irregular, with equalized stress on the syllables. In extrapyramidal disorders and in depression, speech is hypophonic and monotonous, often trailing off with longer phrases.

Stuttering and Cluttering

Common developmental stuttering, or stammering, is familiar to everyone's ear. The rhythm of speech is disturbed by the repetition, prolongation, or arrest of sounds. Acquired stuttering, subtly different from the developmental variety (Helm-Estabrooks 1999), is unusual but can be caused by stroke (Carluer et al. 2000; Grant et al. 1999), traumatic brain injury (Ardila et al. 1999), psychotropic drugs (Brady 1998), and extrapyramidal disease (Benke et al. 2000; Leder 1996). In developmental but not acquired stuttering, involuntary movements of the face and head resembling those of cranial dystonia—such as excessive blinking, forced eye closure, clonic jaw movements, and head tilt—are characteristically seen (Kiziltan and Akalin 1996). Alternatively, such movements can be interpreted as being akin to tics; this view is supported by an increased prevalence of obsessive-compulsive behaviors in persons with developmental stuttering (Abwender et

al. 1998). Rarely, developmental stuttering that had been overcome returns after a brain injury, or developmental stuttering disappears after a brain injury (Helm-Estabrooks 1999).

Cluttering is a disorder of fluency in which discourse, rather than purely articulation, is disturbed by a range of deficits in speech pragmatics, motor control, and attention (Daly and Burnett 1999). Speech output is abnormal because of rapid rate, disturbed prosody, sound transpositions or slips of the tongue, poor narrative skills, and impaired management of the social interaction encompassing speech. Thoughts may be expressed in fragments; words or phrases may be repeated. In sharp contrast to developmental stuttering, patients are characteristically unconcerned about their impairment. Stuttering may be mistakenly diagnosed or occur in association. Rare instances of acquired cluttering have been reported (Thacker and De Nil 1996).

Foreign Accent Syndrome

In 1947, the Scandinavian neurologist Monrad-Krohn (1947) described "dysprosody or altered 'melody of language'" in a patient with a wartime missile injury of the left frontotemporal region. She was a noncombatant, in fact a woman who had never been out of her small Norwegian town. She showed aphasic troubles, mild right-sided signs, and slight personality change. Most strikingly, her speech pattern had changed so that she sounded like a German when she spoke her native Norwegian. A number of similar cases of "foreign accent syndrome" have been described (tabulated in Carbary and Patterson 2000). All showed pathology in the language-dominant hemisphere involving motor or premotor cortex or subjacent white matter; one dextral patient had a foreign accent after a crossed aphemia with right hemisphere infarction (Berthier et al. 1991).

Aprosodia

Ross and Mesulam (1979) reported cases in which right hemisphere lesions led to loss of the affective elements of speech. Analysis of the cases led to recognition of syndromes of loss of prosody in expression and of impaired decoding of prosodic information in speech. Ross (1981) later schematized these syndromes—the "aprosodias"—as mirror images of left hemisphere aphasic syndromes, although others failed to confirm this schema (Cancelliere and Kertesz 1990; Wertz et al. 1998).

Thus, lesions of either the left or the right hemisphere may disturb prosody. Left hemisphere lesions may be marked by dysprosody along with aphasia and cortical dysarthria; right hemisphere lesions may produce alterations in the affective component of speech, sometimes with dysarthria as well (Wertz et al. 1998). Often, disturbed recognition of the affective component of material presented visually is also present in cases of right hemisphere lesions. The examiner must listen to spontaneous speech for prosodic elements; ask the patient to produce statements in various emotional tones, for example, anger, sadness, surprise, and joy; produce such emotional phrasings himself or herself, using a neutral sentence (e.g., "I am going to the store") while turning his or her face away from the patient, and ask the patient to identify the emotion; and ask the patient to reproduce an emotional phrasing the examiner has generated (Ross 1993).

Echolalia

In this phenomenon, the patient repeats the speech of another person automatically, without communicative intent or effect (Ford 1989). Often, the speech repeated is the examiner's, and the phenomenon is immediately apparent, without being specifically elicited. However, at times other verbalizations in the environment are repeated; for example, patients may repeat words overheard from the corridor or the television. Sometimes the patient repeats only the last portion of what he or she hears, beginning with a natural break in the utterance. Sometimes grammatical corrections are made when the examiner deliberately utters an ungrammatical sentence. The patient may reverse pronouns (e.g., "I" for "you"), altering the sentence in a grammatically appropriate way. These corrections and alterations evince intactness of the patient's syntactic capabilities. The completion phenomenon also may be seen, whereby the patient automatically completes a well-known phrase uttered by the examiner: "Roses are red," says the examiner. "Roses are red, violets are blue," responds the patient. Speaking to the patient in a foreign language may elicit obviously automatic echolalic speech (Lecours et al. 1983).

Echolalia is a normal phenomenon in the learning of language in infancy (Lecours et al. 1983). Echolalia in transcortical aphasia marks the intactness of primary language areas in the frontal and temporal lobes, with syntax thus unimpaired but disconnected from control by other language functions. Other underlying disorders include autism, Tourette syndrome, dementia of the frontal type and other degenerative disorders, and startle-reaction disorders (Comings and Comings 1987; Howard and Ford 1992; Snowden and Neary 1993; Stengel 1947). Echolalia in a nonfluent aphasic patient may represent an environmental dependency reaction, akin to imitation behavior (Hadano et al. 1998).

Palilalia

Palilalia is the patient's automatic repetition of his or her own final word or phrase. The volume of the patient's voice trails off, and the rate of speech is festinant. Palilalia occurs with primarily basal ganglion disease (Boller et al. 1973).

Mutism

The term *mutism* should be reserved for the situation "in which a person does not speak and does not make any attempt at spoken communication despite preservation of an adequate level of consciousness" (Departments of Psychiatry and Child Psychiatry 1987, p. 33). The first order of business in examining an alert patient who does not speak is to discover whether the disorder is due to elementary sensorimotor abnormalities involving the apparatus of speech. Such disturbances can be recognized by examining phonation, articulation, and nonspeech movements of the relevant musculature (e.g., swallowing and coughing).

If an elementary disorder is not at fault, the examination proceeds to a search for specific disturbances of verbal communication. Does the patient make any spontaneous attempt at communication through means other than speech? Does the patient gesture? Can the patient write, or, if hemiplegic, can he or she write with the nondominant hand? Can he or she arrange cut-out paper letters or letters from a child's set of spelling toys? Or, if familiar with sign language, can he or she sign?

Some patients with acute vascular lesions restricted to the lower primary motor cortex and the adjacent frontal operculum have transient mutism and then recover through severe dysarthria without agrammatism, a disorder known as aphemia (Schiff et al. 1983). Transcortical motor aphasia features a prominent disturbance of spontaneous speech, occasionally beginning as mutism (Alexander 1989). Damasio and Van Hoesen (1983) described such a patient with a lesion in the dominant supplementary motor area; after recovery, the patient reported that

she lacked the urge to speak. Mutism commonly develops in patients with frontotemporal dementia or primary progressive aphasia (Snowden et al. 1992). A restricted disturbance of verbal communication must be distinguished from a more global disorder of the initiation of activity. At its extreme, the latter is the state of akinetic mutism. Alexander (1999) pointed out that mutism has its "lesser forms": long latencies, terseness, and simplification of utterances.

Abnormalities of Movement

Weakness

Awareness of the findings in nonpyramidal syndromes may help the clinician identify neurobehavioral syndromes associated with cerebral disease outside the primary motor regions. Caplan et al. (1990) described the features of a "nonpyramidal hemimotor" syndrome with caudate nucleus lesions. Patients show clumsiness and decreased spontaneous use of the affected limbs; associated movements are decreased as well. What appears at first glance to be paresis proves to be a slow development of full strength; if coaxed and given time, the patient shows mild weakness at worst. Freund and Hummelsheim (1985) explored the motor consequences of lesions of the premotor cortex. They observed a decrease in spontaneous use of the arm and attributed it to a failure of postural fixation; when supported, the arm showed at worst mild slowing of finger movements. The defect in elevation and abduction of the arm was best demonstrated by asking the patient to swing the arms in a windmill movement, both arms rotating forward or backward; the same defect can be found in cycling movements of the legs, especially backward cycling (Freund 1992). Movement rapidly decomposed when such coordination was required. Pyramidal signs—increased tendon jerks, Babinski's sign, and spasticity—may be absent in patients with these findings. In acute parietal lesions, "motor helplessness" due to loss of sensory input is regularly seen (Ghika et al. 1998).

Disordered Gait

In evaluating gait, attention should be paid to rising from a chair, standing posture, postural reflexes, initiation of gait, stride length and base, and turning (Nutt et al. 1993). Frontal gait disorder is characterized by short, shuffling steps on either a wide or a narrow base, with hesitation at starts and turns. Postural equilibrium is impaired, although not as much as in Parkinson's disease, and the trunk is held upright on stiff, straight legs. Festination is not a feature. This is the gait disorder of subcortical vascular dementia (FitzGerald and Jankovic 1989a; Thompson and Marsden 1987), and it must be distinguished from Parkinson's disease (Kurlan et al. 2000). Stressed gait (e.g., walking heel to toe or on the outer aspects of the feet) may reveal asymmetric posturing of the upper extremity in patients without other signs.

Akinesia

Akinesia has several aspects: delay in the initiation of movement, slowness in the execution of movement, and special difficulty with complex movements. The disturbance is demonstrated by requiring the patient to perform a repeated action, such as tapping thumb to forefinger, or two actions at once. A decrement in amplitude or freezing in the midst of the act is observed. When established, akinesia is unmistakable in the patient's visage and demeanor and in the way he or she sits motionlessly and has trouble arising from the chair. A distinction between parkinsonian akinesia and depressive psychomotor retardation is not easy to make, but the associated features of tremor, rigidity, and postural instability are generally absent in depressive illness (Rogers et al. 1987).

Agitation

The term *agitation* is often misused to refer to the behavior of aggression or the affect of anxiety. "The preferred definition of psychomotor agitation is of a disorder of motor activity associated with mental distress which is characterized by a restricted range of repetitive, non-progressive ('to-and-fro'), non-goal directed activity" (Day 1999, p. 95). In distinction from akathisia, the excessive movement characteristically involves the upper extremities. In some patients with Alzheimer's disease, wandering is associated with depressive and anxiety symptoms and may represent agitation in this cognitively impaired population (Klein et al. 1999; Logsdon et al. 1998).

Roaming, differentiated from wandering by being purposeful and exploratory, is characteristic of frontotemporal dementia (Mendez et al. 1993). In my experience, the excessive activity may be stereotyped, as, for example, the patient who roamed the hospital unit in rectilinear fashion, just so far from each wall with precise turns at each corner.

Akathisia

Motor restlessness accompanied by an urge to move is referred to as akathisia (Sachdev 1995). Although akathisia is most familiar as a side effect of psychotropic drugs, the phenomenon occurs often in idiopathic Parkinson's disease (Comella and Goetz 1994) and occasionally with extensive destruction of the orbitofrontal cortex, as in traumatic brain injury (Stewart 1991) or herpes simplex encephalitis (Brazzelli et al. 1994). In a few cases it has been associated with restricted basal ganglion lesions, even occurring unilaterally with a contralateral lesion (Carrazana et al. 1989; Hermesh and Munitz 1990; Stuppaeck et al. 1995). Akathisia also may occur after withdrawal from dopamine-blocking drugs or as a tardive movement disorder (Lang 1994; Sachdev 1995).

Eliciting the account of subjective restlessness from a psychotic patient may be difficult, but recognizing akathisia and distinguishing it from agitation are important. Complaints specifically referable to the legs are more characteristic of akathisia than of anxiety (Sachdev and Kruk 1994). The patient "marches in place," shifting weight from foot to foot. Seated, the patient may shuffle or tap his or her feet or repeatedly cross his or her legs. When the disorder is severe, the recumbent patient may show myoclonic jerks or a coarse tremor of the legs.

Hypertonus

In spasticity, tone is increased in flexors in the upper extremity and extensors in the lower, but not in the antagonists. The hypertonus shows an increase in resistance followed by an immediate decrease (the clasp-knife phenomenon) and depends on the velocity of the passive movement. This is the typical hemiplegic pattern of hemisphere stroke. In rigidity, tone is increased in both agonists and antagonists throughout the range of motion; the increase is not velocity dependent. This is the characteristic hypertonus of extrapyramidal disease. In paratonia, or *gegenhalten*, increased tone is erratic and depends on the intensity of the imposed movement. This pattern of hypertonus is usually related to extensive brain dysfunction, typically with frontosubcortical involvement. The erratic quality is related to the presence of both oppositional and facilitatory aspects of the patient's motor performance. Beversdorf and Heilman (1998) described a test for facilitatory paratonia: the patient's arm is repeatedly flexed fully at the elbow and extended to 90°; then the examiner's hand is withdrawn at the point of arm extension. In the abnormal response, the patient lifts or even continues to flex and extend the arm. A cogwheel feel to increased muscle tone is not intrinsic to the hypertonus; the cogwheeling in parkinsonism is imparted by postural (not rest) tremor superimposed on rigidity (Findley et al. 1981). In delirium and dementia, the paratonia of diffuse brain dysfunction can be mistaken for extrapyramidal rigidity when the examiner feels cogwheeling, which actually indicates the additional presence of the common tremor of metabolic encephalopathy or postural tremor of some other etiology (Kurlan et al. 2000).

Dystonia

Dystonia has been defined by Fahn et al. (1987) as "sustained muscle contractions, frequently causing twisting and repetitive movements, or abnormal postures" (p. 335). The contractions may be generalized or focal. Typically, the dystonic arm hyperpronates, with a flexed wrist and extended fingers; the dystonic lower extremity shows an inverted foot with plantar flexion. A number of syndromes of focal dystonia are well recognized, such as torticollis, writer's cramp, and blepharospasm with jaw and mouth movements (Meige syndrome). A dystonic pattern of particular interest is oculogyric crisis, in which forced thinking or other psychological disturbance accompanies forced deviation of the eyes (Benjamin 1999; Leigh et al. 1987). Dystonia, including oculogyric crisis, can occur as an acute or tardive effect of dopamine blockade (FitzGerald and Jankovic 1989b; Sachdev 1993; Wojcik et al. 1991). Dystonic movements characteristically worsen with voluntary action and may be evoked only by very specific action patterns. Dystonic movements, especially in an early stage or mild form of the illness, can produce apparently bizarre symptoms, such as a patient who cannot walk because of twisting feet and legs but who is able to run or a patient who can do everything with his or her hands except write. Adding to the oddness is the frequent capacity of the patient to reduce the involuntary movement by using "sensory tricks" (*le geste antagoniste*); in torticollis, for example, the neck contractions that are violent enough to break restraining devices may yield to the patient's simply touching the chin with his or her own finger. Eliciting a history of such tricks or observing the patient's use of them is diagnostic.

Tremor

All tremors are rhythmic, regular oscillating movements around a joint. Three major forms of tremor are distinguished. In rest tremor, the movement is present distally when the limb is supported and relaxed; action reduces the intensity of the tremor. The frequency is usually low, about 4–8 cps. This is the well-known tremor of parkinsonism. Because the amplitude of the tremor diminishes with action, rest tremor is usually less disabling than it might appear. In postural tremor, the outstretched limb oscillates. At times, this can be better visualized by placing a piece of paper over the outstretched hand. Postural tremor is produced by anxiety, by certain drugs (e.g., caffeine, lithium, steroids, and adrenergic agonists), and by hereditary essential tremor. A coarse, irregular, rapid postural tremor is frequently seen in metabolic encephalopathy (Plum and Posner 1980). In intention tremor, the active limb oscillates more prominently as the limb approaches its target during goal-directed movements. This tremor is seen in disease of the cerebellum and its connections. Rubral, or midbrain, tremor is a low-frequency, predominantly unilateral

tremor with rest, postural, and intention components (Samie et al. 1990).

Observing the patient with arms supported and fully at rest, then with arms outstretched, and then with arms abducted to 90° at the shoulders and bent at the elbows, while the hands are held palms down with the fingers pointing at each other in front of the chest, will demonstrate most upper-extremity tremors (Lang 2000). A given patient's organic tremor may vary in amplitude, for example, with anxiety when the patient is aware of being observed. However, anxiety and other factors do not alter tremor frequency. Thus, if the patient's tremor slows or accelerates when the examiner asks him or her to tap slowly or quickly with the opposite limb, hysteria should be suspected (Koller et al. 1989).

Chorea

Chorea is the occurrence of "brief, random, sudden, rapid, arrhythmic, involuntary movements" (Padberg and Bruyn 1986, p. 549) that dance over the patient's body. The patient may incorporate these movements into purposeful ones in an effort to hide the chorea when it is mild. As with dystonia, chorea may become more evident when elicited by gait or other activity. Choreic disturbance of respiratory movements is probably underrecognized, especially in tardive dyskinesia (Ivanovich et al. 1993; Rich and Radwany 1994). Predominantly proximal movements, large in amplitude and violent in force, are called ballistic. Usually, ballism is unilateral and is caused by lesions in the subthalamic nucleus.

Late-onset abnormal movements due to dopamine-blocking drugs—tardive dyskinesia—may be choreic, although the oral movements are best considered stereotypies (Stacy et al. 1993). If the patient has psychosis, the clinician must not assume that chorea is tardive dyskine-

TABLE 1–2.   Tardive dyskinesia (TD) versus Huntington's disease (HD)

	TD	HD
Nature of the movements		
Repetitive stereotypic movements	++	–
Flowing choreic movements	±	++
Sites		
Forehead	–	+
Blepharospasm	±	±
Oro-buccolingual	++	±
Platysma	±	±
Nuchal muscles	±	+
Respiratory	+	±
Trunk, legs	+	++
Additional features		
Oculomotor disturbances, head thrusts	–	++
Impersistence of tongue protrusion	–	++
Improvement of facial movements with tongue protrusion	++	–
Facial dyspraxia	–	++
Dysarthria	–	++
Milkmaid grip	–	++
Body rocking movements	+	±
Marching in place	+	–
Bizarre ataxic gait	–	++
Postural instability	–	++

Note.   ++ = common or characteristic; + = sometimes present; ± = occasionally present;
– = generally absent.
Source.   Adapted from Lang 2000.

sia but must consider a differential diagnosis of diseases that can produce both chorea and psychosis (e.g., Wilson's disease, systemic lupus erythematosus, Huntington's disease, and Fahr's syndrome). Furthermore, abnormal movements similar to those of tardive dyskinesia can be seen in untreated severe psychiatric illness (Fenton et al. 1997; Turner 1992). Lang (2000) tabulated the differential diagnostic features between Huntington's disease and tardive dyskinesia (Table 1–2).

Many elderly dyskinetic patients are edentulous. Koller (1983) reported differences between edentulous dyskinesia and tardive dyskinesia. In the former, abnormal movements of the upper face and limbs were absent, and the tongue lay still in the mouth; tongue protrusion was unimpaired. In contrast, vermicular (wormlike) movements of the tongue inside the mouth are prominent in tardive dyskinesia, and patients are often unable to maintain the tongue protruded.

Myoclonus

Myoclonus is the occurrence of sudden, jerky, shocklike movements arising from the central nervous system (Brown 1999). Myoclonus does not show the continuous, dancelike flow of movement that characterizes chorea. When myoclonus is rhythmic, it differs from tremor in having an interval between individual movements, a "square wave" rather than a "sine wave." The distinction of myoclonus from tic is partly based on subjective features: the tiqueur reports a wish to move, a sense of relief after the movement, and the ability to delay the movement (albeit at the cost of increasing subjective tension) (Lang 1992). Also, tics can be more complex and stereotyped than myoclonic jerks. Myoclonus occurring in a confused patient is usually a feature of toxic-metabolic encephalopathy but should raise the question of nonconvulsive status epilepticus (Rohr-Le Floch et al. 1988; Thomas et al. 1992; Tomson et al. 1992).

Asterixis

Repeated momentary loss of postural tone produces a flapping movement of the outstretched hands originally described in the setting of liver failure but subsequently recognized in many or all states of metabolic encephalopathy and in all muscle groups. Young and Shahani (1986) recommended eliciting it by asking the patient to dorsiflex the index fingers for 30 seconds while the hands and arms are outstretched, with the patient watching to ensure maximum voluntary contraction. The coarse tremor of delirium is a slower version of asterixis. Bilateral asterixis is a valuable sign because it points reliably to a toxic-metabolic confusional state. Asterixis, to my knowledge, has never been described in the "functional" psychoses and is thus pathognomonic for an organic encephalopathy.

Startle

The normal reaction to sudden unexpected auditory stimuli involves eye blink and muscle jerks that are most intense cranially. A rare, usually familial, disorder in which this reflex is disturbed is called hyperexplexia; it features hyperreflexia, hypertonus, and abnormal gait in infancy; myoclonus; and exaggerated startle, frequently causing falls (Brown 1999). Abnormal startle reactions are also seen in posttraumatic stress disorder, Tourette syndrome, some epilepsies, certain culture-bound syndromes such as latah and the "jumping Frenchmen of Maine," brain stem encephalitis, post-anoxic encephalopathy, and hexosaminidase A deficiency (Brown 1999). The stimulus-sensitive myoclonus seen in Creutzfeldt-Jakob disease may not be a true disorder of the startle mechanism (Howard and Ford 1992).

Tic and Compulsions

Tics are sudden jerks, sometimes simple (a blink or a grunt) but sometimes as complex as a well-organized voluntary movement (repeatedly touching an object or speaking a word) (Lees 1985; Lennox 1999). In addition to the important subjective differences noted previously, tics differ from many other abnormal movements in that they may persist during sleep (Lang 2000). (Some myoclonic disorders and some dyskinetic movements may also persist during sleep [Sawle 1999].)

A distinction between complex tics and compulsions rests partly on the subjective experience of the patient (Holzer et al. 1994). Compulsions are taken to be voluntary, but tics may be experienced as deliberate responses to an urge (like scratching because of an itch) or be given a post hoc meaning by the patient, so the distinction may be obscured. Obsessions and compulsions can occur in organic disease (Berthier et al. 1996; Laplane 1994; Weiss and Jenike 2000). Some compulsive behavior may represent utilization behavior rather than activity driven by anxiety (Destée et al. 1990).

Stereotypy and Mannerism

Stereotypies are purposeless and repetitive movements that may be performed in lieu of other motor activity for long periods of time (Lees 1988). Ridley (1994) distinguished stereotypy from perseveration, noting that in the former the amount of one type of behavior is excessive and in the latter the range of behavior is reduced so that behavior is repetitive but not excessive. Stereotypies include movements such as crossing and uncrossing the legs, clasping and unclasping the hands, picking at clothes or at the nails or skin, head banging, and rocking.

Stereotyped movements are seen in schizophrenia, autism, mental retardation, Rett syndrome, Tourette syndrome, neuroacanthocytosis, congenital blindness (but not in those whose blindness is acquired late [Frith and Done 1990; Ridley and Baker 1982]), and numerous other psychopathological states (Stein et al. 1998). They are particularly characteristic of frontotemporal dementia (Neary and Snowden 1996). Many of the abnormal movements of tardive dyskinesia (chewing movements and pelvic rocking) are patterned and repetitive, not random as is chorea, and are best described as stereotypies (Kaneko et al. 1993; Stacy et al. 1993). Amphetamine, cocaine, and levodopa can cause stereotyped movements (Friedman 1994). Stereotypies occur occasionally ipsilateral or contralateral to a motor deficit during the acute phase of stroke (Ghika et al. 1995a; Ghika-Schmidt et al. 1997).

Manneristic movements are purposeful movements carried out in a bizarre way. They may result from the incorporation of stereotypies into goal-directed movements (Lees 1985, 1988).

Catatonia

The syndrome described by Kahlbaum in the last century and incorporated into the concept of dementia praecox by Kraepelin occurs in a wide variety of organic states as well as in the classic functional psychoses (Rogers 1991, 1992). The syndrome can be defined broadly as abnormality of movement or muscle tone associated with psychosis (C.M. Fisher 1989), or more narrowly as "at least one motor sign (cata-

lepsy, posturing, or waxy flexibility) in combination with at least one sign of psychosocial withdrawal or excitement and/ or bizarre repetitious movement (mutism, negativism, impulsiveness, grimacing, stereotypies, mannerisms, command automatism, echopraxia/echolalia or verbigeration)" (Barnes et al. 1986, p. 991). Such signs are common in severe mental disorder (Rogers 1985). Cataleptic postures (waxy flexibility) can occur with contralateral parietal lesions (Ghika et al. 1998; Saver et al. 1993).

Synkinesia and Mirror Movements

Obligatory, congenital bimanual synkinesia ("mirror movements") persisting into adulthood occurs with cervical spine disease, such as Klippel-Feil syndrome, as well as with agenesis of the corpus callosum (Schott and Wyke 1981). When not due to such a malformation, persistent mirror movements are commonly associated with neuropsychiatric disorder, and tests for mirror movements appear in inventories of soft signs (E.Y.H. Chen et al. 1995; Rasmussen 1993). The phenomenon is easily observed by asking the patient to touch, repeatedly and in turn, the fingers to the thumb of each hand; along with watching the active hand for fine motor coordination, the examiner watches the contralateral hand for mirror movements.

Primitive Reflexes

Primitive reflexes (Table 1–3) may be of clinical importance in specific circumstances. E.Y.H. Chen et al. (1995) found the grasp, snout, and palmomental signs infrequently in schizophrenic patients but significantly more commonly than in healthy control subjects. Other investigators also found primitive reflexes more commonly in schizophrenic patients than in control subjects and suggested that the developmental brain abnormality indi-

TABLE 1–3. Primitive reflexes

Name	Stimulus	Abnormal response
Suck	Examiner's knuckle between patient's lips	Any sucking motion
Snout	Minimal pressure of examiner's finger on patient's lips, then drawing away	Puckering of lips
Grasp	Stroking of patient's palm toward fingers while patient is distracted	Flexion of fingers
Avoidance	Same as grasp	Extension of wrist and fingers
Palmomental	Noxious stroking of thenar eminence	Contraction of ipsilateral mentalis muscle
Nuchocephalic	Shoulders of standing patient are briskly turned while eyes are closed	Head remains in initial position
Mouth-opening/ finger-spreading	Patient opens mouth while extended arms are supported by examiner	Spreading and extension of fingers

cated by primitive reflexes and soft signs (see the discussion following) interacts with neuroleptic medication to bring about extrapyramidal side effects (Gupta et al. 1995; Khanna et al. 1994). Primitive reflexes in demented patients may be associated with poorer functional capacity at a given level of cognitive impairment and indicate poor prognosis (Molloy et al. 1991; Mölsä et al. 1995). They are commonly present in patients with cerebrovascular disease (Rao et al. 1999), but they may be more common in frontotemporal dementia than in comparably severe vascular dementia with frontal predominance (Sjögren et al. 1997).

The localizing value of these signs is incompletely understood. To consider them all equally as "frontal release signs" would seem to go beyond the available evidence. The grasp reflex is associated with damage to the supplementary motor area; when the damage is more extensive in the medial frontal cortex, involving the anterior cingulate gyrus, a grope reflex may appear (Hashimoto and Tanaka 1998). Often, it occurs bilaterally with a unilateral lesion (De Renzi and Barbieri 1992). Some less familiar signs such as the nuchocephalic (Jenkyn et al. 1975),

avoidance (Denny-Brown 1958), mouth-opening/finger-spreading (Touwen and Prechtl 1970), and self-grasping (Ropper 1982) signs may prove to be relatively specific or of localizing value.

Soft Signs

Under the rubric of soft signs is grouped a varied set of findings taken to demonstrate impairment in sensorimotor integration and motor control (Sanders and Keshavan 1998) (Table 1–4). A focus on soft signs in psychiatric patients should not blind the examiner to "hard signs" and extrapyramidal signs unrelated to medication in patients with idiopathic psychiatric illness (Caligiuri et al. 1993; Griffiths et al. 1998; Kinney et al. 1993b).

Schizophrenia is unquestionably associated with the finding of an excess of abnormal signs. Such signs seen in adulthood may represent the residua of childhood motor abnormalities (Neumann and Walker 1996; Rosso et al. 2000a). They are independent of neuroleptic treatment (Wolff and O'Driscoll 1999) and are associated with neuropsychological deficits (Arango et al. 1999; Wong et al. 1997), poor treatment response (R.C. Smith et al. 1999), and adverse effects of neurolep-

TABLE 1–4.   Comparison of batteries of soft signs

Element	NES	Modified NES	CNI	Griffiths
Gait and balance				
Casual gait			✓	
Tandem gait	✓	✓	✓	✓
Romberg	✓	✓	✓	✓
Complex movements				
Ring/fist	✓	✓		✓
Fist/edge/palm	✓	✓	✓	✓
Oseretsky (alternating fists)	✓	✓	✓	✓
Finger/thumb opposition	✓		✓	✓
Rhythm tapping	✓		✓	
Tap reproduction	✓	✓		
Dysdiadochokinesia	✓	✓	✓	✓
Extraocular movements				
Visual tracking			✓	✓
Convergence	✓			✓
Gaze persistence	✓		✓	
Other motor				
Drift			✓	
Motor persistence			✓	
Finger-nose	✓		✓	✓
Mirror movements	✓		✓	✓
Synkinesis of head	✓		✓	
Tremor	✓		✓	✓
Choreoathetosis	✓		✓	✓
Sensory				
Audiovisual integration	✓	✓		✓
Stereognosis	✓		✓	✓
Graphesthesia	✓	✓	✓	✓
Face-hand test	✓	✓	✓	✓
Two-point discrimination				
Right-left orientation	✓	✓	✓	✓
Primitive reflexes				
Glabellar	✓		✓	✓
Snout	✓		✓	✓
Palmomental		✓	✓	
Grasp	✓		✓	✓
Suck	✓			✓

Note.   NES = Neurological Evaluation Scale, see Buchanan and Heinrichs 1989. Modified NES, see Sanders et al. 1998. CNI = Cambridge Neurological Inventory, see E.Y.H. Chen et al. 1995. Griffiths, see Griffiths et al. 1998.

tics (Convit et al. 1994). They are present in siblings of schizophrenic persons, implying a relation to genetic risk for the illness (Y.L.R. Chen et al. 2000; Ismail et al. 1998b; Niethammer et al. 2000), although a relation to perinatal injury is possible as well (Cantor-Graae et al. 2000). Although the bulk of studies examine the occurrence of soft signs in schizophrenia, they are not specific for this disorder, being found inter alia in homeless persons (Douyon et al. 1998) as well as in mood disorder (Boks et al. 2000), obsessive-compulsive disorder (Hollander et al. 1990), borderline personality disorder (Gardner et al. 1987), and posttraumatic stress disorder (Gurvits et al. 2000). Thus, the presence of soft signs should be taken as a nonspecific indicator of cerebral dysfunction.

Signs of Callosal Disconnection

The history may disclose features typical of disconnection. Most remarkably, the patient reports behavioral conflict between the hands or merely a sense that the left hand behaves in an "alien" fashion—the "alien hand sign." Not all patients with the alien hand phenomenon have callosal disconnection. A posterior alien hand syndrome seen after noncallosal lesions producing a disturbance of the body schema in addition to abnormal movements has been described (Ay et al. 1998; Bundick and Spinella 2000). The alien hand seen in corticobasal degeneration (Thompson and Marsden 1992) may fit this pattern in some instances; in others it may be more closely akin to the levitation of the upper extremity seen with contralateral parietal lesions (Barclay et al. 1999; Denny-Brown et al. 1952; Mori and Yamadori 1989). Other patients with neurodegenerative disorders and without callosal lesions may have the alien hand syndrome through a combination of deficits involving praxis and proprioception (MacGowan et al. 1997). The phenomenon of directed though unwilled behavior by the hand—the "anarchic hand"—associated with frontal lobe pathology is described later in this chapter.

On examination, the patient with callosal lesions shows an inability to name odors presented to the right nostril. In visual field testing, a hemianopsia appears to be present in each hemifield alter-nately, opposite to the hand the patient uses to point to stimuli. Thus, when the patient is using the right hand, he or she responds only to stimuli in the right hemifield but when using the left, only to the left hemifield.

An apraxia of the left hand can be shown by the usual testing maneuvers. Because verbal information processed in the left hemisphere cannot be transferred to the right, and because the right hemisphere has limited capacity to understand spoken commands, the patient is not able to produce appropriate responses with the left hand to spoken commands. Similarly, writing with the left hand is impossible. For reciprocal reasons, the right hand shows a constructional disorder.

The patient has an anomia for unseen objects felt with the left hand. If the examiner places one of the patient's hands (again unseen) into a given posture, the patient is unable to match the posture with the other hand. Similarly, the patient cannot touch with the left thumb the finger of the left hand that corresponds to the finger of the right hand touched by the examiner, and vice versa.

Orientation

Disorientation is an insensitive and non-specific indicator of organic brain disease. A patient may be unable to give the date or place because of impairment in attention, memory, language, or content of thought. The neuropsychiatrist probes these mechanisms by using more specific tasks.

The pattern of disorientation can have diagnostic significance. Disorientation to place can carry an entirely different significance from disorientation to date (see more discussion in Delusions, "Content of Thought," later in this chapter). Delirious disorientation was distinguished from delusional disorientation in Jacksonian terms by M. Levin (1951, 1956), who pointed out that the delirious patient mistakes the unfamiliar for the familiar—reducing the novel to the automatic—as when the patient reports that the hospital is "a factory," where he or she formerly worked. By contrast, the schizophrenic patient mistakes the familiar for the unfamiliar, as when the patient identifies his or her location as Mars.

Attention

Full alertness with normal attention lies at one end of a continuum, the other end of which is coma. Where the patient is on this continuum can be assessed by observing the reaction to a graded series of probes: entering the room, speaking the patient's name, touching the patient without speaking, shouting, and so on through painful stimulation. The proper recording of the response is by specific notation of the probe and the reaction (e.g., "makes no response to examiner's entrance but orients to examiner's voice; speaks only when shaken by the shoulder").

Deficits occur in the capacity to maintain attention to external stimuli (vigilance), the capacity to attend consistently to internal stimuli (concentration), and the capacity to shift attention from one stimulus to another. Vigilance can be assessed by the patient's capacity to carry out a continuous-performance task; such tasks have been extensively used in the psychological laboratory. In a bedside adaptation, the "A test," the patient is presented with a string of letters, one per second, and is required to signal at each occurrence of the letter *A* (Strub and Black 1988). A single error of omission or of commission is considered an abnormal response. Concentration can be assessed by the patient's capacity to recite the numbers from 20 to 1 or to give the days of the week or the months of the year in reverse order. A pathognomonic error is the intrusion of the ordinary forward

order: "20, 19, 18, 17, 18, 19,..." This amounts to a failure to inhibit the intrusion of the more familiar "set."

Digit span is a classic psychological test of attention, easily performed at the bedside. The examiner recites strings of numbers, slowly, clearly, and without phrasing into chunks. The patient is required to repeat them immediately. Subsequently, the patient can be asked to repeat strings of digits after reversing them in his or her head. The normal forward digit span is usually considered to be a minimum of five. A related task of working memory is asking the patient to alphabetize the letters of the word *world* (Leopold and Borson 1997). Testing working memory by number–letter alternation is discussed later in this chapter (see the section "Screening Batteries and Rating Scales" later in this chapter).

Neglect

The patient who pays no attention to the left side of his or her body and the left side of space is one of the most dramatic phenomena in neuropsychiatry. The bedside clinician can readily identify the patient who entirely ignores one half of space, leaving his or her left arm out of the sleeve of a gown, leaving the left side of breakfast uneaten, and so on. Milder degrees of neglect can be recognized using a line-bisection task (the patient must place an X at the midpoint of a line drawn by the examiner) or a cancellation task (in which the patient crosses out letters or other items for which he or she must search in an array) (Mesulam 2000). Neglect may occur not only in external space but in "representational space" (i.e., the patient may neglect the left half of an imagined object).

Mesulam (1981) constructed a network theory in which the parietal cortex, frontal cortex, and cingulate cortex interact to generate attention to the opposite side of space. Lesions in these cortices produce distinguishable contralateral sensory neglect, directional hypokinesia, and reduced motivational value, respectively.

An inverse syndrome of "acute hemiconcern" was described as occurring after right parietal stroke producing pseudothalamic sensory loss without neglect. The patients transiently concentrated attention on the left side of the body and manipulated it actively (Bogousslavsky et al. 1995).

Hypermetamorphosis

Wernicke coined the term *hypermetamorphosis* to refer to an excessive and automatic attention to environmental stimuli. Klüver and Bucy (1937, 1939) demonstrated this phenomenon in monkeys with bilateral temporal lobectomy; a Klüver-Bucy syndrome can be seen in humans as well (Poeck 1985a).

Memory

Bedside testing of verbal memory can be done briefly and validly (Kopelman 1986). Recall of paragraph-length material after a 45-minute delay may be an ideal test, but recall of a name and address or three words after several minutes is simple and satisfactory (Bowers et al. 1989; Katzman et al. 1983; Kopelman 1986). The improvement of verbal recall with semantic cues implies a disorder of retrieval mechanisms, such as is seen in frontal-subcortical disease (Yuspeh et al. 1998). Similar testing of figural memory at the bedside is also easily done. For example, the "three words–three shapes" test of Weintraub and Mesulam (Weintraub 2000; Weintraub and Mesulam 1985) quickly and simply compares verbal and figural memory side by side. I sometimes ask patients to recall three pointed directions (e.g., up at a 45° angle, to the right, and to the left). Memory failure is a sensitive indicator of attentional dysfunction, in which case the basis is not in memory systems proper.

Language and Praxis

Aphasia

This discussion is a review of what the clinician examines in the patient with an acquired disorder of language (Goodglass and Kaplan 1983).

Spontaneous speech. Although the clinician hears the patient's spontaneous speech during the interview, it is nonetheless essential to listen for a period of time with an ear to language abnormalities. One listens for both fluency—melody, effortfulness, rate, and phrase length—and errors, both of syntax and of word choice (lexicon).

Repetition. Language disorders with spared repetition (or even excessive echolalic repetition) and disproportionately affected repetition both occur. Repetition is tested by offering the patient phrases of increasing length and grammatical complexity. For example, one may start with single words and continue with simple phrases, then invert the phrases into questions, then make up phrases of grammatical function words (e.g., "no ifs, ands, or buts").

Naming. One has already listened for paraphasic errors in the course of the patient's spontaneous speech. Ordinarily, more detailed testing by confrontation naming can be performed by using items at hand: a watch and its parts; parts of the body; shirt, sleeve, or cuff; and so on. One also can ask the patient to name items based on a description (e.g., "What do you call the four-legged animal that barks? What is the vehicle that travels underwater?"). Some patients have extraordinary domain-specific dissociations in naming ability ("category-specific anomia"); for example, the ability to name vegetables may be intact but the ability to name animals devastated (Gainotti 2000).

Comprehension. Preferably the output demands are minimized in testing comprehension, so motor responses should not be required. Asking yes-no questions of progressive difficulty (e.g., "Am I wearing a hat? Is there a tree in the room? Does lunch come before dinner? Is ice cream hotter than coffee?") is simple and is systematized in the Boston Diagnostic Aphasia Examination (BDAE) (Goodglass and Kaplan 1983). Patients with anterior aphasia often have mild disorders of comprehension of syntactically complex material. This can be observed by asking patients to interpret sentences using the passive voice and similarly difficult constructions (e.g., "The lion was killed by the tiger. Which animal was dead?")

Reading. Reading comprehension can be tested conveniently by offering the same stimuli as were used orally. Before diagnosing alexia, one must establish the patient's premorbid literacy. Alexia can be present with no other abnormality of language (alexia without agraphia).

Writing. Writing is most conveniently tested by asking the patient to spontaneously write a short paragraph about his or her illness or being in the hospital. Agraphia is a constant accompaniment of aphasic syndromes, so the writing sample is a good screening test of language function (assuming premorbid literacy). It is a particularly sensitive test in revealing confusional states (Chédru and Geschwind 1972a, 1972b). Similarly, agraphic errors can be seen in writing samples of patients with Alzheimer's disease earlier in the course than aphasic errors in spontaneous speech (Faber-Langendoen et al. 1988; Horner et al. 1988).

Ideomotor Apraxia

Incapacity to perform skilled movements in the absence of elementary sensory or motor dysfunction that explains the defect is known as *apraxia*. Limb-kinetic apraxia amounts to a nonpyramidal clumsiness (Freund and Hummelsheim 1985). Ideational apraxia is discussed later in this chapter. Ideomotor apraxia is discussed here because of its close relationship to language disorders.

Oral apraxia and the left-hand apraxia seen with left hemisphere lesions are revealed by requiring the patient to perform learned movements to command. This means that in the presence of auditory comprehension difficulties, the presence of apraxia is hard to establish. Deficits in motor performance may differ across a number of dimensions: transitive versus intransitive, meaningful versus nonmeaningful, outward-directed versus self-directed, or novel versus overlearned (Leiguarda and Marsden 2000). Furthermore, performance of axial, orofacial, and limb movements may be differentially affected (Alexander et al. 1992). Thus, a screening examination should utilize several tasks that differ in these respects. Disorders of performance of pantomime of transitive movements are predominantly seen in patients with left hemisphere lesions (Leiguarda and Marsden 2000).

For oral apraxia, suitable tests are "Show me how you would blow out a match" or "How do you lick a postage stamp?" For limb apraxia, the patient should demonstrate such movements as waving good-bye, thumbing a ride, using a hammer, comb, or toothbrush, and imitating the examiner's hand positions. Responses in which the patient uses a body part in lieu of the pantomimed object are often considered defective. Thus, if the patient continues to use his or her fingers as the comb despite instruction to pretend he or she is holding a comb, the body-part-as-object response is taken as parapraxic.

Visuospatial Function

Visuospatial Analysis

Abnormalities of visual memory and emotional prosody have already been mentioned as signs of right hemisphere dysfunction. The traditional probes for impairment with regard to spatial relations are drawing and copying tasks. Copying a Greek cross, intersecting pentagons, a figure from the Bender-Gestalt test, or the figures in Mesulam's and Weintraub's three words–three-shapes test (Weintraub 2000), or drawing a clock face serves as a suitable screen; more subtle abnormality may be sought using the Rey Complex Figure (see Chapter 2, Figure 2–3). Copying performance is impaired (although differently) by both left- and right-sided lesions. The complexity of the Rey figure offers the opportunity to assess not only the final performance, but also the patient's strategy. Having the patient change the color of ink several times during the copying process shows the steps taken to produce the final drawing (Milberg et al. 1996). The difference between a piecemeal approach (the patient slavishly copies element by element) and a gestalt approach (the patient grasps the major structures, such as the large rectangle) can be noted, with the former suggesting right-sided disease. Neglect of the left side of the figure likewise strongly suggests right hemisphere disease.

Other tasks probe visuospatial analysis without the same output demand. Elements of neuropsychological instruments can be used, for example, in asking the patient to discern overlapping figures or to identify objects photographed from noncanonical views. Even if vision is impaired, it is possible to test related functions by topographical skills: "If I go from Chicago to New York, is the Atlantic Ocean in front of me, behind me, to my left or right?"

Disorders of Complex Visual Processing

Defects of color vision due to cerebral disease (central achromatopsia) are caused by inferior occipital damage contralateral to the defective field (Damasio et al. 1980). Acquired defects of facial recognition are called prosopagnosia (De Renzi et al. 1994; Ettlin et al. 1992). Equipped with photographs of a few famous people, the bedside examiner can identify clinical cases of prosopagnosia. Some prosopagnostic patients show not only an inability to recognize specific faces (while knowing that they are looking at a face) but also an inability to recognize individual exemplars of other classes of items; such a patient may not be able to identify his or her own car or farm animal (Rizzo 2000). Developmental prosopagnosia is less well studied but may be of relevance in Asperger's syndrome as part of a wider right hemisphere deficit (Kracke 1994).

Isolated defects of topographical skill occur, either on an amnesic or an agnosic basis (Barrash 1998; Luzzi et al. 2000); but usually when one hears of a patient who gets lost in his or her neighborhood or observes a patient having difficulty finding the way to his or her hospital room the impairment is only one element of broader right hemisphere or bilateral dysfunction.

Visual Agnosia

The relative importance of perceptual processes in the agnosias has been debated; certainly, in many cases (the apperceptive agnosias), subtle defects of visual processing can be identified (Farah 1990). The bedside clinician can seek evidence of relatively intact elementary visual processing (e.g., copying the picture of an object may be possible). Although the patient's language is intact (e.g., he or she is able to name the object in the picture from a description or from tactile data), his or her capacity to recognize the object visually—either by naming it or by using it—is strikingly abnormal. Such patients are often markedly impaired in activities of daily living. Like the disorders of complex visual processing described above, visual agnosia results from a ventral lesion of the "what" stream of processing.

Disordered Reaching and Simultanagnosia

Rare patients are unable to guide the movements of the hand and arm by vision (Damasio and Benton 1979; Rondot 1989). This phenomenon, known as optic ataxia, is seen along with apraxia of voluntary gaze (ocular apraxia) and an impairment of the simultaneous perception of multiple objects (simultanagnosia) as Balint's syndrome. If the patient's reaching under visual guidance (within a field of normal vision) is disturbed, arm movement without visual guidance must be examined (e.g., observing the patient, with the patient's eyes closed, dressing, pointing to parts of his or her body, or reaching with the right hand to grasp the outstretched left thumb and vice versa).

Simultanagnosia is detected by asking the patient to describe a visually complex array; the Cookie Theft picture from the BDAE is suitable (Rizzo 2000). Simultanagnosia is a rare and incompletely characterized defect, and its association with optic ataxia and psychic paralysis of gaze is inconstant. Thus, Balint's "syndrome" probably lacks syndromal validity (Rizzo 1993). These disorders result from dorsal lesions of the "where" processing stream. Focal cortical degenerations or Alzheimer's disease may produce dysfunction of posterodorsal or posteroventral cortices with disturbed spatial processing or object recognition (Caselli 2000; Fujimori et al. 1997; Levine et al. 1993; Mendez et al. 1990).

Form of Thought

Thought Disorder

Features of thought disorder in the functional psychoses—poverty of speech, pressure of speech, derailment, tangentiality, incoherence, and so on—have been carefully defined (Andreasen 1979). Cutting and Murphy (1988) differentiated between intrinsic thinking disturbances, including loose associations, concreteness, overinclusiveness, and illogicality; disorders of the expression of thought, including disturbed pragmatics of language; and deficits in real-world knowledge, which can produce odd conversational interchange. Many authors have noted the similarity between the "negative" features of thought disorder and the characteristics of the frontal lobe syndrome. Cutting (1987) contrasted the "positive" features of thought disorder in schizophrenia with the thinking process of delirious patients. The latter was prominently illogical or slowed and impoverished in output; more distinctively, delirious patients gave occasional irrelevant replies amid competent responses. The form of thought in mentally retarded and demented patients has not been well characterized.

Confabulation

The confabulating patient fabricates material in response to the examiner's queries and may tell tales spontaneously as well. Although this disorder is linked with amnesia, elaborate or spontaneous confabulation betokens additional disease outside memory systems, particularly the disturbance of the temporal context of memories that is characteristic of orbitofrontal lesions (Fischer et al. 1995; Kopelman 1999; Ptak and Schnider 1999; Schnider 2000; Schnider and Ptak 1999). Schizophrenic patients produce confabulations in narrative speech, probably because of difficulty suppressing abnormal ideas and insensitivity to context and the listener's expectations (Kramer et al. 1998; Nathaniel-James et al. 1996). Akin to confabulation is a phenomenon Geschwind (1964) called "wild paraphasia." He offered the example of a patient who calls an intravenous pole a Christmas tree decoration. In this case, the failure lies not within language systems but in impaired visual perception as well as in the cerebral apparatus for self-monitoring; disruption of attention in a confusional state is the usual setting (Wallesch and Hundsalz 1994). Delusional memories in psychotic patients appear to be neuropsychologically distinct from confabulation (Kopelman 1999; Kopelman et al. 1995).

Vorbeireden (Vorbeigehen)

Vorbeireden (Vorbeigehen), the symptom of approximate answers, is the defining feature of the Ganser state (Sigal et al. 1992). The patient's responses show that he or she understands the questions, but the lack of knowledge implied by the mistaken replies is implausible (e.g., the patient reports that a horse has three legs). This phenomenon is rare.

Narrative Process in the Interview Setting

Patients who do not have elementary disorders of language function may nonetheless have macrolinguistic deficits. Where words and sentences—lexicon and syntax—are normal, paragraphs and discourse may not be. Patients with right hemisphere disease, despite the adequacy of their lexical-semantic and syntactical performance, have deficits in the capacity to tell a story or recognize the point of a joke (Brownell and Martino 1998; Paradis 1998). These patients rarely give "I don't know" responses, rather they contrive some answer even if implausible; they fail to draw appropriate inferences, especially from emotional data, so that incongruity is

not recognized; and the sense of humor is impaired (Wapner et al. 1981). People with temporal lobe epilepsy or who have had traumatic brain injury show deficits in planning, producing, and monitoring discourse; their narratives may be verbose and inefficient or contain insufficient or irrelevant information, requiring the listener to expend extra effort to understand them (Biddle et al. 1996; Field et al. 2000).

These findings emphasize the value of open-ended inquiries (e.g., "What brings you to the hospital?"), with attention to the patient's discourse taken as a whole as a sign of cerebral function.

Content of Thought

Delusions

Cutting (1987) pointed out that themes of "imminent misadventure to others" and "bizarre happenings in the immediate vicinity" characterize delirium rather than acute schizophrenic psychosis. Misidentification symptoms such as Capgras' and Frégoli's syndromes suggest focal brain dysfunction, especially impairment of facial recognition, and many patients with misidentifications will have right or bilateral frontolimbic lesions (Feinberg 1997). Carefully studied patients with Capgras' and Frégoli's syndromes have shown prominent memory and executive cognitive dysfunction (Feinberg et al. 1999). However, not all patients with misidentification syndromes (or nonsyndromal misidentification phenomena, which are quite common in nonorganic psychosis [Mojtabai 1998]) have a recognizable organic contribution to the disorder (Signer 1994). A number of terms describe patients who, with delusional intensity, mistake their location, including reduplicative paramnesia (Pick 1903), disorientation for place (C.M. Fisher 1982), and délire spatial (spatial delusion) (Vighetto et al. 1985). These patients generally have defects of visuospatial analysis and executive function (Sellal et al. 1996).

Fleminger and Burns (1993) found that the presence of persecutory delusions before the advent of misidentification spoke against evident organic factors, whereas misidentification of place was characteristically of organic origin. Malloy and Richardson (1994) argued that delusions confined to a single topic suggest frontal lobe disorder, but again, as Kopelman et al. (1995) emphasized, by no means can organic disease always be identified. Complex psychotic phenomena, such as first-rank symptoms, are associated with preservation of cognitive capacity (Almeida et al. 1995); patients with dementia show unsystematized abnormal beliefs that often arise ad hoc from situations of cognitive failure.

Hallucinations

Visual hallucinations suggest organic states, especially if auditory hallucinations are absent, but visual hallucinations are common in idiopathic schizophrenia (Bracha et al. 1989; Goodwin et al. 1971). Visual hallucinations without other psychopathology, usually in the presence of ocular disease with visual loss, known as the Charles Bonnet syndrome, are also common, especially in the elderly (Manford and Andermann 1998). The hallucinations are usually vivid images of animals or human beings, and the patient is aware of their unreality. Visual hallucinations in a hemifield blind from cerebral disease are well described (Kölmel 1993). Vivid, elaborate, and well-formed visual hallucinations may occur with disease in the upper brain stem or thalamus (so-called peduncular hallucinosis) (Kölmel 1991). Such hallucinations are often worse in the evening (crepuscular) or when the patient is sleepy, and again the patient is generally aware of their unreality. A dreamlike state

may accompany the hallucinosis. Similar hallucinations occur as hypnagogic phenomena in narcolepsy and in response to dopaminergic drugs in Parkinson's disease, and the brain stem mechanism may be related (C.M. Fisher 1991; Manford and Andermann 1998). Visual hallucinations early in a degenerative dementia suggest a diagnosis of dementia with Lewy bodies (Ballard et al. 1999). A lilliputian character is present in visual hallucinations of various etiologies without apparent specificity (Cohen et al. 1994).

Auditory hallucinations have resulted from pontine lesions (Cambier et al. 1988; Cascino and Adams 1986; Douen and Bourque 1997), with characteristics in some ways similar to peduncular visual hallucinations. Musical hallucinations are associated with hearing impairment, especially in depressed elderly women, and possibly right hemisphere lesions (Keshavan et al. 1992; Pasquini and Cole 1997). Musical hallucinations also occur in schizophrenia (Baba and Hamada 1999). Unilateral auditory hallucinations are characteristically ipsilateral to a deaf (or the more deaf) ear (Almeida et al. 1993).

Olfactory hallucinations, often taken to imply epilepsy or temporal lobe disease, are common in nonorganic psychiatric disorders (Kopala et al. 1994). Palinopsia refers to persisting or recurrent visual images after the stimulus is gone. Responsible lesions are typically parieto-occipital (Norton and Corbett 2000). The analogous phenomenon in auditory experience is palinacousis, which is due to temporal lobe lesions on either side (Jacobs et al. 1973). David (1994) proposed that thought-echo is due to a disturbance in short-term auditory verbal memory (the phonological loop).

Emotion

Assessment of emotion and its modulation is performed by the clinician as a natural part of observing the patient during the examination; in addition, the examiner asks questions about the patient's emotional experience. There is no substitute for extended and sensitive conversation.

Pathological laughter and crying are defined not only by the lack of congruent inner experience but also by their elicitation through nonemotional stimuli (e.g., waving a hand before the patient's face) and by the all-or-none character of the response (Poeck 1985b). These signs, produced by lesions of the descending tracts modulating brain stem centers (Asfora et al. 1989; Ceccaldi et al. 1994), may be on a continuum with the affective dyscontrol, lability, and shallowness that occur in frontal disease or dementia. This latter finding, also called emotionalism, can be defined by increased tearfulness (or, more rarely, laughter) and sudden, unexpected, and uncontrollable tears (Allman 1991; Allman et al. 1990; House et al. 1989). So defined, emotionalism is common, associated with cognitive impairment, and related to left frontal and temporal lesions, but it is not dissociated from the patient's emotional experience or situation. Allman et al. (1992) and Robinson et al. (1993) developed scales for clinician rating of pathological emotion, and Moore et al. (1997) provided a self-report measure. Ross and Stewart (1987) suggested that pathological affect might screen a major depressive syndrome. Thus, faced with pathological affect the examiner should seek not only the signs of pseudobulbar palsy but also the symptoms and signs of melancholia.

A sudden display of laughter—*le fou rire prodromique*—is a rare prodrome to a catastrophic vascular event in the brain stem or thalamus (Ceccaldi and Milandre 1994; Couderq et al. 2000; Wali 1993). Laughing (gelastic) and crying (dacrystic) seizures are unusual (Luciano et al. 1993),

although ictal emotion, especially fear, is common (Williams 1956). Gelastic epilepsy is associated with hypothalamic hamartomas and left-sided lesions (Arroyo et al. 1993), and dacrystic epilepsy is associated with right-sided lesions. Although crying is more common than laughter in pathological affect, laughing seizures are more common than crying seizures (Sackeim et al. 1982). Weeping during an ictus, in fact, suggests pseudoseizure (Walczak and Bogolioubov 1996).

Apathy is the absence or quantitative reduction of affect. It differs from depression; even the slowed, unexpressive depressed patient reports unpleasant emotional experience if carefully questioned. The term *apathy* has been in recent use for the phenomenon called abulia in this chapter. Euphoria, a persistent and unreasonable sense of well-being without the increased mental and motor rates of a manic state, is often alluded to in connection with multiple sclerosis. Actually, euphoria is unusual, and its occurrence almost always signals extensive disease and cognitive impairment (Ron and Logsdail 1989).

Initiation and Organization of Action

The capacity for initiation and organization of action corresponds to a major aspect of the developing concept of executive cognitive function in neuropsychology (Tranel et al. 1994). Disorders of activation, planning, sequencing, self-monitoring, and flexible attention are important causes of functional disability (B.S. Fogel 1994). Moreover, such disturbances may be more evident during clinical examination than during formal neuropsychometric assessment because the structure of the formal assessment replaces the missing capacity of the patient to ignore distracting stimuli and direct and organize action toward adaptive goals.

Abulia

C.M. Fisher (1984) resurrected the old term *abulia* (Berrios and Gili 1995) to describe loss of spontaneity due to cerebral disease, of which the extreme case is akinetic mutism. In a less severe form of abulia, the phenomena include slowness, delayed response, laconic speech, and reduced initiative and effort, the patient perhaps performing only one of a series of requested actions. C.M. Fisher (1968) described a transient but repeated lack of response as "intermittent interruption of behavior." Apathy often accompanies abulia, and in recent years the term *apathy* has come to subsume the disorder of action to which *abulia* has referred as well as the disorder of affect to which *apathy* primarily refers. Laplane and colleagues (Laplane 1994; Laplane et al. 1989) emphasized its occurrence after basal ganglia lesions, with a subjective sense of mental emptiness, in which context obsessive-compulsive phenomena commonly co-occur.

At times, even severe abulia can be overcome by stimuli that elicit automatic responses.

Generating lists of words by categories (e.g., "Name all the animals you can think of," or all modes of transportation, or items one might buy in a supermarket) requires sustained attention to a task, ability to organize an effective search of memory, intact language, and, of course, a certain amount of real-world knowledge. In Alzheimer's disease, generating exemplars for categories is more impaired than generating words beginning with a given letter.

Perseveration

Perseveration refers to the patient's continuing into present activity the elements of previous actions. Luria (1965) devised a number of bedside tasks to probe the programming of action and to reveal perseveration. For example, the patient is asked to form alternately a ring and a fist with his or her hand. Luria noted that in the most characteristic form of abnormality the patient perseverates on one position or the other, even while he or she is correctly saying aloud, "ring-fist-ring-fist." Luria and Homskaya (1963) regarded this disconnection of action from verbal mediation as the essence of frontal dysfunction. A similar but harder task is alternating from fist to edge of hand to palm, or the patient can be asked to alternate repeatedly from outstretched left fist and right palm to outstretched right fist and left palm (the Oseretsky test).

Perseveration can be seen in diseases of various brain regions, but when related to diseases outside frontal regions, it is characteristically limited to a specific modality of processing or response (Goldberg and Bilder 1987). For example, a patient with disease in the temporoparietal language area may make perseverative errors in naming.

Disinhibition

Loss of the capacity for planful action leaves the patient with organic cerebral disease prey to impulses; impulsive behavior is the reverse of the coin of which perseveration is the obverse. The clinician learns about such deficits primarily from the history.

Usually, but not always, the structure of the interview and examination prevents display of impulsive behavior. Few formal tests demonstrate this functional defect. Failure to inhibit reflexive gaze is discussed above. Go/no-go tasks are commonly used to explore the effects of frontal lesions in animals (Drewe 1975). A simple bedside adaptation is a tapping task in which the patient is instructed to tap for one stimulus and to refrain for another: "When I tap once, I want you to tap twice; when I tap twice, you do nothing at all." After a practice trial, a single error of commission represents a failure (Leimkuhler and Mesulam 1985).

Ideational Apraxia

The phenomenon of ideational apraxia is the incapacity to carry out a sequential or ordered set of actions toward a unitary goal in the presence of the necessary objects (Leiguarda and Marsden 2000). For example, the patient may be able to carry out the individual acts involved in preparing a letter to be sent—folding the letter, placing it in the envelope, sealing the envelope—but not be able to do them in the proper order to produce a useful result. Although focal lesions involving the left parietal and frontal cortex may produce ideational apraxia, more often it occurs in association with confusional states or dementia and represents a global disorder of the organization of behavior.

Impersistence

M. Fisher (1956) described the incapacity of certain patients to sustain activities they were quite capable of beginning. The patient with impersistence peeks when asked to do tasks requiring the eyes to be closed or the gaze to be averted. Maintaining eyelid closure, tongue protrusion, mouth opening, and lateral gaze to the left may be the tasks most sensitive to this incapacity (Jenkyn et al. 1977; Kertesz et al. 1985). In most but not all studies, impersistence has been an indicator of right hemisphere disease (De Renzi et al. 1986; Jenkyn et al. 1977; Joynt et al. 1962; Kertesz et al. 1985).

Environment-Driven Responses

An important concept in thinking about dysexecutive syndromes is environmental dependency (Bindschaedler and Assal 1992; Lhermitte 1986). When the organism cannot generate plans for behavior toward self-initiated goals, behavior directed by the environment results. Echolalia, disinhibition, and hypermetamorphosis are discussed above, as is the tendency of the patient with frontal disease to stuff food into the mouth. Visual grasping, manual groping, and the "rush toward rewarding objects" are related "environment-driven responses" (Ghika et al. 1995b). Compulsive reading (Assal 1985), writing (Cambier et al. 1988), and speaking (Tanaka et al. 2000) also fall into this category, but hyperlexia and hypergraphia of this type bear an uncertain relationship to similar phenomena described in limbic epilepsy (Okamura et al. 1993), mental retardation (Jancar and Kettle 1984), and autism (Tirosh and Canby 1993).

Lhermitte et al. (1986) described utilization behavior as an automatic tendency to make use of objects in the environment. Further analysis of this phenomenon demonstrated that unprovoked utilization behavior is unusual (Brazzelli et al. 1994; Shallice et al. 1989). Nonetheless, Lhermitte (1993) found this behavior to be associated with major depression.

Anarchic Hand

The sense of "alienation" of the hand seen in posterior callosal injury is described above. Sometimes, the dramatic manifestation of unwilled acts undertaken by the limb is anatomically and physiologically different. The acts of the "wayward" (G. Goldberg 1987) or "anarchic" (Della Sala et al. 1994) hand are elicited by the environment; they are well organized and recognized as abnormal by the patient. This phenomenon may be due to medial frontal injury with or without callosal involvement and may represent a complex form of grasping or groping; in another sense, it is unilateral utilization behavior (Della Sala et al. 1994; Gasquoine 1993).

Awareness of Deficit

The patient who lacks awareness of a deficit obvious to everyone else is a common phenomenon in neuropsychiatry, one with important implications for treatment. In right-parietal lesions, denial of a left hemiparesis commonly occurs and is called anosognosia (Levine et al. 1991; McGlynn and Schacter 1989; Starkstein et al. 1992). A range of states can be seen, from minimization of the gravity of the deficit (anosodiaphoria) to bizarre denial of ownership of the affected body part or delusional beliefs about it (somatoparaphrenia) (Halligan et al. 1995). More broadly, psychotic patients are regularly unaware of the pathological nature of their perceptions and beliefs and resent attempts to intervene (Amador and David 1998), and the patient with Alzheimer's disease often lacks awareness of the reason his or her spouse wants to visit the doctor (Migliorelli et al. 1995). In Anton's syndrome, the patient is unaware of blindness, typically cortical blindness (Förstl et al. 1993). Patients with tardive dyskinesia are often unaware of the abnormal movements, probably because of a schizophrenic defect state (Collis and Macpherson 1992). The bedside examiner should repeatedly explore the patient's understanding of the nature of the symptoms.

Psychological Management in the Neuropsychiatric Examination

In neuropsychiatry—as in all of medicine—the diagnostic evaluation is also part of the psychological treatment. The interest shown by the examiner, the rapport formed with the patient and the family, and the laying on of hands all form the basis of subsequent treatment and must be attended to from the beginning of the consultation.

A common difficulty for beginners is how to introduce the formal cognitive inquiry. All too often, one hears the examiner apologize for the "silly but routine" questions he or she is about to ask. (One never hears a cardiologist apologize for the silly but routine instrument being applied to the patient's precordium.) This is rarely the best way to gain the patient's full cooperation and best effort. Most of the time, patients report symptoms that can lead naturally (i.e., naturally from the patient's point of view) to a cognitive examination. For example, a patient with depressive symptoms may report trouble concentrating. If the examiner then says, "Let me ask you some questions to check your concentration," the patient is more likely to collaborate and less likely to be offended. Nearly any tasks can then be introduced.

At what point in the interview should this be done? If the initial few minutes of history-taking give reason to suspect substantial cognitive difficulty, one may wish to do at least some of the testing promptly. Not all of the cognitive examination needs to be done at once. Fatigue is an important factor in the cognitive performance of many patients, and long examinations may not elicit their best performance. Caplan (1978) pointed out that variability in performance is characteristic of patients with cerebral lesions and that perseveration may lead to drastic declines as tasks proceed. For this reason, short periods of probing may yield new perspectives on a patient's capacities. Shorter periods of questioning also may help prevent the catastrophic reaction that ensues when a patient's capacities are exceeded. This reaction of agitation and disorganization (Goldstein 1952; Reinhold 1953) is suggestive of organic disease but certainly counterproductive for emotional rapport.

Moreover, for a period after such a reaction, the patient is incapable of tasks that are otherwise within his or her capacities, so the data subsequently collected are limited in their significance.

Who should be present for the diagnostic inquiry? Usually, it is necessary to interview ancillary informants to gather a neuropsychiatric history. Frequently, one discovers that a family member has misjudged the nature or severity of the patient's impairment. Testing the patient in front of the family to reveal impairments allows consensual validation and mutual discussion. This testing requires tact and occasionally requires that the examination be discontinued.

Screening Batteries and Rating Scales

Several investigators have developed brief screening tests of cognitive functioning (Malloy et al. 1997; Nelson et al. 1986; van Gorp et al. 1999). These have the advantages of being repeatable, quantitative, and reliable. They are most useful for the recognition of dementia; focal cognitive syndromes may easily escape detection. The widely used Mini-Mental State Exam (MMSE) (Folstein et al. 1975) has important limitations, notably that executive cognitive dysfunction is not tested. An expansion of the MMSE, called the Modified Mini-Mental State (3MS) (Teng and Chui 1987), which includes elements of executive function, may be more sensitive and specific (Grace et al. 1995). Katzman et al. (1983) offered a particularly simple screening examination for dementia; it consists of questions probing orientation, attention, and memory. Like the MMSE, it serves best as a screen for cortical dementing disorders.

Other instruments may be more appropriate as screens for subcortical disorders.

Power et al. (1995) devised a screening test for HIV-related dementia. Along with a memory task and a test of inhibition of reflexive saccades, it contains timed construction and writing tasks. Even the memory and the timed tasks, without the inhibition task, can identify HIV-related cognitive impairment (Berghuis et al. 1999). A particularly simple screen, also validated in a population of patients with acquired immunodeficiency syndrome (AIDS), is an oral modification of the Trail Making Test Part B, called the Mental Alternation Test (Jones et al. 1993). The patient is asked to alternate between numbers and letters: "1-A, 2-B, 3-C, ..." The number of correct alternations in 30 seconds is the score; incorrect items are not counted. A maximum score would be 52; a cutoff of 14/15 gave a sensitivity of 95% and a specificity of 93% in a population of HIV-positive patients being evaluated for encephalopathy. Grigsby and his colleagues reported on the utility of this measure for assessing information processing and working memory in various other populations (Grigsby and Kaye 1995; Grigsby et al. 1994).

The choice of an appropriate screening instrument thus depends on the population being screened. However, the assessment of executive cognitive dysfunction is of paramount importance in neuropsychiatry, and in all neuropsychiatric populations a screen for cognitive deficit is incomplete without attention to this domain. The sole use of the MMSE or a comparable instrument is insufficient for assessment of the skills required for independent functioning. The Executive Interview (EXIT) is a screening test for executive cognitive dysfunction (Royall et al. 1992). A similar and simpler scale is the Behavioral Dyscontrol Scale (Table 1–5). Both scales show better correlation with functional status, such as the ability to live independently, than the MMSE

TABLE 1–5. Behavioral Dyscontrol Scale

1. Patient taps twice with the dominant hand and once with the nondominant hand, repetitively.
2. Patient taps twice with the nondominant hand and once with the dominant hand, repetitively.
3. Patient squeezes examiner's hand when examiner says "red," does nothing when examiner says "green."
4. If examiner taps twice, patient taps once; if examiner taps once, patient taps twice.
5. Patient alternates between touching the thumb and each finger of dominant hand, in succession, to table top, repetitively.
6. Patient makes a fist with knuckles turned down, places the edge of the extended hand on the table, places the palm on the table, repetitively.
7. Facing the examiner, patient duplicates positions of the examiner's hands, using the same hand as the examiner (i.e., without mirroring). Positions include left fist beside left ear, right index finger pointing to right eye, "T" with left hand vertical and right hand horizontal, left hand on left ear, and fingers of right hand under chin with fingers bent at 90°.
8. Patient alternates counting with recitation of the alphabet through the letter *L*.
9. Examiner rates patient's insight.

Note. All items except rating of insight scored 0 points (failure), 1 point (impaired), or 2 points (normal). Insight is given 0 points (complete inability to judge own performance) to 3 points (intact insight). *Source.* Adapted from Grigsby et al. 1992 and Grigsby et al. 1998.

(Grigsby et al. 1993, 1998; Royall et al. 1993, 2000). Dubois et al. (2000) devised the Frontal Assessment Battery (Figure 1–1) for identifying executive dysfunction at the bedside in several domains in patients with extrapyramidal disorders. Individual items of the scale address motor sequencing, verbal fluency, response inhibition, and other executive functions; the scale requires less than 5 minutes to administer.

Although not yet well validated, it appears promising as a complement to the MMSE or other measures of elementary cognitive functions. Royall and colleagues (Royall et al. 1998, 1999) showed that freehand drawing of a clock is sensitive to executive cognitive dysfunction and can be used as a screening instrument.

Scales for quantifying noncognitive aspects of organic dysfunction also exist. Two instruments of particular interest for neuropsychiatric practice are the Neuropsychiatric Inventory and the Neurobehavioral Rating Scale. The Neuropsychiatric Inventory assesses disturbances, including psychosis, mood and affective disorders, aggression, disinhibition, and aberrant motor activity (Cummings et al. 1994). A screen and metric approach is used; there are 10 screening questions, and supplementary questions to rate frequency and severity are invoked if the screening question is answered affirmatively. A modification allows its use as a questionnaire for relatives or caregivers (Kaufer et al. 2000). The Neurobehavioral Rating Scale is a modification of the well-known Brief Psychiatric Rating Scale, with the addition of items thought relevant initially for a population with head injuries but also appropriate for patients with dementia and other disorders (H.S. Levin et al. 1987; Sultzer et al. 1995). Of interest is a compendium of rating scales for a variety of functional disabilities, many relevant to the neuropsychiatrist (Wade 1992).

Conclusions

The "complete examination" is a figment. No practical examination can include all possible elements. The expert clinician is constantly generating hypotheses and constructing an examination to confirm or refute them (Caplan 1990). The diagnos-

Similarities: "In what way are they alike?"

- banana and orange (in the event of total failure, e.g., "they are not alike," or partial failure, e.g., "both have peel," help the patient by saying, "both a banana and an orange are" but credit 0 for the item; do not help the patient for the two following items)
- table and chair
- tulip, rose, and daisy

Score only category response (fruits, furniture, flower) correct:

    3 correct = 3
    2 correct = 2
    1 correct = 1
    0 correct = 0   [___]

Lexical fluency: "Say as many words as you can beginning with the letter S, any words except surnames or proper nouns." If the patient gives no response during the first 5 seconds, say, "for instance, snake." If the patient pauses 10 seconds, stimulate him by saying, "any word beginning with the letter S." The time allowed is 60 seconds.

Score (word repetitions or variations, surnames, or proper nouns are not counted)

    More than nine words = 3
    Six to nine = 2
    Three to five = 1
    Fewer than three = 0   [___]

Motor series: "Look carefully at what I'm doing." The examiner, seated in front of the patient, performs alone three times with his left hand the series of Luria "fist-edge-palm." "Now, with your right hand do the same series, first with me, then alone." The examiner performs the series three times with the patient, then says to him or her: "Now, do it on your own."

    Six correct consecutive series alone = 3
    At least three correct consecutive series alone = 2
    Fails alone, but performs three correct consecutive series with the examiner = 1
    Cannot perform three correct consecutive series even with the examiner = 0   [___]

Conflicting instructions: "Tap twice when I tap once." To be sure that the patient has understood the instruction, a series of three trials is run: 1-1-1. "Tap once when I tap twice." To be sure that the patient has understood the instruction, a series of three trials is run: 2-2-2. The examiner performs the following series 1-1-2-1-2-2-2-1-1-2.

    No error = 3
    One or two errors = 2
    More than two errors = 1
    Patient taps like the examiner at least four consecutive times = 0   [___]

Go/no-go: "Tap once when I tap once." To be sure that the patient has understood the instruction, a series of three trials is run: 1-1-1. "Do not tap when I tap twice." To be sure that the patient has understood the instruction, a series of three trials is run: 2-2-2. The examiner performs the following series: 1-1-2-1-2-2-2-1-1-2.

    No error = 3
    One or two errors = 2
    More than two errors = 1
    Patient taps like the examiner at least four consecutive times = 0   [___]

FIGURE 1–1. Frontal Assessment Battery.

Source. Reprinted with permission from Dubois B, Slachevsky A, Litvan I, et al.: "The FAB: A Frontal Assessment Battery at Bedside." *Neurology* 55:1621–1626, 2000.

Prehension behavior: The examiner is seated in front of the patient. Place the patient's hands palm up on his or her knees. Without saying anything or looking at the patient, the examiner brings his or her hands close to the patient's hands and touches the palms of both the patient's hands, to see if he or she will spontaneously take them. If the patient takes the hands, the examiner will try again after asking him or her: "Now do not take my hands."

   Patient does not take the examiner's hands = 3

   Patient hesitates and asks what he or she has to do = 2

   Patient takes the hands without hesitation = 1   [___]

   Patient takes the examiner's hand even after being told not to do so = 0   Total =

FIGURE 1–1. Frontal Assessment Battery. *(continued)*

Source. Reprinted with permission from Dubois B, Slachevsky A, Litvan I, et al.: "The FAB: A Frontal Assessment Battery at Bedside." *Neurology* 55:1621–1626, 2000.

tician as historian constantly strives to write the patient's biography: how did this person arrive at this predicament at this time? This biographical endeavor is far more complex than attaching a DSM-IV-TR label to a patient. Diagnosis in neuropsychiatry does not mean the search only for cause, or only for localization, or only for functional capacity. It means, along with those aims, constructing a pathophysiological and psychopathological formulation from cause to effect, from etiological factor to symptomatic complaint or performance. This formulation of pathogenetic mechanisms provides a rational framework for intervention.

Cognitive examination is the traditional psychiatric method for making a nonidiopathic mental diagnosis, and reliance on hard signs on physical examination is the traditional neurological method. The material reviewed in this chapter shows the broad array of tools that can implicate brain impairment in the pathogenesis of mental disorder. The clinician should maximize use of the means available in this difficult task, ideally without interference from disciplinary boundaries.

References

Abwender DA, Trinidad KS, Jones KR, et al: Features resembling Tourette syndrome in developmental stutterers. Brain Lang 62:455–464, 1998

Alexander MP: Frontal lobes and language. Brain Lang 37:656–691, 1989

Alexander MP: Mild traumatic brain injury: pathophysiology, natural history, and clinical management. Neurology 45:1253–1260, 1995

Alexander MP: Disturbances in language initiation: mutism and its lesser forms, in Movement Disorders in Neurology and Psychiatry, 2nd Edition. Edited by Joseph AB, Young RR. Oxford, UK, Blackwell Science, 1999, pp 366–371

Alexander MP, Baker E, Naeser MA, et al: Neuropsychological and neuroanatomical dimensions of ideomotor apraxia. Brain 115:87–107, 1992

Algoed L, Janssens J, Vanhooren G: Apraxia of eyelid opening secondary to right frontal infarction. Acta Neurol Belg 92:228–233, 1992

Allman P: Depressive disorders and emotionalism following stroke. Int J Geriatr Psychiatry 6:377–383, 1991

Allman P, Hope RA, Fairburn CG: Emotionalism following brain damage: a complex phenomenon. Postgrad Med J 66:818–823, 1990

Allman P, Marshall M, Hope T, et al: Emotionalism following stroke: development and reliability of a semi-structured interview. International Journal of Methods in Psychiatric Research 2:125–131, 1992

Almeida OP, Förstl H, Howard R, et al: Unilateral auditory hallucinations. Br J Psychiatry 162:262–264, 1993

Almeida OP, Howard RJ, Levy R, et al: Psychotic states arising in late life (late paraphrenia): the role of risk factors. Br J Psychiatry 166:215–228, 1995

Amador XF, David AS (eds): Insight and Psychosis. Oxford, UK, Oxford University Press, 1998

Andreasen NC: Thought, language, and communication disorders. Arch Gen Psychiatry 36:1315–1321, 1979

Arango C, Bartko JJ, Gold JM, et al: Prediction of neuropsychological performance by neurological signs in schizophrenia. Am J Psychiatry 156:1349–1357, 1999

Ardila A, Niño CR, Pulido E, et al: Episodic psychic symptoms in the general population. Epilepsia 34:133–140, 1993

Ardila A, Rosselli M, Surloff C, et al: Transient paligraphia associated with severe palilalia and stuttering: a single case report. Neurocase 5:435–440, 1999

Arroyo S, Lesser RP, Gordon B, et al: Mirth, laughter and gelastic seizures. Brain 116:757–780, 1993

Arseneault L, Tremblay RE, Boulerice B, et al: Minor physical anomalies and family adversity as risk factors for violent delinquency in adolescence. Am J Psychiatry 157:917–923, 2000

Asfora WT, DeSalles AAF, Abe M, et al: Is the syndrome of pathological laughing and crying a manifestation of pseudobulbar palsy? J Neurol Neurosurg Psychiatry 52: 523–525, 1989

Assal G: Un aspect du comportement d'utilisation: la dépendance vis-à-vis du langage écrit. Rev Neurol (Paris) 141:493–495, 1985

Atre-Vaidya N, Taylor MA, Jampala VC, et al: Psychosensory features in mood disorder: a preliminary report. Compr Psychiatry 35:286–289, 1994

Ay H, Buonanno FS, Price BH, et al: Sensory alien hand syndrome: case report and review of the literature. J Neurol Neurosurg Psychiatry 65:366–369, 1998

Baba A, Hamada H: Musical hallucinations in schizophrenia. Psychopathology 32:242–251, 1999

Ballard C, Holmes C, McKeith I, et al: Psychiatric morbidity in dementia with Lewy bodies: a prospective clinical and neuropathological comparative study with Alzheimer's disease. Am J Psychiatry 156:1039–1045, 1999

Bancaud J, Brunet-Bourgin F, Chauvel P, et al: Anatomic origin of déjà vu and vivid "memories" in human temporal lobe epilepsy. Brain 117:71–90, 1994

Barclay CL, Bergeron C, Lang AE: Arm levitation in progressive supranuclear palsy. Neurology 52:879–882, 1999

Barnes MP, Saunders M, Walls TJ, et al: The syndrome of Karl Ludwig Kahlbaum. J Neurol Neurosurg Psychiatry 49: 991–996, 1986

Barrash J: A historical review of topographical disorientation and its neuroanatomical correlates. J Clin Exp Neuropsychol 20: 807–827, 1998

Bear D, Hermann B, Fogel B: Interictal behavior syndrome in temporal lobe epilepsy: the views of three experts. J Neuropsychiatry Clin Neurosci 1:308–318, 1989

Benjamin S: Oculogyric crisis, in Movement Disorders in Neurology and Neuropsychiatry, 2nd Edition. Edited by Joseph AB, Young RR. Boston, MA, Blackwell Scientific, 1999, pp 92–103

Benke T, Hohenstein C, Poewe W, et al: Repetitive speech phenomena in Parkinson's disease. J Neurol Neurosurg Psychiatry 69:319–325, 2000

Berghuis JP, Uldall KK, Lalonde B: Validity of two scales in identifying HIV-associated dementia. J Acquir Immune Defic Syndr 21:134–140, 1999

Berrios GE, Gili M: Abulia and impulsiveness revisited: a conceptual history. Acta Psychiatr Scand 92:161–167, 1995

Berthier ML, Ruiz A, Massone MI, et al: Foreign accent syndrome: behavioural and anatomic findings in recovered and non-recovered patients. Aphasiology 5:129–147, 1991

Berthier ML, Kulisevsky J, Gironell A, et al: Obsessive-compulsive disorder associated with brain lesions: clinical phenomenology, cognitive function, and anatomic correlates. Neurology 47:353–361, 1996

Beversdorf DQ, Heilman KM: Facilatory paratonia and frontal lobe functioning. Neurology 51:968–971, 1998

Biddle KR, McCabe A, Bliss LS: Narrative skills following traumatic brain injury in children and adults. J Commun Disord 29:447–469, 1996

Bindschaedler C, Assal G: La dépendance à l'égard de l'environnement lors de lésions cérébrales: conduites d'imitation, de préhension et d'utilisation. Schweiz Arch Neurol Psychiatr 143(2):175–187, 1992

Bogousslavsky J, Regli F, Uske A: Thalamic infarcts: clinical syndromes, etiology, and prognosis. Neurology 38:837–848, 1988

Bogousslavsky J, Kumral E, Regli F, et al: Acute hemiconcern: a right anterior parietotemporal syndrome. J Neurol Neurosurg Psychiatry 58:428–432, 1995

Boks MPM, Russo S, Knegtering R, et al: The specificity of neurological signs in schizophrenia: a review. Schizophr Res 43:109–116, 2000

Boller F, Boller M, Denes G, et al: Familial palilalia. Neurology 23:1117–1125, 1973

Bowers D, White T, Bauer RM: Recall of three words after 5 minutes: its relationship to performance on neuropsychological memory tests [abstract]. Neurology 39 (suppl 1):176, 1989

Bracha HS, Wolkowitz OM, Lohr JB, et al: High prevalence of visual hallucinations in research subjects with chronic schizophrenia. Am J Psychiatry 146:526–528, 1989

Brady JP: Drug-induced stuttering: a review of the literature. J Clin Psychopharmacol 18:50–54, 1998

Brazzelli M, Colombo N, Della Sala S, et al: Spared and impaired cognitive abilities after bilateral frontal damage. Cortex 30:27–51, 1994

Brody D, Serby M, Etienne N, et al: Olfactory identification deficits in HIV infection. Am J Psychiatry 148:248–250, 1991

Brown P: Myoclonus, in Movement Disorders in Clinical Practice. Edited by Sawle G. Oxford, UK, Isis Medical Media, 1999, pp 147–157

Brownell H, Martino G: Deficits in inference and social cognition: the effects of right hemisphere brain damage on discourse, in Right Hemisphere Language Comprehension: Perspectives from Cognitive Neuroscience. Edited by Beeman M, Chiarello C. Mahwah, NJ, Erlbaum, 1998, pp 309–328

Bryden MP: Measuring handedness with questionnaires. Neuropsychologia 15:617–624, 1977

Buchanan RW, Heinrichs DW: The Neurological Evaluation Scale (NES): a structured instrument for the assessment of neurological signs in schizophrenia. Psychiatry Res 27:335–350, 1989

Bundick T, Spinella M: Subjective experience, involuntary movement, and posterior alien hand syndrome. J Neurol Neurosurg Psychiatry 68:83–85, 2000

Burke JM, Schaberg DR: Neurosyphilis in the antibiotic era. Neurology 35:1368–1371, 1985

Bushby KMD, Cole T, Matthews JNS, et al: Centiles for adult head circumference. Arch Dis Child 67:1286–1287, 1992

Caligiuri MP, Lohr JB, Jeste DV: Parkinsonism in neuroleptic-naive schizophrenic patients. Am J Psychiatry 150:1343–1348, 1993

Cambier J, Masson C, Benammou S, et al: La graphomanie. Activité graphique compulsive manifestation d'un gliome fronto-calleux. Rev Neurol (Paris) 144:158–164, 1988

Cancelliere AEB, Kertesz A: Lesion localization in acquired deficits of emotional expression and comprehension. Brain Cogn 13:133–147, 1990

Cannon TD, Rosso IM, Hollister JM, et al: A prospective cohort study of genetic and perinatal influences in the etiology of schizophrenia. Schizophr Bull 26:351–366, 2000

Cantor-Graae E, Ismail B, McNeil TF: Are neurological abnormalities in schizophrenic patients and their siblings the result of perinatal trauma? Acta Psychiatr Scand 101:142–147, 2000

Caplan LR: Variability of perceptual function: the sensory cortex as a "categorizer" and "deducer." Brain Lang 6:1–13, 1978

Caplan LR: The Effective Clinical Neurologist. Cambridge, MA, Blackwell Scientific, 1990

Caplan LR, Kelly M, Kase CS, et al: Infarcts of the inferior division of the right middle cerebral artery: mirror image of Wernicke's aphasia. Neurology 36:1015–1020, 1986

Caplan LR, Schmahmann JD, Kase CS, et al: Caudate infarcts. Arch Neurol 47:133–143, 1990

Capstick N, Seldrup J: Obsessional states: a study in the relationship between abnormalities occurring at the time of birth and the subsequent development of obsessional symptoms. Acta Psychiatr Scand 56:427–431, 1977

Carbary TJ, Patterson JP: Foreign accent syndrome following a catastrophic second injury: MRI correlates, linguistic and voice pattern analysis. Brain Cogn 43:78–85, 2000

Carluer L, Marié R-M, Lambert J, et al: Acquired and persistent stuttering as the main symptom of striatal infarction. Mov Disord 15:343–346, 2000

Carrazana E, Rossitch E, Martinez J: Unilateral "akathisia" in a patient with AIDS and a toxoplasmosis subthalamic abscess. Neurology 39:449–450, 1989

Cascino GD, Adams RD: Brainstem auditory hallucinosis. Neurology 36:1042–1047, 1986

Caselli RJ: Visual syndromes as the presenting feature of degenerative brain disease. Semin Neurol 20:139–144, 2000

Ceccaldi M, Milandre L: A transient fit of laughter as the inaugural symptom of capsular-thalamic infarction. Neurology 44:1762, 1994

Ceccaldi M, Poncet M, Milandre L, et al: Temporary forced laughter after unilateral strokes. Eur Neurol 34:36–39, 1994

Chédru F, Geschwind N: Disorders of higher cortical functions in acute confusional states. Cortex 8:395–411, 1972a

Chédru F, Geschwind N: Writing disturbances in acute confusional states. Neuropsychologia 10:343–353, 1972b

Chen EYH, Shapleske J, Luque R, et al: The Cambridge Neurological Inventory: a clinical instrument for assessment of soft neurological signs in psychiatric patients. Psychiatry Res 56:183–204, 1995

Chen YLR, Chen YHE, Mak FL: Soft neurological signs in schizophrenic patients and their nonpsychotic siblings. J Nerv Ment Dis 188:84–89, 2000

Cohen MAA, Alfonso CA, Haque MM: Lilliputian hallucinations and medical illness. Gen Hosp Psychiatry 16:141–143, 1994

Collins SJ, Ahlskog JE, Parisi JE, et al: Progressive supranuclear palsy: neuropathologically based diagnostic clinical criteria. J Neurol Neurosurg Psychiatry 58:167–173, 1995

Collis RJ, Macpherson R: Tardive dyskinesia: patients' lack of awareness of movement disorder. Br J Psychiatry 160:110–112, 1992

Comella CL, Goetz CG: Akathisia in Parkinson's disease. Mov Disord 9:545–549, 1994

Comings DE, Comings BG: A controlled study of Tourette syndrome, IV: obsessions, compulsions, and schizoid behaviors. Am J Med Genet 41:782–803, 1987

Convit A, Volavka J, Czobor P, et al: Effect of subtle neurological dysfunction on response to haloperidol treatment in schizophrenia. Am J Psychiatry 151:49–56, 1994

Couderq C, Drouineau J, Rosier M-P, et al: Fou rire prodromique d'une occlusion du tronc basilaire. Rev Neurol (Paris) 156:281–284, 2000

Cummings JL: Neuropsychiatry of sexual deviations, in Neuropsychiatry and Mental Health Services. Edited by Ovsiew F. Washington, DC, American Psychiatric Press, 1999, pp 363–384

Cummings JL, Mega M, Gray K, et al: The Neuropsychiatric Inventory: comprehensive assessment of psychopathology in dementia. Neurology 44:2308–2314, 1994

Cutting J: The phenomenology of acute organic psychosis: comparison with acute schizophrenia. Br J Psychiatry 151:324–332, 1987

Cutting J, Murphy D: Schizophrenic thought disorder: a psychological and organic interpretation. Br J Psychiatry 152:310–319, 1988

Daly DA, Burnett ML: Cluttering: traditional views and new perspectives, in Stuttering and Related Disorders of Fluency, 2nd Edition. Edited by Curlee RF. New York, Thieme, 1999, pp 222–254

Damasio A, Yamada T, Damasio H, et al: Central achromatopsia: behavioral, anatomic, and physiologic aspects. Neurology 30:1064–1071, 1980

Damasio AR, Benton AL: Impairment of hand movements under visual guidance. Neurology 29:170–178, 1979

Damasio AR, Van Hoesen GW: Emotional disturbances associated with focal lesions of the limbic frontal lobe, in Neuropsychology of Human Emotion. Edited by Heilman KM, Satz P. New York, Guilford, 1983, pp 85–110

Dasco CC, Bortz DL: Significance of the Argyll Robertson pupil in clinical medicine. Am J Med 86:199–202, 1989

David AS: Thought echo reflects the activity of the phonological loop. Br J Clin Psychol 33:81–83, 1994

Day RK: Psychomotor agitation: poorly defined and badly measured. J Affect Disord 55:89–98, 1999

Defazio G, Livrea P, Lamberti P, et al: Isolated so-called apraxia of eyelid opening: report of 10 cases and a review of the literature. Eur Neurol 39:204–210, 1998

Della Sala S, Marchetti C, Spinnler H: The anarchic hand: a fronto-mesial sign, in Handbook of Neuropsychology, Vol 9. Edited by Boller F, Grafman J. Amsterdam, The Netherlands, Elsevier, 1994, pp 233–255

Demirkiran M, Jankovic J, Lewis RA, et al: Neurological presentation of Wilson disease without Kayser-Fleischer rings. Neurology 46:1040–1043, 1996

Denny-Brown D: The nature of apraxia. J Nerv Ment Dis 126:9–32, 1958

Denny-Brown D, Meyer JS, Horenstein S: The significance of perceptual rivalry resulting from parietal lesion. Brain 75:433–471, 1952

Departments of Psychiatry and Child Psychiatry, The Institute of Psychiatry and The Maudsley Hospital London: Psychiatric Examination: Notes on Eliciting and Recording Clinical Information in Psychiatric Patients, 2nd Edition. Oxford, UK, Oxford University Press, 1987

De Renzi E, Barbieri C: The incidence of the grasp reflex following hemispheric lesion and its relation to frontal damage. Brain 115:243–313, 1992

De Renzi E, Gentilini M, Bazolli M: Eyelid movement disorders and motor impersistence in acute hemisphere disease. Neurology 36:414–418, 1986

De Renzi E, Perani D, Carlesimo GA, et al: Prosopagnosia can be associated with damage confined to the right hemisphere: an MRI and PET study and a review of the literature. Neuropsychologia 32:893–902, 1994

Destée A, Gray F, Parent M, et al: Comportement compulsif d'allure obsesionnelle et paralysie supranucléaire progressive. Rev Neurol (Paris) 146:12–18, 1990

Devinsky O, Bear D, Volpe BT: Confusional states following posterior cerebral artery infarction. Arch Neurol 45:160–163, 1988

Douen AG, Bourque PR: Musical auditory hallucinations from Listeria rhombencephalitis. Can J Neurol Sci 24:70–72, 1997

Douyon R, Guzman P, Romain G, et al: Subtle neurological deficits and psychopathological findings in substance-abusing homeless and non-homeless veterans. J Neuropsychiatry Clin Neurosci 10:210–215, 1998

Drewe EA: Go–no go learning after frontal lobe lesions in humans. Cortex 11:8–16, 1975

Dubois B, Slachevsky A, Litvan I, et al: The FAB: a frontal assessment battery at bedside. Neurology 55:1621–1626, 2000

Ellsworth JD, Lawrence MS, Roth RH, et al: D_1 and D_2 dopamine receptors independently regulate spontaneous blink rate in the vervet monkey. J Pharmacol Exp Ther 259:595–600, 1991

Eslinger PJ, Damasio AR, Van Hoesen GW: Olfactory dysfunction in man: anatomical and behavioral aspects. Brain Cogn 1:259–285, 1982

Ettlin TM, Beckson M, Benson DF, et al: Prosopagnosia: a bihemispheric disorder. Cortex 28:129–134, 1992

Faber-Langendoen K, Morris JC, Knesevich JW, et al: Aphasia in senile dementia of the Alzheimer type. Neurology 23:365–370, 1988

Fahn S, Marsden CD, Calne DB: Classification and investigation of dystonia, in Movement Disorders 2. Edited by Marsden CD, Fahn S. London, Butterworths, 1987, pp 332–358

Falconer MA, Wilson JL: Visual field changes following anterior temporal lobectomy: their significance in relation to "Meyer's loop" of the optic radiation. Brain 81:1–14, 1958

Farah MJ: Visual Agnosia: Disorders of Object Recognition and What They Tell Us About Normal Vision. Cambridge, MA, MIT Press, 1990

Feinberg TE: Some interesting perturbations of the self in neurology. Semin Neurol 17:129–135, 1997

Feinberg TE, Eaton LA, Roane DM, et al: Multiple Fregoli delusions after traumatic brain injury. Cortex 35:373–387, 1999

Fenton WS, Blyler CR, Wyatt RJ, et al: Prevalence of spontaneous dyskinesia in schizophrenic and non-schizophrenic psychiatric patients. Br J Psychiatry 171:265–268, 1997

Field SJ, Saling MM, Berkovic SF: Interictal discourse production in temporal lobe epilepsy. Brain Lang 74:213–222, 2000

Findley LJ, Gresty MA, Halmagyi GM: Tremor, the cogwheel phenomenon and clonus in Parkinson's disease. J Neurol Neurosurg Psychiatry 44:534–546, 1981

Fischer RS, Alexander MP, D'Esposito M, et al: Neuropsychological and neuroanatomical correlates of confabulation. J Clin Exp Neuropsychol 17:20–28, 1995

Fisher CM: Intermittent interruption of behavior. Trans Am Neurol Assoc 93:209–210, 1968

Fisher CM: Disorientation for place. Arch Neurol 39:33–36, 1982

Fisher CM: Abulia minor vs. agitated behavior. Clin Neurosurg 31:9–31, 1984

Fisher CM: "Catatonia" due to disulfiram toxicity. Arch Neurol 46:798–804, 1989

Fisher CM: Visual hallucinations on eye closure associated with atropine toxicity. A neurological analysis and comparison with other visual hallucinations. Can J Neurol Sci 18:18–27, 1991

Fisher M: Left hemiplegia and motor impersistence. J Nerv Ment Dis 123:201–218, 1956

FitzGerald PM, Jankovic J: Lower body parkinsonism: evidence for vascular etiology. Mov Disord 4:249–260, 1989a

FitzGerald PM, Jankovic J: Tardive oculogyric crises. Neurology 39:1434–1437, 1989b

Fleminger S, Burns A: The delusional misidentification syndromes in patients with and without evidence of organic cerebral disorder: a structured review of case reports. Biol Psychiatry 33:22–32, 1993

Fletcher WA, Sharpe JA: Tonic pupils in neurosyphilis. Neurology 36:188–192, 1986

Fogel BS: The significance of frontal system disorders for medical practice and health policy. J Neuropsychiatry Clin Neurosci 6:343–347, 1994

Fogel CA, Mednick SA, Michelsen N: Hyperactive behavior and minor physical anomalies. Acta Psychiatr Scand 72:551–556, 1985

Folstein MF, Folstein SE, McHugh PR: Mini-Mental State: a practical method for grading the cognitive state of patients for the clinician. J Psychiatr Res 12:189–198, 1975

Ford RA: The psychopathology of echophenomena. Psychol Med 19:627–635, 1989

Förstl H, Owen AM, David AS: Gabriel Anton and "Anton's symptom": on focal diseases of the brain which are not perceived by the patient (1898). Neuropsychiatry Neuropsychol Behav Neurol 6:1–8, 1993

Freed WJ, Kleinman JE, Karson CN, et al: Eyeblink rates and platelet monoamine oxidase activity in chronic schizophrenic patients. Biol Psychiatry 15:329–332, 1980

Freund H-J: Apraxia, in Diseases of the Nervous System/Clinical Neurobiology, 2nd Edition. Edited by Asbury AK, McKhann GM, McDonald WI. Philadelphia, PA, WB Saunders, 1992, pp 751–767

Freund H-J, Hummelsheim H: Lesions of premotor cortex in man. Brain 108:697–733, 1985

Friedman JH: Punding on levodopa. Biol Psychiatry 36:350–351, 1994

Frith CD, Done DJ: Stereotyped behaviour in madness and in health, in Neurobiology of Stereotyped Behaviour. Edited by Cooper SJ, Dourish CT. Oxford, UK, Clarendon, 1990, pp 232–259

Fujimori M, Imamura T, Yamashita H, et al: The disturbances of object vision and spatial vision in Alzheimer's disease. Dement Geriatr Cogn Disord 8:228–231, 1997

Gainotti G: What the locus of brain lesion tells us about the nature of the cognitive defect underlying category-specific disorders: a review. Cortex 36:539–559, 2000

Gardner D, Lucas PB, Cowdry RW: Soft sign neurological abnormalities in borderline personality disorder and normal control subjects. J Nerv Ment Dis 175:177–180, 1987

Gasquoine PG: Alien hand sign. J Clin Exp Neuropsychol 15:653–667, 1993

Geschwind N: Non-aphasic disorders of speech. Int J Neurol 4:207–214, 1964

Ghika J, Regli F, Assal G, et al: Impossibilité à la fermeture volontaire des paupières: discussion sur les troubles supranucléaires de la fermeture palpébrale à partir de 2 cas, avec revue de la littérature. Schweiz Arch Neurol Psychiatr 139(6):5–21, 1988

Ghika J, Bogousslavsky J, van Melle G, et al: Hyperkinetic motor behaviors contralateral to hemiplegia in acute stroke. Eur Neurol 35:27–32, 1995a

Ghika J, Tennis M, Growden J, et al: Environment-driven responses in progressive supranuclear palsy. J Neurol Sci 130:104–111, 1995b

Ghika J, Ghika-Schmidt F, Bogousslavsky J: Parietal motor syndrome: a clinical description in 32 patients in the acute phase of pure parietal strokes studied prospectively. Clin Neurol Neurosurg 100:271–282, 1998

Ghika-Schmidt F, Ghika J, Regli F, et al: Hyperkinetic movement disorders during and after acute stroke: the Lausanne Stroke Registry. J Neurol Sci 146:109–116, 1997

Gloor P, Olivier A, Quesny LF, et al: The role of the limbic system in experiential phenomena of temporal lobe epilepsy. Ann Neurol 12:129–140, 1982

Goldberg E, Bilder RM: The frontal lobes and hierarchical organization of cognitive control, in The Frontal Lobes Revisited. Edited by Perecman E. Hillsdale, NJ, Erlbaum, 1987, pp 159–187

Goldberg G: From intent to action: evolution and function of the premotor systems of the frontal lobe, in The Frontal Lobes Revisited. Edited by Perecman E. Hillsdale, NJ, Erlbaum, 1987, pp 273–306

Goldstein K: The effect of brain damage on the personality. Psychiatry 15:245–260, 1952

Goodglass H, Kaplan E: The Assessment of Aphasia and Related Disorders, 2nd Edition. Philadelphia, PA, Lea & Febiger, 1983

Goodwin DW, Alderson P, Rosenthal R: Clinical significance of hallucinations in psychiatric disorders: a study of 116 hallucinatory patients. Arch Gen Psychiatry 24:76–80, 1971

Grace J, Nadler JD, White DA, et al: Folstein vs Modified Mini-Mental State Examination in geriatric stroke. Arch Neurol 52:477–484, 1995

Graff-Radford NR, Eslinger PJ, Damasio AR, et al: Nonhemorrhagic infarction of the thalamus: behavioral, anatomic, and physiologic correlates. Neurology 34:14–23, 1984

Grandas F, Esteban A: Eyelid motor abnormalities in progressive supranuclear palsy. J Neural Transm 42 (suppl):33–41, 1994

Grant AC, Biousse V, Cook AA, et al: Stroke-associated stuttering. Arch Neurol 56:624–627, 1999

Griffiths TD, Sigmundsson T, Takei N, et al: Neurological abnormalities in familial and sporadic schizophrenia. Brain 121:191–203, 1998

Grigsby J, Kaye K: Alphanumeric sequencing and cognitive impairment among elderly persons. Percept Mot Skills 80:732–734, 1995

Grigsby J, Kaye K, Robbins LJ: Reliabilities, norms and factor structure of the Behavioral Dyscontrol Scale. Percept Mot Skills 74:883–892, 1992

Grigsby J, Kravcisin N, Ayarbe SD, et al: Prediction of deficits in behavioral self-regulation among persons with multiple sclerosis. Arch Phys Med Rehabil 74:1350–1353, 1993

Grigsby J, Kaye K, Busenbark D: Alphanumeric sequencing: a report on a brief measure of information processing used among persons with multiple sclerosis. Percept Mot Skills 78:883–887, 1994

Grigsby J, Kaye K, Baxter J, et al: Executive cognitive abilities and functional status among community-dwelling older persons in the San Luis Valley Health and Aging Study. J Am Geriatr Soc 46:590–596, 1998

Gualtieri CT, Adams A, Shen CD, et al: Minor physical anomalies in alcoholic and schizophrenic adults and hyperactive and autistic children. Am J Psychiatry 139:640–643, 1982

Gupta S, Andreasen NC, Arndt S, et al: Neurological soft signs in neuroleptic-naive and neuroleptic-treated schizophrenic patients and in normal comparison subjects. Am J Psychiatry 152:191–196, 1995

Gurvits TV, Gilbertson MW, Lasko NB, et al: Neurologic soft signs in chronic posttraumatic stress disorder. Arch Gen Psychiatry 57:181–186, 2000

Gutierrez R, Atkinson JH, Grant I: Mild neurocognitive disorder: needed addition to the nosology of cognitive impairment (organic mental) disorders. J Neuropsychiatry Clin Neurosci 5:161–177, 1993

Gutierrez R, Atkinson JH, Grant I: Corrected tables. J Neuropsychiatry Clin Neurosci 6:76–86, 1994

Hadano K, Nakamura H, Hamanaka T: Effortful echolalia. Cortex 34:67–82, 1998

Halligan PW, Marshall JC, Wade DT: Unilateral somatoparaphrenia after right hemisphere stroke: a case description. Cortex 31:173–182, 1995

Harrison PJ, Pearson RCA: Olfaction and psychiatry. Br J Psychiatry 155:822–828, 1989

Hashimoto R, Tanaka Y: Contribution of the supplementary motor area and anterior cingulate gyrus to pathological grasping phenomena. Eur Neurol 40:151–158, 1998

Helm-Estabrooks N: Stuttering associated with acquired neurological disorders, in Stuttering and Related Disorders of Fluency, 2nd Edition. Edited by Curlee RF. New York, Thieme, 1999, pp 255–268

Hermesh H, Munitz H: Unilateral neuroleptic-induced akathisia. Clin Neuropharmacol 13:253–258, 1990

Hirsch AR: Olfaction in migraineurs. Headache 32:233–236, 1992

Hollander E, Schiffman E, Cohen B, et al: Signs of central nervous system dysfunction in obsessive-compulsive disorder. Arch Gen Psychiatry 47:27–32, 1990

Holzer JC, Goodman WK, McDougle CJ, et al: Obsessive-compulsive disorder with and without a chronic tic disorder: a comparison of symptoms in 70 patients. Br J Psychiatry 164:469–473, 1994

Hopf HC, Müller-Forell W, Hopf NJ: Localization of emotional and volitional facial paresis. Neurology 42:1918–1923, 1992

Horner J, Heyman A, Dawson D, et al: The relationship of agraphia to the severity of dementia in Alzheimer's disease. Arch Neurol 45:760–763, 1988

House A, Dennis M, Molyneux A, et al: Emotionalism after stroke. BMJ 298:991–994, 1989

Howard R, Ford R: From the jumping Frenchmen of Maine to post-traumatic stress disorder: the startle response in neuropsychiatry. Psychol Med 22:695–707, 1992

Hughlings-Jackson J: On right- or left-sided spasm at the onset of epileptic paroxysms, and on crude sensation warnings and elaborate mental states. Brain 3:192–214, 1880/1881

Ismail B, Cantor-Graae E, McNeil TF: Minor physical anomalies in schizophrenic patients and their siblings. Am J Psychiatry 155:1695–1702, 1998a

Ismail B, Cantor-Graae E, McNeil TF: Neurological abnormalities in schizophrenic patients and their siblings. Am J Psychiatry 155:84–89, 1998b

Ismail B, Cantor-Graae E, McNeil TF: Minor physical anomalies in schizophrenia: cognitive, neurological and other clinical correlates. J Psychiatr Res 34:45–56, 2000

Ivanovich M, Glantz R, Bone RC, et al: Respiratory dyskinesia presenting as acute respiratory distress. Chest 103:314–316, 1993

Jacobs L, Feldman M, Diamond SP, et al: Palinacousis: persistent or recurring auditory sensations. Cortex 9:275–287, 1973

Jancar J, Kettle LB: Hypergraphia and mental handicap. J Ment Defic Res 28:151–158, 1984

Jenkyn LR, Walsh DB, Walsh BT, et al: The nuchocephalic reflex. J Neurol Neurosurg Psychiatry 38:561–566, 1975

Jenkyn LR, Walsh DB, Culver CM, et al: Clinical signs in diffuse cerebral dysfunction. J Neurol Neurosurg Psychiatry 40:956–966, 1977

Jones BN, Teng EL, Folstein MF, et al: A new bedside test of cognition for patients with HIV infection. Ann Intern Med 119:1001–1004, 1993

Joynt RJ, Benton AL, Fogel ML: Behavioral and pathological correlates of motor impersistence. Neurology 12:876–881, 1962

Kandel E, Brennan PA, Mednick SA, et al: Minor physical anomalies and recidivistic adult criminal behavior. Acta Psychiatr Scand 79:103–107, 1989

Kaneko K, Yuasa T, Miyatake T, et al: Stereotyped hand clasping: an unusual tardive movement disorder. Mov Disord 8:230–231, 1993

Karson CN, Burns RS, LeWitt PA, et al: Blink rates and disorders of movement. Neurology 34:677–678, 1984

Katzman R, Brown T, Fuld P, et al: Validation of a short orientation-memory-concentration test of cognitive impairment. Am J Psychiatry 140:734–739, 1983

Kaufer DI, Cummings JL, Ketchel P, et al: Validation of the NPI-Q, a brief clinical form of the Neuropsychiatric Inventory. J Neuropsychiatry Clin Neurosci 12:233–239, 2000

Kennard C, Crawford TJ, Henderson I: A pathophysiological approach to saccadic eye movements in neurological and psychiatric disease. J Neurol Neurosurg Psychiatry 57:881–885, 1994

Kertesz A, Nicholson I, Cancelliere A, et al: Motor impersistence: a right-hemisphere syndrome. Neurology 35:662–666, 1985

Keshavan MS, David AS, Steingard S, et al: Musical hallucinations: a review and synthesis. Neuropsychiatry Neuropsychol Behav Neurol 5:211–223, 1992

Khanna R, Damodaran SS, Chakraborty SP: Overflow movements may predict neuroleptic-induced dystonia. Biol Psychiatry 35:491–492, 1994

Kinney DK, Yurgelun-Todd DA, Levy DL, et al: Obstetrical complications in patients with bipolar disorder and their siblings. Psychiatry Res 48:45–56, 1993a

Kinney DK, Yurgelun-Todd DA, Woods BT: Neurological hard signs in schizophrenia and major mood disorders. J Nerv Ment Dis 181:202–204, 1993b

Kiziltan G, Akalin MA: Stuttering may be a type of action dystonia. Mov Disord 11:278–282, 1996

Klein DA, Steinberg M, Galik E, et al: Wandering behavior in community-residing persons with dementia. Int J Geriatr Psychiatry 14(4):272–279, 1999

Klüver H, Bucy PC: Psychic blindness and other symptoms following bilateral temporal lobectomy in rhesus monkeys. Am J Physiol 119:352–353, 1937

Klüver H, Bucy PC: Preliminary analysis of functions of the temporal lobes in monkeys. AMA Archives of Neurology and Psychiatry 42:979–1000, 1939

Kolada SJ, Pitman RK: Eye-head synkinesia in schizophrenic adults during a repetitive visual search task. Biol Psychiatry 18:675–684, 1983

Koller WC: Edentulous orodyskinesia. Neurology 13:97–99, 1983

Koller W, Lang A, Vetere-Overfield B, et al: Psychogenic tremors. Neurology 39:1094–1099, 1989

Kölmel HW: Peduncular hallucinations. J Neurol 238:457–459, 1991

Kölmel HW: Visual illusions and hallucinations. Baillieres Clin Neurol 2:243–264, 1993

Kopala LC, Good KP, Honer WG: Olfactory hallucinations and olfactory identification ability in patients with schizophrenia and other psychiatric disorders. Schizophr Res 12:205–211, 1994

Kopelman MD: Clinical tests of memory. Br J Psychiatry 148:517–525, 1986

Kopelman MD: Varieties of false memory. Cognitive Neuropsychology 16:197–214, 1999

Kopelman MD, Guinan EM, Lewis PDR: Delusional memory, confabulation, and frontal lobe dysfunction: a case study in De Clérambault's syndrome. Neurocase 1:71–77, 1995

Kracke I: Developmental prosopagnosia in Asperger syndrome: presentation and discussion of an individual case. Dev Med Child Neurol 36:873–886, 1994

Kramer S, Bryan KL, Frith CD: "Confabulation" in narrative discourse by schizophrenic patients. Int J Lang Commun Disord 33 (suppl):202–207, 1998

Kurlan R, Richard IH, Papka M, et al: Movement disorders in Alzheimer's disease: more rigidity of definitions is needed. Mov Disord 15:24–29, 2000

Lainhart JE, Piven J, Wzorek M, et al: Macrocephaly in children and adults with autism. J Am Acad Child Adolesc Psychiatry 36:282–290, 1997

Lang AE: Clinical phenomenology of tic disorders: selected aspects. Adv Neurol 58:25–32, 1992

Lang AE: Withdrawal akathisia: case reports and a proposed classification of chronic akathisia. Mov Disord 9:188–192, 1994

Lang AE: Movement disorders: symptoms, in Neurology in Clinical Practice, 3rd Edition. Edited by Bradley WG, Daroff RB, Fenichel GM, et al. Boston, MA, Butterworth-Heinemann, 2000, pp 319–340

Laplane D: Obsessions et compulsions par lésions des noyaux gris centraux. Rev Neurol (Paris) 150:594–598, 1994

Laplane D, Orgogozo JM, Meininger V, et al: Paralysie faciale avec dissociation automatico-volontaire inverse par lesion frontale: son origine corticale. Ses relations avec l'A. M. S. Rev Neurol (Paris) 132:725–734, 1976

Laplane D, Levasseur M, Pillon B, et al: Obsessive-compulsive and other behavioural changes with bilateral basal ganglia lesions: a neuropsychological, magnetic resonance imaging and positron tomographic study. Brain 112:699–725, 1989

Lecours AR, Lhermitte F, Bryans B: Aphasiology. London, Baillière Tindall, 1983

Leder SB: Adult onset of stuttering as a presenting sign in a parkinsonian-like syndrome: a case report. J Commun Disord 29:471–478, 1996

Lees AJ: Tics and Related Disorders. Edinburgh, UK, Churchill Livingstone, 1985

Lees AJ: Facial mannerisms and tics. Adv Neurol 49:255–261, 1988

Leigh RJ, Newman SA, Folstein SE, et al: Abnormal ocular motor control in Huntington's disease. Neurology 33:1268–1275, 1983

Leigh RJ, Foley JM, Remler BF, et al: Oculogyric crisis: a syndrome of thought disorder and ocular deviation. Ann Neurol 22:13–17, 1987

Leiguarda RC, Marsden CD: Limb apraxias: higher-order disorders of sensorimotor integration. Brain 123:860–879, 2000

Leimkuhler ME, Mesulam M-M: Reversible go–no go deficits in a case of frontal lobe tumor. Ann Neurol 18:617–619, 1985

Lennox G: Tics and related disorders, in Movement Disorders in Clinical Practice. Edited by Sawle G. Oxford, UK, Isis Medical Media, 1999, pp 135–146

Leopold NA, Borson AJ: An alphabetical "WORLD": a new version of an old test. Neurology 49:1521–1524, 1997

Levin HS, High WM, Goethe KE, et al: The Neurobehavioural Rating Scale: assessment of the behavioural sequelae of head injury by the clinician. J Neurol Neurosurg Psychiatry 50:183–193, 1987

Levin M: Delirium: a gap in psychiatric teaching. Am J Psychiatry 107:689–694, 1951

Levin M: Thinking disturbances in delirium. AMA Archives of Neurology and Psychiatry 75:62–66, 1956

Levine DN, Calvanio R, Rinn WE: The pathogenesis of anosognosia for hemiplegia. Neurology 41:1770–1781, 1991

Levine DN, Lee JM, Fisher CM: The visual variant of Alzheimer's disease: a clinicopathologic case study. Neurology 43:305–313, 1993

Lezak MD: Subtle sequelae of brain damage: perplexity, distractibility, and fatigue. Am J Phys Med 57:9–15, 1978

Lhermitte F: Human autonomy and the frontal lobes, II: patient behavior in complex and social situations: the "environmental dependency syndrome." Ann Neurol 19:335–343, 1986

Lhermitte F: Les comportements d'imitation et d'utilisation dans les états dépressifs majeurs. Bull Acad Natl Med 177:883–892, 1993

Lhermitte F, Pillon B, Serdaru M: Human autonomy and the frontal lobes, I: imitation and utilization behavior: a neuropsychological study of 75 patients. Ann Neurol 19:326–334, 1986

Lishman WA: Organic Psychiatry: The Psychological Consequences of Cerebral Disorder, 3rd Edition. Oxford, UK, Blackwell Science, 1998

Logsdon RG, Teri L, McCurry SM, et al: Wandering: a significant problem among community-residing individuals with Alzheimer's disease. J Gerontol 53B:294–299, 1998

Lohr JB, Alder M, Flynn K, et al: Minor physical anomalies in older patients with late-onset schizophrenia, early-onset schizophrenia, depression, and Alzheimer's disease. Am J Geriatr Psychiatry 5:318–323, 1997

Luciano D, Devinsky O, Perrine K: Crying seizures. Neurology 43:2113–2117, 1993

Luria AR: Two kinds of motor perseveration in massive injury of the frontal lobes. Brain 88:1–10, 1965

Luria AR, Homskaya ED: Le trouble du role régulateur du langage au cours des lésions du lobe frontal. Neuropsychologia 1:9–26, 1963

Luxon L, Lees AJ, Greenwood RJ: Neurosyphilis today. Lancet 1:90–93, 1979

Luzzi S, Pucci E, Di Bella P, et al: Topographical disorientation consequent to amnesia of spatial location in a patient with right parahippocampal damage. Cortex 36:437–434, 2000

MacGowan DJL, Delanty N, Petito F, et al: Isolated myoclonic alien hand as the sole presentation of pathologically established Creutzfeldt-Jakob disease: a report of two patients. J Neurol Neurosurg Psychiatry 63:404–407, 1997

Malloy PF, Richardson ED: The frontal lobes and content-specific delusions. J Neuropsychiatry Clin Neurosci 6:455–466, 1994

Malloy PF, Cummings JL, Coffey CE, et al: Cognitive screening instruments in neuropsychiatry: a report of the Committee on Research of the American Neuropsychiatric Association. J Neuropsychiatry Clin Neurosci 9:189–197, 1997

Manford M, Andermann F: Complex visual hallucinations. Clinical and neurobiological insights. Brain 121:1819–1840, 1998

Mao C-C, Coull BM, Golper LAC, et al: Anterior operculum syndrome. Neurology 39:1169–1172, 1989

Marsden CD: Wilson's disease. Q J Med 65:959–966, 1987

McGlynn SM, Schacter DL: Unawareness of deficits in neuropsychological syndromes. J Clin Exp Neuropsychol 11:143–205, 1989

McNeil TF, Cantor-Graae E, Ismail B: Obstetric complications and congenital malformation in schizophrenia. Brain Res Rev 31:166–178, 2000

Mendez MF, Mendez MA, Martin R, et al: Complex visual disturbances in Alzheimer's disease. Neurology 40:439–443, 1990

Mendez MF, Selwood A, Mastri AR, et al: Pick's disease versus Alzheimer's disease: a comparison of clinical characteristics. Neurology 43:289–292, 1993

Mendez MF, Foti DJ, Cummings JL: Abnormal oral behaviors in neurological and psychiatric syndromes [abstract]. J Neuropsychiatry Clin Neurosci 7:397, 1995

Mesulam M-M: A cortical network for directed attention and unilateral neglect. Ann Neurol 10:309–325, 1981

Mesulam M-M: Attentional networks, confusional states and neglect syndromes, in Principles of Behavioral and Cognitive Neurology, 2nd Edition. Edited by Mesulam M-M. Oxford, UK, Oxford University Press, 2000, pp 174–256

Migliorelli R, Tesón A, Sabe L, et al: Anosognosia in Alzheimer's disease: a study of associated factors. J Neuropsychiatry Clin Neurosci 7:338–344, 1995

Milberg WP, Hebben N, Kaplan E: The Boston Process Approach to neuropsychological assessment, in Neuropsychological Assessment of Neuropsychiatric Disorders, 2nd Edition. Edited by Grant I, Adams KM. New York, Oxford University Press, 1996, pp 65–86

Mojtabai R: Identifying misidentifications: a phenomenological study. Psychopathology 31:90–95, 1998

Molloy DW, Clarnette RM, McIlroy WE, et al: Clinical significance of primitive reflexes in Alzheimer's disease. J Am Geriatr Soc 39:1160–1163, 1991

Mölsä PK, Marrila RJ, Rinne UK: Long-term survival and predictors of mortality in Alzheimer's disease and multi-infarct dementia. Acta Neurol Scand 91:159–164, 1995

Monrad-Krohn GH: On the dissociation of voluntary and emotional innervation in facial paresis of central origin. Brain 47:22–35, 1924

Monrad-Krohn GH: Dysprosody or altered "melody of language." Brain 70:405–415, 1947

Moore SR, Gresham LS, Bromberg MB, et al: A self report measure of affective lability. J Neurol Neurosurg Psychiatry 63:89–93, 1997

Mori E, Yamadori A: Rejection behaviour: a human homologue of the abnormal behaviour of Denny-Brown and Chambers' monkey with bilateral parietal ablation. J Neurol Neurosurg Psychiatry 52:1260–1266, 1989

Morrell MJ, Sperling MR, Stecker M, et al: Sexual dysfunction in partial epilepsy: a deficit in physiological sexual arousal. Neurology 44:243–247, 1994

Nathaniel-James DA, Foong J, Frith CD: The mechanism of confabulation in schizophrenia. Neurocase 2:475–483, 1996

Neary D, Snowden JS: Fronto-temporal dementia: nosology, neuropsychology, and neuropathology. Brain Cogn 31:176–187, 1996

Nelson A, Fogel BS, Faust D: Bedside cognitive screening instruments: a critical assessment. J Nerv Ment Dis 174:73–83, 1986

Neumann CS, Walker EF: Childhood neuromotor soft signs, behavior problems, and adult psychopathology, in Advances in Clinical Child Psychology. Edited by Ollendick TH, Prinz RJ. New York, Plenum, 1996, pp 173–203

Niethammer R, Weisbrod M, Schiesser S, et al: Genetic influence on laterality in schizophrenia? A twin study of neurological soft signs. Am J Psychiatry 157:272–274, 2000

Norton JW, Corbett JJ: Visual perceptual abnormalities: hallucinations and illusions. Semin Neurol 20:111–121, 2000

Nutt JG, Marsden CD, Thompson PD: Human walking and higher-level gait disorders, particularly in the elderly. Neurology 43:268–279, 1993

Okamura T, Fukai M, Yamadori A, et al: A clinical study of hypergraphia in epilepsy. J Neurol Neurosurg Psychiatry 56: 556–559, 1993

Padberg GW, Bruyn GW: Chorea: differential diagnosis, in Handbook of Neurology, Vol 49: Extrapyramidal Disorders. Edited by Vinken PJ, Bruyn GW, Klawans HL. Amsterdam, The Netherlands, Elsevier, 1986, pp 549–564

Paradis M: The other side of language: pragmatic competence. Journal of Neurolinguistics 11:1–10, 1998

Pasquini F, Cole MG: Idiopathic musical hallucinations in the elderly. J Geriatr Psychiatry Neurol 10:11–14, 1997

PeBenito R, Cracco JB: Congenital ocular motor apraxia. Clin Pediatr 27:27–31, 1988

Penfield W, Robertson JSM: Growth asymmetry due to lesions of the postcentral cerebral cortex. AMA Archives of Neurology and Psychiatry 50:405–430, 1943

Persinger MA, Makarec K: Complex partial epileptic signs as a continuum from normals to epileptics: normative data and clinical populations. J Clin Psychol 49:33–45, 1993

Pick A: Clinical studies, III: on reduplicative paramnesia. Brain 26:260–267, 1903

Pinching AJ: Clinical testing of olfaction reassessed. Brain 100:377–388, 1977

Pine DS, Shaffer D, Schonfeld IS, et al: Minor physical anomalies: modifiers of environmental risks for psychiatric impairment? J Am Acad Child Adolesc Psychiatry 36:395–403, 1997

Plum F, Posner JB: The Diagnosis of Stupor and Coma, 3rd Edition. Philadelphia, PA, FA Davis, 1980

Poeck K: The Kluver-Bucy syndrome in man, in Handbook of Clinical Neurology, Vol 45: Clinical Neuropsychology. Edited by Frederiks JAM. Amsterdam, The Netherlands, Elsevier, 1985a, pp 257–263

Poeck K: Pathological laughter and crying, in Handbook of Clinical Neurology, Vol 45: Clinical Neuropsychology. Edited by Frederiks JAM. Amsterdam, The Netherlands, Elsevier, 1985b, pp 219–225

Power C, Selnes OA, Grim JA, et al: HIV Dementia Scale: a rapid screening test. J Acquir Immune Defic Syndr 8:273–278, 1995

Preti A, Cardascia L, Zen T, et al: Obstetric complications in patients with depression—a population-based case-control study. J Affect Disord 61:101–106, 2000

Ptak R, Schnider A: Spontaneous confabulations after orbitofrontal damage: the role of temporal context confusion and self-monitoring. Neurocase 5:243–250, 1999

Raine A, Brennan P, Mednick SA: Birth complications combined with early maternal rejection at age 1 year predispose to violent crime at age 18 years. Arch Gen Psychiatry 51:984–988, 1994

Rao R, Jackson S, Howard R: Primitive reflexes in cerebrovascular disease: a community study of older people with stroke and carotid stenosis. Int J Geriatr Psychiatry 14: 964–972, 1999

Rasmussen P: Persistent mirror movements: a clinical study of 17 children, adolescents and young adults. Dev Med Child Neurol 35:699–707, 1993

Reinhold M: Human behaviour reactions to organic cerebral disease. Journal of Mental Science 99:130–135, 1953

Remillard GM, Andermann F, Rhi-Sausi A, et al: Facial asymmetry in patients with temporal lobe epilepsy: a clinical sign useful in the lateralization of temporal epileptogenic foci. Neurology 27:109–114, 1977

Rich MW, Radwany SM: Respiratory dyskinesia: an underrecognized phenomenon. Chest 105:1826–1832, 1994

Ridley RM: The psychology of perseverative and stereotyped behaviour. Prog Neurobiol 44:221–231, 1994

Ridley RM, Baker HF: Stereotypy in monkeys and humans. Psychol Med 12:61–72, 1982

Rizzo M: "Balint's syndrome" and associated visuospatial disorders. Baillieres Clin Neurol 2:415–437, 1993

Rizzo M: Clinical assessment of complex visual dysfunction. Semin Neurol 20:75–87, 2000

Roberts RJ, Varney NR, Hulbert JR, et al: The neuropathology of everyday life: the frequency of partial seizure symptoms among normals. Neuropsychology 4:65–85, 1990

Robinson RG, Parikh RM, Lipsey JR, et al: Pathological laughing and crying following stroke: validation of a measurement scale and a double-blind treatment study. Am J Psychiatry 150:286–293, 1993

Rogers D: The motor disorders of severe psychiatric illness: a conflict of paradigms. Br J Psychiatry 147:221–232, 1985

Rogers D: Catatonia: a contemporary approach. J Neuropsychiatry Clin Neurosci 3:334–340, 1991

Rogers D: Motor Disorder in Psychiatry: Toward a Neurological Psychiatry. Chichester, UK, Wiley, 1992

Rogers D, Lees AJ, Smith E, et al: Bradyphrenia in Parkinson's disease and psychomotor retardation in depressive illness. Brain 110:761–776, 1987

Rohr-Le Floch J, Gauthier G, Beaumanoir A: États confusionnels d'origine épileptique: intérêt de l'EEG fait en urgence. Rev Neurol (Paris) 144:425–436, 1988

Ron MA, Logsdail SJ: Psychiatric morbidity in multiple sclerosis: a clinical and MRI study. Psychol Med 19:887–895, 1989

Rondot P: Visuomotor ataxia, in Neuropsychology of Visual Perception. Edited by Brown JW. Hillside, NJ, Erlbaum, 1989, pp 105–119

Ropper AH: Self-grasping: a focal neurological sign. Ann Neurol 12:575–577, 1982

Ross ED: The aprosodias: functional-anatomic organization of the affective components of language in the right hemisphere. Arch Neurol 38:561–569, 1981

Ross ED: Nonverbal aspects of language. Neurol Clin 11:9–23, 1993

Ross ED, Mesulam M-M: Dominant language functions of the right hemisphere? Arch Neurol 36:144–148, 1979

Ross ED, Stewart RS: Pathological display of affect in patients with depression and right frontal brain damage: an alternative mechanism. J Nerv Ment Dis 175:165–172, 1987

Rosso IM, Bearden CE, Hollister JM, et al: Childhood neuromotor dysfunction in schizophrenia patients and their unaffected siblings: a prospective cohort study. Schizophr Bull 26:367–378, 2000a

Rosso IM, Cannon TD, Huttunen T, et al: Obstetric risk factors for early onset schizophrenia in a Finnish birth cohort. Am J Psychiatry 157:801–807, 2000b

Royall DR, Mahurin RK, Gray KF: Bedside assessment of executive cognitive impairment: the executive interview. J Am Geriatr Soc 40:1221–1226, 1992

Royall DR, Mahurin RK, True JE, et al: Executive impairment among the functionally dependent: comparisons between schizophrenic and elderly subjects. Am J Psychiatry 150:1813–1819, 1993

Royall DR, Cordes JA, Polk MJ: CLOX: an executive clock drawing test. J Neurol Neurosurg Psychiatry 64:588–594, 1998

Royall DR, Mulroy AR, Chiodo LK, et al: Clock drawing is sensitive to executive control: a comparison of six methods. J Gerontol 54B:P328–P333, 1999

Royall DR, Chiodo LK, Polk MJ: Correlates of disability among elderly retirees with "subclinical" cognitive impairment. J Gerontol 55A:M541–M546, 2000

Russell RW: Supranuclear palsy of eyelid closure. Brain 103:71–82, 1980

Ryan R, Sunada K: Medical evaluation of persons with mental retardation referred for psychiatric assessment. Gen Hosp Psychiatry 19:274–280, 1997

Sachdev P: Clinical characteristics of 15 patients with tardive dystonia. Am J Psychiatry 150:498–500, 1993

Sachdev P: Akathisia and Restless Legs. Cambridge, UK, Cambridge University Press, 1995

Sachdev P, Kruk J: Clinical characteristics and predisposing factors in acute drug-induced akathisia. Arch Gen Psychiatry 51:963–974, 1994

Sackeim HA, Greenberg MS, Weiman AL, et al: Hemispheric asymmetry in the expression of positive and negative emotions. Arch Neurol 39:210–218, 1982

Samie MR, Selhorst JB, Koller WC: Posttraumatic midbrain tremor. Neurology 40:62–66, 1990

Sanders RD, Keshavan MS: The neurologic examination in adult psychiatry: from soft signs to hard science. J Neuropsychiatry Clin Neurosci 10:395–404, 1998

Sanders RD, Forman SD, Pierri JN, et al: Inter-rater reliability of the neurological examination in schizophrenia. Schizophr Res 29(3):287–292, 1998

Saver J, Greenstein P, Ronthal M, et al: Asymmetric catalepsy after right hemisphere stroke. Mov Disord 8:69–73, 1993

Sawle G: Movement disorders during sleep, in Movement Disorders in Clinical Practice. Edited by Sawle G. Oxford, UK, Isis Medical Media, 1999, pp 159–163

Schachar R: Childhood hyperactivity. J Child Psychol Psychiatry 32:155–191, 1991

Schiff HB, Alexander MP, Naeser MA, et al: Aphemia: clinical-anatomic correlations. Arch Neurol 40:720–727, 1983

Schnider A: Spontaneous confabulations, disorientation, and the processing of "now." Neuropsychologia 38:175–185, 2000

Schnider A, Ptak R: Spontaneous confabulators fail to suppress currently irrelevant memory traces. Nat Neurosci 2:677–681, 1999

Schott GD, Wyke MA: Congenital mirror movements. J Neurol Neurosurg Psychiatry 44:586–599, 1981

Sellal F, Fontaine SF, Van Der Linden M, et al: To be or not to be at home? A neuropsychological approach to delusion for place. J Clin Exp Neuropsychol 18:234–248, 1996

Shallice T, Burgess PW, Schon F, et al: The origins of utilization behavior. Brain 112:1587–1598, 1989

Shaunak S, O'Sullivan E, Kennard C: Eye movements. J Neurol Neurosurg Psychiatry 59:115–125, 1995

Sigal M, Altmark D, Alfici S, et al: Ganser syndrome: a review of 15 cases. Compr Psychiatry 33:124–138, 1992

Signer SF: Localization and lateralization in the delusion of substitution: Capgras symptom and its variants. Psychopathology 27:168–176, 1994

Silberman EK, Post RM, Nurnberger J, et al: Transient sensory, cognitive and affective phenomena in affective illness: a comparison with complex partial epilepsy. Br J Psychiatry 146:81–89, 1985

Silberman EK, Sussman N, Skillings G, et al: Aura phenomena and psychopathology: a pilot investigation. Epilepsia 35:778–784, 1994

Sjögren M, Wallin A, Edman A: Symptomatological characteristics distinguish between frontotemporal dementia and vascular dementia with a dominant frontal lobe syndrome. Int J Geriatr Psychiatry 12:656–661, 1997

Smith G, Vigen V, Evans J, et al: Patterns and associates of hyperphagia in patients with dementia. Neuropsychiatry Neuropsychol Behav Neurol 11:97–102, 1998

Smith RC, Kadewari RP, Rosenberger JR, et al: Nonresponding schizophrenia: differentiation by neurological soft signs and neuropsychological tests. Schizophr Bull 25:813–825, 1999

Snowden JS, Neary D: Progressive language dysfunction and lobar atrophy. Dementia 4:226–231, 1993

Snowden JS, Neary D, Mann DM, et al: Progressive language disorder due to lobar atrophy. Ann Neurol 31:174–183, 1992

Stacy M, Cardoso F, Jankovic J: Tardive stereotypy and other movement disorders in tardive dyskinesias. Neurology 43:937–941, 1993

Starkstein SE, Federoff JP, Price TR, et al: Anosognosia in patients with cerebrovascular lesions: a study of causative factors. Stroke 23:1446–1453, 1992

Steg JP, Rapoport JL: Minor physical anomalies in normal, neurotic, learning disabled, and severely disturbed children. J Autism Child Schizophr 5:299–307, 1975

Stein DJ, Niehaus DJH, Seedat S, et al: Phenomenology of stereotypic movement disorder. Psychiatr Ann 28: 297–312, 1998

Stengel E: A clinical and psychological study of echo-reactions. Journal of Mental Science 93:27–41, 1947

Stevens JR: Disturbances of ocular movements and blinking in schizophrenia. J Neurol Neurosurg Psychiatry 41:1024–1030, 1978a

Stevens JR: Eye blink and schizophrenia: psychosis or tardive dyskinesia. Am J Psychiatry 135:223–226, 1978b

Stewart JT: Akathisia following traumatic brain injury: treatment with bromocriptine. J Neurol Neurosurg Psychiatry 52:1200–1201, 1991

Strub RL, Black FW: The bedside mental status examination, in Handbook of Neuropsychology, Vol I. Edited by Boller F, Grafman J. Amsterdam, The Netherlands, Elsevier, 1988, pp 29–46

Stuppaeck CH, Miller CH, Ehrmann H, et al: Akathisia induced by necrosis of the basal ganglia after carbon monoxide intoxication. Mov Disord 10:229–231, 1995

Sultzer DL, Berisford MA, Gunay I: The neurobehavioral rating scale: reliability in patients with dementia. J Psychiatr Res 29:185–191, 1995

Tanaka Y, Albert ML, Hara H, et al: Forced hyperphasia and environmental dependency syndrome. J Neurol Neurosurg Psychiatry 68:224–226, 2000

Tarrant CJ, Jones PB: Precursors to schizophrenia: do biological markers have specificity? Can J Psychiatry 44:335–349, 1999

Tecoma ES, Laxer KD, Barbaro NM, et al: Frequency and characteristics of visual field deficits after surgery for mesial temporal sclerosis. Neurology 43:1235–1238, 1993

Teicher MH, Glod CA, Surrey J, et al: Early childhood abuse and limbic system ratings in adult psychiatric outpatients. J Neuropsychiatry Clin Neurosci 5:301–306, 1993

Teng EL, Chui HC: The Modified Mini-Mental State (3MS) Examination. J Clin Psychiatry 48:314–318, 1987

Thacker RC, De Nil LF: Neurogenic cluttering. J Fluency Disord 21:227–238, 1996

Thomas P, Beaumanoir A, Genton P, et al: "De novo" absence status of late onset: report of 11 cases. Neurology 42:104–110, 1992

Thompson PD, Marsden CD: Gait disorder of subcortical arteriosclerotic encephalopathy: Binswanger's disease. Mov Disord 2:1–8, 1987

Thompson PD, Marsden CD: Corticobasal degeneration. Baillieres Clin Neurol 1:677–686, 1992

Tinuper P, Plazzi G, Provini F, et al: Facial asymmetry in partial epilepsies. Epilepsia 33:1097–1100, 1992

Tirosh E, Canby J: Autism with hyperlexia: a distinct syndrome? Am J Ment Retard 98:84–92, 1993

Tomson T, Lindbom U, Nilsson BY: Nonconvulsive status epilepticus in adults: thirty-two consecutive patients from a general hospital population. Epilepsia 33:829–835, 1992

Toone BK, Edeh J, Nanjee MN, et al: Hyposexuality and epilepsy: a community survey of hormonal and behavioural changes in male epileptics. Psychol Med 19:937–943, 1989

Touwen BCL, Prechtl HFR: The Neurological Examination of the Child With Minor Nervous Dysfunction. London, Heinemann Medical Books, 1970

Tranel D, Anderson SW, Benton A: Development of the concept of "executive function" and its relationship to the frontal lobes, in Handbook of Neuropsychology, Vol 9. Edited by Boller F, Grafman J. Amsterdam, The Netherlands, Elsevier, 1994, pp 125–148

Trosch RM, Sze G, Brass LM, et al: Emotional facial paresis with striatocapsular infarction. J Neurol Sci 98:195–201, 1990

Turner TH: A diagnostic analysis of the Casebooks of Ticehurst House Asylum, 1845–1890. Psychol Med Monogr Suppl 21:1–70, 1992

van Gorp WG, Marcotte TD, Sultzer DL, et al: Screening for dementia: comparison of three commonly used instruments. J Clin Exp Neuropsychol 21:29–38, 1999

Victor M, Adams RD, Collins GH: The Wernicke-Korsakoff Syndrome and Related Neurological Diseases Due to Alcoholism and Malnutrition, 2nd Edition. Philadelphia, PA, FA Davis, 1989

Vighetto A, Henry E, Garde P, et al: Le délire spatial: une manifestation des lésions de l'hémisphère mineur. Rev Neurol (Paris) 141:476–481, 1985

Waddington JL, O'Callaghan E, Buckley P, et al: Tardive dyskinesia in schizophrenia: relationship to minor physical anomalies, frontal lobe dysfunction and cerebral structure on magnetic resonance imaging. Br J Psychiatry 167:41–45, 1995

Wade DT: Measurement in Neurological Rehabilitation. Oxford, UK, Oxford University Press, 1992

Walczak TS, Bogolioubov A: Weeping during psychogenic nonepileptic seizures. Epilepsia 37:208–210, 1996

Wali GM: "Fou rire prodromique" heralding a brainstem stroke. J Neurol Neurosurg Psychiatry 56:209–210, 1993

Wallesch C-W, Hundsalz A: Language function in delirium: a comparison of single word processing in acute confusional states and probable Alzheimer's disease. Brain Lang 46:592–606, 1994

Walshe JM: Wilson's disease, in Handbook of Clinical Neurology, Vol 49: Extrapyramidal Disorders. Edited by Vinken PJ, Bruyn GW, Klawans HL. Amsterdam, The Netherlands, Elsevier Science, 1986, pp 223–238

Wapner W, Hamby S, Gardner H: The role of the right hemisphere in the apprehension of complex linguistic materials. Brain Lang 14:15–33, 1981

Weinstein DD, Diforio D, Schiffman J, et al: Minor physical anomalies, dermatoglyphic asymmetries, and cortisol levels in adolescents with schizotypal personality disorder. Am J Psychiatry 156:617–623, 1999

Weintraub S: Neuropsychological assessment of mental state, in Principles of Cognitive and Behavioral Neurology, 2nd Edition. Edited by Mesulam M-M. Oxford, UK, Oxford University Press, 2000, pp 121–173

Weintraub S, Mesulam M-M: Mental state assessment of young and elderly adults in behavioral neurology, in Principles of Behavioral Neurology. Edited by Mesulam M-M. Philadelphia, PA, FA Davis, 1985, pp 71–123

Weiss AP, Jenike MA: Late-onset obsessive-compulsive disorder: a case series. J Neuropsychiatry Clin Neurosci 12:265–268, 2000

Weller M: Anterior opercular cortex lesions cause dissociated lower cranial nerve palsies and anarthria but no aphasia: Foix-Chavany-Marie syndrome and "automatic voluntary dissociation" revisited. J Neurol 240:199–208, 1993

Wertz RT, Henschel CR, Auther LL, et al: Affective prosodic disturbance subsequent to right hemisphere stroke: a clinical application. Journal of Neurolinguistics 11:89–102, 1998

Williams D: The structure of emotions reflected in epileptic experiences. Brain 79:29–67, 1956

Wilson SAK: Some problems in neurology: no. 11: pathological laughing and crying. Journal of Neurology and Psychopathology 4:299–333, 1924

Wojcik JD, Falk WE, Fink JS, et al: A review of 32 cases of tardive dystonia. Am J Psychiatry 148:1055–1059, 1991

Wolff A-L, O'Driscoll GA: Motor deficits and schizophrenia: the evidence from neuroleptic-naïve patients and populations at risk. J Psychiatry Neurosci 24:304–314, 1999

Wong AHC, Voruganti LNP, Heslegrave RJ, et al: Neurocognitive deficits and neurological signs in schizophrenia. Schizophr Res 23:139–146, 1997

Young RR, Shahani BT: Asterixis: one type of negative myoclonus. Adv Neurol 43:137–156, 1986

Yuspeh RL, Vanderploeg RD, Kershaw DA: Validity of a semantically cued recall procedure for the Mini-Mental State Examination. Neuropsychiatry Neuropsychol Behav Neurol 11:207–211, 1998

Zametkin AJ, Stevens JR, Pittman R: Ontogeny of spontaneous blinking and of habituation of the blink reflex. Ann Neurol 5:453–457, 1979

The Neuropsychological Evaluation

Diane B. Howieson, Ph.D.

Muriel D. Lezak, Ph.D.

Neuropsychologists assess brain function by making inferences from an individual's cognitive, sensorimotor, emotional, and social behavior. During the early history of neuropsychology, these assessments were often the most direct measure of brain integrity in persons who did not have localizing neurological signs and symptoms and who had problems confined to higher mental functions (Hebb 1942; Teuber 1948). Neuropsychological measures are useful diagnostic indicators of brain dysfunction for many conditions and will remain the major diagnostic modality for some (Bigler 1999; Farah and Feinberg 2000; Jernigan and Hesselink 1987; Lezak 1995; Mesulam 2000). However, diagnosis of brain damage has become increasingly accurate in recent decades as a result of improved visualization of brain structure by computed tomography (CT), magnetic resonance imaging (MRI), and angiography (Frith and Friston 1997; Theodore 1988). Advances in electrophysiologic examination techniques (Caccioppo et al. 2000; Daube 1996; Johnson 1995) and in quantitative and functional neuroimaging have further enriched our understanding of pathological disturbances of the brain (Aine 1995; Binder et al. 1995; Ernst et al. 1999; Frith and Grasby 1995; Levin et al. 1996; Menon and Kim 1999; Papanicolaou 1999). It is even possible to produce precisely placed, reversible "lesions" to study how the remainder of the brain functions without a designated cortical area (Grafman and Wassermann 1999; Walsh and Rushworth 1999). These developments have allowed a shift in the focus of neuropsychological assessment from the diagnosis of possible brain damage to a better understanding of specific brain-behavior relationships and the psychosocial consequences of brain damage.

Indications for Neuropsychological Evaluation

Patients referred to a neuropsychologist for assessment typically fall into one of three groups. The first, and probably largest, group consists of patients with known brain disorders. The more common neurological disorders are cerebrovascular disorders, developmental disorders, traumatic brain injury, Alzheimer's disease and related disorders, Parkinson's disease, multiple sclerosis, Huntington's chorea, tumors, seizures, and infections. Psychiatric disorders also may be associated with brain dysfunction; chief among them are schizophrenia, obsessive-compulsive disorder, and depression.

A neuropsychological evaluation can be useful in defining the nature and severity of resulting behavioral and emotional problems. The assessment provides information about the patient's cognition, personality characteristics, social behavior, emotional status, and adaptation to limitations. The individual's potential for independent living and productive activity can be inferred from these data. Information about the patient's behavioral strengths and weaknesses provides a foundation for treatment planning, vocational training, competency determination, and counseling for both patients and their families (Acker 1989; Diller 2000; Newcombe 1987; Sloan and Ponsford 1995).

The second group of patients is composed of persons with a known risk factor for brain disorder in whom a change in behavior might be the result of such a disorder. In these cases a neuropsychological evaluation might be used both to provide evidence of brain dysfunction and to describe the nature and severity of problems. An individual who has sustained a blow to the head from an automobile accident that produces a brief loss of consciousness, even with no apparent further neurological complications, might experience disruption in cognitive efficiency. On returning to work after 1 week, this individual might be unable to keep up with job demands. After several weeks of on-the-job difficulties, the physician may

refer the patient to a neuropsychologist for evaluation of possible brain injury from the accident. The examiner would look for evidence of problems with divided attention, sustained concentration and mental tracking, and memory, all of which are common findings in the weeks or months following mild head injury (Bennett and Raymonds 1997; Varney and Roberts 1999; Wrightson and Gronwall 1999). The neuropsychologist can advise the patient that these problems frequently occur after head injury and that considerable improvement might be expected during the next month or two. Recommendations about how to structure work activities to minimize both these difficulties and the equally common problem of fatigue provide both aid and comfort to the concerned patient. The neuropsychologist might repeat the examination several months after the injury to see if these predictions held true and to assess the individual's adjustment and possible need for further counseling or other treatment.

A depressed older individual may complain of poor memory, raising concern about a possible illness producing dementia. It is not unusual to observe attention and memory problems in patients such as this based on depression alone. In most cases, the nature and degree of cognitive problems would differentiate the diagnoses.

Many medical conditions can affect brain function (Lezak 1995; Tarter et al. 1988). Brain function can be disrupted by systemic illnesses: endocrinopathies; metabolic and electrolyte disturbances; diseases of the kidney, liver, and pancreas; nutritional deficiencies; and conditions producing decreased blood supply to the brain. The latter include vascular disorders, cardiac disease, pulmonary disease, anemia, and complications of anesthesia or surgery. Age and health habits also must be taken into consideration when evaluating a person's behavioral alterations, since they affect the probability of cerebral disorder (Dubois et al. 1990; Kolb 1989; Perfect and Maylor 2000). In addition, many medicines can disrupt cognition through their subtle effects on alertness, attention, and memory (Blain and Lane 1991; Davison and Hassanyck 1991; Pagliaro and Pagliaro 1998; Stein and Strickland 1998).

In the last group, brain disease or dysfunction is often suspected based on the observation of a change in a person's behavior without an identifiable cause: that is, the patient has no known risk factors for brain disorder and this diagnosis is considered on the basis of exclusion of other diagnoses. Frequently, psychiatrists are asked to evaluate an adult with no previous psychiatric history who has had an uncharacteristic change in behavior or personality and for whom no obvious sources of current emotional distress can be identified. An explanation is sought, since behavior patterns and personality are relatively stable characteristics of adults. The list of differential diagnoses is long and may include a wide variety of brain disorders ranging from metabolic disturbance, vitamin deficiency, endocrine disorder, and heavy metal poisoning to neoplasm, infection, and multiple small strokes. The psychiatric literature contains numerous examples of individuals who were being treated for psychiatric illness before it was discovered that they had brain disease, such as a frontal lobe tumor (R.A. Berg 1988; Fahy et al. 1995; Lesser 1985). The most common application of the neuropsychological evaluation of older adults without obvious risk factors for brain disease is in the early detection of progressive dementia, such as Alzheimer's disease (Howieson et al. 1997; Jacobs et al. 1995; Masur et al. 1994; Morris et al. 1991; Petersen et al. 1994; Rentz and Weintraub 2000).

In cases with no known cause to explain mental deterioration, a search for possible risk factors or other evidence for brain disease is conducted through history taking, performing physical examination, conducting laboratory tests, and interviewing the patient's family or close associates. Even if this search produces no evidence of disease, a diagnostic neuropsychological study might be useful.

The neuropsychological examination of persons with or without known risk factors for brain damage is diagnostically useful if a meaningful pattern of deficits is found. A pattern considered meaningful would be one that may be specific to one, or only a few, diagnoses, such as a pattern of cognitive disruption suggestive of a lateralized or focal brain lesion.

> A man with HIV infection had a two-week history of "feeling odd." He became easily lost, even in familiar settings, and complained of an inability to perform a task as simple as making his sheets "fit the bed." He said that he could not read because he was unable to follow a line consistently across the page. He had stopped working as a barber after giving a poor haircut. He had no established symptoms of his infection. Although he was known to have an appropriate reactive depression related to his infection, his complaints were atypical for depression. A neuropsychological evaluation showed that he had severe and circumscribed visuospatial and constructional deficits, a pattern of cognitive deficits usually associated with right parietal dysfunction. A subsequent MRI scan showed white matter disease involving a large area of the right parietal lobe and several small areas elsewhere in the right hemisphere. A biopsy confirmed the diagnosis of multifocal progressive leukoencephalopathy.

Neuropsychological signs and symptoms that are possible indicators of a pathological brain process are presented in Table 2–1. Positive neuropsychological

TABLE 2–1. Neuropsychological signs and symptoms that are possible indicators of a pathological brain process

Functional class	Symptoms and signs
Speech and language	Dysarthria
	Dysfluency
	Marked change in amount of speech output
	Paraphasias
	Word-finding problems
Academic skills	Alterations in reading, writing, frequent letter or number reversals, calculating, and number abilities
Thinking	Perseveration of speech
	Simplified or confused mental racking, reasoning, and concept formation
Motor	Weakness or clumsiness, particularly if lateralized
	Impaired fine motor coordination (e.g., changes in handwriting)
	Apraxias
	Perseveration of action components
Memory[a]	Impaired recent memory for verbal or visuospatial material or both
	Disorientation
Perception	Diplopia or visual field alterations
	Inattention (usually left-sided)
	Somatosensory alterations (particularly if lateralized)
	Inability to recognize familiar stimuli (agnosia)
Visuospatial abilities	Diminished ability to perform manual skills (e.g., mechanical repairs and sewing)
	Spatial disorientation
	Left-right disorientation
	Impaired spatial judgment (e.g., angulation of distances)
Emotions[b]	Diminished emotional control with temper outburst and antisocial behavior
	Diminished empathy or interest in interpersonal relationships
	Affective changes
	Irritability without evident precipitating factors
	Personality change
Comportment[b]	Altered appetites and appetitive activities
	Altered grooming habits (excessive fastidiousness and carelessness)
	Hyperactivity or hypoactivity
	Social inappropriateness

[a]Many emotionally disturbed persons complain of memory deficits, which most typically reflect the person's self-preoccupation, distractibility, or anxiety rather than a dysfunctional brain. Thus, memory complaints in themselves do not necessarily warrant neuropsychological evaluation.

[b]Some of these changes are most likely to be neuropsychologically relevant in the absence of depression, although they can also be mistaken for depression.

diagnoses are much more likely to be made when risk factors for brain dysfunction exist or signs and symptoms of brain dysfunction are observed than when neuropsychological diagnoses are considered on the basis solely of exclusion of other diagnoses.

One of the greatest challenges for a neuropsychologist is to assess whether patients with psychiatric illness have evidence of an independent underlying brain disorder. Many psychiatric patients without neurological disease have cognitive disruption and behavioral or emotional aberrations. Conversely, neurological disease can present as a psychiatric disorder (Cummings 1999; Skuster et al. 1992). Depressed patients often underperform compared with control subjects on measures of speed of processing, mental flexibility, and executive function (Veiel 1997). Memory impairment is less consistently observed (Basso and Bornstein 1999b; Boone et al. 1995; Palmer et al. 1996), and memory performance may be intact even when memory complaints are present (Dalgleish and Cox 2000; Kalska et al. 1999). Cognitive deficits, including memory, are more common in depressed patients with psychotic features than in those with no psychotic features (Basso and Bornstein 1999a; McKenna et al. 2000). Compared with control subjects, euthymic bipolar patients may have difficulty with attention, memory, abstraction (Denicoff et al. 1999), and executive functions (Ferrier et al. 1999). The degree of cognitive impairment appears to be related to the number of prior episodes (Denicoff et al. 1999; Van Gorp et al. 1998). Although a number of psychological explanations have been proposed, such as self-focused rumination associated with dysphoria (Hertel 1998), the possibility has been raised of an underlying structural abnormality in the neural pathways that modulate mood (Ali et al. 2000; Strakowski et al. 1999).

Role of the Referring Psychiatrist

The referring psychiatrist has the tasks of identifying patients who might benefit from an evaluation, preparing the patient, and formulating referral questions that best define the needed neuropsychological information. A valid evaluation depends on obtaining the patient's best performance. It is nearly impossible to obtain satisfactory evaluations of patients who are uncooperative, fatigued, actively psychotic, seriously depressed, or highly anxious. For example, seriously depressed patients may appear to have dementia and the evaluation may underestimate the individual's full potential (Chaves and Izquierdo 1992; King and Caine 1996; Marcopulos 1989; Yousef et al. 1998). Whenever possible, severely depressed or actively psychotic patients should be referred after there has been clinical improvement, when the results may be more representative of the patient's true ability uncontaminated by reversible emotional or behavioral disturbances.

The Assessment Process

Interview and observation are the chief means by which neuropsychological evaluations are conducted. The interview provides the basis of the evaluation (Christensen 1979; Lezak 1995; Luria 1980; Sbordone 2000). The main purposes are to elicit the patient's and family's complaints, understand the circumstances in which these problems occur, and evaluate the patient's attitude toward these problems. Understanding the range of the patient's complaints, as well as which ones the patient views as most troublesome, contributes to the framework on which the assessment and recommendations are based. A thorough history of complaints and pertinent background is essential.

The presenting problems and the patient's attitude toward them also may provide important diagnostic information. Patients with certain neuropsychological conditions lack awareness of their problems or belittle their significance (Markova and Berrios 2000; Prigatano and Schacter 1991). Many patients with right hemisphere stroke, Alzheimer's disease, and frontal lobe damage are unaware of or unable to appreciate the problems resulting from their brain injury. In the extreme form of right hemisphere stroke, some patients with hemiplegia are unable to comprehend that the left side of their body is part of them, let alone that they cannot use it. In a more muted form, many patients with dementia attribute their memory problems to aging and minimize their significance (see Strub and Black 2000). Conversely, patients, families, or caregivers sometimes attribute problems to brain damage when a careful history suggests otherwise.

The interview provides an opportunity to observe the patient's appearance, attention, speech, thought content, and motor abilities and to evaluate affect, appropriateness of behavior, orientation, insight, and judgment. The interview can provide information about the patient's premorbid intellectual ability and personality, occupational and school background, social situation, and ability to use leisure time.

The tests used by neuropsychologists are simply standardized observation tools that, in many instances, have the added advantage of providing normative data that aid in interpreting the observations. A variety of assessment approaches are available, but they all have in common the goals of determining whether the patient shows evidence of brain dysfunction and identifying the nature of problems detected. The two main approaches are individually tailored examinations and fixed assessment procedures. The former is often referred to as the *hypothesis-testing* approach, because test selection is based on hypotheses about the cause and nature of the brain dysfunction from

information acquired before and during the assessment (Kaplan 1988; Lezak 1995; Milberg et al. 1996). Using this approach, information is obtained about the individual's medical and psychological background and about the patient's activities from the individual and other knowledgeable sources. Hypotheses regarding neuropsychological deficits are generated and tested.

A second approach to neuropsychological testing is to use a fixed battery of tests (Broshek and Barth 2000; Reitan and Wolfson 1993). This approach involves examining the same range of cognitive and behavioral functioning in every individual. It is analogous to a physician conducting a standard physical examination on all patients. These fixed battery examinations frequently last from 6 to 8 hours. The advantage of fixed batteries is that the patient has a fairly broad-based examination. The consistency of the administration procedures and normative data, and the relatively wide range of data, make batteries useful for research purposes. Although these advantages might lure the examiner, this fixed approach does not focus on specific areas of difficulty. In some cases it might be unclear why performance is impaired without additional testing outside of the battery. Time may be wasted in testing areas of cognition or sensorimotor functioning that are not problems, and subtle problems can be overlooked. Tailoring the examination to the patient's requirements rather than using a fixed battery allows the examiner to learn what is needed about the patient with a minimum of time and cost.

Cognitive performance is only one aspect of an assessment. A full evaluation of the individual assesses emotional and social characteristics as well. Many patients with brain injuries have changes in personality, mood, or ability to control emotional states (Heilman et al. 1993;

TABLE 2–2. Ability test classifications expressed as deviations from the mean calculated from the normative sample

Z score range	Percentile	Classification
> +2.0	98–100	Very superior
+1.3 to +2.0	91–97	Superior
+0.67 to +1.3	75–90	High average
−0.66 to +0.66	26–74	Average
−0.67 to −1.3	10–25	Low average
−1.3 to −2.0	3–9	Borderline
< −2.0	0–2	Mentally retarded

Lishman 1997) and problems with social relationships (Dikmen et al. 1996; Lezak 1988a). Depression is a common and sometimes serious complication of brain disease.

The Nature of Neuropsychological Tests

An important component of neuropsychological evaluations is psychological testing, in which an individual's cognitive and often emotional status and executive functioning are assessed. Neuropsychological assessment differs from psychological assessment in its basic assumptions. The latter compares the individual's responses with normative data from a sample of healthy individuals taking the same test (Anastasi and Urbina 1997). The neuropsychological assessment of adults relies on comparisons between the patient's present level of functioning and the known or estimated level of premorbid functioning based on demographically similar individuals and current performance on tests of functions less likely to be affected by brain disorders. Thus, much of clinical neuropsychological assessment involves *intraindividual* comparisons of the abilities and skills under consideration.

The level of competence in different cognitive functions as well as other behav-

iors varies from individual to individual and also within the same individual at different times. This variability also has the characteristics of a normal curve. (See Table 2–2 for interpretations of ability levels based on deviations from the mean and normative sample.)

An individual's score is compared with the normative data, often by calculating a standard or Z score, which describes the individual's performance in terms of statistically regular distances (i.e., standard deviations). In this framework, scores within ±0.66 standard deviation are considered average, since 50% of a normative sample scores within this range. A performance in the below-average direction that is greater than two standard deviations from the mean is usually described as falling in the impaired range because 98% of the normative sample taking the test achieve better scores.

Psychological tests should be constructed to have both reliability and validity (Anastasi and Urbina 1997). The reliability of a test refers to the consistency of test scores when the test is given to the same individual at different times or with different sets of equivalent items. As perfect reliability cannot be achieved for any test, each individual score represents a range of variability, which narrows to the degree that the test's reliability approaches the ideal (Anastasi and Urbina 1997). Tests have validity when they measure what they purport to measure. If a test is designed to measure attention disorders, then patient groups known to have attention deficits should perform more poorly on the test than persons from the population at large. Tests also should be constructed with large normative samples of individuals with similar demographic characteristics, particularly for age and education (Gade et al. 1985; Heaton et al. 1991; Malec et al. 1992). For example, the Wechsler Adult Intelligence Scale–III has normative data for 2,450 adults stratified for age, sex, race, geographic region, occupation, and education according to United States census information (Psychological Corporation 1997). Most tests have much smaller normative samples in the range of 30 to 200 individuals.

Some psychological tests detect subtle deficits better than others. A simple signal detection test of attention, such as crossing out all the letters *A* on a page, is less sensitive a test of attention than a divided attention task, such as crossing out all letters *A* and *C*. Tests involving complex tasks, such as problem solving requiring abstract thinking and cognitive flexibility, are more sensitive than many other cognitive tests at reflecting brain damage, because a wide variety of brain disorders can easily disrupt performance on them. However, other factors such as depression, anxiety, medicine side effects, and low energy level due to systemic illness may also disrupt cognition on these sensitive tests. Therefore, they are sensitive to cognitive disruption but not specific to one type of cognitive disturbance. The specificity of a test in detecting a disorder depends on the overlap between the distributions of the scores of persons who are intact and of the scores of persons who have the disorder (Figure 2–1). The less overlap there is, the more diagnostic the test result. A test that is highly specific, such as the Token Test (Boller and Vignolo

1966; De Renzi and Vignolo 1962), which assesses language comprehension, produces few abnormal test results in nonaphasic persons, that is, few false-positive results. Many neuropsychological tests offer a trade-off between sensitivity and specificity.

Interpretation Principles and Cautions

The interpretation of test performance is based on an assumption that the patient is expected to perform in a particular way on tasks; deviations from expectation require evaluation (Lezak 1986, 1995). Most healthy people perform within a statistically definable range on cognitive tests, and this range of performance levels is considered to be characteristic of healthy people. Deviations below this expected range raise the question of an impairment. A person may have scores in the high average range on many tests except for low average performance in one functional area.

The assumption of deficit is valid in most instances in which one or a set of scores fall significantly below expectations, although a few persons show an unusual variability on cognitive tasks (Matarazzo and Prifitera 1989). Multiple measures involving similar or related abilities increase the reliability of findings. Thus, if a deviant score shows up on one task, other tests requiring similar skills are used to see if the deviant finding persists across tasks. If so, the finding is considered reliable. If similar tasks do not elicit a deviant performance, either the finding was spurious or the additional tasks varied in important features that did not involve the patient's problem area. The need to have multiple measures of many cognitive functions is the reason why neuropsychological examinations may be lengthy.

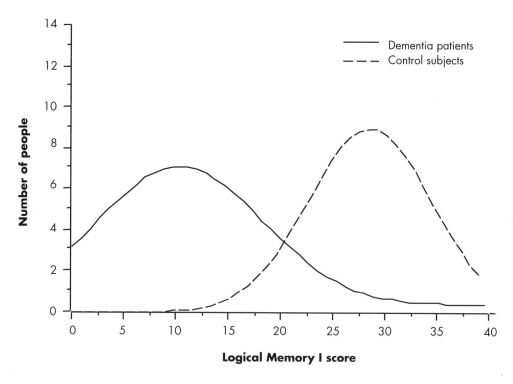

FIGURE 2–1. Distribution of test scores by a group with mild dementia and age-matched control subjects on the Wechsler Memory Scale–Revised Logical Memory I, a story-recall test.

Scores ranging from 15 to 39 occurred in both groups, whereas scores below 15 occurred in only the dementia group. The smaller the areas of overlapping curves, the higher the test specificity.

For meaningful interpretations of neuropsychological test performance, not only do examiners rely on many tests but they search for a performance pattern (test scores plus qualitative features) that makes neuropsychological sense. Because there are few pathognomonic findings in neuropsychology, or in most other branches of medical science for that matter (Sox et al. 1988), a performance pattern often can suggest several diagnoses. For example, a cluster of documented deficits including slowed thinking and mild impairment of concentration and memory is a nonspecific finding associated with a number of conditions: very mild dementia, a mild post-concussion syndrome, mild toxic encephalopathy, depression, and fatigue, to name a few.

Other patterns may be highly specific for certain conditions. The finding of left-sided neglect and visuospatial distortions is highly suggestive of brain dysfunction and specifically occurs with right hemisphere damage. For many neuropsychological conditions, typical deficit patterns are known, allowing the examiner to evaluate the patient's performances in light of these known patterns for a possible match.

The quality of a neuropsychological evaluation depends on many factors. In general, one should beware of conclusions from evaluations in which test scores alone (that is, without information from history, interview, and observations of examination behavior) are used to make diagnostic decisions and of dogmatic statements offered without strongly supportive evidence. It is also important to remember that neuropsychological tests do not measure "brain damage." Rather, the finding of impaired mental functioning implies an underlying brain disorder. It is important to keep in mind that poor performance on neuropsychological tests does not necessarily mean that the patient has a brain disorder. Other possible interpretations may exist.

Major Test Categories

This section presents a brief review of tests used for assessment of major areas of cognition and personality. Many useful neuropsychological tests are not described in this summary. Please refer to *Neuropsychological Assessment*, 3rd edition (Lezak 1995) for a relatively complete review.

Mental Ability

The most commonly used set of tests of general intellectual function of adults in the Western world is contained in the various versions of the Wechsler Intelligence Scales (WIS) (Wechsler 1944, 1955, 1981, 1997a). These batteries of brief tests provide scores on a variety of cognitive tasks covering a range of skills. Each version was originally developed as an "intelligence" test to predict academic and vocational performance of neurologically intact adults by giving an IQ (intelligence quotient) score, which is based on the mean performance on the tests in this battery. The entire test battery is frequently among the tests included in a neuropsychological examination. The individual tests were designed to assess relatively distinct areas of cognition, such as arithmetic, abstract thinking, and visuospatial organization, and thus are differentially sensitive to dysfunction of various areas of the brain. Therefore, this test is

often used to screen for specific areas of cognitive deficits. When given to neuropsychologically impaired persons, the summary IQ scores can be very misleading because individual test scores lowered by specific cognitive deficits, when averaged in with scores relatively unaffected by the brain dysfunction, can result in IQ scores associated with ability levels that represent neither the severity of deficits nor the patient's residual competencies (Lezak 1988b).

For example, a patient with a visuospatial deficit consisting of an inability to appreciate the structure of visual patterns would have difficulty performing the Block Design test, which requires copying pictured designs with blocks. When such a patient performs well above average on other tests, a summation of all the scores would both hide the important data and be lower than the other test scores in the battery would warrant. Therefore, neuropsychologists focus on the pattern of the Wechsler scores rather than the summed or average performance on all the tests in the battery.

A similar battery for assessing children is the Wechsler Intelligence Scale for Children–III (WISC-III) (Wechsler 1991). It contains tests similar to those in the Wechsler Adult Intelligence Scale–III but appropriate for ages 6–16 years.

Language

Lesions to the hemisphere dominant for speech and language, which is the left hemisphere in 95%–97% of right-handed persons and 60%–70% of left-handed persons (Corballis 1991; Strauss and Goldsmith 1987), can produce any of a variety of disorders of symbol formulation and use, the aphasias (see Mendez and Cummings, Chapter 6, in this volume). Although many aphasiologists argue against attempting to classify all patients into one of the standard aphasia syndromes because of individual differences, persons with aphasia tend to be grouped according to whether the main disorder is in language comprehension (receptive aphasia), expression (expressive aphasia), repetition (conduction aphasia), or naming (anomic aphasia). Many comprehensive language assessment tests are available, such as the Multilingual Aphasia Examination (Benton and Hamsher 1989). Comprehensive aphasia test batteries are best administered by speech pathologists or other clinicians with special training in this field. These batteries usually include measures of spontaneous speech, speech comprehension, repetition, naming, reading, and writing.

Attention and Mental Tracking

A frequent consequence of brain disorders is slowed thinking and impaired ability for focused behavior (Gronwall and Sampson 1974; Van Zomeren and Brouwer 1994). Damage to the brain stem or diffuse damage involving the cerebral hemispheres can produce a variety of attentional deficits, and attentional deficits are common in neuropsychiatric disorders.

Many neuropsychological assessments will include measures of these abilities. The Wechsler scales contain several. The Digit Span test measures attention span or short-term memory for numbers by assessing forward digit repetition. The task also measures backward digit repetition, which is a more demanding task requiring concentration and mental tracking. It is not uncommon for severely brain-damaged patients to perform poorly only on the backward repetition portion of this test. Because Digits Forward and Digits Backward measure different functions, assessment data for each should be given separately. The Digit Symbol test also requires concentration and both motor and mental speed for successful perfor-

mance. The patient must accurately and rapidly code numbers into symbols.

Another commonly used measure of concentration and mental tracking is the Trail Making Test (Armitage 1946). In the first part of this test (Part A), the patient is asked to draw rapidly and accurately a line connecting in sequence a random display of numbered circles on a page. The level of difficulty is increased in the second part (Part B) by having the patient again sequence a random display of circles, this time alternating numbers and letters (Figure 2–2). This test requires concentration, visual scanning, and flexibility in shifting cognitive sets and, as such, it is among those that are most sensitive to the presence of brain injury (Crockett et al. 1988; Spreen and Benton 1965; Van Zomeren and Brouwer 1994). However, it shares with other highly sensitive tests vulnerability to many other kinds of deficits such as motor slowing, which could be based on peripheral factors such as nerve damage, and diminished visual acuity. It is also sensitive to educational deprivation and cannot be used with persons not accustomed to the alphabet as known in Western countries.

In cases of subtle brain injury, assessment sensitivity can be increased by selecting a more difficult measure of concentration and mental tracking in which material must be held in mind while information is manipulated for the performance of such complex cognitive activities as comprehension, learning, and reasoning. Performance on the orally administered WIS Arithmetic test provides information about attention deficits, as it requires intact auditory attention span and mental tracking for success. When patients perform poorly on the Arithmetic test, the examiner must determine whether the failure results from attentional deficits or lack of arithmetic skills.

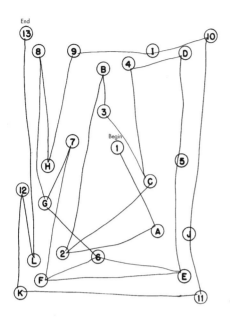

FIGURE 2–2. Trail Making Test (Armitage 1946) Part B performance by a 61-year-old man with normal-pressure hydrocephalus.
Two types of errors are demonstrated: erroneous sequencing (1→A→2→C) and failure to alternate between numbers and letters (D→5→E→F).

The ability to hold information in mind while performing a mental task is called working memory (Baddeley 1994). As such, working memory requires attention and short-term memory. The Self Ordered Pointing Task (Petrides and Milner 1982; Spreen and Strauss 1998) instructs patients to point to one item in a set ranging from 6 to 18 varied items. On each trial, in which the positions of the items are randomly changed, patients are told to point to a different item that they have not previously pointed to, and then another, until they had pointed to all the items. The successful performance of this working memory task depends on keeping in mind which items have already been eliminated.

Another example of a difficult attentional task is the Paced Auditory Serial Addition Test (PASAT) (Gronwall 1977; Gronwall and Sampson 1974). The patient is required to add consecutive pairs of numbers rapidly under an interference condition. As numbers are presented at a fixed rate, the patient must always add the last two numbers presented and ignore the number that represents the last summation. For example, if the numbers "3–5–2–7" are presented, the patient must respond "8" after the number 5, and then "7" after the number 2, and then "9." It is a difficult test of divided attention because of the strong tendency to add the last number presented to the last summation. The level of difficulty can be heightened by speeding up the rate of presentation of numbers.

Memory

Memory is another cognitive function frequently impaired by brain disorders (see Stern and Sackeim, Chapter 7, in this volume). Many diffuse brain injuries produce general impairments in abilities for new learning and retention. Many focal brain injuries also produce memory impairment; left hemisphere lesions are most likely to produce primarily verbal memory deficits, whereas visuospatial memory impairments tend to be associated with right hemisphere lesions (Milner 1978; Ojemann and Dodrill 1985). Memory impairment often is a prominent feature of herpes encephalitis, Huntington's chorea, Korsakoff's syndrome, hypoxia, closed head injury, and a variety of neurological degenerative diseases such as Alzheimer's disease (Baddeley et al. 1995; Butters and Miliotis 1985; Kapur 1988; Mayes 2000).

In most cases of brain injury, memory for information learned before the injury is relatively preserved compared with new learning. For this reason, many patients with memory impairment will perform relatively well on tests of fund of information or recall of remote events. However, amnesic disorders can produce a retrograde amnesia, with loss of memory extending weeks, months, or years before the onset of the injury. Electroconvulsive therapy can also produce retrograde amnesia (Squire et al. 1975). The retrograde amnesia of Huntington's chorea or Korsakoff's syndrome can go back for decades (Butters and Miliotis 1985; Cermak 1982). In rare cases, a patient will have retrograde amnesia without significant anterograde amnesia, that is, new learning ability remains intact (Kapur et al. 1996; Reed and Squire 1998). Isolated retrograde amnesia may include amnesia for autobiographical events (Della Sala et al. 1993; Evans et al. 1996; Kapur 1997; Levine et al. 1998). However, cases of amnesia for personal identity often have a psychogenic cause (Hodges 1991).

The Wechsler Memory Scale (WMS) batteries (Wechsler 1987, 1997b) are the most commonly used set of tests of new learning and retention in the United States. These batteries are composed of a variety of tests measuring free recall or recognition of both verbal and visual material. In addition, these tests include measures of recall of personal information and attention, concentration, and mental tracking. Several of the tests provide measures of both immediate and delayed (approximately 30 minutes) recall.

Other memory tests frequently used include word-list learning tasks, such as the Rey Auditory Verbal Learning Test (Lezak 1995; Rey 1964; Schmidt 1996) or the California Verbal Learning Test (Delis et al. 1983, 1986, 1987), and visuospatial tasks such the Complex Figure Test (Mitrushina et al. 1999; Osterrieth 1944; Rey 1941; Spreen and Strauss 1998). When patients are unable to produce verbal responses or use their preferred hand for producing drawings, recognition memory tests requiring a simple "yes" or "no" response are useful. Representative of these learning tests are the Continuous

Visual Memory Test (Trahan and Larrabee 1988) and the Recognition Memory Test (Warrington 1984).

Perception

Perception arising from any of the sensory modalities can be affected by brain disease. Perceptional inattention (sometimes called neglect) is one of the major perceptual syndromes because of its frequency in association with focal brain damage (Bisiach and Vallar 1988; Heilman et al. 2000b; Lezak 1994; Rafal 2000). This phenomenon involves diminished or absent awareness of stimuli in one side of personal space by a patient with an intact sensory system. Unilateral inattention is often most prominent immediately after acute-onset brain injury such as stroke. Most commonly seen is left-sided inattention associated with right hemisphere stroke.

The most commonly used forms of perceptual tests assess perceptual discrimination among similar stimuli. These visual tests may include discrimination of geometric forms, angulation, color, faces, or familiar objects (Lezak 1995; McCarthy and Warrington 1990; Newcombe and Ratcliff 1989). Some perceptual tasks assess the patient's perceptual synthesis ability. The Hooper Visual Organization Test (Hooper 1958) presents line drawings of familiar objects in fragmented, disarranged pieces and asks for the name of each object. Many of these tests can also be administered in tactile version (Craig 1985; Van Lancker et al. 1989; Varney 1986). Frequently used tactile tests include form recognition and letter or number recognition (Reitan and Wolfson 1993).

Another important area of perceptual assessment is recognition of familiar visual stimuli. Although the syndromes are rare and often occur independently of one another, a brain injury can produce an inability to recognize visually familiar objects (visual object agnosia) or faces (prosopagnosia) (Benson 1989; Damasio et al. 1989; McCarthy and Warrington 1990). Assessment involves testing the recognition—often in the form of naming—of real objects or representations of objects, sometimes in a masked or distorted form. The WIS batteries include a perceptual task in which the subject must identify missing features of line drawings of familiar objects.

Praxis

Many patients with left hemisphere damage have at least one form of apraxia, and apraxia is common in progressed stages of Alzheimer's disease, Parkinson's disease, Pick's disease, and progressive supranuclear palsy (Dobigny-Roman et al. 1998; Fukui et al. 1996; Leiguarda et al. 1997). Inability to perform the required sequence of motor activities is not based on motor weakness. Rather, the deficit is in planning and carrying out the required activities (De Renzi et al. 1983; Heilman et al. 2000a; Jason 1990) and is associated with disruption of neural representations for extrapersonal (e.g., spatial location) and intrapersonal (e.g., hand position) features of movement (Haaland et al. 1999). Tests for apraxia assess the patient's ability to reproduce learned movements of the face or limbs. These learned movements can include the use of objects (usually pantomime use of objects) and gestures (Goodglass and Kaplan 1987; Rothi et al. 1997; Strub and Black 2000), or sequences of movements demonstrated by the examiner (Christensen 1979; Haaland and Flaherty 1984).

Constructional Ability

Although constructional problems were once considered a form of apraxia, more recent analysis has shown that the underlying deficits involve impaired apprecia-

tion of one or more aspects of spatial relationships. These can include distortions in perspective, angulation, size, and distance judgment. Thus, unlike apraxias, the problem is not an inability to draw lines or assemble constructions, but rather misperceptions and misjudgments involving spatial relationships. Neuropsychological assessments may include any of a number of measures of visuospatial processing. Patients may be asked to copy geometric designs, such as the Complex Figure (Mitrushina et al. 1999; Osterrieth 1944; Rey 1941; Spreen and Strauss 1998) presented in Figure 2–3 or one of the alternate forms (Loring et al. 1988; Meador et al. 1993; Taylor 1979). The WIS battery includes constructional tasks involving reconstructing designs with blocks and assembling puzzle pieces (Wechsler 1944, 1955, 1981, 1997a). Lesions of the posterior cerebral cortex cause the greatest difficulty with constructions, and right hemisphere lesions produce greater deficits than left hemisphere lesions (Benton and Tranel 1993).

Conceptual Functions

Tests of concept formation measure aspects of thinking including reasoning, abstraction, and problem solving. Conceptual dysfunction tends to occur with serious brain injury regardless of site. Most neuropsychological tests require that simple conceptual functioning be intact. For example, reasoning skills are required for the successful performance of most WIS tests: Comprehension assesses commonsense verbal reasoning and interpretation of proverbs; Similarities measures ability to make verbal abstractions by asking for similarities between objects or concepts; Arithmetic involves arithmetic problem solving; Picture Completion requires perceptual reasoning; Picture Arrangement examines sequential reasoning for thematic pictures; Block Design and Object

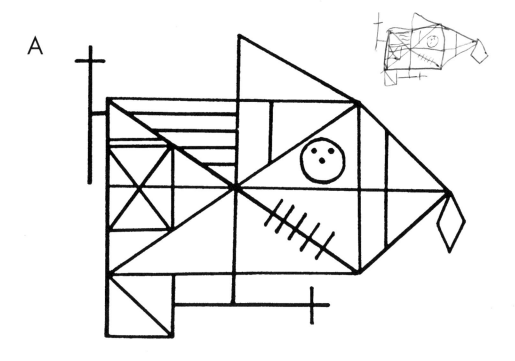

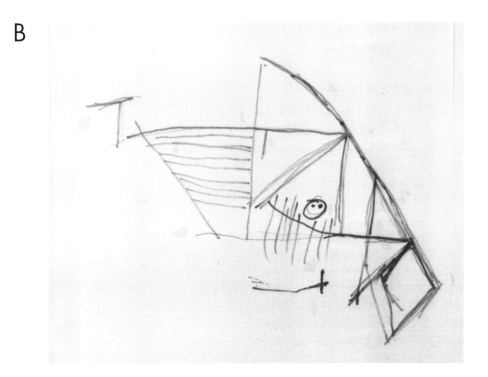

FIGURE 2–3.   Rey Complex Figure (*Panel A*) and copy (*Panel B*) drawn by a 42-year-old, right-handed man who had a right frontoparietal stroke 4 days before this examination.

The copy shows the patient's neglect of the left and lower portions of the figure, a strong perseverative tendency, and visuospatial fragmentation.

Assembly test visuospatial analysis and problem solving of block designs and puzzles; and Matrix Reasoning depends on pattern, spatial, and numerical relationships.

Other commonly used tests of concept formation include the Category Test (Halstead 1947) and the Wisconsin Card Sorting Test (WCST) (E.A. Berg 1948; Grant and Berg 1948; Spreen and Strauss 1998). These tests measure concept formation, hypothesis testing, problem solving, and flexibility of thinking. The Category Test presents patterns of stimuli and requires the patient to figure out a principle or concept that is true for each item within the set based on feedback about the correctness of each response. The patient is told that the correct principle may be the same for all sets or different for each set. For example, the correct principle in one set is position (first, second, etc.) of the stimulus on the page, whereas for another it is the number of items on the page.

Executive Functions

Executive functions include abilities to formulate a goal, to plan, to carry out goal-directed plans effectively, and to monitor and self-correct spontaneously and reliably (Lezak 1982). These are difficult tasks for many patients with frontal lobe or diffuse brain injuries (Luria 1980). Yet they are essential for fulfilling most adult responsibilities and maintaining socially appropriate conduct. Tasks that best assess executive functions are tests of planning and/or are open-ended tests that permit the patient to decide how to perform the task and when it is complete. The Bender-Gestalt (Bender 1938), a favorite old neuropsychological test, requires foresight to arrange nine drawings on a single page so that space is well used. Another type of test that requires planning is a maze. The patient must plan an exit from the maze, which involves foresight to minimize trial-and-error behavior. The Tower of London (Shallice 1982) and Tower of Hanoi tests also assess planning and foresight, as disks are moved from stack to stack to reach a stated goal. Patients with frontal lobe lesions have particular difficulty with planning tests (Carlin et al. 2000; Goel and Grafman 1995). Other tasks that rely heavily on planning for successful completion are multistep tasks calling for decision making or priority-setting abilities. Few neuropsychological tests are specifically designed to assess these aspects of behavior, yet many complex tasks depend on this analysis.

One example of a priority-setting task is the Twenty Questions test, which is known as a popular game. In the test version (Laine and Butters 1982), the patient is shown an array of 48 drawings of familiar objects and told to identify the one the examiner is thinking of by asking only "yes/no" questions. The goal is to identify the specified objects with as few questions as possible. The quality of the questions asked varies according to the number of objects they include or exclude as a possible target. Many patients with frontal lobe injuries begin questioning with low-priority questions or even by asking whether the target is a specific object (Upton and Thompson 1999). Frontal lobe injury patients also can have difficulty with the conceptual requirement of the test, because high-priority questions are more abstract. Detoxified alcoholics also have difficulty on this task (Laine and Butters 1982).

Inertia presents one of the most difficult assessment problems for neuropsychologists. There are few open-ended tests that measure initiation or ability to carry out purposeful behavior. By their very nature, most tests are structured and require little initiation by the patient (Lezak 1982). Examples of less structured tests include the Tinkertoy Test, in which the patient decides what to build and how to design it (Bayless et al. 1989; Lezak 1982). Because there are few rules, the patient's level of productivity on this task typically reflects his or her level of productivity in the real world (Lezak 1995). Tests of verbal fluency are used to measure initiation of concepts and persistence on a task. Patients are asked to name as many items as they can in a category, such as animals, or produce as many words as they can beginning with a specified letter of the alphabet (Mitrushina et al. 1999; Spreen and Strauss 1998). These tasks are performed best if the examinee initiates effective and varied strategies.

Motor Functions

Neuropsychological tests can supplement the neurological examination of motor functions by providing standardized measures of motor activities. Normative data have been acquired for commonly measured functions such as grip strength and finger tapping; more complex tests of fine motor coordination include tests that require patients to rapidly place pegs in holes, such as the Grooved Pegboard Test (Mitrushina et al. 1999) and the Purdue Pegboard Test (Spreen and Strauss 1998). These tests examine absolute performance as well as comparing the preferred hand against the nonpreferred hand to measure the possibility of lateralized motor deficit.

Personality and Emotional Status

Many tests devised to measure psychological distress or psychiatric illness have been used with persons with brain disorders. The Symptom Check List 90–Revised (SCL-90-R) (Derogatis 1983) is a self-report of symptoms associated with psychiatric disorders when they occur at high frequency levels. The MMPI (Dahlstrom et al. 1975; Hathaway and McKinley 1951; Welsh and Dahlstrom 1956) and the revised version, called the MMPI-2 (Butcher 1989; Butcher and Pope 1990; Butcher et al. 1989), have been used extensively with patients with brain disorders (Chelune et al. 1986; Dahlstrom et al. 1975; Mueller and Girace 1988). In general, these patients tend to have elevated MMPI and MMPI-2 profiles, which may reflect the relatively frequent incidence of emotional disturbance (Filskov and Leli 1981), their accurate reporting of symptoms and deficits (Lezak 1995), or their compromised ability to read or understand the test questions. Elevations in scales Hs, Hy, and Sc are common because many "neurological" symptoms appear on these scales (Alfano et al. 1990; Cripe 1999; Gass 1992; Gass and Apple 1997). The interpretation of data from persons with brain disorders must take into account the contributions of neurological symptoms, the patient's emotional reactions to the condition, and the patient's premorbid personality.

Many attempts have been made to use the MMPI to differentiate diagnoses of psychiatric and neurological illness. Results generally have been unsatisfactory, probably because of the extreme variety of brain disorders and their associated problems (Alfano et al. 1990; Lezak 1995; Mueller and Girace 1988). Not surprisingly, the MMPI also has been an inefficient instrument for localizing cerebral lesions (Lezak 1995).

Neuropsychologists are frequently asked to evaluate "psychological overlay" or functional complaints. The diagnostic problem occurs because some individuals may be financially motivated to establish injuries related to work or accidents for which financial compensation may be sought. In addition, some individuals receive emotional or social rewards for invalidism, leading to malingering and functional disabilities. It is difficult to establish with complete certainty that a person's complaints are functional. To add to the complexity of the diagnosis, patients with established brain injury sometime embellish their symptoms, wittingly or unwittingly, so that the range of problems may represent a combination of true deficits and exaggeration. The clinician usually must search for a combination of factors that would support or discredit a functional diagnosis. General factors include evidence of inconsistency in history, reporting of symptoms, or test performance; the individual's emotional predisposition; the probability of secondary gain; and the patient's emotional reactions to his or her complaints, such as the classic *la belle indifférence*.

Psychological tests may be helpful in establishing evidence of exaggeration of symptoms. Responses to the MMPI and MMPI-2 validity scales (L, F, and K) can provide information about the patient's cooperativeness while taking this test and the likelihood that symptoms are exaggerated—or minimized. Because people faking brain damage tend to exaggerate poor performance on testing, another useful diagnostic approach has been the Symptom Validity Test (Pankratz 1979). The fundamental procedure is that the patient's complaints are examined by forcing a response to a simple, two-alternative problem. Using many trials, the examiner can calculate the likelihood that the performance deviates from chance. The validity of memory complaints is tested by the Hiscock and Hiscock Digit Memory Test (Hiscock et al. 1994) by requiring the patient to recall a short series of numbers using a forced-choice, two-item recognition task and by the Test of Memory Malingering (TOMM) by asking the patient to choose which pictures had been shown to them previously using a similar forced-choice technique (Spreen and Strauss 1998; Tombaugh 1996).

Treatment and Planning

Examination findings are used to assess an individual's strengths and weaknesses and to formulate treatment interventions (Lezak 1987; Raskin and Mateer 1999; Sohlberg and Mateer 1989). Clinical interventions vary according to the individual's specific needs. Many patients with brain disorders have primary or secondary emotional problems for which psychotherapy or counseling is advisable. However, brain-injured patients frequently have problems that require special consideration. Foremost among these problems are cognitive rigidity, impaired learning ability, and diminished self-awareness, any one of which may limit the patient's adaptability and capacity to benefit from rehabilitation. Therefore, neuropsychological evaluations provide important information about treatment possibilities and strategies. The evaluation is also used to consider patients' ability for independence in society and their educational or vocational potential.

References

Acker MB: A review of the ecological validity of neuropsychological tests, in The Neuropsychology of Everyday Life: Assessment and Basic Competencies. Edited by Tuppert DE, Cicerone KD. Boston, MA, Kluwer, 1989, pp 19–55

Aine CJ: A conceptual overview and critiques of functional neuroimaging techniques in humans, I: MRI/FMRI and PET. Crit Rev Neurobiol 9:229–309, 1995

Alfano DP, Finlayson AJ, Stearns GM, et al: The MMPI and neurologic dysfunction: profile configuration and analysis. Clin Neuropsychol 4:69–79, 1990

Ali SO, Denicoff KD, Altshuler LL, et al: A preliminary study of the relation of neuropsychological performance to neuroanatomic structures in bipolar disorder. Neuropsychiatry Neuropsychol Behav Neurol 13:20–28, 2000

Anastasi A, Urbina S: Psychological Testing. Upper Saddle River, NJ, Prentice-Hall, 1997

Armitage SG: An analysis of certain psychological tests used for the evaluation of brain injury. Psychol Monogr 60(277):1–48, 1946

Baddeley A: Working memory: the interface between memory and cognition, in Memory Systems 1994. Edited by Schacter DL, Tulving E. Cambridge, MA, MIT Press, 1994, pp 351–367

Baddeley AD, Wilson BA, Watts FN (eds): Handbook of Memory Disorders. Chichester, UK, Wiley, 1995

Basso MR, Bornstein RA: Neuropsychological deficits in psychotic versus nonpsychotic unipolar depression. Neuropsychology 13: 69–75, 1999a

Basso MR, Bornstein RA: Relative memory deficits in recurrent versus first-episode major depression on a word-list learning task. Neuropsychology 13:557–563, 1999b

Bayless JD, Varney NR, Roberts RJ: Tinker Toy Test performance and vocational outcome in patients with closed head injuries. J Clin Exp Neuropsychol 11:913–917, 1989

Bender L: A visual motor gestalt test and its clinical use. American Orthopsychiatric Association Research Monographs (No 3), 1938

Bennett T L, Raymonds MJ: Special issue: mild brain injury. Appl Neuropsychol 4, 1997

Benson DF: Disorders of visual gnosis, in Neuropsychology of Visual Perception. Edited by Brown JW. New York, IRBN Press, 1989, pp 59–76

Benton AL, Hamsher K de S: Multilingual Aphasia Examination. Iowa City, IA, AJA Associates, 1989

Benton AL, Tranel D: Visuoperceptual, visuospatial, and visuoconstructive disorders, in Clinical Neuropsychology, 3rd Edition. Edited by Heilman KM, Valenstein E. New York, Oxford University Press, 1993, pp 461–497

Berg EA: A simple objective test for measuring flexibility in thinking. J Gen Psychol 39:15–22, 1948

Berg RA: Cancer, in Medical Neuropsychology. Edited by Tarter RE, Van Thiel DH, Edwards KL. New York, Plenum, 1988, pp 265–290

Bigler ED: Neuroimaging in mild TBI, in The Evaluation and Treatment of Mild Traumatic Brain Injury. Edited by Varney NR, Roberts RJ. Hillsdale, NJ, Erlbaum, 1999, pp 63–80

Binder JR, Rao SM, Hammeke TA, et al: Lateralized human brain language systems demonstrated by task subtraction functional magnetic resonance imaging. Arch Neurol 52:593–601, 1995

Bisiach E, Vallar G: Hemineglect in humans, in Handbook of Neuropsychology, Vol 1. Edited by Boller F, Grafman J. Amsterdam, The Netherlands, Elsevier, 1988, pp 195–222

Blain PG, Lane RJM: Neurological disorders, in Textbook of Adverse Drug Reactions, 4th Edition. Edited by Davies DM. Oxford, UK, Oxford University Press, 1991, pp 535–566

Boller F, Vignolo LA: Latent sensory aphasia in hemisphere-damaged patients: an experimental study with the Token Test. Brain 89:815–831, 1966

Boone KB, Lesser IM, Miller BL, et al: Cognitive functioning in older depressed outpatients: relationship of presence and severity of depression to neuropsychological test scores. Neuropsychology 9:390–398, 1995

Broshek DK, Barth JT: The Halstead-Reitan Neuropsychological Test Battery, in Neuropsychological Assessment in Clinical Practice. Edited by Groth-Marnet G. New York, Wiley, 2000, pp 223–262

Butcher JN: User's Guide for the MMPI-2 Minnesota Report: Adult Clinical System. Minneapolis, MN, National Computer Systems, 1989

Butcher JN, Pope KS: MMPI-2: a practical guide to clinical, psychometric, and ethical issues. Independent Practitioner 10: 20–25, 1990

Butcher JN, Dahlstrom WG, Graham JR, et al: Minnesota Multiphasic Personality Inventory: (MMPI-2): Manual for Administration and Scoring. Minneapolis, MN, University of Minnesota Press, 1989

Butters J, Miliotis P: Amnesic disorders, in Clinical Neuropsychology, 2nd Edition. Edited by Heilman KM, Valenstein E. New York, Oxford University Press, 1985, pp 403–451

Caccioppo JT, Tassinary LG, Bernston GG: Handbook of Psychophysiology. New York, Cambridge University Press, 2000

Carlin D, Bonerba J, Phipps M, et al: Planning impairments in frontal lobe dementia and frontal lobe lesion patients. Neuropsychologia 38:655–665, 2000

Cermak LS (ed): Human Memory and Amnesia. Hillsdale, NJ, Erlbaum, 1982

Chaves ML, Izquierdo I: Differential diagnosis between dementia and depression: a study of efficiency increment. Acta Neurol Scand 85:378–382, 1992

Chelune GJ, Ferguson W, Moehle K: The role of standard cognitive and personality tests in neuropsychological assessment, in Clinical Application of Neuropsychological Test Batteries. Edited by Incagnoli T, Goldstein G, Golden CJ. New York, Plenum, 1986, pp 75–119

Christensen A-L: Luria's Neuropsychological Investigation Test, 2nd Edition. Copenhagen, Denmark, Munksgaard, 1979

Corballis MC: The Lopsided Ape. New York, Oxford University Press, 1991

Craig JC: Tactile pattern perception and its perturbations. J Acoust Soc Am 77:238–246, 1985

Cripe LI: Use of the MMPI with mild closed head injury, in The Evaluation and Treatment of Mild Traumatic Brain Injury. Edited by Varney NR, Roberts RJ. Hillsdale, NJ, Erlbaum, 1999, pp 291–314

Crockett D, Tallman K, Hurwitz T, et al: Neuropsychological performance in psychiatric patients with or without documented brain dysfunction. Int J Neurosci 41:71–79, 1988

Cummings JL: Principles of neuropsychiatry: towards a neuropsychiatric epistemology. Neurocase 5:181–188, 1999

Dahlstrom WG, Welsh GS, Dahlstrom LE: An MMPI Handbook, Vol 1: Clinical Interpretation, Revised. Minneapolis, MN, University of Minnesota Press, 1975

Dalgleish R, Cox SG: Mood and memory, in Memory Disorders in Psychiatric Practice. Edited by Berrios GE, Hodges JR. New York, Cambridge University Press, 2000, pp 34–46

Damasio AR, Tranel D, Damasio H: Disorders of visual recognition, in Handbook of Neuropsychology, Vol 2. Edited by Boller F, Grafman J. Amsterdam, The Netherlands, Elsevier, 1989, pp 317–332

Daube J: Clinical Neurophysiology. Philadelphia, PA, FA Davis, 1996

Davison K, Hassanyck F: Psychiatric disorders, in Textbook of Adverse Drug Reactions, 4th Edition. Edited by Davies DM. Oxford, UK, Oxford University Press, 1991, pp 601–642

Delis DC, Kramer JH, Kaplan E, et al: California Verbal Learning Test, Form II (Research Edition). San Antonio, TX, Psychological Corporation, 1983

Delis DC, Kramer JH, Kaplan E, et al: California Verbal Learning Test. San Antonio, TX, Psychological Corporation, 1986

Delis DC, Kramer JH, Kaplan E, et al: California Verbal Learning Test, Form II (Research Edition). San Antonio, TX, Psychological Corporation, 1987

Della Sala S, Laiacona M, Spinnler H, et al: Autobiographical recollection and frontal damage. Neuropsychologia 31:823–839, 1993

Denicoff KD, Ali SO, Mirsky AF, et al: Relationship between prior course of illness and neuropsychological functioning in patients with bipolar disorder. J Affect Disord 56:67–73, 1999

De Renzi E, Vignolo LA: The Token Test: a sensitive test to detect disturbances in aphasics. Brain 85:665–678, 1962

De Renzi E, Faglioni P, Lodesani M, et al: Performance of left brain–damaged patients on imitation of single movements and motor sequences. Cortex 19:333–343, 1983

Derogatis LR: Symptom Checklist 90–Revised (SCL-90-R). Towson, MD, Clinical Psychometric Research, 1983

Dikmen S, Machamer J, Savoie T, et al: Life quality outcome in head injury, in Neuropsychological Assessment of Neuropsychiatric Disorders, 2nd Edition. Edited by Grant I, Adams KM. New York, Oxford University Press, 1996, pp 552–576

Diller L: Poststroke rehabilitation practice guidelines, in International Handbook of Neuropsychological Rehabilitation. Edited by Christensen A-L, Uzzell BP. New York, Kluwer Academic/Plenum, 2000, pp 167–182

Dobigny-Roman N, Dieudonne-Moinet B, Verny M, et al: Ideomotor apraxia test: a new test of imitation of gestures for elderly people. Eur J Neurol 5:571–578, 1998

Dubois B, Pillon B, Sternic N, et al: Age-induced cognitive deficit in Parkinson's disease. Neurology 40:38–41, 1990

Ernst T, Chang L, Itti L, et al: Correlation of regional cerebral blood flow from perfusion MRI and SPECT in normal subjects. Magn Reson Imaging 17:349–354, 1999

Evans JJ, Breen EK, Antoun N, et al: Focal retrograde amnesia for autobiographical events following cerebral vasculitis: a connectionist account. Neurocase 2:1–11, 1996

Fahy ST, Carey TG, Oswens JM, et al: Psychiatric presentation of frontal meningiomas. Ir J Psychol Med 12:61–63, 1995

Farah MJ, Feinberg TE (eds): Patient-Based Approaches to Cognitive Neuroscience. Cambridge, MA, MIT Press, 2000

Ferrier IN, Stanton BR, Kelly TP, et al: Neuropsychological function in euthymic patients with bipolar disorder. Br J Psychiatry 175:246–251, 1999

Filskov SB, Leli DA: Assessment of the individual in neuropsychological practice, in Handbook of Clinical Neuropsychology. Edited by Filskov SB, Boll TJ. New York, Wiley-Interscience, 1981, pp 545–576

Frith CD, Friston KJ: Studying brain function with neuroimaging, in Cognitive Neuroscience. Edited by Rugg MD. Cambridge, MA, Cambridge University Press, 1997, pp 169–195

Frith CD, Grasby PM: rCBF studies of prefrontal function and their relevance to psychosis, in Positron Emission Tomography and Neurobehavior. Edited by Baron JC. Amsterdam, The Netherlands, Elsevier, 1995, pp 383–403

Fukui T, Sugita K, Kawamura M, et al: Primary progressive apraxia in Pick's disease: a clinicopathologic study. Neurology 47:467–473, 1996

Gade A, Mortensen EL, Udensen H, et al: On the importance of control data and background variables in the evaluation of neuropsychological aspects of brain functioning, in Neurobehavioral Methods in Occupational and Environmental Health. Environmental Health Series. Copenhagen, Denmark, World Health Organization, 1985, pp 91–96

Gass CS: MMPI-2 interpretation of patients with cerebrovascular disease: a correction factor. Arch Clin Neuropsychol 7:17–27, 1992

Gass CS, Apple C: Cognitive complaints in closed-head injury: relationship to memory test performance and emotional disturbance. J Clin Exp Neuropsychol 19:290–299, 1997

Goel V, Grafman J: Are the frontal lobes implicated in "planning" functions? interpreting data from the Tower of Hanoi. Neuropsychologia 33:623–642, 1995

Goodglass H, Kaplan E: Boston Diagnostic Aphasia Examination (BDAE), 2nd Edition. Philadelphia, PA, Lea & Febiger, 1987

Grafman J, Wassermann E: Transcranial magnetic stimulation can measure and modulate learning and memory. Neuropsychologia 37:159–167, 1999

Grant DA, Berg EA: A behavioral analysis of degree of reinforcement and ease of shifting to new responses on a Weigl-type card-sorting problem. J Exp Psychol 38:404–411, 1948

Gronwall DMA: Paced auditory serial-addition task: a measure of recovery from concussion. Percept Mot Skills 44:367–373, 1977

Gronwall DMA, Sampson H: The Psychological Effects of Concussion. Auckland, New Zealand, University Press, 1974

Haaland KY, Flaherty D: The different types of limb apraxia made by patients with left vs. right hemisphere damage. Brain Cogn 3:370–384, 1984

Haaland KY, Harrington DL, Kneight RT: Spatial deficits in ideomotor limb apraxia. A kinematic analysis of aiming movements. Brain 122:1169–1182, 1999

Halstead WC: Brain and Intelligence. Chicago, IL, University of Chicago Press, 1947

Hathaway SR, McKinley JC: The Minnesota Multiphasic Personality Inventory Manual, Revised. New York, Psychological Corporation, 1951

Heaton RK, Grant I, Matthews CG: Comprehensive Norms for an Expanded Halstead-Reitan Battery: Demographic Corrections, Research Findings, and Clinical Applications. Odessa, FL, Psychological Assessment Resources, 1991

Hebb DO: The effect of early and late brain injury upon test scores, and the nature of normal adult intelligence. Proc Am Philos Soc 85: 275–292, 1942

Heilman KM, Bowers D, Valenstein E: Emotional disorders associated with neurological disease, in Clinical Neuropsychology, 3rd Edition. Edited by Heilman KM, Valenstein E. New York, Oxford University Press, 1993, pp 461–497

Heilman KM, Watson RT, Rothi LJG: Disorders of skilled movement, in Patient-Based Approaches to Cognitive Neuroscience. Edited by Farah MJ, Feinberg TE. Cambridge, MA, MIT Press, 2000a, pp 335–343

Heilman KM, Watson RT, Valenstein E: Neglect I: clinical and anatomic issues, in Patient-Based Approaches to Cognitive Neuroscience. Edited by Farah MJ, Feinberg TE. Cambridge, MA, MIT Press, 2000b, pp 115–123

Hertel PT: Relation between rumination and impaired memory in dysphoric moods. J Abnorm Psychol 107:166–172, 1998

Hiscock CK, Branham JD, Hiscock M: Detection of feigned cognitive impairment: the two-alternative forced-choice method compared with selected conventional tests. Journal of Psychopathology and Behavioral Assessment 16:95–110, 1994

Hodges JR: Transient Amnesia: Clinical and Neuropsychological Aspects. London, WB Saunders, 1991

Hooper HE: The Hooper Visual Organization Test Manual. Los Angeles, CA, Western Psychological Services, 1958

Howieson DB, Dame A, Camicioli R, et al: Cognitive markers preceding Alzheimer's dementia in the healthy oldest old. J Am Geriatr Soc 45:584–589, 1997

Jacobs D, Sana M, Dooneief G, et al: Neuropsychological detection and characterization of preclinical Alzheimer's disease. Neurology 45:957–962, 1995

Jason GW: Disorders of motor function following cortical lesions: review and theoretical considerations, in Cerebral Control of Speech and Limb Movements. Edited by Hammond GR. Amsterdam, The Netherlands, Elsevier, 1990, pp 141–168

Jernigan TL, Hesselink JR: Human brain-imaging: basic principles and applications in psychiatry, in Psychiatry. Edited by Michels R, Cavenar JO. Philadelphia, PA, JB Lippincott, 1987, pp 1–9

Johnson RJ: Event-related brain potentials and cognition, in Handbook of Neuropsychology, Vol 10. Edited by Boller F, Grafman J. Amsterdam, The Netherlands, Elsevier, 1995, pp 3–327

Kalska H, Punamaki RL, Makinen-Belli T, et al: Memory and metamemory functioning among depressed patients. Appl Neuropsychol 6:96–107, 1999

Kaplan E: A process approach to neuropsychological assessment, in Clinical Neuropsychological and Brain Function: Research, Measurement, and Practice. Edited by Boll T, Bryant BK. Washington, DC, American Psychological Association, 1988, pp 125–167

Kapur N: Memory Disorders in Clinical Practice. London, Butterworth, 1988

Kapur N: How can we best explain retrograde amnesia in human memory disorder? Memory 5:115–129, 1997

Kapur N, Scholey K, Moore E, et al: Long-term retention deficits in two cases of disproportionate retrograde amnesia. J Cogn Neurosci 8:416–434, 1996

King DA, Caine ED: Cognitive impairment and major depression: beyond the pseudodementia syndrome, in Neuropsychological Assessment of Neuropsychiatric Disorders, 2nd Edition. Edited by Grant I, Adams KM. New York, Oxford University Press, 1996, pp 200–217

Kolb B: Preoperative events and brain damage: a commentary, in Preoperative Events: Their Effects on Behavior Following Brain Damage. Edited by Schulkin J. New York, Erlbaum, 1989, pp 305–311

Laine M, Butters N: A preliminary study of problem solving strategies of detoxified long-term alcoholics. Drug Alcohol Depend 10:235–242, 1982

Leiguarda RC, Pramstaller PP, Merello M, et al: Apraxia in Parkinson's disease, progressive supranuclear palsy, multiple system atrophy and neuroleptic-induced parkinsonism. Brain 120:75–90, 1997

Lesser RP: Psychogenic seizures, in Recent Advances in Epilepsy. Edited by Pedley TA, Meldrum BS. New York, Churchill Livingstone, 1985, pp 273–293

Levin JM, Ross MH, Harris G, et al: Applications of dynamic susceptibility contrast magnetic resonance imaging in neuropsychiatry. Neuroimage 4:S147–162, 1996

Levine B, Black SE, Cabeza R, et al: Episodic memory and the self in a case of isolated retrograde amnesia. Brain 121:1951–1973, 1998

Lezak MD: The problem of assessing executive functions. Int J Psychol 17:281–297, 1982

Lezak MD: An individual approach to neuropsychological assessment, in Clinical Neuropsychology. Edited by Logue PE, Schear JM. Springfield, IL, Charles C Thomas, 1986, pp 29–49

Lezak MD: Assessment for rehabilitation planning, in Neuropsychological Rehabilitation. Edited by Meier M, Benton AL, Diller L. Edinburgh, UK, Churchill Livingstone, 1987, pp 41–58

Lezak MD: Brain damage is a family affair. J Clin Exp Neuropsychol 10:111–123, 1988a

Lezak MD: IQ: R.I.P. J Clin Exp Neuropsychol 10:351–361, 1988b

Lezak MD: Domains of behavior from a neuropsychological perspective: the whole story, in Integrative Views of Motivation, Cognition, and Emotion. Nebraska Symposium on Motivation. Edited by Spaulding WD. Lincoln, NE, University of Nebraska Press, 1994, pp 23–55

Lezak MD: Neuropsychological Assessment, 3rd Edition. New York, Oxford University Press, 1995

Lishman WA: Organic Psychiatry, 3rd Edition. Oxford, UK, Blackwell Scientific, 1997

Loring DW, Lee GP, Meador KJ: Revising the Rey-Osterrieth: rating right hemisphere recall. Arch Clin Neuropsychol 3:239–247, 1988

Luria AR: Higher Cortical Functions in Man, 2nd Edition. New York, Basic Books, 1980

Malec JF, Ivnik R, Smith G, et al: Mayo's older Americans' normative studies: utility of corrections for age and education for the WAIS-R. Clin Neuropsychol 6:31–47, 1992

Marcopulos BA: Pseudodementia, dementia, and depression: test differentiation, in Testing Older Adults: A Reference Guide for Geropsychological Assessments. Edited by Hunt T, Lindley CJ. Austin, TX, Pro-Ed, 1989, pp 70–91

Markova IS, Berrios GE: Insight into memory deficits, in Memory Disorders in Psychiatric Practice. Edited by Berrios GE, Hodges JR. New York, Cambridge University Press, 2000, pp 34–46

Masur D, Sliwinsi M, Lipton R, et al: Neuropsychological prediction of dementia and the absence of dementia in healthy elderly persons. Neurology 44:1427–1432, 1994

Matarazzo JD, Prifitera A: Subtest scatter and premorbid intelligence: lessons from the WAIS-R standardization sample. J Consult Clin Psychol 1:186–191, 1989

Mayes AR: Selective memory disorders, in The Oxford Handbook of Memory. Edited by Tulving E, Craik FIM. Oxford, UK, Oxford University Press, 2000, pp 427–440

McCarthy RA, Warrington EK: Cognitive Neuropsychology: A Clinical Introduction. San Diego, CA, Academic Press, 1990

McKenna PJ, McKay AP, Laws K: Memory in functional psychosis, in Memory Disorders in Psychiatric Practice. Edited by Berrios GE, Hodges JR. New York, Cambridge University Press, 2000, pp 234–267

Meador KJ, Moore EE, Nichols OL: The role of cholinergic systems in visuospatial processing and memory. J Clin Exp Neuropsychol 15:832–842, 1993

Menon RS, Kim SG: Spatial and temporal limits in cognitive neuroimaging with fMRI. Trends Cogn Sci 3:207–216, 1999

Mesulam M-M: Principles of Behavioral and Cognitive Neurology, 2nd Edition. New York, Oxford University Press, 2000

Milberg WP, Hebben N, Kaplan E: The Boston approach to neuropsychological assessment, in Neuropsychological Assessment of Neuropsychiatric Disorders, 2nd Edition. Edited by Grant I, Adams KM. New York, Oxford University Press, 1996, pp 58–80

Milner B: Clues to the cerebral organization of memory, in Cerebral Correlates of Conscious Experience. Edited by Buser PA, Raugeul-Buser A. INSERM Symposium No 6. Amsterdam, The Netherlands, Elsevier North-Holland, 1978, pp 139–153

Mitrushina MN, Boone KB, D'Elia LF: Handbook of Normative Data for Neuropsychological Assessment. New York, Oxford University Press, 1999

Morris J, McKeel D Jr, Storandt M, et al: Very mild Alzheimer's disease: informant-based clinical, psychometric, and pathologic distinction for normal aging. Neurology 41:469–478, 1991

Mueller SR, Girace M: Use and misuse of the MMPI, a reconsideration. Psychol Rep 63:483–491, 1988

Newcombe F: Psychometric and behavioral evidence: scope, limitations, and ecological validity, in Neurobehavioral Recovery From Head Injury. Edited by Levin HS, Grafman J, Eisenberg HM. New York, Oxford University Press, 1987, pp 129–145

Newcombe F, Ratcliff G: Disorders of visuospatial analysis, in Handbook of Neuropsychology, Vol 2. Edited by Boller F, Grafman J. Amsterdam, The Netherlands, Elsevier, 1989, pp 333–356

Ojemann GA, Dodrill CB: Verbal memory deficits after left temporal lobectomy for epilepsy. J Neurosurg 62:101–107, 1985

Osterrieth PA: Le test de copie d'une figure complex. Archives de Psychologie 30:206–356, 1944

Pagliaro LA, Pagliaro AM: Psychologists' Neuropsychotropic Drug Reference. Philadelphia, PA, Brunner/Mazel, 1998

Palmer BW, Boone KB, Lesser IM, et al: Neuropsychological deficits among older depressed patients with predominantly psychological or vegetative symptoms. J Affect Disord 41:17–24, 1996

Pankratz L: Symptom validity testing and symptom retraining: procedures for the assessment and treatment of functional sensory deficits. J Consult Clin Psychol 47:409–410, 1979

Papanicolaou AC: Fundamentals of Functional Brain Imaging. Lisse, The Netherlands, Swets & Zeitlinger, 1999

Perfect TJ, Maylor EA (eds): Models of Cognitive Aging. Oxford, UK, Oxford University Press, 2000

Petersen R, Smith G, Ivnik R, et al: Memory function in very early Alzheimer's disease. Neurology 42:867–872, 1994

Petrides M, Milner B: Deficits on subject-ordered tasks after frontal- and temporal-lobe lesions in man. Neuropsychologia 20:249–262, 1982

Prigatano GP, Schacter DL (eds): Awareness of Deficit After Brain Injury. New York, Oxford University Press, 1991

Psychological Corporation: WAIS-III and WMS-III Technical Manual. San Antonio, TX, Psychological Corporation, 1997

Rafal RD: Neglect II: cognitive neuropsychological issues, in Patient-Based Approaches to Cognitive Neuroscience. Edited by Farah MJ, Feinberg TE. Cambridge, MA, MIT Press, 2000, pp 115–123

Raskin SA, Mateer CA: Neuropsychological Management of Mild Traumatic Brain Injury. New York, Oxford University Press, 1999

Reed JM, Squire LR: Retrograde amnesia for facts and events: findings from four new cases. J Neurosci 18:3943–3954, 1998

Reitan RM, Wolfson D: The Halstead-Reitan Neuropsychological Test Battery: Theory and Clinical Interpretation, 2nd Edition. Tucson, AZ, Neuropsychology Press, 1993

Rentz DM, Weintraub S: Neuropsychological detection of early probable Alzheimer's disease, in Early Diagnosis of Alzheimer's Disease. Edited by Scinto LFM, Daffner KR. Totowa, NJ, Humana Press, 2000, pp 169–189

Rey A: L'examen psychologique dans les cas d'encephalopathie traumatique. Archives de Psychologie 28(112):286–340, 1941

Rey A: L'examen clinique en psychologie. Paris, Presses Universitaires de France, 1964

Rothi LJG, Raymer AM, Heilman KM: Limb praxis assessment, in Apraxia: The Neuropsychology of Action. Edited by Rothi LJG, Heilman KM. Hove, UK, Psychology Press, 1997, pp 61–73

Sbordone RJ: The assessment interview in clinical neuropsychology, in Neuropsychological Assessment in Clinical Practice. Edited by Groth-Marnat G. New York, Wiley, 2000, pp 94–126

Schmidt M: Rey Auditory Verbal Learning Test (RAVLT): A Handbook. Los Angeles, CA, Western Psychological Services, 1996

Shallice T: Specific impairments of planning. Philos Trans R Soc Lond B Biol Sci 298:199–209, 1982

Skuster DZ, Digre KB, Corbett JJ: Neurologic conditions presenting as psychiatric disorders. Psychiatr Clin North Am 15:311–333, 1992

Sloan S, Ponsford J: Assessment of cognitive difficulties following TBI, in Traumatic Brain Injury. Rehabilitation for Everyday Adaptive Living. Edited by Ponsford J. Hillsdale, NJ, Erlbaum, 1995, pp 65–101

Sohlberg MM, Mateer CA: Introduction to Cognitive Rehabilitation. New York, Guilford, 1989

Sox HC, Blatt MA, Higgins MC, et al: Medical Decision Making. Boston, MA, Butterworths, 1988

Spreen O, Benton AL: Comparative studies of some neuropsychological tests for cerebral damage. J Nerv Ment Dis 140:323–333, 1965

Spreen O, Strauss E: A Compendium of Neuropsychological Tests, 2nd Edition. New York, Oxford University Press, 1998

Squire LR, Slater PC, Chase PM: Retrograde amnesia: temporal gradient in very long-term memory following electroconvulsive therapy. Science 187:77–79, 1975

Stein RA, Strickland TL: A review of the neuropsychological effects of commonly used prescription medicines. Arch Clin Neuropsychol 13:259–284, 1998

Strakowski SM, Del Bello MP, Sax KW, et al: Brain magnetic resonance imaging of structural abnormalities in bipolar disorder. Arch Gen Psychiatry 56:254–260, 1999

Strauss E, Goldsmith SM: Lateral preferences and performance on non-verbal laterality tests in a normal population. Cortex 23:495–503, 1987

Strub RL, Black FW: The Mental Status Examination in Neurology. Philadelphia, PA, FA Davis, 2000

Tarter RE, Edwards KL, Van Thiel DH: Perspective and rationale for neuropsychological assessment of medical disease, in Medical Neuropsychology. Edited by Tarter RE, Van Thiel DH, Edwards KL. New York, Plenum 1988, pp 1–10

Taylor LB: Psychological assessment of neurosurgical patients, in Functional Neurosurgery. Edited by Rasmussen T, Marino R. New York, Raven, 1979, pp 165–180

Teuber H-L: Neuropsychology, in Recent Advances in Diagnostic Psychological Testing. Edited by Harrower MR. Springfield, IL, Charles C Thomas, 1948

Theodore WH: Clinical neuroimaging, in Frontiers of Neuroscience, Vol 4. Edited by Theodore WH. New York, Alan R Liss, 1988, pp 1–9

Tombaugh TN: Test of Memory Malingering (TOMM). New York, Multi Health Systems, 1996

Trahan DE, Larrabee GJ: Continuous Visual Memory Test. Odessa, FL, Psychological Assessment Resources, 1988

Upton D, Thompson PJ: Twenty questions task and frontal lobe dysfunction. Arch Clin Neuropsychol 14: 203–216, 1999

Van Gorp WG, Altshuler L, Theberge DC, et al: Cognitive impairment in euthymic bipolar patients with and without prior alcohol dependence. A preliminary study. Arch Gen Psychiatry 55:41–46, 1998

Van Lancker DR, Dreiman J, Cummings J: Voice perception deficits: neuroanatomical correlates of phonagnosia. J Clin Exp Neuropsychol 11:665–674, 1989

Van Zomeren AH, Brouwer WH: Clinical Neuropsychology of Attention. New York, Oxford University Press, 1994

Varney NR: Somesthesis, in Experimental Techniques in Human Neuropsychology. Edited by Hannay HJ. New York, Oxford University Press, 1986, pp 212–237

Varney NR, Roberts RJ (eds): The Evaluation and Treatment of Mild Traumatic Brain Injury. Hillsdale, NJ, Erlbaum, 1999

Veiel HO: A preliminary profile of neuropsychological deficits associated with major depression. J Clin Exp Neuropsychol 19:587–603, 1997

Walsh V, Rushworth M: A primer of magnetic stimulation as a tool for neuropsychology. Neuropsychologia 37:125–135, 1999

Warrington EK: Recognition Memory Test. Windsor, UK, NFER-Nelson, 1984

Wechsler D: The Measurement of Adult Intelligence, 3rd Edition. Baltimore, MD, Williams & Wilkins, 1944

Wechsler D: WAIS Manual. New York, Psychological Corporation, 1955

Wechsler D: WAIS-R Manual. New York, Psychological Corporation, 1981

Wechsler D: Wechsler Memory Scale–Revised Manual. San Antonio, TX, Psychological Corporation, 1987

Wechsler D: WISC-III Manual. Wechsler Intelligence Scale for Children–III. New York, Psychological Corporation, 1991

Wechsler D: WAIS-III. Administration and Scoring Manual. San Antonio, TX, Psychological Corporation, 1997a

Wechsler D: WMS-III. Administration and Scoring Manual. San Antonio, TX, Psychological Corporation, 1997b

Welsh GS, Dahlstrom WG (eds): Basic Readings on the MMPI in Psychology and Medicine. Minneapolis, MN, University of Minnesota Press, 1956

Wrightson P, Gronwall D: Mild Head Injury. Oxford, UK, Oxford University Press, 1999

Yousef G, Ryan WJ, Lambert T, et al: A preliminary report: a new scale to identify the pseudodementia syndrome. Int J Geriatr Psychiatry 13:389–399, 1998

CHAPTER 3

Clinical Imaging in Neuropsychiatry

Robin A. Hurley, M.D.

L. Anne Hayman, M.D.

Katherine H. Taber, Ph.D.

Neuropsychiatry, as a subspecialty, developed to assess and treat patients with cognitive or emotional disturbances due to brain dysfunction. This concept could not have evolved without the influence of brain imaging. In the short time span of one century, imaging technology has advanced from a primitive skull X ray to real-time pictures of brain changes as we perform a task or feel an emotion such as sadness or happiness. Future imaging contributions will not only be in the diagnostic arena but also in estimating the course of illness and treatment response and in the development of new neurotransmitter-specific medications.

Currently, brain imaging is divided into two categories: functional and structural (Table 3–1). Functional imaging of the brain measures changes related to neuronal activity. The most common functional imaging techniques utilize indirect measures, such as blood flow, metabolism, or oxygen extraction. Functional imaging

techniques include single photon emission computed tomography (SPECT), positron emission tomography (PET), functional magnetic resonance imaging (fMRI), magnetic resonance spectroscopy (MRS), and magnetoencephalography (MEG). These techniques and their application to neuropsychiatry are discussed in Chapter 4 of this book. Structural imaging is defined as information gathered regarding the physical constitution of the brain at any one point in time and is not dependent on thought, motor activity, or mood. It includes both anatomic and pathologic studies. Computed tomography (CT) and magnetic resonance imaging (MRI) are the standard tools. However, recent advances have broadened the range of information that can be obtained clinically. For example, xenon-enhanced computed tomography (Xe/CT) is available on the newer CT scanners, providing a way to identify structural lesions once hidden from view.

TABLE 3–1. Brain imaging modalities

Type of imaging	Parameter measured
Anatomic and pathologic	
Computed tomography (CT)	Tissue density
Xenon-enhanced computed tomography (Xe/CT)	Xenon concentration in blood
Magnetic resonance imaging (MRI)	Many properties of tissue (T1 and T2 relaxation times, spin density, magnetic susceptibility, water diffusion, blood flow)
Functional (brain activation)	
Positron emission tomography (PET)	Radioactive tracers in blood or tissue
Single photon emission computed tomography (SPECT)	Radioactive tracers in blood or tissue
Functional magnetic resonance imaging (fMRI)	Deoxyhemoglobin levels in blood
Magnetoencephalography (MEG)	Magnetic fields induced by neuronal discharges
Magnetic resonance spectroscopy (MRS)	Metabolite concentrations in tissue
Tomographic electroencephalography	Summed neuronal discharges

What Can Be Learned From Structural Imaging

Soon after the advent of CT and MRI, scientists began to image patients with psychotic and mood disorders hoping to demonstrate concrete proof that these illnesses were indeed brain disorders and not conditions of "weak personalities" or "poor parenting." Initial studies in the classic conditions of bipolar disorder, major depression, and schizophrenia met with disappointing results—with, at most, nonspecific findings that occur in many disease states (i.e., ventricular enlargement or generalized atrophy). As neuropsychiatry matures, so is the knowledge that can be attained from structural images. Researchers studying conditions such as cerebral vascular accidents, ruptured aneurysms, traumatic brain injury, and multiple sclerosis were among the first to document that psychiatric symptoms do occur as a result of brain injury; that emotion, memory, and thought pro-

cessing happen by way of tracts or circuits (Mega and Cummings 1994); and that indeed many patients do have subtle lesions that account for their symptoms. Not only has this information led to a further understanding of brain function, but it has provided prognostic information for patients and has led to treatment plan changes.

In an era when cost containment and third-party review has restricted the physician's ability to provide service, it is imperative that the practicing neuropsychiatrist understand structural imaging as a helpful tool and be able to explain why it is *essential* in the workup of a patient with psychiatric symptoms. This chapter focuses on the basic concepts of CT and MRI, advancing technology, and normal imaging anatomy related to the "brain circuits" that affect one's emotion or thought processing. The chapter also contains selected examples to illustrate where structural imaging can provide valuable clinical information. The chapter does not cover all psychiatric conditions in which there are imaging findings, but it does provide the tools to understand the available scientific literature that documents those conditions. (Examples of recent review articles that cover selected neuropsychiatric conditions and their imaging findings are Chakos et al. 1998; Weight and Bigler 1998.)

General Principles for Neuropsychiatric Imaging

Early studies in the 1980s promoted the limited use of CT scanning in psychiatric patients only after focal neurological findings had been developed (Larson et al. 1981). Studies of the late 1980s and 1990s encouraged a wider use of diagnostic CT in psychiatric patients (Beresford et al. 1986; Kaplan et al. 1994; Weinberger 1984). With the advent of utilization review and cost containment in the late 1990s, once again more narrow criteria were proposed that recommended use of CT only when reversible pathology was suspected (Branton 1999; Schemmer et al. 1999). Others strongly debate these criteria, including the authors of this chapter.

An excellent review of this controversy can be found in an article by Rauch and Renshaw (1995). They propose six categories of psychiatric patients in whom imaging should be performed: those with new-onset psychosis; those with delirium or dementia of unknown cause; and those with acute mental status changes associated with either abnormal findings on neurological examination, brain injury of any kind (traumatic or "organic"), or age greater than 50. We propose slightly wider criteria (Table 3–2). These are based on several factors: 1) rapid advances in clinical imaging allow identification of once-hidden lesions; 2) clinical experience indicates that patients with symptoms outside

the "clinical norms" for a working diagnosis often have brain lesions that will explain the presentation; and 3) an identified brain lesion can change treatment plans, medication choices for targeted symptoms, and prognosis. For example, a patient with poststroke mania might best be treated with sodium valproate rather than lithium, as lithium could increase confusion or cognitive impairment in such a patient.

TABLE 3–2. Clinical indications for imaging in psychiatric patients

Psychiatric symptoms outside "clinical norms"
Dementia or cognitive decline
Traumatic brain injury
New-onset mental illness after age 50
Initial psychotic break
Alcohol abuse
Seizure disorders with psychiatric symptoms
Movement disorders
Autoimmune disorders
Eating disorders
Poison or toxin exposure
Catatonia
Focal neurological signs

Practical Considerations

Ordering the Examination

The neuroradiologist needs very clear clinical information on the imaging request form (not just "rule out pathology" or "new-onset mental status changes"). If a lesion is suspected in a particular location, the neuroradiologist should be informed of this or given enough clinical data for selection of the best imaging method and parameters to view suspicious areas. The clinician should ask the neuroradiologist about any special imaging techniques that may enhance visualization of the limbic circuits (see "Common Pulse Sequences" later in this chapter). The neuroradiologist and technical staff also need information on the patient's current condition (e.g., delirious, psychotic, easily agitated, paranoid). This may eliminate difficulties with patient management during the scan.

Contrast-Enhanced Studies

When ordering CT or MRI, the physician can request that an additional set of images be gathered after intravenous administration of a contrast agent. This process, although using different physical principles for CT or MRI (see later sections for full discussion), is required for identification of lesions that are the same signal intensity as surrounding brain tissue. Contrast agents travel in the vascular system and normally do not cross into the brain parenchyma because they cannot pass through the blood-brain barrier (BBB). The BBB is formed by tight junctions in the capillaries that serve as a structural barrier and function like a plasma membrane. The ability of a substance to pass through these junctions depends on several factors, including the substance's affinity for plasma proteins, its lipophilic nature, and its size. (An excellent review of the physiology of the BBB and the basics of contrast enhancement can be found in Sage et al. 1998.)

In some disease processes, the BBB is broken or damaged. As a result, contrast agents can diffuse into brain tissue. Pathologic processes in which the BBB is disrupted include autoimmune diseases, infections, and tumors. Contrast enhancement can also be useful in the case of vascular abnormalities (such as arteriovenous malformations and aneurysms), although the contrast agent remains intravascular. When ordering the imaging procedure, the neuropsychiatrist should be mindful to request a study with contrast enhancement if one of the above disease states is suspected.

Patient Preparation

The psychiatrist should always explain the procedure to the patient shortly beforehand, being mindful to mention the loud noises of the scanner (MRI), the tightly enclosing imaging coil (MRI), and the requirement for absolute immobility during the test (MRI and CT). Both the body and head are secured with tight wraps to minimize movement during scanning. If the psychiatrist suspects that the patient may become agitated or be unable to remain still for the length of the examination, then sedation may be necessary. A clinician may select a regimen that he or she is familiar and comfortable with. We have found that for patients with agitation and psychosis, a sedating antipsychotic with lorazepam 1–2 mg intramuscularly 30 minutes before scanning usually works well in a physically healthy nongeriatric adult.

Understanding the Scan

The neuropsychiatrist should review the scan and radiology report with the neuroradiologist. It is important to remember that the radiographic view places the patient's right on the reader's left and the patient's left on the reader's right. The first points to observe on a scan are the demographics: the hospital name; the date; the scanner number; and the patient's name, age, sex, and identification number. It is also important to note whether the scan was done with or without contrast enhancement. If an MRI has been obtained, the weighting parameters are important. The locations of these factors on CT and MRI scans are illustrated later in the chapter. Next, the neuropsychiatrist should ask the neuroradiologist to point out the normal anatomic markers and any pathology observed on the films. Prior understanding of the limbic system anatomy is essential and is reviewed in the unabridged chapter by Hurley et al. 2002.

Computed Tomographic Imaging

The first computed tomographic image, obtained in 1972, required 9 days to collect the data and more than 2 hours to process on a mainframe computer (Orrison 1995). The scanners of today can capture a slice in one half second (Figure 3–1). With the use of multiple detectors, several slices can be acquired simultaneously. Thus, with multislice imaging, CT scans of the entire brain can be completed in less than 17 seconds (B.R. Westerman, unpublished communication, May 2000). Newer CT technologies that are just beginning to be applied to neuropsychiatric patients include three-dimensional helical (spiral) CT and Xe/CT.

Technical Considerations

Standard Two-Dimensional CT

Like a conventional radiograph, CT uses an X-ray tube as a source of photons. When a conventional radiograph is acquired, the photons directly expose X-ray film. When a CT image is acquired, the photons are collected by detectors. The latest generation of CT scanners split the X-ray beam and add multiple detectors, allowing collection of multiple slices simultaneously ("multislice scanners"). These data are relayed to a computer that places the data in a two-dimensional grid that is then printed on X-ray film or viewed on monitor (Rauch and Renshaw 1995). CT scans deliver a clinically insignificant cumulative dose of about 5 rads localized to the head. To avoid even this small dose of radiation to the lens of the eye, CT scans are angled parallel to a line drawn between the orbit and the external auditory meatus (referred to as the *orbitomeatal line*). Although there is no appreciable radiation deposited outside the head, a lead apron is often placed over the abdomen of a pregnant woman during a head CT.

The patient lies on a table that is advanced between acquisition of each CT slice. To acquire each CT slice, a beam of photons rotates around the head. As the photons pass through the head, some are absorbed by the tissues of the head. Detectors located opposite the beam source measure the attenuation of the photons (Figure 3–2). Thus, the CT images of the brain record tissue density as measured by the variable attenuation of X-ray photons. High-density tissues such as bone appear white, indicating an almost complete absorption of the X rays (high attenuation). Air has the lowest rate of attenuation (or absorption of radiation) and appears black. The appearance of other tissues is given in Table 3–3.

Modern CT scanners can generate brain images that range from 0.5 to 10 mm in thickness, with 3–5 mm used most commonly. The slice thickness of a CT image is an important variable in clinical scanning. Thinner slices allow visualization of smaller lesions. However, the thinnest sections have less contrast (i.e., the signal intensity difference between gray and white matter is less) because the signal:noise ratio is lower. It also takes longer to complete the examination because more slices must be acquired. Thus there is more chance of patient motion degrading the images. The longer scan time also decreases the number of patients that can be examined in a day. Thicker sections (or slices) have greater contrast, but smaller lesions may be missed. There is also a greater incidence of artifacts due to increased volume averaging. This is particularly true in the base of the skull, and this may obscure brain stem and mesial temporal structures. See Figure 3–3 for other scan parameters that affect image quality.

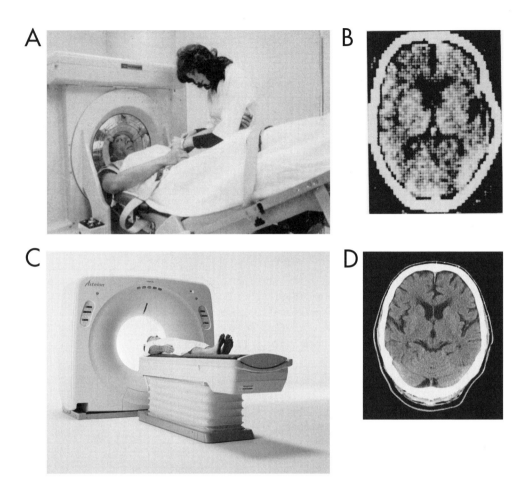

FIGURE 3–1.   Computed tomography then and now.

A first-generation computed tomography (CT) scanner (*Panel A*), circa 1975, created crude brain images (*Panel B*) that still were superior to other imaging techniques available at the time. In 1986, helical (or spiral) CT was patented. This technique significantly increased scan speed and expanded the application of CT into new areas. In 1998, the multislice CT scanner (*Panel C*) was introduced. Multislice CT opens new possibilities for more efficient health care, better diagnoses, earlier disease detection, and cost reduction. Multislice CT has been hailed as the biggest advancement in medical imaging of the 1990s (Diagnostic Imaging January 2000). Modern CT scanners produce images of much higher resolution (*Panel D*) than early CT images.

Source.   Panel C, photograph of Aquilion Multi scanner courtesy of Toshiba America Medical Systems, Inc. Panel D, image courtesy of Toshiba America Medical Systems, Inc., and Delta County Memorial Hospital, Delta, CO.

Three-Dimensional CT (Single-Slice and Multislice Helical CT)

As CT imaging became an integral part of medical diagnostics, faster and more advanced technologies were invented. The 1990s brought the clinical introduction of helical (spiral) CT, in which slip rings allow continuous scanning of a patient. This is much faster than the older "scan—stop—move the table and reset the detector—scan again" sequence used for standard two-dimensional CT (Figure 3–4). In addition, there is less radiation exposure, and less contrast agent is needed. More images can be collected before the X-ray beam must be shut down for cooling. Two-dimensional images can be reconstructed in any plane of section

TABLE 3–3. Relative gray-scale appearance on a noncontrast computed tomography scan

Tissue	Appearance
Bone	White
Calcified tissue	White
Clotted blood	White[a]
Gray matter	Light gray
White matter	Medium gray
Cerebrospinal fluid	Nearly black
Water	Nearly black
Air	Black

[a]Becomes isointense to brain as clot ages approximately 1–2 weeks.

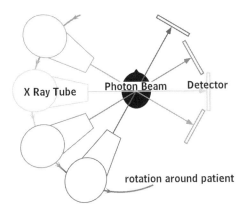

FIGURE 3–2. Schematic of conventional computed tomography X-ray tube and detector.

Note the simultaneous circular movement of both devices about the head.

For a color version of this figure, please see the color insert at the back of this book.

from the acquired three-dimensional data set. Three-dimensional reconstructions can also be done in as little as 2 minutes (Figure 3–5).

Initially, single-slice helical CT was principally useful in body scanning. It had limited use in the brain due to skull thickness (i.e., it produced grainy images that did not discriminate between gray and white matter very well) (Bahner et al. 1998; Coleman and Zimmerman 1994). Applications for the head included evaluations of pediatric patients (thinner cranium), adult carotid stenosis, aneurysms, arteriovenous malformations, vessel occlusions in acute stroke, and as a tool for intravenous angiography (Coleman and Zimmerman 1994; Kuszyk et al. 1998; Schwartz 1995). The newest helical CT scanners provide images of similar quality to the standard single-slice CT (Kuntz et al. 1998). Three-dimensional reconstruction is still available for use in stereotactic neurosurgery planning and vascular evaluations (Katada 1999; Moringlane et al. 1997).

Xenon-Enhanced CT

Although officially labeled a functional imaging technique, xenon-enhanced CT (Xe/CT) allows identification of structural lesions that may be invisible on CT and MRI. Xe/CT uses stable xenon gas as a contrast agent because it is radiodense and lipid soluble. After obtaining baseline standard CT images, the patient inhales a mixture of xenon (26%–33%) and oxygen. A second set of images is then collected in which the distribution of the xenon shows regional blood flow, allowing areas of abnormality to be identified.

Xe/CT has evolved to allow more routine clinical use as technical advances have lessened the side effects and permit repeated imaging. However, in 2001, the FDA withdrew xenon's status as a "grandfathered" x-ray contrast agent. At present, the FDA-required studies to reacquire approval are under way. Approval is anticipated shortly. Currently, the images can be computed in seconds. At the diluted concentration mentioned above, transient side effects of xenon inhalation include euphoria, dysphoria, sedation, nausea, and apnea (reversible with instructions to breathe). Advantages of Xe/CT over other methods of imaging blood flow include

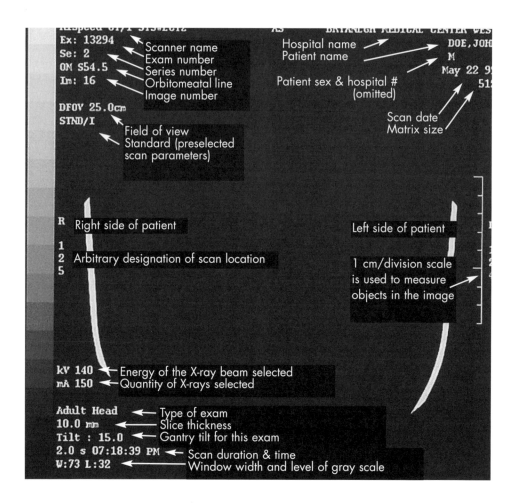

FIGURE 3–3. Computed tomography header information and arbitrary gray scale.

Explanations for abbreviations used on the image are also included.

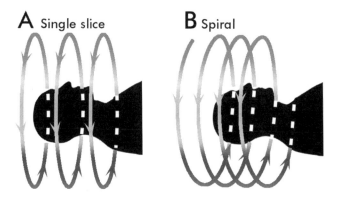

FIGURE 3–4. Schematic of computed tomography (CT) scanning path.

Panel A. Conventional CT. *Panel B.* Helical (spiral) CT. Note the continuous overlapping helical path in spiral CT.

For a color version of this figure, please see the color insert at the back of this book.

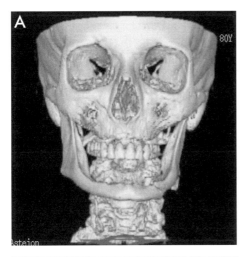

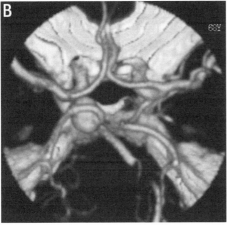

FIGURE 3–5. Three-dimensional reconstruction from helical computed tomography (CT).

Current CT scanners can acquire extremely detailed data sets in a matter of seconds. The data can be viewed as three-dimensional volume images from any desired angle. Reconstructions of bone (*Panel A*) are valuable both for diagnosis and for surgical planning. CT angiography, such as this view of an aneurysm in the circle of Willis (*Panel B*), is capable of displaying vessels from any angle. Since scanning is very rapid and noninvasive, such examinations may be performed in place of conventional angiograms. **For a color version of this figure, please see the color insert at the back of this book.**
Source.   Images courtesy of Toshiba America Medical Systems, Inc.

lack of radiation or radiotracer exposure, good image resolution, and direct anatomic correlation. It is inexpensive (the technique adds less than $100 per study), can be repeated frequently (e.g., after a drug challenge), and adds no more than 10 minutes to the total examination time.

Clinical indications for Xe/CT are slowly emerging. Currently, the technique has proved advantageous in discovering hidden lesions not evident on standard imaging. Patients whose clinical symptoms do not fit the classic historical picture for the working diagnosis should therefore be considered for Xe/CT. Taber et al. reported a case of a patient whose diagnoses were changed from probable Alzheimer's disease and major depression to dementia secondary to a cerebrovascular accident. In that particular case, treatment plans were then altered (Taber et al. 1999). Examples of a normal CT and companion Xe/CT scan in a different stroke patient are given in Figure 3–6.

Contrast Agents

The administration of intravenous iodinated contrast medium immediately before obtaining a CT scan greatly improves the detection of many brain lesions that are isodense on noncontrast CT. Contrast agents are useful when there is a breakdown of the BBB. Under normal circumstances, the BBB does not allow passage of contrast medium into the extravascular spaces of the brain. When there is a break in this barrier, the contrast agent enters the damaged area and collects in or around the lesion. The *increased* density of the contrast agent will appear as a white area on the scan. Without a companion noncontrast CT scan, preexisting dense areas (calcified or hemorrhagic) might be mistaken for contrast-enhanced lesions. In difficult cases, a double dose of contrast agent may be used to improve detection of lesions with minimal BBB impairment.

Currently there are two types of iodinated CT contrast agents: ionic or high

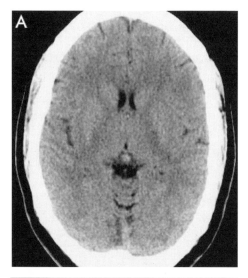

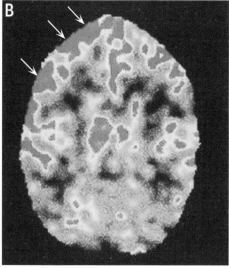

FIGURE 3–6. Imaging of acute stroke in a 52-year-old woman who presented with left-sided weakness.

Computed tomographic (CT) images acquired 1.5 hours after onset (*Panel A*) were normal. Companion xenon-enhanced CT images (*Panel B*) showed luxury perfusion on the right (arrows), indicating that the area of the stroke had already reperfused. Magnetic resonance images acquired the next day were normal. **For a color version of this figure, please see the color insert at the back of this book.**

Source. Images courtesy of Ben Taub General Hospital, Houston, TX.

osmolality and nonionic or low osmolality. Both types are associated with allergic reactions, and contraindications for both

exist. Allergic reactions to contrast agents are defined by two types in two time frames: anaphylactoid or nonanaphylactoid (chemotoxic) and immediate or delayed. The recent literature debates the true incidence of all of these (Federle et al. 1998; Jacobs et al. 1998; Oi et al. 1997; Yasuda and Munechika 1998). Immediate reactions occur within 1 hour of injection; delayed reactions occur within 7 days but usually within 24 hours. Anaphylactoid reactions include hives, rhinitis, bronchospasm, laryngeal edema, hypotension, and death. Chemotoxic reactions include nausea, vomiting, warmth or pain at the injection site, hypotension, tachycardia, and arrhythmias (Cohan et al. 1998a; Federle et al. 1998). The overall mortality rate from ionic dyes is reported to be 1 per 12,000–170,000 (average is 1/100,000), with severe reactions occurring in 1 per 1,000 patients (Cohan et al. 1998b; Jacobs et al. 1998). The rates for severe reactions to nonionic dyes are significantly lower (1–2 per 10,000 examinations) (Cohan et al. 1998c). Currently, average rates for milder reactions are 5%–25% for ionic agents and 1%–5% for nonionic agents (Federle et al. 1998; Jacobs et al. 1998; Yasuda and Munechika 1998). The ionic agents are significantly less expensive, but they are very rarely used because of the greater risk of allergic reactions (see Table 3–6 later in this chapter for the cost of both the scan and contrast media).

The American College of Radiology standards recommend the use of nonionic dye in patients with histories of previous significant contrast media reactions; any previous serious allergic reaction to any material; asthma; sickle cell disease; diabetes; renal insufficiency (creatinine ≥ 1.5 mg/dL); cardiac diseases; inability to communicate; geriatric age; or other debilitating health problems (Cohan et al. 1998d; Halpern et al. 1996). Patients who are receiving dialysis or who have histories of milder reactions to shellfish require the use of nonionic dyes when contrast CT is unavoidable. The older ionic agents are not used in these patients.

Extravasation (leakage of the contrast dye at the injection site) is generally a mild problem associated with some stinging or burning. However, in infrequent cases, patients have developed tissue ulceration or necrosis. If a patient has had a previous episode of extravasation, then nonionic dye should be used, as it is associated with fewer reactions.

Other areas of caution include patients with histories of anaphylaxis. These patients should be considered for other types of imaging, rather than contrast-enhanced CT. If contrast-enhanced CT is necessary, then premedication with steroids and antihistamines and the use of nonionic dye are recommended. Metformin, an oral antihyperglycemic agent, must be withheld before iodinated dye is given. It can be restarted after 48 hours with laboratory evidence of normal renal function. Metformin can cause lactic acidosis, especially in patients with a history of renal or hepatic dysfunction, alcohol abuse, or cardiac disease (Cohan et al. 1998d).

Magnetic Resonance Imaging

In 1946, the phenomenon of nuclear magnetic resonance was discovered. The discovery led to the development of a powerful new technique for studying matter by using radio waves together with a static magnetic field. This development, combined with other important insights and emerging technologies in the 1970s, led to the first magnetic resonance image of a living patient. By the 1980s, commercial MRI scanners were becoming more common. Although the physics that make MRI possible are complex, a grasp of the basic principles will help the clinician understand the results of the imaging examination and explain this procedure to anxious patients.

Physical Principles

Reconstructing an Image

Clinical MRI is based on manipulating the small magnetic field around the nucleus of the hydrogen atom (proton), a major component of water in soft tissue. To make a magnetic resonance image of a patient's soft tissues, the patient must be placed inside a large magnet. The strength of the magnet is measured in teslas (T). A high-field clinical system has a field strength of 1.5 T. (More powerful systems are often used in research settings.) A mid-field system is generally 0.5 T, and low-field units range from 0.1 to 0.5 T.

The magnetic field of the MRI scanner slightly magnetizes the hydrogen atoms in the body, changing their alignment. The stronger the magnetic field, the more magnetized the hydrogen atoms in tissue become and the more signal they will produce. The stronger signal available with 1.5-T systems allows higher-resolution images to be collected. However, this increased detail is costly, because high-field systems are more expensive than mid- or low-field systems. Also, many patients feel uncomfortable while lying inside these huge enclosing magnets (Figure 3–7A). Open-design magnets are now available that help the patient feel less confined (Figure 3–7B).

To create a magnetic resonance image, the patient's hydrogen atoms are exposed to a carefully calculated series of radio frequency (RF) pulses while the patient is within the scanner's magnetic field. These RF pulses cause changes in the magnetization of the hydrogen atoms. This changing magnetic field generates tiny electric signals that are picked up by a receiver

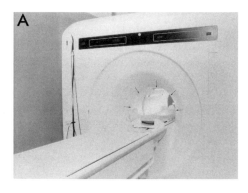

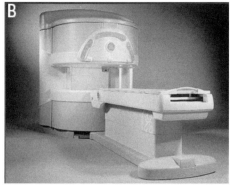

Figure 3–7. Magnetic resonance scanners.

Panel A. High-field (1.5-T) magnetic resonance scanner. Note the relatively small circular opening (arrows). *Panel B.* An open-design scanner allows greater access to the patient and reduces the likelihood of claustrophobia.
Source. Photographs of Signa scanner (Panel A) and Signa OpenSpeed scanner (Panel B) courtesy of GE Medical Systems.

placed close to the area being scanned (the imaging coil). A head coil that closely encloses the head, allowing maximal signal reception, is used to obtain brain images.

The scanner's computer converts these signals into a spatial map, the magnetic resonance image. This conversion requires parceling information into blocks that form a square (or sometimes rectangular) grid. The size of each block (commonly called a voxel or a pixel in the final two-dimensional image) in the grid is important. If the blocks are too large, they will contain many types of tissue and will not

have the desired spatial resolution. If the blocks are too small, there will not be enough signal in each to form an image.

The scanner's computer places signals in each block using a two-step process that makes each block slightly different from all other blocks. First the computer alters the magnetic field strength in each succeeding row of blocks by applying a magnetic field gradient across the tissue (the *read gradient*). This difference in magnetic field strength changes the frequency of the signal from each row in the image, hence the term *frequency-encoding direction* (Figure 3–8A). The number of frequency bands the computer divides the signal into determines the number of rows that will form the image (most commonly 256 or 512). Thus, each row represents a different frequency (measured in hertz).

The second step separates the signals in the other direction to superimpose columns over the rows (Figure 3–8B). A *phase gradient* is applied across the columns to speed up (or slow down) the radio waves that form the signal, hence the term *phase-encoding direction*. The individual measurement, called a *view*, has to be repeated multiple times, with the phase gradient increased each time. This process takes up most of the scan time. The number of *phase-encoding steps* determines the number of columns in the image. It is selectable and is usually set at 192 or 256. The computer uses the combination of the exact frequency and phase of each component radio wave from the signal to assign it to the correct block within the grid, thus forming the image (Figure 3–8C). The technologist can apply read and phase gradients in any direction, but they must remain perpendicular to each other to form a grid and thereby create the magnetic resonance image.

The magnetic field gradients needed to acquire the image are created by huge coils of wire embedded in the magnet.

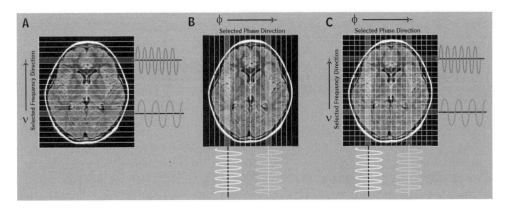

FIGURE 3–8. Origin of the imaging grid.

Panel A. Sample magnetic resonance image is overlaid with rows created by a read (frequency-encoding) gradient. *Panel B.* Sample magnetic resonance image is overlaid with columns created by a phase gradient. *Panel C.* Sample magnetic resonance image is overlaid with the grid created by the frequency and phase gradients. The computer uses the combination of frequency and phase to identify the signal from each block in the grid. **For a color version of this figure, please see the color insert at the back of this book.**

TABLE 3–4. Acquisition parameter ranges for different pulse sequences (given in milliseconds)

Acquisition parameter	Pulse sequence		
	T1-weighted	**T2-weighted**	**Spin density–weighted**
Repetition time (TR)	400–800	3,000–5,000	3,000–5,000
Echo time (TE)	10–20	60–120	10–20

These are driven with large-current audio amplifiers similar to those used for musical concerts. The gradients must be switched on and off very rapidly. This creates loud noises during the scan and may distress the unprepared patient.

Common Pulse Sequences

The combination of RF and magnetic field pulses used by the computer to create the image is called the *pulse sequence*. Pulse sequences have been developed that result in images sensitive to different aspects of the hydrogen atom's behavior in a high magnetic field. Thus each image type contains unique information about the tissue. A pulse sequence is repeated many times to form an image (see previous section).

The pulse sequence used most commonly in clinical MRI is the *spin echo* (SE) sequence. Many centers now use a faster variant of this sequence, the *fast spin echo* (FSE). These pulse sequences emphasize different tissue properties by varying two factors. One is the time between applying each repetition of the sequence, referred to as the *repetition time* or *time to recovery* (TR). The other is the time at which the receiver coil collects signal after the RF pulses have been given. This is called the *echo time* or *time until the echo* (TE). The ranges of TR and TE that result in commonly used types of magnetic resonance images are listed in Table 3–4. A summary of the expected imaging appearance of various tissues on commonly used types of magnetic resonance images is given in Table 3–5.

TABLE 3–5.   Relative gray scale values present in tissues visible on magnetic resonance imaging scans (noncontrast enhanced)

Tissue	Pulse sequence		
	T1-weighted	**T2-weighted**	**Spin density–weighted**
Bone	Black	Black	Black
Calcified tissue	Variable, usually gray	Variable, usually gray	Variable, usually gray
Gray matter	Medium gray	Medium gray	Light gray
White matter	Light gray	Dark gray	Medium gray
Cerebrospinal fluid	Black	White	Gray
Water	Black	White	Gray
Air	Black	Black	Black
Pathology (excluding blood)	Gray	White	White
Blood			
Acute	Dark gray	Black	Light gray
Subacute	White	White	White

Images collected using a short TR and short TE are most heavily influenced by the T1 relaxation times of the tissues and so are called *T1 weighted* (T1W). Figure 3–9 shows a T1-weighted set of brain images. Note the sharply marginated boundaries between the brain (light gray) and cerebrospinal fluid (CSF) (black). Traditionally, this type of image is considered best for displaying anatomy.

Images collected using a long TR and a long TE are most heavily influenced by the T2 relaxation times of tissues and so are called *T2 weighted* (T2W). Figure 3–10 shows a set of T2-weighted images of the same brain. This type of image is best for displaying pathology, which most commonly appears bright, often similar in intensity to CSF. A very useful variant on the T2-weighted scan, called a *fluid-attenuated inversion recovery* (FLAIR) image, allows the intense signal from CSF to be nullified. This makes pathology near CSF-filled spaces much easier to see (Arakia et al. 1999; Bergin et al. 1995; Brant-Zawadzki et al. 1996; Rydberg et al. 1994). Figure 3–11 shows a set of FLAIR images. We have found this method of

MRI to be extremely useful in neuropsychiatric imaging (Figure 3–12).

If a long TR and a short TE are used, the image is most sensitive to the concentration of hydrogen atoms, also called the proton density or spin density. Thus, these images are called *spin density weighted* (SDW). The striking contrast between brain tissue and CSF seen on the T1-weighted and T2-weighted images is not present. The mild T2 weighting of this type of image makes fiber tracts easy to see.

The next most commonly used pulse sequence in clinical imaging is the *gradient echo* (GE or GRE) sequence. In this type of image acquisition, a gradient reversal rather than an RF pulse is used to generate the echo. As a result, this technique is very sensitive to anything in the tissue causing magnetic field inhomogeneity, such as hemorrhage or calcium. These images are sometimes called *susceptibility weighted* because differences in magnetic susceptibility between tissues cause magnetic field inhomogeneity and signal loss. As a result, gradient echo images have artifacts at the interfaces between tissues with very different magnetic susceptibility, such as bone

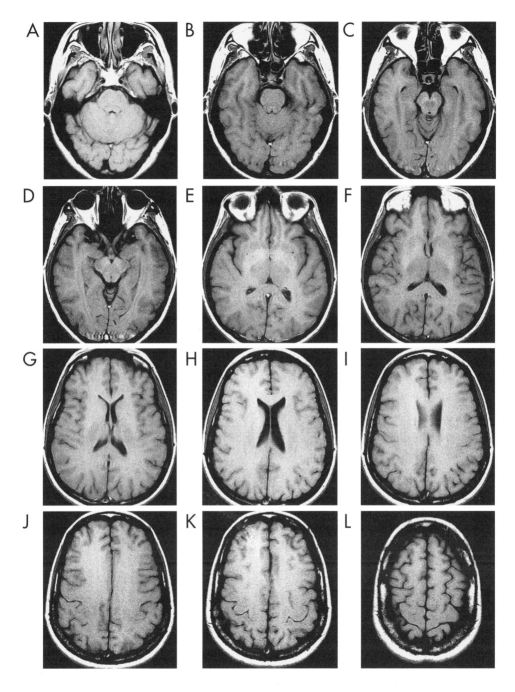

FIGURE 3–9. Serial axial T1-weighted magnetic resonance images of a normal adult brain.
Source. Images courtesy of GE Medical Systems.

and brain. The artifacts at the skull base are sometimes severe. Other scan parameters also affect image quality. These parameters are indicated in Figure 3–13.

New Pulse Sequences

Several types of pulse sequences that are sensitive to other aspects of tissue state are being tested for clinical work. One

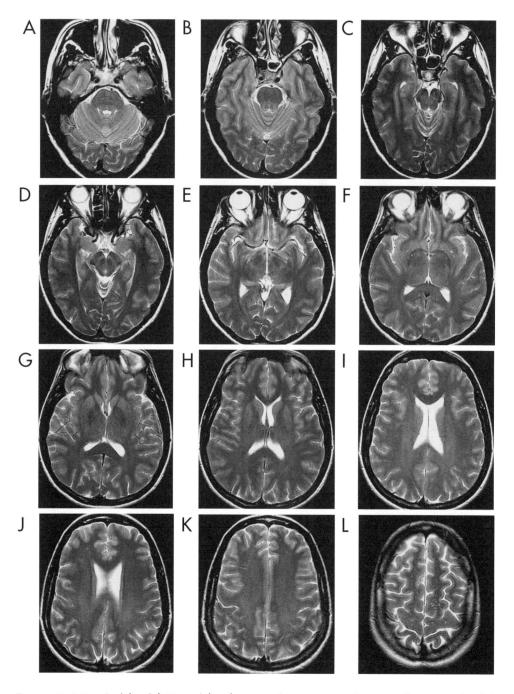

FIGURE 3–10. Serial axial T2-weighted magnetic resonance images of a normal adult brain.

Source. Images courtesy of GE Medical Systems.

method is sensitive to interactions between free protons (unbound water in tissue) and bound protons (water bound to macromolecules such as those in myelin membranes) (Hanyu et al. 1999; Tanabe et al. 1999). This type of magnetic

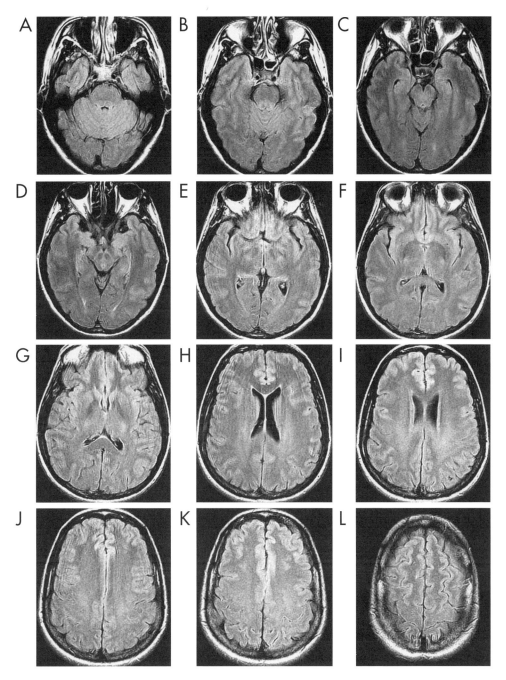

FIGURE 3–11. Serial axial fluid-attenuated inversion recovery (FLAIR) magnetic resonance images of a normal adult brain.
Source. Images courtesy of GE Medical Systems.

resonance image, called a magnetization transfer (MT) image, may be able to differentiate white matter lesions due to different causes and thus provide insight into pathologic processes (Hanyu et al. 1999; Tanabe et al. 1999). Another method of MRI is sensitive to the speed of water diffusion. Diffusion-weighted (DW) MRI

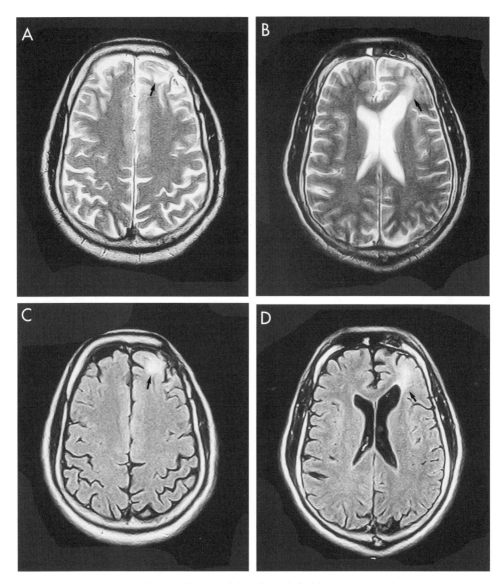

FIGURE 3–12.   Comparison of T2-weighted and fluid-attenuated inversion recovery (FLAIR) magnetic resonance imaging (MRI).

MRI scans of a 36-year-old man who presented for admission with nausea, vomiting, and hyponatremia. Two days later the patient was agitated, sexually inappropriate, and wandering incoherently. Neuropsychiatric work-up revealed status epilepticus. Subsequent MRI demonstrated a previous left frontal traumatic brain injury. Although the injury is visible on T2-weighted images (A and B), the extent of the injury is much more easily appreciated on the FLAIR images (C and D).

may be able to visualize areas of stroke in the critical first few hours after onset. It may be that in the future, a combination of some of these newer methods of MRI will provide important information for differential diagnosis.

Contrast Agents

The first experimental contrast-enhanced magnetic resonance image was made in 1982 using a gadolinium complex, gadolinium-diethylenetriamine pentaacetic

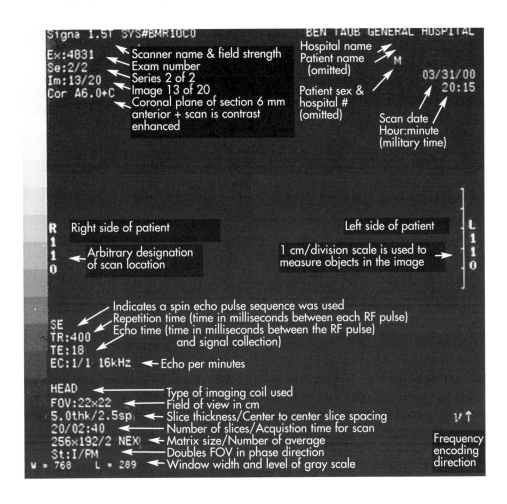

FIGURE 3–13.   Magnetic resonance imaging header information and arbitrary gray scale. Explanations for abbreviations used on the image are also included.

acid (Gd-DTPA), now called gadopentetate dimeglumine. Six years later gadopentetate dimeglumine was approved as an intravenous contrast agent for human clinical MRI scans (Wolf 1991). See Table 3–6 for the cost of both MRI and contrast agent.

Metal ions such as gadolinium are quite toxic to the body if they are in a free state. To make an MRI contrast agent, the metal ion is attached to a very strong ligand (such as DTPA) that prevents any interaction with surrounding tissue. This allows the gadolinium complex to be excreted intact by the kidneys. Three gadolinium-based contrast agents are currently in common use: gadopentetate dimeglumine (Magnevist, Berlex Laboratories), gadodiamide (Omniscan, Amersham Health), and gadoteridol (ProHance, Bracco Diagnostics) (Shellock and Kanal 1999). These agents are administered intravenously, whereupon they distribute to the vascular compartment and then diffuse throughout the extracellular compartment (Mitchell 1997).

Gadolinium is a metal ion that is highly paramagnetic, with a natural magnetic field 657 times greater than that of the hydrogen atom. Unlike the iodinated contrast agents used in CT, the currently used clinical MRI contrast agents are not

TABLE 3–6.   Factors considered when choosing computed tomography (CT) or magnetic resonance imaging (MRI) examination

Clinical considerations	CT	MRI
Availability	Universal	Limited
Sensitivity	Good	Superior
Resolution	1.5 mm	1.5 mm
Average examination time	1 minute	30–45 minutes
Plane of section	Axial only	Any plane of section
Conditions for which it is the preferred procedure	Acute hemorrhage Calcified lesions Screening examination Bone injury	All subcortical lesions Poison or toxin exposure Demyelinating disorders Eating disorders Examination requiring anatomic detail, especially temporal lobe Any condition best viewed in nonaxial plane
Contraindications	History of anaphylaxis or severe allergic reaction (contrast-enhanced CT) Creatinine ≥ 1.5 mg/dL (contrast-enhanced CT) Metformin administration on day of scan (contrast-enhanced CT)	Any magnetic metal in the body, including surgical clips and sutures Implanted electrical, mechanical, or magnetic devices Claustrophobia History of welding (requires skull films before MRI) Pregnancy (legal contraindication)
Cost to patient per scan without contrast medium[a]	~$230	~$550
Cost to patient per single dose of contrast medium[a]	~$60 nonionic	~$110

[a]Costs are regionally variable. Please consult imaging sources in your area for current figures.

imaged directly. Rather, the presence of the contrast agent changes the T1 and T2 properties of hydrogen atoms (protons) in nearby tissue (Runge et al. 1997). Like CT contrast agents, MRI contrast agents do not enter the brain under normal conditions because they cannot pass through the BBB. When there is damage to the BBB, these agents accumulate in tissue around the breakdown. The effect of this accumulation is most easily seen on a T1-weighted scan, where it results in an increase in signal (seen as a white or bright area; see Figure 3–14) (Runge et al. 1997).

On a worldwide basis, 30%–40% of MRI studies include contrast enhancement (Shellock and Kanal 1999). The total incidence of adverse side effects appears to be less than 3%–5%, with any single type of side effect occurring in fewer than 1% of patients (Runge et al. 1997; Shellock and Kanal 1999). Immediate reactions at the injection site include warmth or a burning sensation, pain, and local edema. Delayed reactions (including erythema, swelling, and pain) appear 1–4 days after the injection. Immediate systemic reactions include nausea (sometimes vomiting) and headache. Anaphylactoid reactions have been

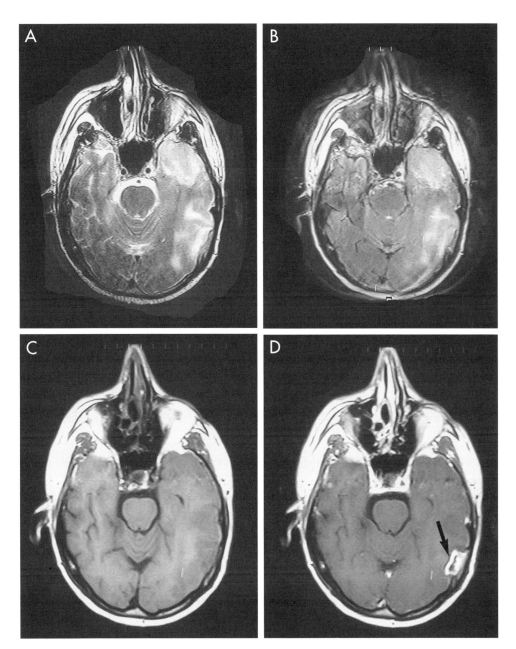

FIGURE 3–14. Contrast-enhanced magnetic resonance imaging of a 69-year-old man who presented with acute confusion and status post a generalized tonic-clonic seizure.

Sequential imaging revealed a left temporal mass, most probably an astrocytoma (infiltrating type). The tumor is more easily seen on T2-weighted (*Panel A*) and fluid-attenuated inversion recovery (*Panel B*) images than on T1-weighted images (*Panel C*). After administration of contrast medium (*Panel D*), an area of blood-brain barrier breakdown within the tumor becomes visible (arrow).

reported, particularly in patients with a history of allergic respiratory disease. The incidence of these reactions appears to be somewhere between 1 and 5 in 500,000.

These agents can be used even in a patient with severe renal disease, provided there is some renal output. This allows contrast-enhanced MRI scans to be obtained in dialysis patients. (For a more extensive review of the biosafety aspects of MRI contrast agents, see Shellock and Kanal 1999.)

Many new MRI contrast agents are under development (Earls and Bluemke 1999; Mitchell 1997). Some link metal ions (gadolinium, manganese) with a structure that allows them to be directed toward specific tissues. Another approach uses specially formulated iron oxide particles (superparamagnetic iron oxide). These alter T2 relaxation more than T1 and are imaged using T2-weighted and gradient echo sequences. Still other efforts are directed toward developing MRI of specific receptors (Nunn et al. 1997). As new contrast agents become available for MRI of the brain, the range of applications in neuropsychiatry may well expand.

Safety and Contraindications

To date, there appear to be no permanent hazardous effects from short-term exposure to magnetic fields and RF pulses generated in clinical MRI scanners (Price 1999). Volunteers scanned using systems with very high field strength (4 T) have reported effects including headaches, dizziness, and nausea (Shellock and Kanal 1991). With very intense gradients it is possible to directly stimulate peripheral nerves, but this is not a concern at clinical field strengths (Bourland et al. 1999; Hoffmann et al. 2000).

There are, however, important contraindications to the use of MRI (see Table 3–6 for summary). The magnetic field can damage electrical, mechanical, or magnetic devices implanted in or attached to the patient. Pacemakers can be damaged by programming changes, possibly inducing arrhythmias. Currents can develop within the wires, leading to burns, fibrillation, or movement of the wires or the pacemaker unit itself. Cochlear implants,

dental implants, magnetic stoma plugs, bone-growth stimulators, and implanted medication-infusion pumps can all be demagnetized or injure the patient by movement during exposure to the scanner's magnetic field. In addition, metallic implants, shrapnel, bullets, or metal shavings within the eye (e.g., from welding) can conduct a current and/or move, injuring the eye. All of these devices distort the magnetic resonance image locally and may decrease diagnostic accuracy. Metallic objects near the magnet can be drawn into the magnet at high speed, injuring the patient or staff (Price 1999; Shellock and Kanal 1991).

Although there is no evidence of damage to the developing fetus, most authorities recommend caution. Judgment should be exercised when considering MRI of a pregnant woman. When possible, express written consent might be obtained from the patient, especially in the first trimester (Shellock and Kanal 1991).

Difficulties have also been encountered when a patient requires physiologic monitoring during the procedure. Several manufacturers have developed MRI-compatible respirators and monitors for blood pressure and heart rate. If these are not available, then the standard monitoring devices must be placed at least 8 feet from the magnet. Otherwise, the readout may be altered or the devices may interfere with obtaining the MRI scan.

MRI Versus CT

The choice of imaging modality should be based on the anatomy and/or pathology that one desires to view (see Table 3–6). CT is used as an inexpensive screening examination. There are also a few conditions best viewed with CT. These include calcification, acute hemorrhage, and any

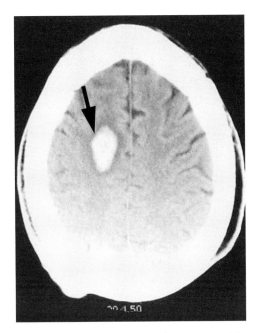

FIGURE 3–15. Computed tomographic image of a 56-year-old man taking warfarin who presented with left-sided weakness a few hours after being involved in a motorcycle accident.

He experienced a brief loss of consciousness after the accident. Note the well-visualized area of hyperdense hemorrhage (arrow).

bone injury, as these pathologies are not yet reliably imaged with MRI (Figure 3–15). However, in the vast majority of cases, MRI is the preferred modality. The image resolution is much higher, more types of pathology are visible, and the brain can be imaged in any plane of section. For example, subcortical lesions are consistently better visualized with MRI because of the greater gray-white contrast and the ability to image in planes other than axial (Figure 3–16). Demyelination due to poison exposure or autoimmune disease (such as multiple sclerosis) is also seen significantly better on MRI, especially when many small lesions are present (Figure 3–17). MRI does not produce the artifacts from bone that are seen in CT, so all lesions near bone (i.e., brain stem, posterior fossa, pituitary, hypothalamus) are

better visualized on MRI. Most temporal lobe structures, especially the hippocampal formation and amygdala, are most easily evaluated using the coronal and sagittal planes of section, rather than axial.

Normal Imaging Anatomy

It is essential for the practicing neuropsychiatrist to have a basic understanding of the cortical and subcortical anatomy involved in thought, memory, and emotion if he or she is to use information gathered from imaging. This includes sufficient knowledge to identify these structures on CT and MRI in the various planes of section. In addition, the neuropsychiatrist must have the ability to identify clinical scenarios that warrant imaging investigation for lesions (e.g., traumatic brain injury, stroke, poison/toxin exposure). (Please see the unabridged chapter by Hurley et al. 2002.)

References

Arakia Y, Ashikaga R, Fujii K, et al: MR fluid-attenuated inversion recovery imaging as routine brain T2-weighted imaging. Eur J Radiol 32:136–143, 1999

Bahner ML, Reith W, Zuna I, et al: Spiral CT vs incremental CT: is spiral CT superior in imaging of the brain? Eur Radiol 8:416–420, 1998

Beresford TP, Blow FC, Hall RCW, et al: CT scanning in psychiatric inpatients: clinical yield. Psychosomatics 27:105–112, 1986

Bergin PS, Fish DR, Shorvon SD, et al: Magnetic resonance imaging in partial epilepsy: additional abnormalities shown with the fluid attenuated inversion recovery (FLAIR) pulse sequence. J Neurol Neurosurg Psychiatry 58:439–443, 1995

Bourland JD, Nyenhuis JA, Schaefer DJ: Physiologic effects of intense MR imaging gradient fields. Neuroimaging Clin N Am 9:363–377, 1999

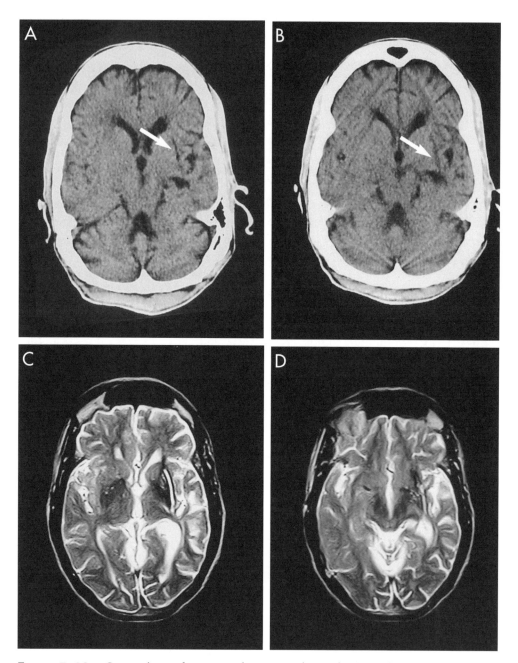

FIGURE 3–16. Comparison of computed tomography and T2-weighted magnetic resonance imaging.

Images of a 69-year-old man who presented status post a generalized tonic-clonic seizure. Abnormal areas indicative of subcortical ischemia are evident on the conventional CT images (*Panel A* and *Panel B*, arrows). Areas of ischemic injury and old hemorrhage as well as normal anatomy are much better visualized on T2-weighted magnetic resonance images (*Panel C* and *Panel D*).

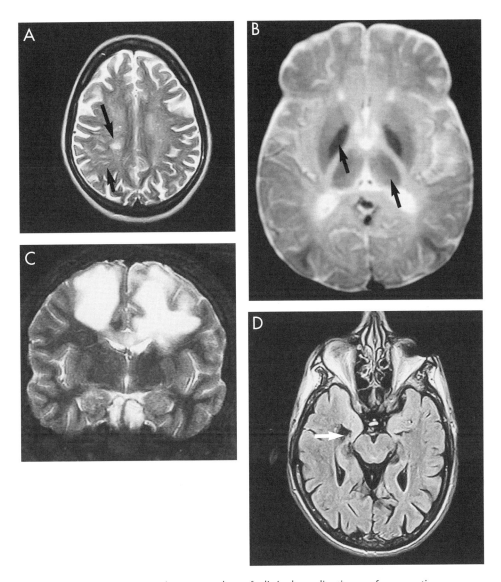

FIGURE 3–17. Representative examples of clinical applications of magnetic resonance imaging (MRI).

Panel A. MRI of a 23-year-old woman with multiple sclerosis. Note the characteristic ovoid, hyperintense demyelinating lesions (arrows). *Panel B.* MRI of an 18-year-old woman with chronic severe toluene abuse. Note the global demyelination and hypointense signal in the globus pallidus and to a lesser extent in the thalamus (arrows). *Panel C.* MRI of a 10-year-old girl with acute disseminated encephalomyelitis. Note the extensive white matter damage as indicated by the hyperintense signal in both medial frontal lobes. *Panel D.* MRI of a 49-year-old man with mesial temporal sclerosis secondary to traumatic brain injury. Note the dilation of the tip of the right temporal horn due to volume loss in the surrounding temporal lobe structures (arrow).

Brant-Zawadzki M, Atkinson D, Detrick M, et al: Fluid-attenuated inversion recovery (FLAIR) for assessment of cerebral infarction. Initial clinical experience in 50 patients. Stroke 27:1187–1191, 1996

Branton T: Use of computerized tomography by old age psychiatrists: an examination of criteria for investigation of cognitive impairment. Int J Geriatr Psychiatry 14: 567–571, 1999

Chakos MH, Esposito S, Charles C, et al: Clinical applications of neuroimaging in psychiatry. Magn Reson Imaging Clin N Am 6:155–164, 1998

Cohan RH, Matsumoto JS, Quagliano PV: Adverse effects, in Manual on Contrast Media, 4th Edition. Edited by Cohan RH, Matsumoto JS, Quagliano PV. Reston, VA, American College of Radiology, 1998a, pp 4–7

Cohan RH, Matsumoto JS, Quagliano PV: Incidence, in Manual on Contrast Media, 4th Edition. Edited by Cohan RH, Matsumoto JS, Quagliano PV. Reston, VA, American College of Radiology, 1998b, p 8

Cohan RH, Matsumoto JS, Quagliano PV: Letter of correction for incidence, in Manual on Contrast Media, 4th Edition. Edited by Cohan RH, Matsumoto JS, Quagliano PV. Reston, VA, American College of Radiology, 1998c

Cohan RH, Matsumoto JS, Quagliano PV: Manual on Contrast Media, 4th Edition. Reston, VA, American College of Radiology, 1998d

Coleman LT, Zimmerman RA: Pediatric craniospinal spiral CT: current applications and future potential. Semin Ultrasound CT MR 15:148–155, 1994

Earls JP, Bluemke DA: New MR imaging contrast agents. Magn Reson Imaging Clin N Am 7:255–273, 1999

Federle MP, Willis LL, Swanson DP: Ionic versus nonionic contrast media: a prospective study of the effect of rapid bolus injection on nausea and anaphylactoid reactions. J Comput Assist Tomogr 22:341–345, 1998

Halpern JD, Hopper KD, Arredondo MG, et al: Patient allergies: role in selective use of nonionic contrast material. Radiology 199:359–362, 1996

Hanyu H, Asano T, Sakurai H, et al: Magnetization transfer ratio in cerebral white matter lesions of Binswanger's disease. J Neurol Sci 166:85–90, 1999

Hoffmann A, Faber SC, Werhahn KJ, et al: Electromyography in MRI—first recordings of peripheral nerve activation caused by fast magnetic field gradients. Magn Reson Med 43(4):534–539, 2000

Hurley RA, Hayman LA, Taber KH: Clinical imaging in neuropsychiatry, in The American Psychiatric Publishing Textbook of Neuropsychiatry and Clinical Neurosciences, 4th Edition. Edited by Yudofsky SC, Hales RE. Washington, DC, American Psychiatric Publishing, 2002, pp 245–283

Jacobs JE, Birnbaum BA, Langlotz CP: Contrast media reactions and extravasation: relationship to intravenous injection rates. Radiology 209:411–416, 1998

Kaplan H, Sadock B, Grebb J: The brain and behavior, in Kaplan and Sadock's Synopsis of Psychiatry. Behavioral Sciences Clinical Psychiatry, 7th Edition. Edited by Kaplan H, Sadock BJ, Graff JA. Baltimore, MD, Williams & Wilkins, 1994, pp 112–125

Katada K: Current status and future prospects of multislice CT; moving toward the ideal x-ray CT system. Toshiba Medical Review 71:1–11, 1999

Kuntz R, Skalej M, Stefanou A: Image quality of spiral CT versus conventional CT in routine brain imaging. Eur J Radiol 26:235–240, 1998

Kuszyk BS, Beauchamp NJJ, Fishman EK: Neurovascular applications of CT angiography. Semin Ultrasound CT MR 19:394–404, 1998

Larson EB, Mack LA, Watts B, et al: Computed tomography in patients with psychiatric illnesses: advantage of a "rule-in" approach. Ann Intern Med 95:360–364, 1981

Mega MS, Cummings JL: Frontal-subcortical circuits and neuropsychiatric disorders. J Neuropsychiatry Clin Neurosci 6:358–370, 1994

Mitchell DG: MR imaging contrast agents—what's in a name? J Magn Reson Imaging 7:1–4, 1997

Moringlane JR, Bartylla K, Hagen T, et al: Stereotactic neurosurgery planning with 3-D spiral CT-angiography. Minim Invasive Neurosurg 40:83–86, 1997

Nunn AD, Linder KE, Tweedle MF: Can receptors be imaged with MRI agents? Q J Nucl Med 41:155–162, 1997

Oi H, Yamazaki H, Matsushita M: Delayed vs immediate adverse reactions to ionic and non-ionic low-osmolality contrast media. Radiat Med 15:23–27, 1997

Orrison WW: Introduction to brain imaging, in Functional Brain Imaging. Edited by Orrison WW Jr, Levine JD, Sanders JA, et al. St. Louis, MO, Mosby-Year–Book, 1995, pp 1–12

Price RR: The AAPM/RSNA physics tutorial for residents. MR imaging safety considerations. Radiological Society of North America. Radiographics 19:1641–1651, 1999

Rauch SL, Renshaw PF: Clinical neuroimaging in psychiatry. Harv Rev Psychiatry 2:297–312, 1995

Runge VM, Muroff LR, Wells JW: Principles of contrast enhancement in the evaluation of brain diseases: an overview. J Magn Reson Imaging 7:5–13, 1997

Rydberg JN, Hammond CA, Grimm RC, et al: Initial clinical experience in MR imaging of the brain with a fast fluid-attenuated inversion-recovery pulse sequence. Radiology 193:173–180, 1994

Sage MR, Wilson AJ, Scroop R: Contrast media and the brain. The basis of CT and MR imaging enhancement. Neuroimaging Clin N Am 8:695–707, 1998

Schemmer DS, Siekierski M, Steiner M: CT of the brain: how useful is it in general psychiatry? (letter). Can J Psychiatry 44:929, 1999

Schwartz RB: Helical (spiral) CT in neuroradiologic diagnosis. Radiol Clin North Am 33:981–995, 1995

Shellock FG, Kanal E: Policies, guidelines, and recommendations for MR imaging safety and patient management. SMRI Safety Committee. J Magn Reson Imaging 1:97–101, 1991

Shellock FG, Kanal E: Safety of magnetic resonance imaging contrast agents. J Magn Reson Imaging 10:477–484, 1999

Taber KH, Zimmerman JG, Yonas H, et al: Applications of xenon CT in clinical practice: detection of hidden lesions. J Neuropsychiatry Clin Neurosci 11:423–425, 1999

Tanabe JL, Ezekiel F, Jagust WJ, et al: Magnetization transfer ratio of white matter hyperintensities in subcortical ischemic vascular dementia. AJNR Am J Neuroradiol 20:839–844, 1999

Weight DG, Bigler ED: Neuroimaging in psychiatry. Psychiatr Clin North Am 21:725–759, 1998

Weinberger DR: Brain disease and psychiatric illness: when should a psychiatrist order a CAT scan? Am J Psychiatry 141:1521–1527, 1984

Wolf GL: Paramagnetic contrast agents for MR imaging of the brain, in MR and CT Imaging of the Head, Neck, and Spine. Edited by Latchaw RE. St. Louis, MO, Mosby-Year–Book, 1991, pp 95–108

Yasuda R, Munechika H: Delayed adverse reactions to nonionic monomeric contrast-enhanced media. Invest Radiol 33:1–5, 1998

CHAPTER 4

Functional Neuroimaging in Psychiatry

James C. Patterson II, M.D., Ph.D.

Kathryn J. Kotrla, M.D.

The practice of psychiatry alleviates a staggering array of symptoms that result from disorders of thought, mood, and behavior. The pathophysiologic processes producing these symptoms are poorly understood, making it difficult to understand the neurobiological basis for psychiatric illnesses, or predict the best treatment intervention. Fortunately, functional neuroimaging techniques allow scientists and clinicians to look inside the human brain and attempt to see the human mind.

Currently, functional neuroimaging methods are mostly restricted to scientific investigations. Day-to-day clinical practice, with a few exceptions, is unlikely to benefit from any of the functional imaging techniques outlined below. Nevertheless, results from functional neuroimaging are shaping our understanding about many neuropsychiatric conditions.

Abnormal activity in specific brain areas that is associated with any psychiatric symptom or disorder that results in abnormal behavior is theoretically measurable. In addition, the changes in concentration of various brain chemicals associated with these disorders can be determined, specific neurotransmitter receptors can be labeled, and the effects of psychotropic medication can be studied in vivo, all with functional neuroimaging. Such results lead to hypotheses about the neuroanatomic and neurochemical substrate for psychiatric conditions.

This chapter provides an overview of the techniques themselves, how they are used to understand normal brain functioning, and what has been learned about neuropsychiatric disorders. It provides a foundation to evaluate the information from functional neuroimaging, so that the practicing psychiatrist can assess research findings that affect clinical practice.

Functional Neuroimaging Concepts

There are various ways to image the functional activity of the living human brain. One approach uses radioactivity to measure brain metabolism, blood flow, or neurotransmitter receptors via positron emission tomography (PET) or single photon emission computed tomography (SPECT). Another avenue to investigate the brain's function applies magnetic resonance imaging (MRI) techniques to produce various types of functional images without the use of radioactivity. Functional magnetic resonance imaging (fMRI) uses blood oxygenation levels to estimate neural activation, whereas a technique known as arterial spin tagging (AST) can estimate cerebral blood flow. Local chemical concentrations can be examined with magnetic resonance spectroscopy (MRS), and evaluation of white matter integrity is done via a process known as diffusion-weighted imaging. Yet another technique, magnetoencephalography (MEG), involves looking at the minute magnetic fluctuations associated with regional brain activity.

All these techniques give us a general idea of neuronal activity in localized regions of the brain. Active neurons expend maximal energy at their synapses, causing localized increases in metabolic demands and glucose consumption (Schwartz et al. 1979). As metabolism increases, blood flow increases concordant with (or greater than) the increased energy demand (Fox et al. 1988). PET using radiolabeled glucose images changes in synaptic metabolism, whereas PET using (^{15}O)water, SPECT, fMRI, and AST use direct and indirect measures of blood flow to follow changes in synaptic activity.

When a functional brain image shows changes in regional metabolism or blood flow, this is due to the activity of afferent synapses in that area. The neuronal cell bodies that have altered their firing rate may lie in nearby cortex or in distant locations. The afferent input may come from inhibitory or excitatory synapses, so it is possible that decreased blood flow to a region in the frontal cortex, for example, may be due to decreased inhibitory inputs, leading to increased firing of those frontal output neurons. Conversely, increased blood flow may reflect increased inhibitory inputs, functionally quieting the area's output (Nadeau and Crosson 1995). This means that when a change in activity in an area is reported, this is a composite picture of the firing of local and distant afferent neurons. How this alters the area's output is an unknown. Because of this, studies that examine the connectivity of regions are important. Various types of statistical analyses are beginning to be used to examine connectivity. These techniques look at not just what changes occur in a given location, but how the regions are related to one another in terms of activity within a network.

Functional neuroimaging provides a way to examine patterns of brain activity during complex cognitive processes and emotions. In fact, its remarkable sensitivity is both an advantage and a disadvantage. Although virtually any brain function can be imaged, uncontrolled (and undesired) mental activities and moods compose part of that functional image. This is particularly troublesome in studies done at rest, in which results reflect incoming sensory stimuli and internal thoughts and feelings (Andreasen et al. 1995). The rest state may differ significantly between neuropsychiatrically ill patients and healthy volunteers, as the baseline mood, thoughts, or response to scanning may be distinct for the two populations. To control for the rest state, many functional neuroimaging studies are performed while the participant is doing a task, thereby engaging specific brain systems or neural networks. In addition, recent work in studies of "rest" shows that there is a consistent network that is active when the body is not expressing behavior (Binder et al. 1999), and this network overlaps significantly with brain regions that are pathological in many psychiatric disorders.

Each functional neuroimaging technique has advantages and limitations. The techniques differ in repeatability, which determines whether participants are imaged at rest or during tasks. They differ in spatial resolution, which limits how easily activity is localized to specific brain regions. They differ in sensitivity, and this influences which brain processes are observable. Of practical importance, they differ in price and availability, which affects who gets imaged. PET imaging has been the most expensive and difficult to find outside an academic research institution; however, it is becoming more prevalent as the technology becomes less expensive and more common and as clinical uses expand. A review of the techniques allows the practicing psychiatrist to understand what conclusions can be drawn from each one.

Functional Neuroimaging Techniques

Positron Emission Tomography

Theory

PET is named from its use of positron-emitting isotopes to image brain functioning. Positron-emitting isotopes are very short-lived radioactive entities including oxygen-15 (^{15}O), nitrogen-13 (^{13}N), carbon-11 (^{11}C), and fluorine-18 (^{18}F). The radioactive isotopes are incorporated into specific molecules to study cerebral metabolism, blood flow, and neuroreceptors. Most commonly used are (^{15}O)water for cerebral blood flow studies or [^{18}F]fluoro-deoxyglucose (FDG) to image metabolism (Berman and Weinberger 1991; Nadeau and Crosson 1995).

Radioactive agents are intravenously injected into the subject, whose head is positioned within a radiation detector. The radioactive isotope decays within the brain, releasing a positron. The positron travels a short distance and collides with an electron, resulting in the emission of two photons that travel at 180° to each other at the speed of light. The photons are detected at the opposite sides of the head simultaneously, and the location of the emitting positron can thus be calculated (Berman and Weinberger 1991).

Cerebral Blood Flow and Metabolism

(^{15}O)water and FDG are the two mainstays of PET and have quite different properties. (^{15}O)water provides a measure of cerebral blood flow and has a half-life of about 2 minutes (Saha et al. 1994). Because of the short half-life, up to 8–10 scans can be performed during a single imaging session. This allows experimenters to image multiple conditions, as participants can perform different tasks during the 8–10 scans (Nadeau and Crosson 1995).

FDG is actively taken up by the glucose transport mechanism into cells and is phosphorylated to FDG-6-phosphate by hexokinase. This remains trapped intracellularly because it is not a glycolytic substrate. Scanning produces a measure of glucose metabolism; because most brain energy use is synaptic, a map of regional glucose use indicates neural activity (Saha et al. 1994).

FDG uptake requires about 30 minutes, a relatively long time for functional neuroimaging. Often, brain images are obtained during a resting state or during the same task lasting 30 minutes. The relatively long imaging time limits the number of brain states imaged. Because of radiation exposure, each participant can be studied only two to four times a year (Berman and Weinberger 1991).

Neurotransmitters and Receptors

PET also images neurotransmitters and their receptors. See Table 4–1 for a listing of various ligands and their use. Although they are not specifically listed in the table, PET radiotracers have also been made by attaching a radioactive carbon to pharmacologically active compounds like deprenyl and fluoxetine (George et al. 1996).

Advantages and Limitations

PET imaging is extremely valuable to clinical neuroscience. (^{15}O)water PET has been used extensively to understand normal brain functioning because participants are imaged during several conditions. Both (^{15}O)water and FDG PET are widely used for research on neuropsychiatric illnesses. Such usefulness has led to the development of sophisticated methods for data acquisition and analysis, which improve the reliability and credibility of PET information.

However, PET images lack the spatial resolution and anatomical details needed to specifically identify smaller areas of brain activity. Technical constraints limit the theoretical resolution of PET to about 4 mm (Messa et al. 1995), although data are often blurred 1.5 to 2 times the spatial resolution of the image (Friston et al. 1995) to diminish the influence of individual neuroanatomic variability. To localize brain activity, the image from an individual may be converted into a standardized, stereotactic space such as Talair-

ach space (Talairach and Tournoux 1988). Data from many individuals are grouped to uncover areas of activation. Alternatively, computer programs can register PET scans with high-resolution MRI scans of the same participant. Areas of PET activation are then localized using the structural brain image. Each of these techniques has its own pitfalls, and it is best to consider whether one wants across-subject examinations that can be generalized to a population, or within-subject analyses that have more internal accuracy. For example, if a patient with an ill-defined brain tumor has a functional image study done to locate regions of neoplasm or inflammation in the brain, this can be overlaid on the subject's MRI to provide precise localization of the functional changes. However, if a population of schizophrenic patients was the topic of study, across-subject analysis would be optimal.

Because of the short-half lives of positron-emitting isotopes, PET must be performed near the cyclotron that produces them. Thus, PET has been exclusively performed near research centers and therefore has not enjoyed wide clinical use. However, regional cyclotrons that can deliver isotopes (with the exception of the short-half-life ^{15}O-labeled isotopes) to nearby PET scanners are becoming more common, making it possible to have a PET scanner at regional and private hospitals. Many types of clinical PET scans are now covered by some health insurance plans, mainly for cancer evaluations.

Also, the use of radioactivity inherently limits the number of scans that can be done within a single individual, so longitudinal studies or studies in children are ethically difficult. Despite these limitations, PET has made substantial inroads into understanding normal brain functioning and investigating abnormalities in neuropsychiatric populations.

TABLE 4–1. Radioligands used in positron emission tomography

Common name	Radiolabel	Labeling target	Citation
Water	^{15}O	Cerebral blood flow	
Fluorodeoxyglucose (FDG)	^{18}F	Cerebral metabolism	
Dihydrotetrabenazine (DTBZ)	^{11}C	Vesicular monoamine transporter	Henry and Scherman 1989
Fluorodopa	^{18}F	Dopamine neurons	Seeman and Seeman 1988
β-CIT	^{11}C	Dopamine transporter	Muller et al. 1993
RTI-32	^{11}C	Dopamine transporter	Wilson et al. 1996
NNC112	^{11}C	D_1 receptor	Halldin et al. 1998
NNC756	^{11}C	D_1 receptor	Rinne et al. 1996
SCH23390	^{11}C or ^{76}Br	D_1 receptor	Seeman and Seeman 1988
Spiperone	$^{18}F, ^{11}C, ^{76}Br$	D_2 receptor	Seeman and Seeman 1988
Fluorethylspiperone	^{18}F	D_2 receptor	Seeman and Seeman 1988
Raclopride	^{11}C	D_2 receptor	Seeman and Seeman 1988
Benperidol, bromperidol, brombenperidol	$^{18}F, ^{75}Br$	D_2 receptor	Seeman and Seeman 1988
Haloperidol	^{18}F	D_2 receptor	Seeman and Seeman 1988
Pimozide	^{11}C	D_2 receptor	Seeman and Seeman 1988
N-methylspiroperidol	^{18}F or ^{11}C	D_2 receptor	Seeman and Seeman 1988
Epidepride	^{11}C	D_2 receptor	Langer et al. 1999
FLB 457	^{11}C	D_2 receptor	Farde et al. 1997
Nemonapride YM-09151–2	^{11}C	D_2 receptor	Tanji et al. 1998
N-methylspiperone	^{11}C	5-HT$_2$ and D_2 receptors	Berman and Weinberger 1991
Deprenyl	^{11}C	Monoamine oxidase	George et al. 1996
Fluoxetine	^{11}C	Serotonin transporter	George et al. 1996
(+)McN5652	^{11}C	Serotonin transporter	Szabo et al. 1996
α-Methyl-tryptophan	^{11}C	Serotonin synthesis rate	Muzik et al. 1997
WAY-100635	^{11}C	5-HT$_{1A}$ receptor	Pike et al. 1996
CPC0222	^{11}C	5-HT$_{1A}$ receptor	Houle et al. 1997
Setoperone	^{18}F	5-HT$_{2A}$ receptor	Blin et al. 1990
Altanserin	^{18}F	5-HT$_{2A}$ receptor	Crouzel et al. 1992
Flumazenil	^{11}C	Benzodiazepine receptor	Saha et al. 1994
N1′-(methyl) naltrindole	^{11}C	Delta opioid receptor	Madar et al. 1996
6-deoxy-6-β-fluoronaltrexone	^{18}F	Opioid receptor	Cohen et al. 1997
Carfentanil	^{11}C	μ-selective opioid receptor	Frost et al. 1985
Diprenorphine	^{11}C	Non-μ opioid receptor	Jones et al. 1988

TABLE 4–1. Radioligands used in positron emission tomography *(continued)*

Common name	Radiolabel	Labeling target	Citation
PMP	^{11}C	Acetylcholinesterase	Kuhl et al. 1999
Nicotine	^{11}C	Nicotinic cholinergic receptor	Cumming et al. 1999
NMPB	^{11}C	Muscarinic cholinergic receptor	Asahina et al. 1998
Xanomeline, and the analog butylthio-TZTP	^{11}C	Muscarinic cholinergic receptor	Farde et al. 1996

Single Photon Emission Computed Tomography

Theory

SPECT also uses radioactive compounds to image brain activity. Like PET, SPECT derives its name from the type of radioisotope involved, compounds that produce only one photon per disintegration. The radioisotopes are readily available from commercial sources. This makes SPECT available in most clinical centers. However, because SPECT imaging depends on a single photon being released, its spatial resolution is less than that of PET.

Cerebral Blood Flow

SPECT produces both quantitative and qualitative measures of cerebral blood flow. The most common radioligand used to produce qualitative measures of brain perfusion is [^{99m}Tc]hexamethylpropylene amine oxime (HMPAO). After it is intravenously injected, it is accumulated by endothelial cell membranes within several minutes. It concentrates in proportion to regional cerebral blood flow (rCBF) (Reba 1993), and its activity may remain constant for up to 24 hours (Saha et al. 1994). Because of this, participants can be injected during very controlled conditions, away from the noise and anxiety of the scanning room. A snapshot of the relative cerebral perfusion during this controlled period is obtained when the participant is scanned up to several hours

later (Saha et al. 1994). Another available radioligand is [^{99m}Tc]ethyl cysteinate dimer (ECD). Although this ligand produces less extracerebral uptake, it also has some dramatically different patterns of uptake within the cerebrum compared with HMPAO (Patterson et al. 1997). Many other studies also find differences between these two tracers. This indicates that there may be differences in uptake based on the ligand, and therefore variance in activity patterns may result not only from changes in brain activity but also from the radioligand being used.

SPECT resolution is limited to around 10 mm by the technique itself. Also, for perfusion studies with HMPAO, only a limited number of scans can be done in a subject because of the relatively long half-life of the radioisotope. Likewise, if multiple scans are desired, for example during multiple tasks, they must be performed after delays of several days to allow for isotope washout (Nadeau and Crosson 1995).

Advantages and Limitations

SPECT is clinically available for a qualitative measure of cerebral perfusion. It may be beneficial in diagnosing dementing illnesses. Areas of relative hypoperfusion, corresponding to neuronal degeneration, are visually apparent. SPECT is also used for research. Many studies done in the late 1980s and early 1990s analyzed SPECT scans using regions of interest (ROIs) and used a cerebellar region as the "control" region. This is because it was thought at the time that the cerebellum had little to do with cognition. Over the past few years, it has become apparent that the cerebellum is very actively involved in cognitive processes (see, e.g., Gao et al. 1996). Many new studies find either cerebellar activity in normal subjects, or cerebellar pathology in studies of mental disorders, thus older SPECT evaluations that use the cerebellum as a control site must be interpreted with this in mind. Even older studies that used (^{133}Xe) SPECT (one of the original radiolabeled tracers used for brain imaging) suffer from very limited spatial resolution, making localization of brain activity difficult. [^{99m}Tc]HMPAO SPECT has limited repeatability, so many studies are done at rest. Although SPECT has contributed to the understanding of neuropsychiatric illnesses, it is a less precise tool than PET because of its significantly lower temporal and spatial resolution.

Functional Magnetic Resonance Imaging

Theory

Functional MRI couples the exquisite spatial resolution of structural MRI with the ability to image areas related to neural activity. It does this noninvasively, without the use of radioactive agents. When a localized region of brain tissue becomes active, it uses oxygen and glucose and produces certain metabolic byproducts. In these areas of increased neural activity, the metabolism and blood flow increase with the increased energy demands. The cerebrovascular physiology of the brain is such that local blood flow and volume increase to supply the needed fuel and remove the metabolic waste products. Although the exact mechanism remains to be determined, many scientists believe that the supply of oxygen is much greater than what neurons utilize. This results in

an actual increase in the concentration of oxygenated hemoglobin compared with deoxygenated hemoglobin in areas of neural activity. Oxygenated hemoglobin is less paramagnetic and has increased intensity (looks brighter) compared with deoxygenated hemoglobin on images created with T_2-weighted pulse sequences. fMRI uses this blood oxygen–level dependent (BOLD) effect to image changes in neural activity (Kwong et al. 1992).

Advantages and Limitations

Because fMRI requires no radiation and can be completely noninvasive, a participant can be imaged multiple times. This allows patients to be imaged during different clinical states, or before and after pharmacologic, psychotherapeutic, or behavioral treatments to determine how treatment interventions affect cerebral functioning. It also removes ethical constraints about imaging children and adolescents with psychiatric illnesses. In addition, fMRI is performed in standard, clinically available 1.5-T magnetic resonance scanners. In theory, it can be implemented at any of the numerous sites that have a magnetic resonance scanner.

Although fMRI provides precise neuroanatomic localization, it also means that minor subject movements introduce artifacts that impair the ability to appreciate neural activity. Moreover, relying on the oxygenation status of endogenous hemoglobin molecules produces very small changes in signal intensity, on the order of 1%–5%. This makes it very difficult to appreciate the true signal associated with neural activity above the background noise of ongoing brain activity.

Magnetic Resonance Spectroscopy

Theory

MRS is performed in the same scanners as structural and functional MRI. However, by altering the scanning parameters, the signal represents chemical entities from brain areas. The response of an atom in a magnetic field is characteristic, based on the number and nature of its subatomic particles, as well as its unique molecular environment. Spectra are obtained that are characteristic for nuclei within certain molecules (McClure et al. 1995). This principle is employed in MRS to study the concentration of brain metabolites. Typically, spectra are obtained from a number of nuclei, including hydrogen-1 (^{1}H), carbon-13 (^{13}C), sodium-23 (^{23}Na), lithium-7 (^{7}Li), and phosphorus-31 (^{31}P).

In psychiatry, investigators are primarily using ^{1}H and ^{31}P MRS. Proton (^{1}H) spectroscopy can distinguish *N* aspartate (NAA), creatine and phosphocreatine, and phosphatidylcholine. Signals can be obtained from glutamate, glutamine, γ-aminobutyric acid, lactate, and inositol phosphates, although these signals may be difficult to adequately resolve (Narayana and Jackson 1991). NAA is found in neurons and is absent in most glial cell lines. Decreases in NAA may reflect a diminished number or density of neurons; NAA levels decrease proportionate to the brain loss in neurodegenerative disorders (Maier 1995; Renshaw et al. 1995). Creatine and phosphocreatine are important energy substrates, and phosphatidylcholine is an important component of cell membranes (Narayana and Jackson 1991).

MRS with ^{31}P detects the relative tissue concentrations of certain phosphorus metabolites, including those involved in energy and phospholipid metabolism (Waddington et al. 1990). Resonances are obtained from the precursors and breakdown products of membrane phospholipids (phosphomonoesters and phosphodiesters, respectively), which uncover potential abnormalities in membrane turnover. To reflect energy metabolism, ^{31}P MRS senses phosphocreatine, adenosine triphosphate, adenosine diphosphate, and inorganic orthophosphate; intracellular pH can also be assessed (Pettegrew et al. 1991).

Advantages and Limitations

MRS is notable for its noninvasiveness, repeatability, and ability to provide information about membrane and metabolic moieties. It has successfully imaged abnormalities in areas of tumor growth and ischemia. Comparisons have been made of the concentrations of substances between healthy brains and brains with neuropsychiatric abnormalities. It may prove ideal for longitudinal studies. However, it has limited spatial resolution, although this is improving. Also, for molecules present in low concentration, like receptor sites, PET is superior because it uses radiolabeled ligands (Moonen et al. 1990).

Limitations of Functional Neuroimaging

Many neuropsychiatric conditions are investigated with functional neuroimaging techniques, and general themes are emerging about the neuroanatomic location of these illnesses. However, much work remains to be done to clarify the neurobiology of psychiatric symptoms. Currently, seeking global differences in brain blood flow or metabolism between patients and control subjects yields mixed results. The most consistent finding in this regard is in patients with thyroid abnormalities. In this population, thyroid-stimulating hormone levels have been found to inversely correlate with global flow. More consistent findings emerge by imaging the participant during a task that taps into a particular neural network.

Many factors can produce inconsistent findings when evaluating brain activity in a given patient population. First, patients sharing a diagnostic label can be very heterogeneous. For example, patients with schizophrenia can have paranoid schizophrenia with mainly positive symptoms, or disorganized schizophrenia with mainly negative symptoms. The same can be said of a diagnosis of major depressive disorder. It is also possible that distinct pathophysiologic processes (with different patterns of brain activity) can lead to expression of very similar symptoms.

Other biases can easily affect results as well. Different research sites may attract particular subtypes of psychiatric disorders, and different criteria for inclusion and exclusion may bias the population. Often, studies are done with small numbers of subjects. When this is combined with several of the confounds listed above, as well as a small main effect within the data, results can vary significantly and thus may not be representative of the population being studied. The subjects' medication state, whether they are imaged during an acutely or chronically ill state or during a state of remission, even what time of day they are imaged, can all affect the resulting patterns of brain activity. Also, many studies of neuropsychiatric patients are performed at rest, which means that thoughts and feelings during the scan are imaged. Individuals respond idiosyncratically to the scanning environment; this may be more pronounced when comparing patients with volunteers. Different research groups allow variable stimuli during a resting scan. Some participants are imaged with their eyes closed and their ears plugged; others can see and hear the ambient environment. As mentioned earlier, recent work has shown consistent patterns of activity during rest (Binder et al. 1999) as well as in sleep (Nofzinger et al. 1999, 2000), and this activity is present in some of the same regions that are affected in many psychiatric disorders.

Lastly, independent research groups differ in the techniques used. PET, SPECT, fMRI, and MRS have all been applied to neuropsychiatric populations, and these methods have variable anatomical resolution and repeatability. Even when groups use the same general method, the scanners used vary in their resolution, sensitivity, and quality of images. Once the data are acquired, researchers choose a variety of methods for data analysis. All these variables can result in conflicting neuroimaging results.

Despite these problems, functional neuroimaging has provided tantalizing insights into neuropsychiatric conditions. Perhaps as the technology advances further, it will be possible to image an individual, understand the function and dysfunction within specific neural networks, and determine how the brain responds to treatment interventions.

State Versus Trait Markers in Neuroimaging Studies of Mental Disorders

From the standpoint of longitudinal studies of brain function in a given disorder, it is difficult to know whether there are brain perfusion changes before there is phenotypic expression (disease symptoms) of those changes. Most patients do not have functional brain imaging done *before* they get sick; they get scans as a result of the disease process being expressed. Thus, little is known about what changes in perfusion might be occurring before diagnosis. Some studies are beginning to look at family members of mentally ill patients to look for possible "trait" markers, but this type of study is in its infancy (Blackwood et al. 1999). After an ill patient has had functional imaging performed, and has then been treated and gotten well, additional scans can be obtained. Comparison of these brain scans in two different *states* within the same patient or patient population is quite useful. This provides information about brain regions or networks that are affected by the disease process. Regions of abnormal activity during illness that normalize during remission are generally considered to be "state" markers, whereas regions that remain constantly abnormal irrespective of the wellness of the subject are "trait" markers of the illness being studied. A good example of this is the subgenual anterior cingulate cortex in familial depression, which remains hypoperfused even during states of remission from depression (Drevets et al. 1997). It is possible, at least in theory, that trait markers like these can predict illness, if subjects at risk are screened for the disease.

Neuropsychiatric Disorders

Autism

Children with pervasive developmental disorder exhibit many problematic symptoms. Social interaction is impaired, language is delayed, and stereotyped motor behaviors and a marked need for sameness are common. Although structural neuroanatomic abnormalities are reported in autism, results from functional neuroimaging studies to date have been inconsistent. This may be due to technical limitations, difficulty conceptualizing the illness, or the heterogeneity of the disorder itself. Fortunately, with SPECT ligand studies, fMRI, and MRS, there is every reason to hope for clearer answers about the neuroanatomic and neurobiological basis of autism.

Using FDG PET, the resting cerebral metabolism of autistic men was higher than that of control subjects (Horwitz et al. 1988; Rumsey et al. 1985). In contrast, [^{99m}Tc]HMPAO SPECT of four autistic adult men showed decreased perfusion throughout the brain and focal decreases in the right temporal and bilateral frontal lobes. However, the control volunteers were not matched for IQ or gender to the autistic patients (George et al. 1992). In six autistic children, reduced perfusion was noted in the temporal and parietal lobes, but again, control subjects were not IQ matched to the patients (Mountz et al. 1995). In addition, in resting PET and SPECT studies, no abnormalities in cerebral blood flow or metabolism were found in autistic children (De Volder et al. 1987; Zilbovicius et al. 1992) or adults (Herold et al. 1988).

Matching on IQ is critical, since any abnormalities noted should be associated with autism as opposed to general mental retardation. For example, when children with autism were compared with age-matched control subjects with developmental disabilities and attention deficit/hyperactivity disorder (ADHD), blood flow to the frontal and temporal lobes in the autistic children was reduced. The blood flow to these areas was positively correlated with the developmental level (and IQ), underscoring the need to assess IQ when evaluating functional neuroimaging results (Hashimoto et al. 2000).

When SPECT was used to compare autistic children with nonautistic children of similar age and IQ, decreased perfusion was found in the bilateral insula, superior temporal gyri, left inferior frontal gyrus, and left middle frontal gyrus. Moreover, specific symptoms were associated with blood flow patterns. Impairments in communication and social interaction were positively correlated with blood flow in the left medial prefrontal cortex and the anterior cingulate gyrus, whereas an obsessive desire for sameness was positively correlated with blood flow in the right medial temporal region (Ohnishi et al. 2000). Abnormalities in the anterior cingulate gyrus were also noted in an MRI and PET study of autistic adults comparing them with gender- and age-matched control subjects, in which the dorsal anterior cingulate gyrus was reduced in volume and metabolism in autism (Haznedar et al. 1997).

Using proton MRS, reduced NAA was found in the cerebellums of children with autism, consistent with neuropathological reports of reduced cerebellar Purkinje and granule cells in the cerebellar cortex in autism (Chugani et al. 1999).

The serotonin system has been investigated in autistic children using a PET tracer for serotonin synthesis. Neurochemical abnormalities were seen in boys with autism in the network connecting the dentate nucleus of the cerebellum, the thalamus, and the prefrontal cortex (Chugani et al. 1997). This pathway is important in motor learning and higher cognitive functions, including language (R.A. Muller et al. 1998).

Two pilot studies investigated auditory functions and language in a small number of autistic adults compared with non-IQ-matched control subjects. (^{15}O)water PET revealed a trend toward reduced auditory cortex but increased left anterior cingulate gyrus activations in autism when listening to tones. Autistic individuals showed a significant reversal of normal left dominance and cerebellar dentate nuclear activation when listening to sentences. Repeating sentences caused reduced blood flow in the prefrontal cortex of healthy individuals but not in autistic individuals. When required to generate sentences, the autism group showed reduced activation of the left thalamus and possibly the prefrontal cortex, again implicating abnormalities in the dentate-thalamo-cortical pathway that had been implicated in disordered serotonin synthesis (R.A. Muller et al. 1998, 1999).

Since social interactions are universally impaired in autism, even with spared IQ, a recent fMRI study imaged nine males with Asperger's syndrome or autism, and compared them with age-, gender-, and IQ-matched control subjects. Participants viewed faces with neutral, happy, or angry expressions. Individuals with autism did not activate the right fusiform gyrus (the cortical area that processes faces), left amygdala, or left cerebellum when processing emotional expressions (Critchley et al. 2000).

One novel approach has been to use fMRI to study individuals with autism during a task at which they are superior to healthy control subjects. One of these tasks is the Embedded Figures Task, in which a participant is asked to find a simple shape embedded in a more complex one. Six individuals with autism or Asperger's syndrome were matched to control subjects by age, gender, handedness, and IQ. Both groups activated the middle and inferior temporal gyri, the supramarginal gyrus, inferior frontal gyrus, and middle occipital gyrus to perform the task. However, the control subjects showed significantly greater response in bilateral dorsal parietal cortex and right dorsolateral prefrontal cortex, whereas the autistic group showed more activation in the right occipital cortex extending to the inferior temporal gyrus (Ring et al. 1999). This suggests that individuals with autism use a more posterior and "local" approach to processing complex visual information, rather than at the global level by activating the prefrontal cortex.

These recent studies offer the potential to explore specific neural networks linking the cerebellum, thalamus, striatum, limbic system, and prefrontal cortex, and to determine the association between discrete networks and the symptoms expressed under the global diagnosis of autism.

Attention Deficit/ Hyperactivity Disorder

ADHD is characterized by hyperactivity, disordered attention, and impulsivity. Although this disorder begins in childhood, symptoms may persist into adulthood. In adults with ADHD performing an auditory continuous-attention task, brain metabolism showed a generalized reduction, with focal decreases in the premotor and superior prefrontal areas (Zametkin et al. 1990). In adolescents with ADHD, regional metabolic decreases were uncovered in the left anterior frontal and right temporal lobes (Zametkin et al. 1993). A more recent study evaluated adult patients with ADHD during a working memory task (Schweitzer et al. 2000). The data found that patients had a relative lack of task-related activity in frontal regions while having more extrastriate activity. This indicates a defect in engaging frontal regions for use in difficult executive tasks, while having to use more visual imagery to make up for this. The cerebral basis of attention has been fairly well studied with PET and fMRI (see the section "Attention" in the unabridged chapter by Patterson and Kotrla 2002). Brain areas with abnormal metabolism in ADHD correspond to regions involved in attention in healthy volunteers. This was remarkably well demonstrated by two studies done using fMRI. In the first, adult ADHD patients failed to activate the cognitive/attention division of the anterior cingulate gyrus during the Counting Stroop task compared with a group of matched control subjects. Instead the patients with ADHD activated a different network, including the insula, striatum, and thalamus (Bush et al. 1999). The second study examined children with ADHD during a motor response inhibition task and found less activity in regions of the medial pre-frontal cortex bordering the cingulate attentional region. This region is important in directing motor responses (Rubia et al. 1999).

One of the fundamental underlying dysfunctions in ADHD is thought to be within the dopamine system. Most drugs that are effective in treating ADHD (e.g., stimulants) work by blocking reuptake of dopamine by the dopamine transporter. Two studies done with radiolabeled ligands have been performed to evaluate dopamine's involvement in this disorder. The first was a SPECT study that used [123I]Altropane to examine dopamine transporter density in adults with ADHD. Dougherty and colleagues saw a 70% increase in dopamine transporter density in the striatum of adults with ADHD compared with control subjects (Dougherty et al. 1999). Another study done using the PET radioligand [18F]fluorodopa found a 48% increase of dopa accumulation in the right midbrain of children (medication-free for 2 weeks) with ADHD compared with control subjects. Furthermore, the degree of accumulation of radiolabeled dopa in the right midbrain correlated with the severity of ADHD symptoms in the patients (Ernst et al. 1999). These studies are complementary, as overproduction of dopamine in the midbrain could be related to increased reuptake of dopamine in the striatum.

Anxiety and Panic Disorders

Panic disorder is defined by spontaneous panic attacks, discrete episodes of intense fear with accompanying somatic symptoms. A review of the functional imaging literature related to panic disorder has been published (Goddard and Charney 1997). In panic disorder, the intravenous infusion of sodium lactate can precipitate a panic attack, and patients with panic disorder produce excessive amounts of blood lactate in response to a variety of metabolic challenges. MRS offers a noninvasive measure of brain lactate. It was used to compare a small number of panic disorder patients with healthy control subjects during hyperventilation. Brain lactate level rose significantly more in patients with panic disorder (Dager et al. 1995). Another MRS investigation used ^{31}P MRS to examine high-energy phosphate metabolism in the frontal lobes of patients with panic disorder (Shioiri et al. 1996). This study found phosphocreatine asymmetry with levels on the left greater than those on the right, consistent with previous findings of perfusion asymmetry in this disorder. In another resting state examination, unmedicated females with panic disorder were compared with control subjects in a PET study of metabolism using FDG. This work found increased activity at rest in the hippocampus and the parahippocampal gyrus on the left side, but decreased activity in the inferior parietal and posterior temporal regions on the right (Bisaga et al. 1998). The presence of panic disorder was confirmed after performance of the scan by measuring lactate level. Other studies have also found abnormalities in the hippocampus. Another PET study that also used FDG examined metabolism in medicated, stable responders and found abnormal asymmetry in the orbitofrontal and hippocampal regions (Nordahl et al. 1998). To summarize, many studies of panic disorder implicate the limbic system as playing a role in this disease.

Obsessive-Compulsive Disorder

Obsessive-compulsive disorder (OCD) is characterized by unwanted, persistent, repetitive thoughts and the performance of ritualistic behaviors. This disorder is associated with a number of neurological conditions, including Sydenham's chorea, Tourette syndrome, postencephalitic Parkinson's disease, and bilateral globus pallidus lesions (Insel 1992). These conditions all involve dysfunction in the basal ganglia, suggesting a neuroanatomic basis for OCD.

The basal ganglia are involved in fine motor control, habit learning, and behavior selection. Five separate parallel circuits connect areas of cortex with the striatum and thalamus. The role these circuits play in behavior and cognition depends on their unique cortical connections. Functional neuroimaging has implicated dysfunction in three of these circuits in OCD. There is a dorsolateral prefrontal circuit that may play a role in memory functions. A lateral orbitofrontal circuit projects to the ventral caudate nucleus; lesions in animals result in an inability to switch behavioral routines. An anterior cingulate circuit involves cortex, ventral striatum, and limbic structures such as the hippocampus, amygdala, and overlying mesial temporal cortex. Animal studies have been insufficient to delineate a role for this circuit (Alexander et al. 1986), although the limbic connections suggest an affective component.

Using resting FDG PET, OCD patients were shown to have increased metabolism in the caudate and orbitofrontal gyri (Baxter et al. 1987, 1988). Patients with childhood-onset OCD shared this abnormality and additionally had evidence of increased prefrontal and cingulate metabolism (Swedo et al. 1989).

Treatment interventions alter the abnormal metabolic patterns. FDG PET during a continuous-performance task was performed on OCD patients before and after treatment with clomipramine. With clomipramine, metabolism in the basal ganglia and orbitofrontal cortex decreased to a level comparable to that seen in healthy volunteers; clinical improvement correlated with the normalized caudate and orbitofrontal metabolism (Benkelfat et al. 1990).

In a resting SPECT study, OCD patients had increased mesial-frontal perfusion, which normalized with fluoxetine treatment (Hoehn-Saric et al. 1991). A resting FDG PET study looked at changes in cerebral metabolism after OCD patients responded to treatment with either fluoxetine or behavior therapy. With either intervention, responders showed normalized caudate metabolism (Baxter et al. 1992). In a group of patients with childhood-onset OCD, successful treatment was associated with normalization of metabolism in the orbitofrontal cortex (Swedo et al. 1992).

In one of the earliest fMRI studies of this disorder, symptom provocation was used to induce pathological activity in patients with OCD. Abnormally increased brain activity was found in the orbitofrontal cortex and in the anterior cingulate, anterior temporal, and insular regions (Breiter et al. 1996). A further symptom-provocation study was done using PET to examine rCBF in three different anxiety disorders (OCD, simple phobia, and posttraumatic stress disorder). In compiling the results of this evaluation, the researchers looked at pooled data from all three diagnoses and again found increased orbitofrontal and insular activity. However, they also found increased rCBF in the striatum and brain stem, and the brain stem foci correlated with subjective anxiety scores (Rauch et al. 1997).

Gilles de la Tourette Syndrome

Tourette syndrome is defined by intrusive, impulsive motor acts, including tics and vocalizations. The association between Tourette syndrome and OCD is well established. The two have a high comorbidity and may result from the same genetic basis.

SPECT scans were performed at rest on 50 patients with Tourette syndrome, who were compared with healthy participants. Patients showed reduced perfusion in the left caudate nucleus, anterior cingulate cortex, and left dorsolateral prefrontal cortex, although the latter hypoperfusion was likely associated with depression (Moriarty et al. 1995). In this initial study, the neural circuits that are abnormal in Tourette syndrome are those involved in the initiation, continuation, and inhibition of actions, similar to findings in OCD. Another study performed in twins discordant for severity of Tourette syndrome symptoms found that there was a high correlation between a symptom index and the degree of $[^{123}I]$3-iodo-6-methoxybenzamine (IBZM) binding in the head of the caudate nucleus (Wolf et al. 1996). This indicated that the quantity of dopamine type 2 (D_2) receptor binding in the head of the caudate nucleus may be related to the severity of Tourette syndrome.

Within this group of studies, there are inconsistencies. Not every research group finds altered metabolism or perfusion in the same brain region. Such inconsistencies are perhaps not surprising in that these groups use different scanning methods with different spatial resolution. In addition, some groups have participants rest with eyes open, others with eyes closed; some groups have participants performing a sustained-attention task. Also, for the before-and-after-treatment studies, OCD patients were studied while taking different medications and after treatments that ranged in duration from 10 weeks to 1 year. These differences, too, could significantly affect the functional neuroimaging results (Insel 1992). What is remarkable is the consistency with which specific cortico-basal ganglia-thalamo-cortical circuits are implicated, particularly those involving the orbitofrontal, cingulate, and prefrontal cortices and the caudate nucleus.

Mood Disorders

Mood disorders are particularly heterogeneous. Mood states encompass a wide range of severity and may or may not include psychosis. Some patients experience significant cognitive impairment, whereas others do not. Some patients do not respond to intervention; others experience discrete episodes of illness and return to premorbid functioning after treatment. The etiologic bases for these different types of illness may be varied and likely involve both genetic vulnerability and responses to difficult life events.

Coupled with the heterogeneity of the illnesses is the variability in patient populations recruited, length and stage of illness, number of patients in a given study, medication state, imaging technique, imaging state (resting vs. performing a task), and method of data analysis. Some studies have taken the approach of looking at mood disorders across diagnostic categories to search for common abnormalities. Others examine not just a specific illness but a subset of patients within that illness, for example, unmedicated patients with major depressive disorder, acute onset, without cognitive deficits. Both approaches provide useful information about brain regions related to pathological mood states.

Despite these many variables, there is some consensus about the cerebral basis of mood disorders. There have been several reviews of the functional imaging findings in mood disorders (Drevets 1998, 1999; Soares and Mann 1997). There seems to be an underlying network of regions implicated in most studies of depressed patients. Although this network is almost always involved, the actual regions and the direction of change in a given region vary based on several factors. This network includes the medial prefrontal cortex, orbitofrontal cortex, perigenual cingulate cortex, posterior cingulate cortex, amygdala, and extended amygdala. Of note, this same network of cortical and subcortical regions is involved in many anxiety disorders. Furthermore, another network that is active in executive functioning includes the dorsolateral prefrontal cortex; this network is frequently involved in mood disorders.

When unipolar depressed patients with similar severity of depressive symptoms were compared based on the presence or absence of pseudodementia, patients with cognitive impairment showed reduced flow in the left medial prefrontal cortex and increased flow in the cerebellum. Compared with healthy control subjects, depressed patients showed decreased flow in the dorsolateral prefrontal cortex, left anterior cingulate cortex, and right insula (Dolan et al. 1992).

Likewise, specific symptom complexes are associated with blood flow patterns. Psychomotor agitation was associated with increased flow in the posterior cingulate and inferior parietal cortices. Psychomotor retardation and mood disturbance were correlated with decreased flow in the left dorsolateral prefrontal cortex and left angular gyrus. Decreased blood flow in the medial prefrontal cortex was associated with increasing cognitive impairment (Bench et al. 1993), and decreased metabolism in the nearby subgenual anterior cingulate cortex has been related to familial mood disorders, both unipolar and bipolar (Drevets et al. 1997).

The involvement of the frontal cortex in depression is strengthened by a study in which 10 unipolar depressed patients were imaged using resting FDG PET before and after treatment. Improved mood was associated with increases in metabolism in the prefrontal and anterior cingulate cortices (Mayberg et al. 1997). A follow-up study showed that nondepressed patients with provoked dysphoric mood and depressed patients recovered from depression had inverse relationships with brain activity in the subgenual anterior cingulate and dorsolateral prefrontal cortices (Mayberg et al. 1999).

Regional differences between depressed and nondepressed participants included decreased [^{99m}Tc]HMPAO uptake in bilateral orbitofrontal, inferotemporal, and parietal areas (Lesser et al. 1994). A PET comparison between predominantly unipolar depressed patients and healthy volunteers showed that the depressed group had decreased flow in specific brain regions, including the left dorsolateral prefrontal cortex, the left angular gyrus, and the left anterior cingulate gyrus; increased flow was found in the left posterior cingulate gyrus (Bench et al. 1993). A [^{99m}Tc]HMPAO resting SPECT study found hypoperfusion in the inferior frontal, anterior temporal, and anterior cingulate cortices in patients with refractory depression (Mayberg et al. 1994).

Not all studies find reductions in frontal blood flow or metabolism. In fact, many studies show relative increases in flow in the ventral and medial orbitofrontal regions of patients with acute untreated, unmedicated major depression, coupled with changes in activity in the dorsolateral prefrontal cortex. The majority of studies examining this illness report changes either bilaterally or localized to the left side. Using (^{15}O)water PET, it was shown that depressed patients had increased left ventrolateral frontal blood flow and increased blood flow in the left amygdala (Drevets et al. 1992). Interestingly, patients in remission showed normalized frontal flow but continued elevations in the amygdala (Drevets et al. 1992), indicating possible state versus trait differences. FDG PET likewise found increased metabolism in the orbitofrontal lobes, along with decreased metabolism in the dorsolateral frontal and parietal cortices of unipolar depressed patients (Biver et al. 1994). This study suggests that distinct regions of frontal cortex may play different roles in depression.

Furthermore, an fMRI study of depressed patients and nondepressed control subjects measured brain activity in a task viewing sadness-laden film clips (Beauregard et al. 1998). Patients with depression had significantly greater activity in the left medial prefrontal cortex and right cingulate gyrus than did control subjects. Another report of pathology in this same network came from an examination of regional perfusion using PET. Depressed patients were compared with healthy control subjects in a study examining flow changes in response to performance feedback on a task. Unlike the nondepressed subjects, the depressed patients did not activate the ventromedial orbitofrontal cortex and medial caudate nucleus (Elliott et al. 1998).

There has also been recent work on receptor activity and function in depression. Both the serotonin receptor and transporter have been studied. The 5-hydroxytryptamine (serotonin) type 1A (5-HT$_{1A}$) receptor has been of interest to psychiatrists, as modulation of this presynaptic autoreceptor may play a role in both anxiolytic and antidepressant efficacy. A study that examined this receptor in depressed patients found significantly decreased binding potential for the PET radioligand [^{11}C]WAY-100635 in both regions examined (dorsal raphe, mesiotemporal cortex). However, more widespread decreases were thought to be present, as post hoc examination revealed decreased binding potential in other regions as well (Drevets et al. 1999). Another study did look at the 5-HT$_{1A}$ receptor across the entire brain, and indeed found significantly decreased binding potential (Sargent et al. 2000).

This study also examined the effect of antidepressant treatment and, surprisingly, found no difference in binding potential between patients treated with antidepressant (paroxetine) and those who were not treated. Furthermore, the study found no difference between those who responded to treatment and those who did not.

An evaluation of the brain stem serotonin transporter was carried out with $[^{123}I]2\beta$-carbomethoxy-3β-(4-iodophenyl)tropane, a cocaine analog with specific binding to the serotonin and dopamine transporters (Malison et al. 1998). Because there appear to be no dopamine transporters in the brain stem, this radioligand was used to study the serotonin reuptake pump in this region. Decreased specific binding of the radioligand to the serotonin transporter was found in the brain stem, indicating likely decreased numbers of receptors there. The serotonin type 2 (5-HT_2) receptor has also been examined with PET. $[^{18}F]$setoperone was used to examine this receptor in patients with depression before treatment and 3 weeks after treatment with a tricyclic antidepressant (Attar-Levy et al. 1999). These researchers found a trend toward lower specific binding in untreated depressed patients compared with control subjects. Specific binding also decreased with antidepressant treatment, coincident with binding of the receptor by the antidepressant and/or modulation.

Bipolar Disorder

Patients in the manic phase of bipolar disorder are often difficult to study due to their illness, and thus there are only a few examinations of patients in this state. However, those that report on this disorder also find pathological activity in many of the same regions found in unipolar depression. Two recent PET studies examined regional cerebral perfusion in three groups of subjects: medicated patients with bipolar mania, medicated euthymic patients with bipolar disorder, and healthy control subjects. The researchers examined activity across these three groups during the resting state and during a word-generation task (word generation minus word repetition) (Blumberg et al. 1999, 2000). During the word-generation task, the researchers found decreased activity in the right prefrontal cortex of the manic patients compared with either the euthymic patients or control subjects. In addition, manic patients compared with euthymic patients at rest had decreased activity in the right posterior orbitofrontal cortex and decreased activity in the left ventromedial prefrontal cortex compared with the psychiatrically healthy subjects. In the manic patients compared with euthymic patients, increased activity was found in the left caudate nucleus and left dorsal anterior cingulate gyrus, with trends to increased activity in the right dorsal and ventral anterior cingulate gyrus. Another examination of patients with familial mood disorders (either unipolar or bipolar) found decreased subgenual anterior cingulate activity, regardless of the mood state (Drevets et al. 1997). Medicated patients with stable bipolar disorder who were withdrawn from lithium treatment and then became manic developed relative increases in the dorsal anterior cingulate gyrus and the left orbitofrontal cortex (Goodwin et al. 1997).

In summary, mood disorders appear to be associated with changes in specific networks involving prefrontal cortical and limbic regions. The specific regions affected may be linked to specific clinical symptoms. Different regions or subsections of the affected networks are likely involved in different diagnoses and/or stages of the illness. Interestingly, inducing transient sadness in healthy volunteers increases blood flow to orbitofrontal regions, areas that show flow decreases in some depressed patients and flow increases in others. This further implicates the orbitofrontal cortex as being an integral part of a network that controls mood.

Schizophrenia

Functional neuroimaging studies in schizophrenia are arguably the most advanced in neuropsychiatry. These techniques are used to explore many aspects of the illness, including schizophrenia subtypes, response to antipsychotic treatment, neurotransmitter systems involved, cognitive networks affected, symptom-related pathology, and others. What appears likely is that schizophrenia is not caused by dysfunction in one brain area. Rather, there is abnormal modulation of, and/or abnormal activity in, the networks linking subcortical regions, the cerebellum, and frontal, parietal, and temporal cortices.

The Dopamine Hypothesis

Functional neuroimaging allows direct and indirect tests of hypotheses about the etiology of schizophrenia. PET is particularly well suited to obtaining images that show the distribution and density of dopamine and other receptors. The dopamine hypothesis of schizophrenia maintains that the illness results from an abnormality of the brain dopaminergic system. This is suggested because all antipsychotic medications have the ability to block D_2 receptors, and their efficacy as antipsychotics is typically correlated with the degree of D_2 blockade, at least with the typical antipsychotics. This has been directly investigated using PET and dopaminergic ligands in many studies.

Although a twofold to threefold increase in D_2 receptor density in the striatum has been reported in neuroleptic-naïve schizophrenic patients (Wong et al. 1986), this finding has not been replicated in several

studies in which normal densities of D_2 receptors were found in schizophrenic patients (Farde et al. 1987, 1990; Nordstrom et al. 1995). A more recent study was done after a 3-week medication washout in patients classified as treatment nonresponders and in treatment-responsive patients. The cerebral metabolic response induced by a single dose of antipsychotic medication distinguished between treatment responders and nonresponders (Bartlett et al. 1998). Kapur and others examined this issue as well, using $[^{11}C]$raclopride as a probe of D_2 receptor occupancy (Kapur et al. 2000a). Patients with schizophrenia were given either 1.0 or 2.5 mg of haloperidol in a double-blind fashion, and measurements were taken 2 weeks later. The relationship between occupancy at the D_2 receptor and clinical response, extrapyramidal side effects, and prolactin levels in 22 patients with first-episode schizophrenia was examined. The patients showed a wide range of D_2 receptor occupancy, from 38% to 87%. However, the magnitude of receptor binding was directly related to clinical response, side effects, and serum prolactin levels. A clinical response was found when receptor occupancy was greater than 65%, but extrapyramidal side effects were not apparent until 78% occupancy. Hyperprolactinemia was intermediate between these two levels, associated with 72% occupancy. Given the wide range in variability in D_2 receptor binding and this narrow therapeutic window, this PET study demonstrates the difficulty in optimal titration of haloperidol dose across a patient population. This may not be true for the newer atypical antipsychotics, however. One SPECT study using $[^{123}I]$IBZM examined dopamine receptor binding in the presence of either a low dose (5 mg) or a high dose (20 mg) of olanzapine. The researchers found significant differences in D_2 binding at the two doses, but no clinically significant differences in ratings, symptoms, or extrapyramidal symptoms (Raedler et al. 1999). Quetiapine, on the other hand, had markedly different patterns of D_2 blockade. Using $[^{11}C]$raclopride as a measure of D_2 binding, quetiapine was found to cause transient blockade of the D_2 receptor 2–3 hours after administration, at levels up to approximately 60%, that would then slowly decrease over time (Kapur et al. 2000b).

In summary, it appears likely from all these reports that dopamine plays a central role in schizophrenia. Radioligand studies like the ones reviewed here are helping to shed light on clinically relevant questions regarding this disorder.

Cognitive Dysmetria

One recent model of schizophrenia attempts to unify rather than divide the disorder based on varied presentations and is founded on the common thread that all individuals with schizophrenia have cognitive deficits. This model implicates cerebellar abnormalities in schizophrenia and is consistent with increasing information about the role of the cerebellum in cognitive function. The idea of "cognitive" dysmetria posits that cerebellar dysfunction is involved in the schizophrenic patient's uncoordinated thought processes, similar to the uncoordinated motor deficits seen with lesions in motor-related portions of the cerebellum (Andreasen et al. 1999). There have been multiple recent studies that indicate the cerebellum is involved in the pathophysiology of schizophrenia. Functional MRI using an injected contrast agent showed increased cerebellar blood flow in persons with schizophrenia, and lower than normal flow in patients with bipolar disorder (Loeber et al. 1999).

Studies Performed Using Cognitive Tasks

By imaging participants during the performance of tasks, cerebral activity patterns reflect a state with less variability due to random, task-independent thought processes. Schizophrenic individuals invariably show dysfunction within frontal-parietal-temporal networks, regardless of the task used.

Attention. In a group of 79 medication-free schizophrenic patients, FDG PET was done during a continuous-performance test. The PET results were then compared with clinical symptoms. Patients with reality distortion and patients with negative symptoms had decreased activity in the anterior cingulum/mesial frontal area. Negative symptoms were associated with hyperfrontality (Schroder et al. 1995).

In another PET study done using (^{15}O)water, performance on a single-trial Stroop task was used to measure attention in 14 patients compared with 15 healthy subjects. The researchers found that patients with schizophrenia (chronic, stable, medicated) made more errors and had less activation in the right anterior cingulate gyrus during color naming in the color-incongruent part of the task (Carter et al. 1997). This was consistent with their hypothesis of deficits of attention in schizophrenic patients, as well as the many other studies that find pathophysiology in this subsystem.

Memory. Unmedicated schizophrenic patients were compared with matched healthy volunteers during ^{133}Xe SPECT while performing verbal and facial recognition tasks. Although the control subjects showed areas of specific regional activation during both tasks, patients with schizophrenia showed diffuse increases in the task. During the facial task, control subjects showed activation in the frontal pole and in the precentral, postcentral, and anterior temporal regions; during the verbal task, control subjects had increased blood flow in the dorsolateral prefrontal, premotor, precentral, and postcentral regions (Gur et al. 1994). Patients did not activate as much as control subjects and showed activation in different brain regions, namely the left frontal pole and the anterior temporal and occipital temporal regions.

A recent study of memory retrieval examined three sets of subjects: control subjects, schizophrenic individuals with the deficit syndrome, and schizophrenic individuals without the deficit syndrome (Heckers et al. 1999). They found that patients with primary negative symptoms recruited hippocampal regions equally as well as patients without deficit symptoms. The difference was found in bilateral regions of the prefrontal cortex, where there was significantly less activity in schizophrenic patients with deficit syndrome, consistent with many of the previous studies that found decreased prefrontal cortex activity with this disorder. It is interesting to note here that, despite the difference in prefrontal rCBF, performance in the recall task was not different between the deficit and nondeficit subtypes of schizophrenia.

Language. During a PET cerebral blood flow study, healthy control subjects and schizophrenic patients were imaged during verbal tasks. In one task, words beginning with a certain letter (e.g., *A*, apple) were generated by the participant every 5 seconds; in another, given words were simply repeated. From work with healthy control subjects during word generation, activation was expected in the dorsolateral prefrontal cortex, cingulate cortex, and superior temporal cortex. Schizophrenic patients showed activation in the same areas as the control subjects; however, they may have needed to activate a greater region of the dorsolateral prefrontal cortex to perform the task and did not show the expected decrease in the superior temporal cortex (Frith et al. 1995). This supports the idea that the neural networks linking the frontal and temporal cortices function abnormally in schizophrenia.

Executive function. Executive functions include assessment of the environment, planning behavior, and generating novel responses, areas of particular difficulty for schizophrenic individuals. The Wisconsin Card Sorting Test (WCST) is an abstract reasoning test that taps executive functions. In it, a card is matched to one of four possible choices; participants must decide whether to match on color, object shape, or number of objects on the card. They must remember which responses are correct and periodically alter which aspect of the card is the right response. When newly diagnosed patients with schizophrenia or schizophreniform disorder were compared with healthy volunteers using [^{99m}Tc]HMPAO SPECT, they activated a neural network including the frontal, parietal, and temporal cortices. To underscore the advantage of imaging during a task, no perfusion differences were seen at rest (Rubin et al. 1991). Conversely, in an fMRI working memory task (Sternberg Item Recognition Paradigm), schizophrenic patients showed greater activation in the left dorsolateral prefrontal cortex than did a group of healthy control subjects, despite worse performance on the task per se (Manoach et al. 1999). Further examination by the same group revealed striatal activation only in the patients, indicating possible frontostriatal dysfunction (Manoach et al. 2000).

Importantly, it does not appear to be an abstract task per se that results in abnormal blood flow patterns. Rather, it appears to be dependent on which neural network is involved in the task. A different abstract reasoning task, the Ravens

Progressive Matrices (RPM), requires participants to complete missing parts of abstract designs. Using ^{133}Xe SPECT, healthy volunteers showed increased blood flow primarily to posterior cortical areas, including parietal and parieto-occipital cortices. The same pattern was seen in medication-free chronic schizophrenic patients (Berman et al. 1988).

Additional work in schizophrenic individuals performing a working memory task evaluated changes in brain activity related to switching from classic to atypical antipsychotic medication (Honey et al. 2000). This fMRI study found increased prefrontal and parietal cortical activation in patients taking risperidone on a verbal working memory task compared with a group of patients taking classic antipsychotics, consistent with less mesocortical D_2 blockade with this drug.

MRS in Schizophrenia

MRS provides information about the chemical composition of brain areas with functional abnormalities in schizophrenia. ^{31}P MRS has been used to investigate membrane components and high-energy phosphate compounds in the left dorsolateral prefrontal cortex of drug-naïve patients with first-episode schizophrenia, patients with chronic schizophrenia, and healthy control subjects. All patients with schizophrenia, whether acute, drug-naïve, or chronic, showed decreased levels of phosphomonoesters, building blocks for cell membranes. First-episode, drug-naïve schizophrenic patients had increased levels of phosphodiesters, membrane breakdown products (Pettegrew et al. 1991), which were not found in newly diagnosed medicated or long-term medicated patients (Stanley et al. 1995). It appears that membrane breakdown products are increased early in the course of schizophrenia, whereas membrane precursors are reduced throughout the illness (Pette-

grew et al. 1993; Stanley et al. 1995). This leads to speculation that schizophrenia involves an exaggeration of normal dendritic remodeling and pruning (Maier 1995). However, other groups have reported increased phosphodiesters even in chronic patients and have not replicated the reduction in phosphomonoesters (Deicken et al. 1994).

Using ^{1}H MRS, abnormalities were found in the ratio of NAA, a marker of neuronal integrity to either creatine or choline in chronic schizophrenic patients. ROIs were drawn in multiple brain regions, but only in the mesial temporal lobe and dorsolateral prefrontal cortices did patients show reduced NAA (Bertolino et al. 1995). This has been replicated in both temporal lobes in patients with schizophrenia and in a mixed group of bipolar and schizophrenic patients (Renshaw et al. 1995; Yurgelun-Todd et al. 1993). This fits well with PET and SPECT results finding abnormalities in the neural networks linking the frontal, parietal, and temporal lobes. However, as with many of these techniques, there are inconsistencies. One study investigated the left frontal and temporal lobes of a mixed group of patients with first-episode and chronic schizophrenia; differences in NAA were found only in the left frontal lobes of male patients (Buckley et al. 1994). A recent study involving a cognitive-activation task in schizophrenic patients discovered a strong correlation between dorsolateral prefrontal NAA and activation of the cortical network involved in working memory (Figure 4–1) (Bertolino et al. 2000). Further work with this technique in the dorsolateral prefrontal cortex has found that patients with the deficit syndrome of schizophrenia have lower NAA in this region than do other patients or control subjects (Delamillieure et al. 2000). Another study looking only at the thalamus found significantly

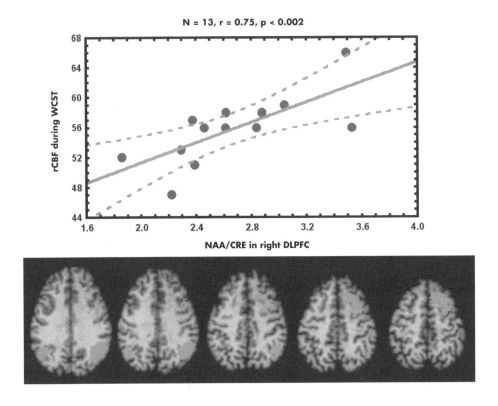

FIGURE 4–1. Correlations between metabolite ratios for the dorsolateral prefrontal cortex (DLPFC) of 13 schizophrenic patients and blood flow activation during performance of the Wisconsin Card Sorting Test (WCST).

The bottom part of the figure shows the brain locations of maximal positive correlations between blood flow activation during the WCST and the ratio of N-acetyl aspartate to creatine (NAA/CRE). The top portion shows the correlations between NAA/CRE and regional cerebral blood flow (rCBF) in the DLPFC.

For a color version of this figure, please see the color insert at the back of this book.

Source.   Reprinted with permission from Bertolino A, Esposito G, Callicott JH, et al.: "Specific Relationship Between Prefrontal Neuronal N-Acetylaspartate and Activation of the Working Memory Cortical Network in Schizophrenia." *American Journal of Psychiatry* 157:26–33, 2000.

decreased NAA bilaterally in patients with schizophrenia (Deicken et al. 2000). In summary, these MRS studies of schizophrenia are consistent with brain areas implicated in schizophrenia, both from postmortem and other in vivo imaging studies.

White Matter Integrity: Diffusion Tensor Imaging

New technological advances in MRI make it possible to study white matter tracts with MRI. By studying the diffusion

anisotropy in water around white matter, these tracts can be traced. There have been several studies in schizophrenic individuals indicating that white matter regions of the brain are pathological. A study looked at this property of white matter in a group of five patients with schizophrenia and also in six control subjects (Buchsbaum et al. 1998). The researchers studied the prefrontal cortex and striatum using PET and found that the patients had less correlation between metabolic rates in the two regions than the control subjects, indicating less connectivity. Indeed, the white matter tracts connecting the two regions also had significantly lower diffusion anisotropy, agreeing with the PET findings, supplying twofold evidence for decreased connectivity between the striatum and prefrontal cortex. Another study used magnetization transfer imaging as an indicator of myelin and axonal integrity (Foong et al. 2000). In this study, white matter abnormalities were found in the temporal lobes of patients with schizophrenia. In contrast to these two studies, an evaluation of white matter integrity using diffusion tensor imaging found widespread differences in a group of schizophrenic patients (Lim et al. 1999).

Conclusions

The various functional neuroimaging modalities make possible the study of the activity of the living human brain. With these techniques, we are able to determine the neural networks underlying the psychiatric illnesses that afflict our patients and families. The future holds great promise for this field and provides an open door to investigate the neurobiological bases for these disorders, disease and symptom heterogeneity, and treatment responsiveness. Many of these studies are going on now, and the mysteries of the mind and brain's function may someday be understood with much more clarity.

References

Alexander GE, DeLong MR, Strick PL: Parallel organization of functionally segregated circuits linking basal ganglia and cortex. Annu Rev Neurosci 9:357–381, 1986

Andreasen NC, O'Leary DX, Cizadlo T, et al: Remembering the past: two facets of episodic memory explored with positron emission tomography. Am J Psychiatry 152:1576–1585, 1995

Andreasen NC, Nopoulos P, O'Leary DS, et al: Defining the phenotype of schizophrenia: cognitive dysmetria and its neural mechanisms. Biol Psychiatry 46:908–920, 1999

Asahina M, Suhara T, Shinotoh H, et al: Brain muscarinic receptors in progressive supranuclear palsy and Parkinson's disease: a positron emission tomographic study. J Neurol Neurosurg Psychiatry 65:155–163, 1998

Attar-Levy D, Martinot JL, Blin J, et al: The cortical serotonin2 receptors studied with positron-emission tomography and [18F]-setoperone during depressive illness and antidepressant treatment with clomipramine. Biol Psychiatry 45(2):180–186, 1999

Bartlett EJ, Brodie JD, Simkowitz P, et al: Effect of a haloperidol challenge on regional brain metabolism in neuroleptic-responsive and nonresponsive schizophrenic patients. Am J Psychiatry 155:337–343, 1998

Baxter LR Jr, Phelps ME, Mazziotta JC, et al: Local cerebral glucose metabolism rates in obsessive-compulsive disorder. Arch Gen Psychiatry 44:211–218, 1987

Baxter LR Jr, Schwartz JM, Mazziotta JC, et al: Cerebral glucose metabolic rates in nondepressed patients with obsessive-compulsive disorder. Am J Psychiatry 145: 1560–1563, 1988

Baxter LR Jr, Schwartz JM, Bergman KS, et al: Caudate glucose metabolic rate changes with both drug and behavior therapy for obsessive-compulsive disorder. Arch Gen Psychiatry 49:681–689, 1992

Beauregard M, Leroux JM, Bergman S, et al: The functional neuroanatomy of major depression: an fMRI study using an emotional activation paradigm. Neuroreport 9:3253–3258, 1998

Bench CJ, Friston KJ, Brown RG, et al: Regional cerebral blood flow in depression measured by positron emission tomography: the relationship with clinical dimensions. Psychol Med 23:579–590, 1993

Benkelfat C, Thomas TE, Semple WE, et al: Local cerebral glucose metabolic rates in obsessive-compulsive disorder. Arch Gen Psychiatry 47:840–848, 1990

Berman KF, Weinberger DR: Functional localization in the brain schizophrenia, in American Psychiatric Press Review of Psychiatry, Vol 10. Edited by Tasman A, Goldfinger SM. Washington, DC, American Psychiatric Press, 1991, pp 24–59

Berman KF, Illowsky BP, Weinberger DR: Physiological dysfunction of dorsolateral prefrontal cortex in schizophrenia, IV: further evidence for regional and behavioral specificity. Arch Gen Psychiatry 45: 616–622, 1988

Bertolino A, Nawroz S, Mattay VS, et al: Multislice proton magnetic resonance spectroscopic imaging in schizophrenia: regional reduction of a marker of neuronal density (abstract). Abstr Soc Neurosci 21: 260, 1995

Bertolino A, Esposito G, Callicott JH, et al: Specific relationship between prefrontal neuronal N-acetylaspartate and activation of the working memory cortical network in schizophrenia. Am J Psychiatry 157:26–33, 2000

Binder JR, Frost JA, Hammeke TS, et al: Conceptual processing during the conscious resting state: a functional MRI study. J Cogn Neurosci 11(1):80–93, 1999

Bisaga A, Katz JL, Antonini A, et al: Cerebral glucose metabolism in women with panic disorder. Am J Psychiatry 155:1178–1183, 1998

Biver F, Goldman S, Delvenne V, et al: Frontal and parietal metabolic disturbances in unipolar depression. Biol Psychiatry 36: 381–388, 1994

Blackwood DH, Glabus MF, Dunan J, et al: Altered cerebral perfusion measured by SPECT in relatives of patients with schizophrenia. Correlations with memory and P300. Br J Psychiatry 175:357–366, 1999

Blin J, Sette G, Fiorelli M, et al: A method for the in vivo investigation of the serotonergic 5-HT2 receptors in the human cerebral cortex using positron emission tomography and 18F-labeled setoperone. J Neurochem 54:1744–1754, 1990

Blumberg HP, Stern E, Ricketts S, et al: Rostral and orbital prefrontal cortex dysfunction in the manic state of bipolar disorder. Am J Psychiatry 156:1986–1988, 1999

Blumberg HP, Stern E, Martinez D, et al: Increased anterior cingulate and caudate activity in bipolar mania. Biol Psychiatry 48(11):1045–1052, 2000

Breiter HC, Rauch SL, Kwong KK, et al: Functional magnetic resonance imaging of symptom provocation in obsessive-compulsive disorder. Arch Gen Psychiatry 53:595–606, 1996

Buchsbaum MS, Tang CY, Peled S, et al: MRI white matter diffusion anisotropy and PET metabolic rate in schizophrenia. Neuroreport 9:425–430, 1998

Buckley PF, Moore C, Long H, et al: ^{1}H-Magnetic resonance spectroscopy of the left temporal and frontal lobes in schizophrenia: clinical, neurodevelopmental, and cognitive correlates. Biol Psychiatry 36: 792–800, 1994

Bush G, Frazier JA, Rauch SL, et al: Anterior cingulate cortex dysfunction in attention-deficit/hyperactivity disorder revealed by fMRI and the Counting Stroop. Biol Psych 45:1542–1552, 1999

Carter CS, Mintun M, Nichols T, et al: Anterior cingulate gyrus dysfunction and selective attention deficits in schizophrenia: [^{15}O]H$_2$O PET study during single-trial Stroop task performance. Am J Psychiatry 154:1670–1675, 1997

Chugani DC, Muzik O, Rothermel R, et al: Altered serotonin synthesis in the dentatothalamocortical pathway in autistic boys. Ann Neurol 42:666–669, 1997

Chugani DC, Sundram BS, Behen M, et al: Evidence of altered energy metabolism in autistic children. Prog Neuropsychopharmacol Biol Psychiatry 23:635–641, 1999

Cohen RM, Andreason PJ, Doudet DJ, et al: Opiate receptor avidity and cerebral blood flow in Alzheimer's disease. J Neurol Sci 148:171–180, 1997

Critchley HD, Daly EM, Bullmore ET, et al: The functional neuroanatomy of social behavior: changes in cerebral blood flow when people with autistic disorder process facial expressions. Brain 123:2203–2212, 2000

Crouzel C, Guillaume M, Barre L, et al: Ligands and tracers for PET studies of the 5-HT system—current status. Int J Rad Appl Instrum B 19: 857–870, 1992

Cumming P, Yokoi F, Chen A, et al: Pharmacokinetics of radiotracers in human plasma during positron emission tomography. Synapse 34:124–134, 1999

Dager SR, Strauss WL, Marro KI, et al: Proton magnetic resonance spectroscopy investigation of hyperventilation in subjects with panic disorder and comparison subjects. Am J Psychiatry 152:666–672, 1995

Deicken RF, Calabrese G, Merrin EL, et al: ^{31}Phosphorus magnetic resonance spectroscopy of the frontal and parietal lobes in chronic schizophrenia. Biol Psychiatry 36:503–510, 1994

Deicken RF, Johnson C, Eliaz Y, et al: Reduced concentrations of thalamic N-acetylaspartate in male patients with schizophrenia. Am J Psychiatry 157:644–647, 2000

Delamillieure P, Fernandez J, Constans JM, et al: Proton magnetic resonance spectroscopy of the medial prefrontal cortex in patients with deficit schizophrenia: preliminary report. Am J Psychiatry 157:641–643, 2000

De Volder A, Bol A, Michel C, et al: Brain glucose metabolism in children with the autistic syndrome: positron tomography analysis. Brain Dev 9:581–587, 1987

Dolan RJ, Bench CJ, Brown RG, et al: Regional cerebral blood flow abnormalities in depressed patients with cognitive impairment. J Neurol Neurosurg Psychiatry 55:768–773, 1992

Dougherty DD, Bonab AA, Spencer TJ, et al: Dopamine transporter density in patients with attention deficit hyperactivity disorder. Lancet 354:2132–2133, 1999

Drevets WC: Functional neuroimaging studies of depression: the anatomy of melancholia. Annu Rev Med 49:341–361, 1998

Drevets WC: Prefrontal cortical-amygdalar metabolism in major depression. Ann N Y Acad Sci 877:614–637, 1999

Drevets WC, Videen TO, Price JL, et al: A functional anatomical study of unipolar depression. J Neurosci 12:3628–3641, 1992

Drevets WC, Price JL, Simpson JR, et al: Subgenual prefrontal cortex abnormalities in mood disorders. Nature 386:824–827, 1997

Drevets WC, Frank E, Price JC, et al: PET imaging of serotonin 1A receptor binding in depression. Biol Psychiatry 46(10): 1375–1387, 1999

Elliott R, Sahakian BJ, Michael A, et al: Abnormal neural response to feedback on planning and guessing tasks in patients with unipolar depression. Psychol Med 28:559–571, 1998

Ernst M, Zametkin AJ, Matochik JA, et al: High midbrain [18F]DOPA accumulation in children with attention deficit hyperactivity disorder. Am J Psychiatry 156:1209–1215, 1999

Farde L, Wiesel F, Hall H, et al: No D$_2$ receptor increase in PET study of schizophrenia. Arch Gen Psychiatry 44:671–672, 1987

Farde L, Wiesel F-A, Stone-Elander S, et al: D$_2$ dopamine receptors in neuroleptic-naive schizophrenic patients. Arch Gen Psychiatry 47:213–219, 1990

Farde L, Suhara T, Halldin C, et al: PET study of the M1-agonists [11C]xanomeline and [11C]butylthio-TZTP in monkey and man. Dementia 7:187–195, 1996

Farde L, Suhara T, Nyberg S, et al: A PET-study of [11C]FLB 457 binding to extrastriatal D$_2$-dopamine receptors in healthy subjects and antipsychotic drug-treated patients. Psychopharmacology 133:396–404, 1997

Foong J, Maier M, Barker GJ, et al: In vivo investigation of white matter pathology in schizophrenia with magnetisation transfer imaging. J Neurol Neurosurg Psychiatry 68: 70–74, 2000

Fox PT, Raichle ME, Mintun MA, et al: Nonoxidative glucose consumption during focal physiologic neural activity. Science 241:462–464, 1988

Friston KJ, Holmes A, Poline J-B, et al: Detecting activations in PET and fMRI: levels of inference and power. Neuroimage 4:223–235, 1995

Frith CD, Friston KJ, Herold S, et al: Regional brain activity in chronic schizophrenic patients during the performance of a verbal fluency task. Br J Psychiatry 167:343–349, 1995

Frost JJ, Wagner HN, Dannals RF, et al: Imaging opiate receptors in the human brain by positron tomography. J Comput Assist Tomogr 9:231–236, 1985

Gao JH, Parsons LM, Bower JM, et al: Cerebellum implicated in sensory acquisition rather than motor control. Science 272:545–547, 1996

George MS, Costa DC, Kouris K, et al: Cerebral blood flow abnormalities in adults with infantile autism. J Nerv Ment Dis 180:413–417, 1992

George MS, Ketter TA, Kimbrell TA, et al: What functional imaging has revealed about the brain basis of mood and emotion, in Advances in Biological Psychiatry, Vol 2. Edited by Panksepp J. Greenwich, CT, JAI Press, 1996, pp 63–113

Goddard AW, Charney DS: Toward an integrated neurobiology of panic disorder. J Clin Psychiatry 58 (suppl 2):4 –11, 1997

Goodwin GM, Cavanagh JTO, Glabus MF, et al: Uptake of 99mTc-exametazime shown by single photon emission computed tomography before and after lithium withdrawal in bipolar patients: associations with mania. Br J Psychiatry 170:426–430, 1997

Gur RE, Jaggi JL, Shtasel DL, et al: Cerebral blood flow in schizophrenia: effects of memory processing on regional activation. Biol Psychiatry 35:3–15, 1994

Halldin C, Foged C, Chou YH, et al: Carbon-11-NNC 112: a radioligand for PET examination of striatal and neocortical D1-dopamine receptors. J Nucl Med 39: 2061–2068, 1998

Hashimoto T, Sasaki M, Fukumizu M, et al: Single-photon emission computed tomography of the brain in autism: effect of the developmental level. Pediatr Neurol 23:416–420, 2000

Haznedar MM, Buchsbaum MS, Metzger M, et al: Anterior cingulated gyrus volume and glucose metabolism in autistic disorder. Am J Psychiatry 154:1047–1050, 1997

Heckers S, Goff D, Schacter DL, et al: Functional imaging of memory retrieval in deficit vs nondeficit schizophrenia. Arch Gen Psychiatry 56:1117–1123, 1999

Henry JP, Scherman D: Radioligands of the vesicular monoamine transporter and their use as markers of monoamine storage vesicles. Biochem Pharmacol 38:2395–2404, 1989

Herold S, Frackowiak RSJ, LeCouteur A, et al: Cerebral blood flow and metabolism of oxygen and glucose in young autistic adults. Psychol Med 18:823–831, 1988

Hoehn-Saric R, Pearlson GD, Harris GJ, et al: Effects of fluoxetine on regional cerebral blood flow in obsessive-compulsive patients. Am J Psychiatry 148:1243–1245, 1991

Honey GD, Bullmore ET, Soni W, et al: Differences in frontal cortical activation by a working memory task after substitution of risperidone for typical antipsychotic drugs in patients with schizophrenia. Proc Natl Acad Sci U S A 96:13432–13437, 2000

Horwitz B, Rumsey JM, Grady CL, et al: The cerebral metabolic landscape in autism: intercorrelations of regional glucose utilization. Arch Neurol 45:749–755, 1988

Houle S, Wilson AA, Inaba T, et al: Imaging 5-HT1A receptors with positron emission tomography: initial human studies with [11C]CPC-222. Nucl Med Commun 18:1130–1134, 1997

Insel TR: Toward a neuroanatomy of obsessive-compulsive disorder. Arch Gen Psychiatry 49:739–744, 1992

Jones AK, Luthra SK, Maziere B, et al: Regional cerebral opioid receptor studies with ^{11}C diprenorphine in normal volunteers. J Neurosci Methods 23:121–129, 1988

Kapur S, Zipursky R, Jones C, et al: A positron emission tomography study of quetiapine in schizophrenia. Arch Gen Psychiatry 57:553–559, 2000a

Kapur S, Zipursky R, Jones C, et al: Relationship between dopamine D_2 occupancy, clinical response, and side effects: a double-blind PET study of first-episode schizophrenia. Am J Psychiatry 157:514–520, 2000b

Kuhl DE, Koeppe RA, Minoshima S, et al: In vivo mapping of cerebral acetylcholinesterase activity in aging and Alzheimer's disease. Neurology 52:691–699, 1999

Kwong KK, Belliveau JW, Chesler DA, et al: Dynamic magnetic resonance imaging of human brain activity during primary sensory stimulation. Proc Natl Acad Sci U S A 89:5675–5679, 1992

Langer O, Halldin C, Dolle F, et al: Carbon-11 epidepride: a suitable radioligand for PET investigation of striatal and extrastriatal dopamine D_2 receptors. Nucl Med Biol 26:509–518, 1999

Lesser IM, Mena I, Boone KB, et al: Reduction of cerebral blood flow in older depressed patients. Arch Gen Psychiatry 51:677–686, 1994

Lim KO, Hedehus M, Moseley M, et al: Compromised white matter tract integrity in schizophrenia inferred from diffusion tensor imaging. Arch Gen Psychiatry 56:367–374, 1999

Loeber RT, Sherwood AR, Renshaw PF, et al: Differences in cerebellar blood volume in schizophrenia and bipolar disorder. Schizphr Res 37:81–89, 1999

Madar I, Lever JR, Kinter CM, et al: Imaging of delta opioid receptors in human brain by N1′ -([11C]methyl)naltrindole and PET. Synapse 24:19–28, 1996

Maier M: In vivo magnetic resonance spectroscopy: applications in psychiatry. Br J Psychiatry 167:299–306, 1995

Malison RT, Price LH, Berman R, et al: Reduced brain serotonin transporter availability in major depression as measured by [123I]-2 beta-carbomethoxy-3 beta-(4-iodophenyl)tropane and single photon emission computed tomography. Biol Psychiatry 44(11):1090–1098, 1998

Manoach DS, Press DZ, Thangaraj V, et al: Schizophrenic subjects activate dorsolateral prefrontal cortex during a working memory task, as measured by fMRI. Biol Psychiatry 45: 1128–1137, 1999

Manoach DS, Gollub RL, Benson ES, et al: Schizophrenic subjects show aberrant fMRI activation of dorsolateral prefrontal cortex and basal ganglia during working memory performance. Biol Psychiatry 48:99–109, 2000

Mayberg HS, Lewis PJ, Regenold W, et al: Paralimbic hypoperfusion in unipolar depression. J Nucl Med 35:929–934, 1994

Mayberg HS, Brannan SK, Mahurin RK, et al: Cingulate function in depression: a potential predictor of treatment response. Neuroreport 8:1057–1061, 1997

Mayberg HS, Liotti M, Brannan SK, et al: Reciprocal limbic-cortical function and negative mood: converging PET findings in depression and normal sadness. Am J Psychiatry 156(5):675–682, 1999

McClure RJ, Kanfer JN, Panchalingam K, et al: Magnetic resonance spectroscopy and its application to aging and Alzheimer's disease. Neuroimaging Clin N Am 5:69–86, 1995

Messa C, Fazio F, Costa DC, et al: Clinical brain radionuclide imaging studies. Semin Nucl Med 25:111–143, 1995

Moonen CTW, van Zijl PCM, Frank JA, et al: Functional magnetic resonance imaging in medicine and physiology. Science 250:53–61, 1990

Moriarty J, Campos Costa D, Schmitz B, et al: Brain perfusion abnormalities in Gilles de la Tourette's syndrome. Br J Psychiatry 167:249–254, 1995

Mountz JM, Tolbert LC, Lill DW, et al: Functional deficits in autistic disorder: characterization by technetium-99m-HMAO and SPECT. J Nucl Med 36:1156–1162, 1995

Muller L, Halldin C, Farde L, et al: [11C] beta-CIT, a cocaine analogue. Preparation, autoradiography and preliminary PET investigations. Nucl Med Biol 20(3):249–255, 1993

Muller RA, Chugani DC, Behen ME, et al: Impairment of dentate-thalamo-cortical pathway in autistic men: language activation data from positron emission tomography. Neurosci Lett 245:1–4, 1998

Muller RA, Behen ME, Rothermel RD, et al: Brain mapping of language and auditory perception in high-functioning autistic adults: a PET study. J Autism Dev Disord 29:19–31, 1999

Muzik O, Chugani DC, Chakraborty P, et al: Analysis of [C-11]alpha-methyl-tryptophan kinetics for the estimation of serotonin synthesis rate in vivo. J Cereb Blood Flow Metab 17:659–669, 1997

Nadeau SE, Crosson B: A guide to the functional imaging of cognitive processes. Neuropsychiatry Neuropsychol Behav Neurol 8:143–162, 1995

Narayana PA, Jackson EF: Image-guided in vivo proton magnetic resonance spectroscopy in human brain. Cur Sci 61:340–351, 1991

Nofzinger EA, Nichols TE, Meltzer CC, et al: Changes in forebrain function from waking to REM sleep in depression: preliminary analyses of [18F]FDG PET studies. Psychiatry Res 91:59–78, 1999

Nofzinger EA, Price JC, Meltzer CC, et al: Towards a neurobiology of dysfunctional arousal in depression: the relationship between beta EEG power and regional cerebral glucose metabolism during NREM sleep. Psychiatry Res 98:71–91, 2000

Nordahl TE, Stein MB, Benkelfat C, et al: Regional cerebral metabolic asymmetries replicated in an independent group of patients with panic disorder. Biol Psychiatry 44:998–1006, 1998

Nordstrom A-L, Farde L, Eriksson L, et al: No elevated D_2 dopamine receptors in neuroleptic-naive schizophrenic patients revealed by positron emission tomography and [11C]N-methylspiperone. Psychiatry Res 61:67–83, 1995

Ohnishi T, Matsuda H, Hashimoto T, et al: Abnormal regional cerebral blood flow in childhood autism. Brain 123:1838–1844, 2000

Patterson JC, Kotrla KJ: Functional neuroimaging in psychiatry, in The American Psychiatric Publishing Textbook of Neuropsychiatry and Clinical Neurosciences, 4th Edition. Edited by Yudofsky SC, Hales RE. Washington, DC, American Psychiatric Publishing, 2002, pp 285–321

Patterson JC, Early TS, Martin A, et al: Computerized SPECT image analysis using statistical parametric mapping: comparison of ^{99m}Tc-radiolabeled exametazime and bicisate tracers. J Nucl Med 38:1721–1725, 1997

Pettegrew JW, Keshavan MS, Panchalingam K, et al: Alterations in brain high-energy phosphate and membrane phospholipid metabolism in first-episode, drug-naive schizophrenics. Arch Gen Psychiatry 48:563–568, 1991

Pettegrew JW, Keshavan MS, Minshew NJ: 31P nuclear magnetic resonance spectroscopy: neurodevelopment and schizophrenia. Schizophr Bull 19:35–53, 1993

Pike VW, McCarron JA, Lammertsma AA, et al: Exquisite delineation of 5-HT1A receptors in human brain with PET and [carbonyl-11 C]WAY-100635. Eur J Pharmacol 301:R5–R7, 1996

Raedler TJ, Knable MB, Lafargue T, et al: In vivo determination of striatal dopamine D_2 receptor occupancy in patients treated with olanzapine. Psychiatry Res 90:81–90, 1999

Rauch SL, Savage CR, Alpert NM, et al: The functional neuroanatomy of anxiety: a study of three disorders using positron emission tomography and symptom provocation. Biol Psychiatry 42:446–452, 1997

Reba RC: PET and SPECT: opportunities and challenges for psychiatry. J Clin Psychiatry 54 (11 suppl):26–32, 1993

Renshaw PF, Yurgelun-Todd DA, Tohen M, et al: Temporal lobe proton magnetic resonance spectroscopy of patients with first-episode psychosis. Am J Psychiatry 152:444–446, 1995

Ring HA, Baron-Cohen S, Wheelwright S, et al: Cerebral correlates of preserved cognitive skills in autism: a functional MRI study of Embedded Figures Task performance. Brain 122:1305–1315, 1999

Rinne JO, Hublin C, Partinen M, et al: Striatal dopamine D1 receptors in narcolepsy: a PET study with [11C]NNC 756. J Sleep Res 5:262–264, 1996

Rubia K, Overmeyer S, Taylor E, et al: Hypofrontality in attention deficit hyperactivity disorder during higher-order motor control: a study with functional MRI. Am J Psychiatry 156:891–896, 1999

Rubin P, Holm S, Friberg L, et al: Altered modulation of prefrontal and subcortical brain activity in newly diagnosed schizophrenia and schizophreniform disorder. Arch Gen Psychiatry 48:987–995, 1991

Rumsey JM, Duara R, Grady C, et al: Brain metabolism in autism. Resting cerebral glucose utilization rates as measured with positron emission tomography. Arch Gen Psychiatry 42:448–455, 1985

Saha GB, MacIntyre WJ, Go RT: Radiopharmaceuticals for brain imaging. Semin Nucl Med 24:324–349, 1994

Sargent PA, Kjaer KH, Bench CJ, et al: Brain serotonin1A receptor binding measured by positron emission tomography with [11C]WAY-100635: effects of depression and antidepressant treatment. Arch Gen Psychiatry 57:174–180, 2000

Schroder J, Buchsbaum MS, Siegel BV, et al: Structural and functional correlates of subsyndromes in chronic schizophrenia. Psychopathology 28:38–45, 1995

Schwartz WJ, Smith CB, Davidsen L, et al: Metabolic mapping of functional activity in the hypothalamo-neurohypophysial system of the rat. Science 205:723–725, 1979

Schweitzer JB, Faber TL, Grafton ST, et al: Alterations in the functional anatomy of working memory in adult attention deficit hyperactivity disorder. Am J Psychiatry 157:278–280, 2000

Seeman MV, Seeman P: Psychosis and positron tomography. Can J Psychiatry 33:299–306, 1988

Shioiri T, Tadafumi K, Murashita J, et al: High-energy phosphate metabolism in the frontal lobes of patients with panic disorder detected by phase-encoded 31P-MRS. Biol Psychiatry 40:785–793, 1996

Soares JC, Mann JJ: The functional neuroanatomy of mood disorders. J Psychiatr Res 31:393–432, 1997

Stanley JA, Williamson PC, Drost DJ, et al: An in vivo study of the prefrontal cortex of schizophrenic patients at different stages of illness via phosphorus magnetic resonance spectroscopy. Arch Gen Psychiatry 52:399–406, 1995

Swedo SE, Schapiro MB, Grady CL, et al: Cerebral glucose metabolism in childhood-onset obsessive-compulsive disorder. Arch Gen Psychiatry 46:518–523, 1989

Swedo SE, Pietrini P, Leonard HL, et al: Cerebral glucose metabolism in childhood-onset obsessive-compulsive disorder. Revisualization during pharmacotherapy. Arch Gen Psychiatry 49:690–694, 1992

Szabo Z, Kao PF, Mathews WB, et al: Positron emission tomography of 5-HT reuptake sites in the human brain with C-11 McN5652 extraction of characteristic images by artificial neural network analysis. Behav Brain Res 73:221–224, 1996

Talairach J, Tournoux P: Co-planar Stereotaxic Atlas of the Human Brain. Stuttgart, Germany, Thieme, 1988

Tanji H, Nagasawa H, Araki T, et al: PET study of striatal fluorodopa uptake and dopamine D2 receptor binding in a patient with juvenile parkinsonism. Eur J Neurol 5: 243–248, 1998

Waddington JL, O'Callaghan E, Larkin C, et al: Magnetic resonance imaging and spectroscopy in schizophrenia. Br J Psychiatry 157:56–65, 1990

Wilson AA, DaSilva JN, Houle S: In vivo evaluation of [11C]- and [18F]-labelled cocaine analogues as potential dopamine transporter ligands for positron emission tomography. Nucl Med Biol 23:141–146, 1996

Wolf SS, Jones DW, Knable MB, et al: Tourette syndrome: prediction of phenotypic variation in monozygotic twins by caudate nucleus D_2 receptor binding. Science 273(5279): 1225–1227, 1996

Wong DF, Wagner HN Jr, Tune LE, et al: Positron emission tomography reveals elevated D_2-dopamine receptors in drug-naive schizophrenics. Science 234:1558–1563, 1986

Yurgelun-Todd DA, Renshaw PF, Waternaux CM, et al: ^{1}H spectroscopy of the temporal lobes in schizophrenic and bipolar patients. Society of Magnetic Resonance in Medicine 12th Annual Meeting Abstracts 3:1539, 1993

Zametkin AJ, Nordahl TE, Gross M, et al: Cerebral glucose metabolism in adults with hyperactivity of childhood onset. N Engl J Med 323:1361–1366, 1990

Zametkin AJ, Liebenauer LL, Fitzgerald GA, et al: Brain metabolism in teenagers with attention-deficit hyperactivity disorder. Arch Gen Psychiatry 50:333–340, 1993

Zilbovicius M, Garreau B, Tzourio N, et al: Regional cerebral blood flow in childhood autism: a SPECT study. Am J Psychiatry 149:924–930, 1992

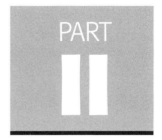

PART

II

Neuropsychiatric Symptomatologies

Neuropsychiatric Aspects of Delirium

Paula T. Trzepacz, M.D.

David J. Meagher, M.D.,
M.R.C.Psych., M.Sc. (Neuroscience)

Michael G. Wise, M.D.

Delirium is a commonly occurring neuropsychiatric syndrome primarily, but not exclusively, characterized by impairment in cognition, which causes a "confusional state." Delirium is a state of consciousness between normal alertness and awakeness and stupor or coma (Figure 5–1). Delirium may have a rapid, robust onset replete with many symptoms, or it may be preceded by subclinical delirium with more insidious changes such as alterations in sleep or aspects of cognition. Precise clinical delineation between severe delirium and stupor is difficult when the delirium presents hypomotorically. It is generally believed that coming out of coma involves a period of delirium before normalcy is achieved.

Because there is a wide variety of underlying etiologies for delirium—identification of which is part of clinical management—it is considered a syndrome and not a unitary disorder. It may, however, represent dysfunction of a final common neural pathway that leads to its characteristic symptoms. Its broad constellation of symptoms includes not only the diffuse cognitive deficits implicit for its diagnosis but also disturbances of thought, sleep, and behavior (see Table 5–1).

Unlike most other psychiatric disorders, delirium symptoms typically fluctuate in intensity over a 24-hour period. During this characteristic waxing and waning of symptoms, relative lucid or quiescent periods often occur.

Although delirium in children has not been as well studied as delirium in adults, the symptoms appear to be the same (Platt et al. 1994b; Prugh et al. 1980). Documentation of delirium symptoms in preverbal children or noncommunicative adults is difficult. In these patients, there is a need for more reliance on inference and observation of changed or unusual behaviors, for example, inferring hallucinations or recording changes in the sleep-wake cycle.

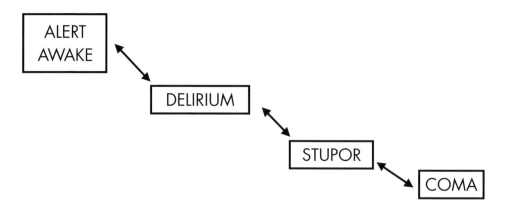

FIGURE 5–1.   Continuum of level of consciousness.

Delirium is the accepted term to denote acute disturbances of global cognitive function as defined in both DSM-IV and ICD-10 research classification systems (American Psychiatric Association 1994; World Health Organization 1992). Unfortunately, different terms are used by physicians from different disciplines, who associate its occurrence with specific clinical settings. Examples of these terms are *intensive care unit (ICU) psychosis, hepatic encephalopathy, toxic psychosis,* and *posttraumatic amnesia.* These terms inappropriately suggest the existence of independent psychiatric disorders for each etiology rather than acknowledging delirium as a unitary syndrome. The term *delirium* subsumes these many other terms, and its use will enhance medical communication and diagnosis as well as research.

Differential Diagnosis

The presence of delirium is frequently not detected in clinical practice. Between one-third and two-thirds of cases are missed across a range of therapeutic settings and by a variety of specialists, including psychiatrists and neurologists (Johnson et al. 1992). Nonrecognition is not merely the result of labeling delirium using one of its synonyms (e.g., "acute confusion") but represents an actual failure to recognize both the symptoms and diagnosis of delirium and is reflected in poorer outcomes (Rockwood et al. 1994). Poor detection rates in part reflect that delirium is an inherently fluctuating neuropsychiatric disorder involving multiple cognitive and noncognitive disturbances that confer great clinical variability.

The stereotyped image of delirium in an agitated psychotic patient does not represent the majority of patients with delirium, who have either mixed or hypoactive symptom profiles (Meagher and Trzepacz 2000). The hypoactive presentation is less appreciated because the quiet, untroublesome patient is often presumed to have intact cognition and is more easily overlooked in the time-pressurized technological environment of modern medicine. Detection can be improved by routinely assessing cognitive function, improving awareness of the varied presentations of delirium, and using one of the screening instruments for delirium currently available (Rockwood et al. 1994), such as the Confusion Assessment Method (CAM) (Inouye et al. 1990) (see the section "Delirium Assessment Instruments" later in this chapter).

TABLE 5–1. Signs and symptoms of delirium

Diffuse cognitive deficits
- Attention
- Orientation (time, place, person)
- Memory (short- and long-term; verbal and visual)
- Visuoconstructional ability
- Executive functions

Temporal course
- Acute/abrupt onset
- Fluctuating severity of symptoms over 24-hour period
- Usually reversible
- Subclinical syndrome may precede and/or follow the episode

Psychosis
- Perceptual disturbances (especially visual), including illusions, hallucinations, metamorphopsias
- Delusions (usually paranoid and poorly formed)
- Thought disorder (tangentiality, circumstantiality, loose associations)

Sleep-wake disturbance
- Fragmented throughout 24-hour period
- Reversal of normal cycle
- Sleeplessness

Psychomotor behavior
- Hyperactive
- Hypoactive
- Mixed

Language impairment
- Word-finding difficulty/dysnomia/paraphasia
- Dysgraphia
- Altered semantic content
- Severe forms can mimic expressive or receptive aphasia

Altered or labile affect
- Any mood can occur, usually incongruent to context
- Anger or increased irritability common
- Hypoactive delirium often mislabeled as depression
- Lability (rapid shifts) common
- Unrelated to mood preceding delirium

Delirium has a wide differential diagnosis. It can be mistaken for dementia, depression, primary or secondary psychosis, anxiety and somatoform disorders, and, particularly in children, behavioral disturbance (Table 5–2). Accurate diagnosis requires close attention to symptom profile, temporal onset, and results of tests (e.g., cognitive, laboratory, electroencephalographic). Given that delirium can be the presenting feature of serious medical illness, any patient experiencing a sudden deterioration in cognitive function should be investigated for possible delirium. Urinary tract infections in nursing home patients commonly present as delirium.

The most difficult differential diagnosis for delirium is dementia, the other cause of generalized cognitive impairment. Indeed, end-stage dementia has been described as a chronic delirious state. The distinction is clouded by the increasing recognition of a form of dementia that bears close resemblance to delirium: Lewy body dementia, which fluctuates in severity and involves prominent psychotic symptoms (e.g., visual hallucinations). The overlap between delirium and dementia extends beyond symptom profile; any cognitive impairment, including dementia, is a potent predisposing factor for the development of delirium. Consequently, delirium and dementia have high comorbidity rates, especially in the elderly, and up to two-thirds of cases of delirium occur superimposed on preexisting cognitive impairment (Wahlund and Bjorland 1999). Delirium is 2–3.5 times more common in patients with dementia than in nondemented control subjects (Erkinjuntti et al. 1986; Jitapunkul et al. 1992). The risk of delirium appears to be greater in Alzheimer's disease of late onset and in dementia of vascular origin compared with other dementias, perhaps reflecting the rela-

TABLE 5–2. Differential diagnosis of delirium

	Delirium	Dementia	Depression	Schizophrenia
Onset	Acute	Insidious[a]	Variable	Variable
Course	Fluctuating	Often progressive	Diurnal variation	Variable
Reversibility	Usually[b]	Not usually	Usually but can be recurrent	No, but has exacerbations
Level of consciousness	Impaired	Clear until late stages	Generally unimpaired	Unimpaired (perplexity in acute stage)
Attention/ memory	Inattention, poor memory	Poor memory without marked inattention	Poor attention, memory intact	Poor attention, memory intact
Hallucinations	Usually visual; can be auditory, tactile, gustatory, olfactory	Can be visual or auditory	Usually auditory	Usually auditory
Delusions	Fleeting, fragmented, and usually persecutory	Paranoid, often fixed	Complex and mood congruent	Frequent, complex, systematized, and often paranoid

[a]Except for large strokes.
[b]Can be chronic (paraneoplastic syndrome, central nervous system adverse events of medications, severe brain damage).

tively widespread neuronal disturbance associated with these conditions (Robertsson et al. 1998).

Despite this substantial overlap, delirium and dementia can be reliably distinguished by a combination of careful history taking and interviewing for onset of the symptom profile and clinical investigation. The tendency for abrupt onset and fluctuating course are highly characteristic of delirium. In addition, level of consciousness and attention are markedly disturbed in delirium but remain relatively intact in uncomplicated dementia. Dementia patients often have nocturnal disturbances of sleep, whereas in delirium there are varying degrees of disruption of the sleep-wake cycle, including fragmentation and sleeplessness. Overall, the presentation of delirium does not seem to be greatly altered by the presence of dementia, and delirium symptoms dominate the

clinical picture when they co-occur (Trzepacz et al. 1998).

A range of investigative tools can facilitate the differentiation of delirium and dementia in clinical practice. Both the Delirium Rating Scale (DRS) (Trzepacz and Dew 1995), which allows assessment of delirium symptom severity, and the Cognitive Test for Delirium (CTD) (Hart et al. 1996), an instrument specifically designed to assess cognition in delirious ICU patients, can be used to help differentiate the conditions. Although abnormalities of the electroencephalogram (EEG) are common to both delirium and dementia, diffuse slowing occurs more frequently (81% vs. 33%) and favors a diagnosis of delirium. Electroencephalographic slowing occurs later in the course of most degenerative dementias, although slowing occurs sooner with viral and prion dementias. The percentage of theta activity on quantitative EEGs allows differentiation of delirium from dementia (Jacobson and Jerrier 2000).

Hypoactive delirium is frequently mistaken for depression (Nicholas and Lindsey 1995). Some symptoms of major depression occur in delirium (e.g., psychomotor slowing, sleep disturbances, irritability). However, in major depression, symptom onset tends to be less acute and mood disturbances typically dominate the clinical picture, with any cognitive impairments of depression resembling a mild subcortical dementia: "depressive pseudodementia." Delirium can be precipitated by dehydration or malnutrition in severely depressed patients who are unable to maintain food or fluid intake. The distinction of delirium from depression is particularly important because, in addition to delayed treatment, some antidepressants have anticholinergic activity (paroxetine and tricyclics) that can aggravate delirium. Conversely, the overactive, disinhibited profile of some delirious patients can closely mimic similar disturbances encountered in patients with agitated depression or mania. The most severe mania ("Bell's mania") includes cognitive impairment and mimics delirium.

Abnormalities of thought and perception can occur in both delirium and schizophrenia, but they are more fluctuant and fragmentary in delirium. Delusions in delirium are rarely as fixed or complex as in schizophrenia, and first-rank symptoms are uncommon (Cutting 1987). Unlike in schizophrenia, hallucinations in delirium tend to be visual rather than auditory. Consciousness, attention, and memory are generally less impaired in schizophrenia, with the exception of the pseudodelirious picture that can occur due to marked perplexity in the acute stage of illness. Careful examination, coupled with EEG and/or an instrument such as the DRS, generally distinguishes delirium from these functional disorders.

Epidemiology

Delirium can occur at any age, although it is unfortunately understudied in children and adolescents. In contrast, most epidemiologic studies focus on the elderly, who are at higher risk to develop delirium than younger adults. This is likely because of changes that occur in the brain with aging. These changes include decreased cholinergic activity, often referred to as "reduced brain reserve." The frequent occurrence of central nervous system (CNS) disorders (e.g., stroke, hypertensive and diabetic vessel changes, tumor, dementia) in the elderly further increases their vulnerability to delirium. These facts will also present a serious challenge for physicians and medical personnel in the future because the world's population is aging at a dramatic rate.

Most studies of the incidence and prevalence of delirium report general hospital populations consisting of either referral samples or consecutive admissions to a given service. A wide range of percentages has been found in studies. Specific patient populations (e.g., elderly patients who have undergone hip surgery) may be responsible for disparate rates reported in studies. In addition, not all studies employ sensitive and specific diagnostic and measurement techniques, possibly resulting in overestimates or underestimates of the true occurrence of delirium. The review by Fann (2000) of (mostly) prospective studies found an incidence range from 3% to 42% and a prevalence range from 5% to 44% in hospitalized patients. Up to 60% of nursing home patients over 65 years old may be delirious when assessed cross-sectionally (Sandberg et al. 1998). In addition, 10%–15% of elderly persons are delirious when admitted to a hospital and another 10%–40% are diagnosed with delirium during the hospitalization. Table 5–3 describes several studies of the incidence and prevalence of delirium in which DSM diagnostic criteria or rating scales were used. A clinical rule of thumb seems to be that, on average, approximately a fifth of general hospital patients have delirium sometime during hospitalization.

Morbidity and Mortality

Delirium is associated with high rates of morbidity and mortality. Whether the mortality risk is increased during the index admission, at long-term follow-up, or both is not completely clear. It is not known whether the increased mortality rate is 1) solely attributable to the physiological perturbations due to the underlying causes of delirium, 2) attributable to indirect effects on the body related to perturbations of neuronal (or neuronal-endocrine-immunological) function during delirium, or 3) attributable to damaging effects on the brain from neurochemical abnormalities associated with delirium (e.g., similar to glutamate surges after stroke). Furthermore, delirious patients cannot fully cooperate with their medical care or participate in rehabilitative programs during hospitalization. Their behaviors can even directly reduce the effectiveness of procedures meant to treat their medical problems (e.g., removing tubes and intravenous lines, climbing out of bed), which adds to morbidity and possibly to further physiological injury and mortality.

Methodological inconsistencies and shortcomings affect the interpretation of studies of mortality risk associated with delirium. Some do not compare delirium to control groups, most do not address the effects of treatment, many include comorbid dementia, many do not control for severity differences in medical comorbidity, most do not address effects of advanced age as a separate risk factor, and rarely are specific delirium rating instruments utilized. Prospective application of DSM criteria by qualified clinicians, attention to whether the sample is incident or prevalent, identification of biases related to referral samples, and whether or not follow-up mortality rates are cumulative to include the original sample size are also important issues that vary across study designs.

Mortality rates during index hospitalization for a delirium episode range from 4% to 65% (Cameron et al. 1987; Gustafson et al. 1988) depending on the study design and population. One study found significant differences in index mortality rate among motoric subtypes, with the lowest rate (10%) in hyperalert patients compared with hypoalert patients (38%) and mixed cases (30%) (Olofsson et al. 1996). When delirium present on admission was excluded, the index mortality rate for incident cases was as low as about 1.5% (Inouye et al. 1999). Index mortality rates for delirium did not differ significantly from those of nondelirious control subjects in some studies (Forman et al. 1995; George et al. 1997; Gustafson et al. 1988; Inouye et al. 1998, 1999; Kishi et al. 1995), whereas it did in others (Cameron et al. 1987; Jitapunkul et al. 1992; Pompeii et al. 1994; Rabins and Folstein 1982; van Hemert et al. 1994). Many studies of longer-term follow-up of delirium mortality rates (more than 3 months after discharge) do find worse mortality rates in delirium groups. Excessive mortality in some reports was attributed to greater age (Gustafson et al. 1988; Huang et al. 1998; Kishi et al. 1995; Trzepacz et al. 1985; Weddington 1982), more serious medical problems (Cole and Primeau 1993; Jitapunkul et al. 1992;

TABLE 5–3. Epidemiology of delirium using established criteria[a]

Reference	N	Type of patient	Frequency, %	Prevalence, %	Incidence, %
Erkinjuntti et al. 1986	2,000	Medical, age 55 or older		15	
Cameron et al. 1987	133	Medical, age 32–97		11.3	4.2
Gustafson et al. 1988	111	Femoral neck fracture, age 65 or older			
		Before surgery	33		
		After surgery	42		
Rockwood 1989	80	Medical, age 65 or older		16	10.4
Johnson et al. 1990	235	Medical, age 70 or older		16	5
Francis et al. 1990	229	Medical, age 70 or older		15.7	7.3
Schor et al. 1992	325	Medical/surgical, age 65 or older		11	31
Rockwood 1993	168	Geriatric		18	7
Marcantonio et al. 1994a	134	Postsurgical (elective noncardiac)			9
Pompeii et al. 1994[b]	432	Medical/surgical, age 65 or older		5	10
	323	Medical/surgical, age 70 or older		15	12
Inouye and Charpentier 1996	196	Consecutive admissions, age 70 or older		5	18
	312	Consecutive admissions, age 70 or older		2	15
O'Keeffe and Lavan 1997	225	Acute case geriatric		18	29
Inouye et al. 1998	727	Consecutive admissions, age 65 or older		12	
Lawlor et al. 2000	104	Consecutive admissions with advanced cancer, age 62±11.9 years		42.3	45
Brauer et al. 2000	571	Admissions with hip fracture, age 69–101			
		Delirium at time of admission (4)		1	
		Developed delirium before surgery (16)			4
		Delirium day of surgery (5)			1
		Developed delirium after surgery (29)			5

[a]DSM-III, DSM-III-R, DSM-IV criteria or delirium assessment instruments.

[b]Lower rates in this study may be explained by exclusion of patients with severe cognitive impairment.

Source. Reprinted from Wise MG, Gray KF, Seltzer B: "Delirium, Dementia, and Amnestic Disorders," in *American Psychiatric Press Textbook of Psychiatry*, 3rd Edition. Edited by Hales RE, Yudofsky SC, Talbott JA. Washington, DC, American Psychiatric Press, 1999, p. 31. Used with permission.

Magaziner et al. 1989; Trzepacz et al. 1985), and dementia (Cole and Primeau 1993; Gustafson et al. 1988). Other researchers did not find cancer as an explanation for higher mortality rates (Rabins and Folstein 1982), whereas studies comparing only cancer inpatients did find significantly poorer survival in delirium patients compared with control subjects (Lawlor et al. 2000; Minagawa et al. 1996). Manos and Wu (1997) found no differences in delirium mortality rates between medical and postoperative groups after 3.5 years. Inouye et al. (1998) found that delirium significantly increased mortality risk even after controlling for age, sex, dementia, activities of daily living (ADL) level, and APACHE II (Knaus et al. 1985) scores in a prospective study of medically hospitalized elderly persons when using the CAM for delirium diagnosis.

Morbidity associated with delirium during an index episode is easily appreciated in terms of human suffering by patients and caregivers, although this is less easily measured. One study found more complications in the delirium group during index hospitalization, including decubitus ulcers, feeding problems, and urinary incontinence (Gustafson et al. 1988). Effects on hospital length of stay (LOS), "persistence" of cognitive impairment, increased rate of institutionalization, and reduced ambulation and/or ADL level have been reported.

Significantly increased LOS associated with delirium has been reported in many studies (Forman et al. 1995; Francis et al. 1990; Gustafson et al. 1988; Hales et al. 1988; Levkoff et al. 1992; Pompeii et al. 1994; R.I. Thomas et al. 1988) and as a trend toward significance in one (Inouye et al. 1998). In contrast, others have not found an increased LOS (Cole et al. 1994; George et al. 1997; Jitapunkul et al. 1992; Rockwood 1989). However, a meta-analysis of eight studies (Cole and Primeau 1993) does support both numerical and statistical differences between delirium and control groups' LOS.

Decreased independent living status and increased rate of institutionalization during follow-up after a delirium episode were found in many studies (Cole and Primeau 1993; George et al. 1997; Inouye et al. 1998). Reduction in ambulation and/or ADL level at follow-up is also commonly reported (Francis and Kapoor 1992; Gustafson et al. 1988; Inouye et al. 1998; Minagawa et al. 1996; Murray et al. 1993). Delirium also has an impact in nursing home settings, where incident cases are associated with poor 6-month outcome including behavioral decline, initiation of physical restraints, greater risk of hospitalization, and increased mortality rate (Murphy 1999).

One controversial matter is so-called persistent cognitive impairment at longer-term follow-up, which some (Levkoff et al. 1992) suggest represents damage from the delirium episode affecting future brain function. Many interpret persisting cognitive deficits as being more related to "diminished brain reserve" or preexisting dementia that has simply progressed over time (Francis and Kapoor 1992; Koponen et al. 1994). Dementia may go unrecognized at the time of the delirium index episode and is a key risk factor for the occurrence of delirium; often they are comorbid. In nursing home patients, better cognitive function at baseline was associated with better outcome from delirium (Murphy 1999). This finding lends support to the notion that impaired brain reserve is an important predelirium factor that needs to be taken into account in any longitudinal outcome assessments. Therefore, carefully designed longitudinal research is needed to help clarify this issue. It is necessary to gather premorbid cognitive functioning data and to administer neuropsychological tests over time that are designed to detect and differentiate patterns of dementia that could have existed before the delirium and may be progressive. Detection of cognitive deficit patterns among elderly persons that do not match those associated with either Alzheimer's disease or vascular, frontal, or other dementing processes or the medical insults experienced could then suggest separate delirium-induced damage. Alternatively, longitudinal postdelirium cognitive assessments of younger adults who are not at risk for dementia could help answer this question.

In summary, although the mechanism is not understood, the presence of delirium does indeed appear to be an adverse prognostic sign that is associated with substantial morbidity and an increased risk for mortality, extending well beyond the index hospitalization. To what extent aggressive treatment of both the delirium and its comorbid medical problems would reduce morbidity and mortality is not well studied, but such treatment makes good clinical sense.

Reversibility of a Delirium Episode

Delirium has traditionally been distinguished from dementia by virtue of acute onset, fluctuating severity level, symptom profile, and reversibility. In most cases it is reversible, except in terminal illness or particular examples of severe brain injury. Whether delirium itself causes permanent damage is under debate.

Bedford's (1957) landmark study of delirium indicated that approximately 5% of patients were still "confused" at 6-month follow-up, but more recent studies suggest that persistent disturbances may be more frequent following an episode of delirium. Levkoff et al. (1994), in a 6-

month longitudinal study of DSM-III-R (American Psychiatric Association 1987) diagnosed delirium in elderly patients, found that almost one-third of patients still had delirium, with a majority still having some of its features (orientation difficulties, emotional lability, and sleep disturbances). However, dementia patients had not been excluded from this study. Full resolution of delirium symptoms at hospital discharge of elderly patients may be the exception rather than the rule (Levkoff et al. 1992; Rockwood 1993). However, these studies do not fully account for the role of underlying etiologies, treatment received, preexisting cognitive impairment, or even fiscal constraints promoting premature discharge. Kopnonen et al.'s (1994) 5-year longitudinal study of delirium in the elderly found persistence and progression of symptoms to be attributed more to the underlying dementia than to the previous delirium episode. Camus et al. (2000) found that preexisting dementia was associated with partial or no recovery from delirium in hospitalized elderly persons at 3-week follow-up. Kolbeinsson and Jonsson (1993) found that delirium was complicated by dementia at follow-up in 70% of cases. Thus, "persistent" deficits may instead reflect an underlying disorder and not the delirium.

The relationship between delirium and "persistent symptoms" at follow-up may be explained by an index episode of delirium being an actual risk factor, rather than a cause or marker, for other causes of cognitive impairment. Rockwood et al. (1999) reported an 18% annual incidence of dementia in patients with delirium—more than 3 times higher risk than incidence in nondelirious patients when the confounding effects of comorbid illness severity and age were adjusted for. Camus et al. (2000), in a cross-sectional study of consecutive psychogeriatric admissions,

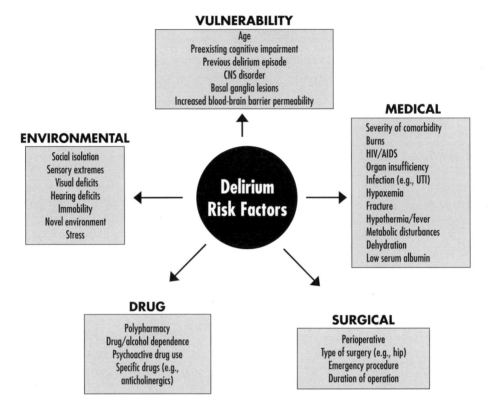

FIGURE 5–2. Delirium risk factors.

AIDS = acquired immune deficiency syndrome; CNS = central nervous system; HIV = human immunodeficiency virus; UTI = urinary tract infection.

found that the only factor significantly linked to incomplete symptom resolution in delirium was the presence of preexisting cognitive impairment.

To date, the roles of unrecognized prior cognitive impairment, delirium treatment exposure, and the possibility that certain etiologies may be associated with persistence of cognitive impairment have not been fully accounted for in studies. Nonetheless, the concept of delirium as an inherently reversible condition is being increasingly questioned. Terminology is also difficult regarding when chronic delirium becomes dementia and whether the experience of an index episode of delirium, perhaps by virtue of a neurotoxic or kindling effect, may alter the threshold for further episodes of delirium or contribute to the development of dementia.

Risk Factors for Delirium

Delirium is particularly common during hospitalization when there is a confluence of both predisposing factors (vulnerabilities) and precipitating factors. A number of patient-related, illness, pharmacologic, and environmental factors have been identified as being relevant risk factors for delirium, as illustrated in Figure 5–2. Although certain factors are more relevant in certain settings, age, preexisting cognitive impairment, severe comorbid illness, and medication exposure are particularly robust predictors of delirium risk across a range of populations (Inouye et al. 1999).

Stress-vulnerability models for the occurrence of delirium have been long recognized. Henry and Mann (1965) described "delirium readiness." More recent models of causation involve cumulative interactions between predisposing (vulnerability) factors and precipitating insults (Inouye and Charpentier 1996; O'Keeffe and Lavan 1996). If baseline vulnerability is low, patients are very resistant to the development of delirium despite exposure to significant precipitating factors, whereas if baseline vulnerability is high, delirium is likely even in response to minor precipitants. Tsutsui et al. (1996), for example, found that in patients over 80 years old, delirium occurred in 52% after emergency surgery and in 20% after elective procedures, whereas no case of delirium was noted in patients under age 50 undergoing either elective or emergency procedures. It is generally believed that the aged brain is more vulnerable to delirium, in part related to structural/degenerative changes as well as altered neurochemical flexibility. Children are also considered to be at higher risk for delirium, possibly related to structural and chemical brain development.

O'Keeffe and Lavan (1996) stratified patients into four levels of delirium risk based on the presence of three factors (chronic cognitive impairment, severe illness, elevated serum urea level) and found that the risk of delirium increased as these factors accumulated. Similarly, Inouye and Charpentier (1996) developed a predictive model that included four predisposing factors (cognitive impairment, severe illness, visual impairment, and dehydration) and five precipitating factors (more than three medications added, catheterization, use of restraints, malnutrition, any iatrogenic event). These predicted a 17-fold variation in the relative risk of developing delirium. Although the value of reducing risk factors appears self-evident, many risk factors may simply be markers of general morbidity, and there-

fore studies demonstrating preventive impact are important.

Inouye et al. (1999) studied the impact of preventive measures aimed at minimizing six of the risk factors identified in their previous work with hospitalized elderly persons (Inouye et al. 1993). Standardized protocols to address cognitive impairment, sleep deprivation, immobility, visual impairment, hearing impairment, and dehydration resulted in significant reductions in the number and duration of delirium episodes.

Polypharmacy and drug intoxication/ withdrawal may be the most common causes of delirium, and drug use is also a risk factor (Hales et al. 1988; Trzepacz et al. 1985). Benzodiazepines, opiates, and drugs with anticholinergic activity have a particular association with delirium (Brown 2000; Marcantonio et al. 1994b). Many drugs (and their metabolites) can unexpectedly contribute to delirium due to unrecognized anticholinergic effects. It is therefore important to minimize drug exposure, especially when facing high-risk periods such as the perioperative phase.

There has been relatively little study of risk factors for delirium in children and adolescents despite a general belief that children are especially vulnerable to delirium. Thiamine deficiency is an underappreciated cause of and/or risk factor for delirium in pediatric intensive care and oncology patients (Seear et al. 1992) and nonalcoholic elderly patients (O'Keeffe et al. 1994).

van der Mast and Fekkes (2000) proposed that surgery induces immune activation and a physical stress response. This is composed of increased limbic-hypothalamic-pituitary-adrenocortical axis activity, low T3 syndrome, and alterations of blood-brain barrier permeability. Increased blood-brain barrier permeability is a risk factor for delirium, as occurs in uremia. A large multicenter study found age, duration of anesthesia, lower educational level, second operation, postoperative infection, and respiratory complications to be predictors of postoperative cognitive impairment. However, this study revealed little about possible pathophysiological mechanisms for impairment because delirium risk was not linked to hypoxemia, hypotension, or use of specific anesthetic agents or procedures (Moller et al. 1998).

Low serum albumin is an important risk factor at any age and may signify poor nutrition, chronic disease, or liver or renal insufficiency. Hypoalbuminemia results in a greater bioavailability of many drugs that are transported in the bloodstream by albumin, which in turn is associated with an increased risk of side effects including delirium (Dickson 1991; Trzepacz and Francis 1990). This increased biological drug activity occurs within the therapeutic range and is not recognized because increased levels of free drug are not separately reported in assays.

Diagnosis and Assessment

Diagnosis

Diagnostic criteria for delirium first appeared in DSM-III (American Psychiatric Association 1980). Thus, early clinical reports and research were affected by this lack of diagnostic specificity. Symptom rating scales for delirium began to appear around the time of DSM-III.

DSM-IV-TR (American Psychiatric Association 2000) has five categories of delirium; the criteria are the same for each category except the one for etiology. The categories are delirium due to 1) a general medical condition (Table 5–4), 2) substance intoxication, 3) substance withdrawal, 4) multiple etiologies, and 5) not otherwise specified.

DSM-III, DSM-III-R, and DSM-IV

TABLE 5–4. DSM-IV-TR diagnostic criteria for delirium due to a general medical condition

A. Disturbance of consciousness (i.e., reduced clarity of awareness of the environment) with reduced ability to focus, sustain, or shift attention.
B. A change in cognition (such as memory deficit, disorientation, language disturbance) or the development of a perceptual disturbance that is not better accounted for by a preexisting, established, or evolving dementia.
C. The disturbance develops over a short period of time (usually hours to days) and tends to fluctuate during the course of the day.
D. There is evidence from the history, physical examination, or laboratory findings that the disturbance is caused by the direct physiological consequences of a general medical condition.

Source. Reprinted from the *Diagnostic and Statistical Manual of Mental Disorders*, 4th Edition, Text Revision. Washington, DC, American Psychiatric Association, 2000. Copyright 2000, American Psychiatric Association. Used with permission.

include efforts to further clarify the major criterion describing altered state of consciousness. This criterion has been considered as either inattention or "clouding of consciousness." The latter term is obfuscating because the elements of consciousness that are altered are not specified, nor is it clear how "clouding" differs from "level" of consciousness. Attentional disturbance distinguishes delirium from dementia where the first criterion is memory impairment. Attentional disturbances in delirium range from general, nonspecific reduction in alertness (may be nicotinic cholinergic, histaminergic, or adrenergic) to decreased selective focusing or sustaining of attention (may be muscarinic cholinergic). The contribution of attentional deficits to the altered awareness that occurs in delirium is insufficient by itself to account for other prominent symptoms—formal thought disorder, language and sleep-wake cycle disturbances, and other cognitive-perceptual deficits.

The characteristic features of the temporal course of delirium—acute onset and fluctuation of symptoms—have constituted a separate criterion in each of the last three editions of DSM. Temporal features assist in distinguishing delirium from dementia, and most clinicians consider them to be important in making a diagnosis.

Cognitive Assessment

Because delirium is primarily a cognitive disorder, bedside assessment of cognition is critical to proper diagnosis. All cognitive domains are affected—orientation, attention, short-term and long-term memory, visuoconstructional ability, and executive functions (the latter are poorly studied in delirium)—even though attentional deficits are most specifically emphasized in DSM. Pattern and timing of deficits assist in differential diagnosis from dementias and amnestic disorders. Use of bedside screening tests such as the Mini-Mental State Exam (MMSE) is clinically important to document the presence of a cognitive disorder, although the MMSE alone is insufficient to distinguish delirium from dementia (Trzepacz et al. 1988a). The MMSE is easy for many people (ceiling effect) and has a limited breadth of items, particularly for prefrontal executive and right hemisphere functions.

The CTD (Hart et al. 1996) is a more recent bedside test designed specifically for delirious patients, who are often unable to speak or write in a medical setting. The CTD correlates highly with the MMSE ($r = 0.82$) in delirium patients and was performable in 42% of ICU patients in whom the MMSE was not. It has two equivalent forms that correlate highly ($r = 0.90$) in dementia patients, which makes it better

suited for repeated measurements. However, it correlates less well with symptom rating scales for delirium that also include noncognitive symptoms—for example, the Medical College of Virginia Nurses Rating Scale for Delirium (Hart et al. 1996) ($r = -0.02$) or the Delirium Rating Scale–Revised-98 (DRS-R-98) (Trzepacz et al. 2001) ($r = -0.62$). The CTD has many nonverbal (nondominant hemisphere) items and includes abstraction questions.

Manos (1997) found that the Clock Drawing Test is a useful screen for cognitive impairment in medically ill patients, but it does not discriminate between delirium and dementia.

Delirium Assessment Instruments

Diagnostic criteria are important in diagnosing delirium, and cognitive tests are useful to document cognitive impairment. Rating a range of delirium symptoms, however, requires other methods. More than 10 instruments have been proposed to assess symptoms of delirium (Trzepacz 1994b) for screening, diagnosis, or symptom severity rating. However, only a few of these have been used broadly.

The CAM is probably the most widely used delirium screening tool in general hospitals (Inouye et al. 1990). It is based on DSM-III-R criteria and requires the presence of three of four cardinal symptoms of delirium. It is intended for use by nonpsychiatric clinicians in hospital settings and is useful for case finding, although nurses' ratings were much less sensitive than those done by physicians (1.00 vs. 0.13) when compared with an independent physician's DSM-III-R diagnosis (Rolfson et al. 1999). One study (Rockwood 1993) suggested that lower specificity and sensitivity are a trade-off for its simplicity, although in other studies it performed well compared with physicians' diagnoses in short-term hospital settings. It has not been well studied for its ability to distinguish delirium from dementia, depression, or other psychiatric disorders. The CAM appears to be useful to screen elderly emergency room patients for delirium (Monette et al. 2001). Based on a geriatrician's interview, comparison between ratings from the geriatrician interviewer and an observing lay person revealed interrater reliability of 0.91, sensitivity of 0.86, and specificity of 1.00. A recent extension of the CAM is the CAM-ICU (Ely et al. 2001), aimed at use in severely medically ill patients. It uses specific adjunctive tests and standardized administration to enhance reliability and validity.

The DRS (Trzepacz et al. 1988a) is a 10-item scale assessing a breadth of delirium features and can function both to clarify diagnosis and to assess symptom severity, due to its hierarchical nature (Trzepacz 1999a; van der Mast 1994). It is probably the most widely used delirium rating scale and has been translated into Italian, French, Spanish, Korean, Japanese, Mandarin Chinese, Dutch, Swedish, German, Portuguese, and a language of India for international use. It is generally used by those who have some psychiatric training. The DRS has high interrater reliability and validity even compared with other psychiatric patient groups, and it distinguishes delirium from dementia. However, because of some of its items it does not function as well for frequent repeated measurements, and thus it has been modified by some researchers to a 7- or 8-item subscale. In one study (Treloar and MacDonald 1997), the DRS and CAM diagnosed delirium patients with a high level of agreement ($\kappa = 0.81$).

The Memorial Delirium Assessment Scale (MDAS) is a 10-item severity rating scale for use after a diagnosis of delirium has been made (Breitbart et al. 1997). It was intended for repeated ratings within a 24-hour period, as occurs in treatment studies. The MDAS does not include items for temporal onset and fluctuation of symptoms, which are characteristic symptoms that help to distinguish delirium from dementia. The MDAS correlated highly with the DRS ($r = 0.88$) and the MMSE ($r = -0.91$). The Japanese version of the MDAS was validated in 37 elderly patients with either delirium, dementia, mood disorder, or schizophrenia and was found to distinguish among them ($P < 0.0001$), with a mean score of 18 in the delirium group (Matsuoka et al. 2001). It correlated reasonably well with the DRS Japanese version ($r = 0.74$) and the Clinician's Global Rating of Delirium ($r = 0.67$), and less well with the MMSE ($r = -0.54$).

The DRS-R-98 is a substantially revised version of the DRS that addresses the shortcomings of the DRS (Trzepacz et al. 2001). It allows for repeated measurements and includes separate/new items for language, thought processes, motor agitation, motor retardation, and five cognitive domains. The DRS-R-98 has 16 items, with 3 diagnostic items separable from 13 severity items. Severity for a broad range of symptoms known to occur in delirium is described using standard phenomenological definitions, without a priori assumptions about which symptoms occur more frequently. The total scale is used for initial evaluation of delirium to allow discrimination from other disorders. The DRS-R-98 total score ($P < 0.001$) distinguished delirium from dementia, schizophrenia, depression, and other medical conditions during blind ratings, with sensitivities ranging from 91% to 100% and specificities from 85% to 100%, depending on the cutoff score chosen. It has high internal consistency (Cronbach's alpha $= 0.90$), correlates well with the DRS ($r = 0.83$) and the CTD ($r = -0.62$), and has high interrater reli-

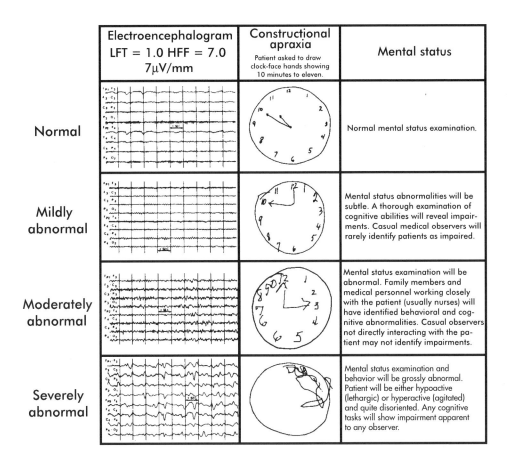

Electroencephalogram LFT = 1.0 HFF = 7.0 7μV/mm	Constructional apraxia Patient asked to draw clock-face hands showing 10 minutes to eleven.	Mental status
Normal		Normal mental status examination.
Mildly abnormal		Mental status abnormalities will be subtle. A thorough examination of cognitive abilities will reveal impairments. Casual medical observers will rarely identify patients as impaired.
Moderately abnormal		Mental status examination will be abnormal. Family members and medical personnel working closely with the patient (usually nurses) will have identified behavioral and cognitive abnormalities. Casual observers not directly interacting with the patient may not identify impairments.
Severely abnormal		Mental status examination and behavior will be grossly abnormal. Patient will be either hypoactive (lethargic) or hyperactive (agitated) and quite disoriented. Any cognitive tasks will show impairment apparent to any observer.

FIGURE 5–3. Comparison of electroencephalogram, constructional apraxia, and mental status.

ability (intraclass correlation coefficient [ICC] = 0.99). Translations are already under way for Japanese, Korean, Greek, Portuguese, Danish, Dutch, German, Norwegian, and Spanish versions.

Electroencephalography

In the 1940s, Engel and Romano (1944, 1959; Romano and Engel 1944) first wrote a series of classic papers that described the relationship of delirium, as measured by cognitive impairment, to electroencephalographic slowing. In their seminal work, they showed an association between abnormal electrical activity of the brain and the psychiatric symptoms of delirium; the reversibility of both of these

conditions; the ubiquity of electroencephalographic changes for different underlying disease states; and improvement in electroencephalography background rhythm that paralleled clinical improvement. Figure 5–3 demonstrates the progression of cognitive impairment, using the Clock Drawing Test, coupled with increasing degree of electroencephalographic slowing to illustrate this relationship.

Working with burn patients, Andreasen et al. (1977) showed that the time course of electroencephalographic slowing could precede or lag behind overt clinical symptoms of delirium, although sensitive delirium symptom ratings were not used.

TABLE 5–5.　Electroencephalographic patterns in patients with delirium

Electroencephalographic finding	Comment	Causes
Diffuse slowing	Most typical delirium pattern	Many causes, including anticholinergicity, posttraumatic brain injury, hepatic encephalopathy, hypoxia
Low-voltage fast activity	Typical of delirium tremens	Alcohol withdrawal; benzodiazepine intoxication
Spikes/polyspikes, frontocentral	Toxic ictal pattern (nonconvulsive)	Hypnosedative drug withdrawal; tricyclic and phenothiazine intoxication
Left/bilateral slowing or delta bursts; frontal intermittent rhythmic delta	Acute confusional migraine	Usually in adolescents
Epileptiform activity, frontotemporal or generalized	Status with prolonged confusional states	Nonconvulsive status and complex partial status epilepticus

Electroencephalographic dominant posterior rhythm, along with serum albumin and the Trail Making Test Part B, distinguished delirious from nondelirious cirrhosis patients in another study (Trzepacz et al. 1988b). Although generalized slowing is the typical electroencephalographic pattern for both hypoactive and hyperactive presentations of delirium and for most etiologies of delirium, delirium tremens is associated with low-voltage fast activity (Kennard et al. 1945), making it an important exception. An animal model for delirium using atropine found similar electroencephalographic slowing in rats as in humans that were associated over time with worsened cognitive function (maze performance) (Leavitt et al. 1994; Trzepacz et al. 1992).

Electroencephalographic characteristics in delirium include slowing/dropout of the dominant posterior rhythm, diffuse theta or delta waves (i.e., slowing), poor organization of background rhythm, and loss of reactivity of the EEG to eye opening and closing (Jacobson and Jerrier

2000). Similarly, quantitative electroencephalography (QEEG) in delirium shows parallel findings affecting slowing of power bands' mean frequency.

Table 5–5 describes different electroencephalographic patterns that can be seen clinically in delirium. Although diffuse slowing is the most common presentation, false-negative results occur when a person's characteristic dominant posterior rhythm does not slow sufficiently to drop from the alpha to the theta range, thereby being read as normal despite the presence of abnormal slowing for that individual. (Generally, a change of more than 1 Hz from an individual's baseline is considered abnormal.) Comparison with prior baseline EEGs is often helpful to document that slowing has in fact occurred. Less commonly, but nonetheless important, an EEG may detect focal problems, such as ictal and subictal states or a previously unsuspected tumor that presents with prominent confusion. These include toxic ictal psychosis, nonconvulsive status, and complex partial status epilepticus (Drake and Coffey 1983; Trzepacz 1994a) or focal lesions (Jacobson and Jerrier 2000). New-onset complex partial seizures are underappreciated in the elderly, related to ischemic damage (Sundaram and Dostrow 1995). Jacobson and Jerrier (2000) warned that it can be difficult to distinguish delirium from drowsiness and light sleep unless the technologist includes standard alerting procedures during the EEG. In most cases, EEGs are not needed to make a clinical diagnosis of delirium, instead being used when seizures are suspected or differential diagnosis is difficult, such as in schizophrenic patients with medical illness.

More recent advances in electroencephalographic technologies have expanded our knowledge. Using spectral analysis of delirious elderly patients (about 75% of whom also had dementia), Koponen et al. (1989b) found significant reductions of alpha percentage, increased theta and delta activity, and slowing of the peak and mean frequencies. All of these findings are consistent with electroencephalographic slowing. The study also found a correlation between the severity of cognitive decline and the length of the patient's hospital stay, on one hand, and the degree of electroencephalographic slowing, on the other. Using QEEG, Jacobson et al. (1993a) could distinguish delirious from nondelirious individuals using the relative power of the alpha frequency band and could distinguish delirious from demented patients using theta activity and the relative power of the delta band. Serial EEGs of delirious patients showed associations between the relative power of the alpha band and cognitive ability, whereas in demented patients, the absolute power of the delta band was associated with cognitive changes (Jacobson et al. 1993b). QEEG could replace conventional electroencephalography for delirium assessment in the future (Jacobson and Jerrier 2000).

Evoked potentials may also be abnormal in delirium, suggesting thalamic or subcortical involvement in the production of symptoms. Metabolic causes of delirium precipitate abnormalities in visual, auditory, and somatosensory evoked potentials (Kullmann et al. 1995; Trzepacz 1994a), whereas somatosensory evoked potentials are abnormal in patients whose delirium is due to posttraumatic brain injury, suggesting damage to the medial lemniscus. In general, normalization of evoked potentials parallels clinical improvement, although evoked potentials are not routinely recorded for clinical purposes.

EEGs and evoked potentials in children with delirium show patterns similar to those in adults, with diffuse slowing on EEG and increased latencies of evoked potentials (J. A. Katz et al. 1988; Prugh et al. 1980; Ruijs et al. 1993, 1994). The degree of slowing on EEGs and evoked potentials recorded serially over time in children and adolescents correlates with the severity of delirium and with recovery from delirium (Foley et al. 1981; Montgomery et al. 1991; Onofrj et al. 1991).

Phenomenology

Symptoms

Wolff and Curran's (1935) classic descriptive study of 106 consecutive dysergastic reaction (delirium) patients is still consistent with modern notions of delirium symptoms. More recent reports, however, suffer from inconsistent terminology, unclear definitions of symptoms, and underutilization of standardized symptom assessment tools. This makes it difficult to compare symptom incidences across studies and patient etiologic populations. Nearly all studies are cross-sectional, so we lack an understanding of how various symptoms change over the course

TABLE 5–6. Delirium symptom frequencies reported in studies (not all symptoms reported in all studies)

Symptom	Frequencies from various studies (%)
Disorientation	43, 78, 80, 88, 100
Attentional deficits	17, 62, 100
Clouded consciousness	58, 65, 100
Diffuse cognitive deficits	77
Memory impairment	64, 90
Language deficits	41, 47, 62, 76, 93
Disorganized thinking	95
Sleep-wake cycle disturbance	25, 49, 77, 95, 96
Hallucinations/perceptual disturbance	24, 35, 41
Delusions	18, 19, 25, 68
Affective lability	43, 63
Psychomotor changes	38, 53, 55, 92, 93

of an episode. Even whether sleep disruption occurs as a heralding symptom of delirium is not clear from the limited work in this area.

Despite across-study inconsistencies (Table 5–6) for symptom frequencies, it does appear that certain symptoms appear more often than others, consistent with the proposal that there are core symptoms in delirium irrespective of etiology (Trzepacz 1999b, 2000). Figure 5–4 illustrates how multiple etiologies for delirium may "funnel" into a final common neural pathway (Trzepacz 1999b, 2000) so that the phenomenological expression becomes similar despite a breadth of different physiologies. This also implies that certain brain circuits and neurotransmitter systems are more affected (see the section "Neuropathophysiology" later in this chapter) (Trzepacz 1994a, 1999b, 2000). Candidates for "core" symptoms include attentional deficits, memory

impairment, disorientation, sleep-wake cycle disturbance, thought process abnormalities, motoric alterations, and language disturbances, whereas "associated" or noncore symptoms would include perceptual disturbances (illusions, hallucinations), delusions, and affective changes (Trzepacz 1999b). The presence of associated symptoms might suggest the involvement of specific etiologies that are associated with specific physiologies or with individual differences in brain circuitry and vulnerability. Characteristic diagnostic features of delirium, such as altered state of consciousness (called "clouding" by some) and fluctuation of symptom severity over a 24-hour period, may be epiphenomena and not symptoms per se.

Memory impairment occurs often in delirium, affecting both short-term and long-term memory, although most reports have not distinguished between types of memory impairment. In subclinical hepatic encephalopathy, attention is intact but nonverbal memory is impaired, suggesting that these cognitive functions may be differentially affected with delirium (Tarter et al. 1988). In delirium due to posttraumatic brain injury, procedural and declarative memory are impaired, and procedural memory improves first (Ewert et al. 1985). Patients are usually amnestic for some or all of their delirium episodes.

Language disturbances in delirium include dysnomia, paraphasias, impaired comprehension, dysgraphia, and word-finding difficulties. In extreme cases, language resembles a fluent dysphasia. Incoherent speech or speech disturbance is reported commonly. Dysgraphia was once believed to be specific to delirium (Chedru and Geschwind 1972). A more recent comparison with writing samples from patients with other psychiatric disorders revealed that dysgraphia was not specific (Patten and Lamarre 1989). It appears

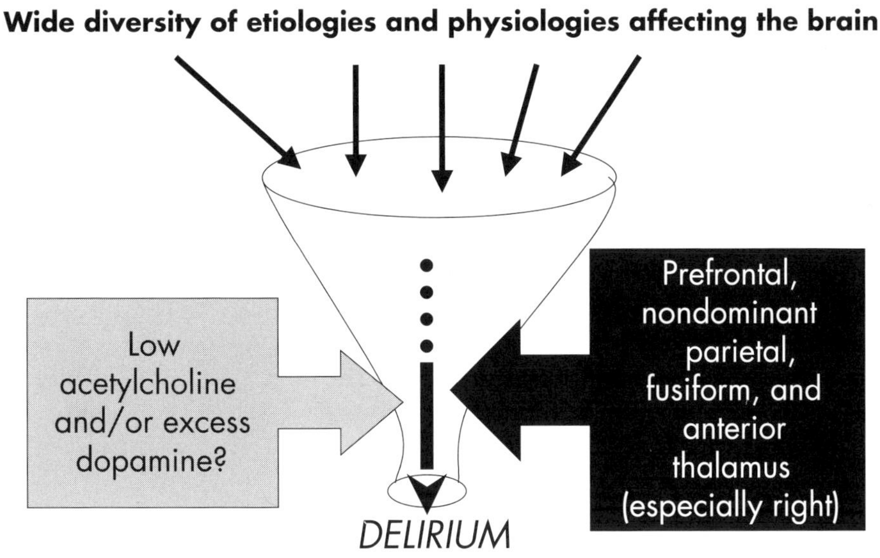

Wide diversity of etiologies and physiologies affecting the brain

FIGURE 5–4. Delirium final common pathway.

that the semantic content of language is a more differentiating feature of delirium.

Disorganized thinking was found in 95% of patients in one study (Rockwood 1993) and was also noted by Cutting (1987) to be different from schizophrenic thought processes. However, very little work has been done to characterize thought process disorder in patients with delirium, which clinically ranges from tangentiality and circumstantiality to loose associations.

Disturbances of the sleep-wake cycle are common in patients with delirium. Sleep-wake cycle disturbances may underlie fluctuations in the severity of symptoms during a 24-hour period. Sleep disturbances range from napping and nocturnal disruptions to a more severe disintegration of the normal circadian cycle. The extent to which sleep-wake cycle disturbance confounds the hyperactive-hypoactive subtyping of delirium is not known.

The type of perceptual disturbance and delusion distinguishes delirium from schizophrenia (Cutting 1987). Hallucina-tions, illusions, other misperceptions, and delusions occur less frequently in delirium than do "core" symptoms. Clinically, the occurrence of visual (as well as tactile, olfactory, and gustatory) hallucinations heightens the likelihood of an identifiable medical problem, although primary psychiatric disorders occasionally present with visual misperceptions. Visual hallucinations range from patterns or shapes to complex and vivid animations, which may vary according to which part of the brain is being affected (Trzepacz 1994a). Persecutory delusions that are poorly formed (not systematized) are the most common type in delirium, although other types can occur (e.g., somatic or grandiose). Delusions do not seem to be a result of cognitive impairment per se.

Affective lability that changes within minutes is characteristic of delirium. It takes many forms (e.g., anxious, apathetic, angry, dysphoric), changes from one type to another without obvious relationship to the context (i.e., incongruent), and is usually not under good self-control.

Motoric Subtypes

Numerous delirium subtyping schema have been suggested, including those based on putative underlying neuropathophysiology, etiology, and symptom profile (Trzepacz 1994a). Motorically defined subgroups have been most studied. Although not all delirious patients express a motoric change, different presentations of psychomotor activity have been recognized for centuries.

Lipowski (1990) combined these concepts under the umbrella of delirium and described three motoric subtypes: "hyperactive," "hypoactive," and "mixed." Definitions of motoric subtypes are subjectively described, not standardized, and include nonmotoric behavioral features such as disturbances of speech, emotion, thinking, and perception. Using such definitions, motoric subtypes have similar degrees of overall cognitive impairment and electroencephalographic slowing (Koponen et al. 1989b; Ross 1991), but they differ for some nonmotoric symptoms. Delusions, hallucinations, mood lability, speech incoherence, and sleep disturbances may be more frequent in hyperactive patients (Meagher and Trzepacz 2000; Ross et al. 1991). Waxing and waning of symptom severity and sleep-wake cycle abnormalities complicate understanding motoric subtypes, as well as reliance on subjective and retrospective reports of behavior over 24-hour periods. There is wide variation among reports of relative frequencies of motoric subtypes (Table 5–7), even when alcohol withdrawal cases are excluded. Objective motor activity level monitoring is needed.

To date, clinical studies have not provided convincing evidence that motoric subtypes have distinct neurobiological underpinnings. The delirium symptom profile of patients with localized cerebral insults does not reliably link specific motoric subtypes to lesions at particular cerebral sites. Moreover, studies of cognition and EEG indicate that both hypoactive and hyperactive delirium are associated with comparable disturbances. Alcohol withdrawal delirium, which is generally hyperactive, is associated with increased beta electroencephalographic activity, but all other causes of delirium are typically associated with diffuse electroencephalographic slowing, regardless of motoric presentation (Trzepacz 1994a). Similarly, functional neuroimaging studies of delirium indicate increased cerebral blood flow in alcohol withdrawal delirium (Hemmingsen et al. 1988), whereas other causes are associated with reductions in global or frontal cerebral blood flow irrespective of motoric subtype (Trzepacz 1994a).

Disturbances of cholinergic systems are the neurochemical aberration most consistently linked to delirium. Evidence from animal studies and normal human volunteers suggests that reduced cholinergic activity is associated with relative hyperactivity, but studies measuring possible markers of CNS cholinergic function in delirium, such as serum anticholinergic activity and cerebrospinal fluid (CSF) somatostatin-like immunoreactivity, have not supported this possibility. Similarly, arguments have been made for involvement of other neurochemical systems (dopamine, serotonin, γ-aminobutyric acid [GABA], histamine), but more study is needed (Meagher and Trzepacz 2000).

Patients with a hyperactive subtype experience better outcomes after an episode of delirium in the form of shorter LOS, lower mortality rates, and a higher rate of full recovery (Kobayashi et al. 1992; Liptzin and Levkoff 1992; Olofsson et al. 1996; Reyes et al. 1981). However, these differences may reflect neuropathophysiological underpinnings, underlying causes, recognition rates, and/or treat-

TABLE 5–7. Studies of frequency of motoric subtypes in delirium

Study	Motoric definition	Hyper %	Hypo %	Mixed %	None %
Koponen et al. 1989a	Lipowski description	38	13	49	—
Koponen et al. 1989b	Lipowski description	31	14	55	—
Ross et al. 1991	Visual analog scale	68	32	—	14
Liptzin and Levkoff 1992	Liptzin and Levkoff criteria	15	19	52	—
Kobayashi et al. 1992	Lipowski description	79	6	15	—
Platt et al. 1994a	Psychomotor item of DRS	37	46	17	—
Uchiyama et al. 1996	Clinical observation	80	20	—	—
Meagher et al. 1996	Liptzin and Levkoff criteria	30	24	46	—
Olofsson et al. 1996	Clinical observation	71	18	11	—
O'Keeffe and Lavan 1999	DAS score during initial 48 hours	21	29	43	7
Okamoto et al. 1999	DSI item	73	—	27	—
Camus et al. 2000	Own checklist	46	26	27	—

Note. Comorbid dementia was not excluded, nor was effect of drug treatment accounted for in most of these studies.
DRS = Delirium Rating Scale; DAS = Delirium Assessment Scale; DSI = Delirium Symptom Inventory.

ment practices. Underdetection is especially common in hypoactive patients. Even when the influence of earlier detection or more active investigation is negated by active screening, hypoactive cases may still have a poorer outcome (O'Keeffe and Lavan 1999). Meagher et al. (1996) found that use of psychotropic medication and supportive environmental ward strategies were more closely linked to level of hyperactivity rather than to the degree of cognitive disturbance. In contrast, Olofsson et al. (1996) reported better outcome in patients with hyperactive delirium but noted that they received less haloperidol than nonhyperactive patients. O'Keeffe and Lavan (1999) reported greater use of neuroleptics and shorter hospital stays in hyperactive patients but linked this to less severe illness at the onset of delirium and a lower incidence of hospital-acquired infections and bedsores in those who were hyperactive. Still other work has found similar outcomes in the different motoric groups (Camus et al. 2000). The precise relationship between motoric subtype, treatment exposure, and outcome therefore remains uncertain.

Clinical experience and one study found comparable efficacy for haloperidol in treating both hypoactive and hyperactive delirious medical patients (Platt et al. 1994a). Uchiyama et al. (1996) found better rates of response to mianserin in delirium with hyperactive motoric presentation compared with hypoactive motoric profile, perhaps related to its sedating effects.

Etiologies of Delirium

Delirium can be caused by a wide variety of etiologies alone or in combination (Table 5–8). These include primary cerebral disorders, systemic disturbances that affect cerebral function, drug/toxin expo-

sure (including intoxication and withdrawal), and a range of factors that can contribute to delirium but have an uncertain role as etiologic factors by themselves (psychological/environmental factors). For an etiology to be considered causal, it should be a recognized possible cause of delirium and should be temporally related in onset and course to delirium presentation, and the delirium should not be better accounted for by other factors.

In studies in which the possibility of multiple etiologies has been considered, between two and six possible causes are typically identified (Breitbart et al. 1996; Francis et al. 1990; Meagher et al. 1996; O'Keeffe 1999; Trzepacz et al. 1985), with a single etiology identified in fewer than 50% of cases (Camus et al. 2000; O'Keeffe 1999; Olofsson et al. 1996). Multiple-etiology delirium is more frequent in the elderly and those with terminal illness.

Some causes are more frequently encountered in particular populations. Drugs and polypharmacy commonly cause or contribute to delirium, especially in the elderly (T.M. Brown 2000). Drug-related causes are more commonly reported in psychiatric populations. Delirium in children and adolescents involves the same categories of etiologies as in adults, although specific causes may differ. Delirium related to illicit drugs is more common in younger populations, whereas that due to prescribed drugs and polypharmacy is more common in older populations. Cerebral hypoxia is common at age extremes, with chronic obstructive airway disease, myocardial infarction, and stroke common in older patients and hypoxia due to foreign body inhalation, drowning, and asthma more frequent in younger patients. Poisonings are also more common in children than in adults, whereas children and the elderly both have high rates of delirium related to head trauma—

TABLE 5–8. Etiologies of delirium

Drug intoxication
  Alcohol
  Sedative-hypnotic
  Opiate
  Psychostimulant
  Hallucinogenic
  Inhalants
  Industrial poisons
  Prescribed or over-the-counter drug
Drug withdrawal
  Alcohol
  Sedative-hypnotic
  Opiate
  Psychostimulants
  Prescribed drug
Metabolic/endocrine disturbance
  Volume depletion/volume overload
  Acidosis/alkalosis
  Hypoxia
  Uremia
  Anemia
  Avitaminosis (B_1, B_6, B_{12}, folate)/
    hypervitaminosis (A, D)
  Hypoglycemia/hyperglycemia
  Hypoalbuminemia/hyperalbuminemia
  Bilirubinemia
  Hypocalcemia/hypercalcemia
  Hypokalemia/hyperkalemia
  Hyponatremia/hypernatremia
  Hypomagnesemia/hypermagnesemia
  Hypophosphatemia
  Hypothyroidism/hyperthyroidism
  Hypoparathyroidism/hyperparathyroidism
  Cushing's syndrome
  Addison's disease
  Hypopituitarism
  Hyperinsulinoma
  Metabolic disorders (porphyria, carcinoid
    syndrome)
Traumatic brain injury
Seizures

Neoplastic disease
  Intracranial primary/metastasis/meningeal
  Carcinomatosis
  Extracranial primary/paraneoplastic syndrome
Intracranial infection
  Meningitis
  Encephalitis
  Abscess
  Neurosyphilis
  Human immunodeficiency virus
Systemic infection
  Bacteremia
  Sepsis
  Fungal
  Protozoal
  Viral
Cerebrovascular disorder
  Transient ischemic attack
  Subarachnoid hemorrhage
  Stroke
  Subdural hemorrhage
  Subdural hematoma
  Cerebral edema
  Cerebral aneurysm
  Hypertensive encephalopathy
  Intraparenchymal hemorrhage
  Cerebral vasculitis
Organ insufficiency
  Cardiac/pulmonary/hepatic/renal/pancreatic
Other central nervous system etiologies
  Parkinson's disease
  Huntington's disease
  Multiple sclerosis
  Wilson's disease
  Hydrocephalus
Other systemic etiologies
  Heat stroke
  Hypothermia
  Radiation
  Electrocution
  Postoperative state
  Immunosuppression
  Fractures

bicycle accidents in children and falls in the elderly.

Once the diagnosis of delirium is made, a careful and thorough, though priori-

tized, search for causes must be conducted. Ameliorations of specific underlying causes are important in resolving delirium, although this should not preclude treatment of the delirium itself, which can reduce symptoms even before underlying medical causes are rectified (Breitbart et al. 1996).

Treatment of Delirium

After the diagnosis of delirium is made, the process of identifying and reversing suspected causes begins. Rapid treatment is important because of the high morbidity and mortality rates associated with delirium. Treatments include medication, environmental manipulation, and patient and family psychosocial support (American Psychiatric Association 1999). However, there is no drug with a U.S. Food and Drug Administration (FDA) indication for the treatment of delirium, and double-blind, placebo-controlled studies are lacking. The American Psychiatric Association (APA) Practice Guidelines on treatment of delirium note the need for such research (American Psychiatric Association 1999).

The use of orienting techniques (e.g., calendars, night-lights, and reorientation by staff) and familiarizing the patient with the environment (e.g., with photographs of family members) are sometimes comforting, although it is important to remember that environmental manipulations alone do not reverse delirium (S.D. Anderson 1995; American Psychiatric Association 1999). It has also been suggested that diurnal cues from natural lighting reduce sensory deprivation and incidence of delirium (Wilson 1972), although sensory deprivation alone is insufficient to cause delirium (Frances 1993).

Pharmacologic treatment with a neuroleptic agent (dopamine D_2 antagonist) is the clinical standard of delirium treatment. Benzodiazepines are generally reserved for delirium due to ethanol or

sedative-hypnotic withdrawal; lorazepam or clonazepam (the latter for alprazolam withdrawal) is often used. Some use lorazepam as an adjunctive medication with haloperidol in severe cases of delirium or when extra assistance with sleep is needed.

The cholinergic deficiency hypothesis of delirium suggests that treatment with a cholinergic enhancer drug could be therapeutic. Physostigmine reverses anticholinergic delirium (Stern 1983), but its side effects (seizures) and short half-life make it unsuitable for routine clinical treatment of delirium. Tacrine was also shown to reverse central anticholinergic syndrome (Mendelson 1977), although it has not been studied formally. Three case reports found that donepezil improved delirium in postoperative state, comorbid Lewy body dementia, and comorbid alcohol dementia (Burke et al. 1999; Wengel et al. 1998, 1999).

Psychostimulants can worsen delirium—probably via increased dopaminergic activity—and have not been recommended when a depressed mood is present (J.A. Levenson 1992; Rosenberg et al. 1991). Whether a combination of a D_2 blocker and a stimulant could treat hypoactive delirium is under study.

Mianserin, a serotonergic tetracyclic antidepressant, has been used in Japan for delirium in elderly medical and postsurgical cohorts, administered either orally or as a suppository. Several open-label studies found reductions in DRS scores similar to those seen when using haloperidol (J. Nakamura et al. 1995, 1997a, 1997b; Uchiyama et al. 1996). The efficacy of mianserin was theorized to be due to its effect on the sleep-wake cycle and/or to its weak D_2 receptor antagonism in conjunction with blockade of postsynaptic serotonin type 2 (5-HT_2), presynaptic α-adrenergic, and histamine type 1 (H_1) and type 2 (H_2) receptor blockade.

A single 8-mg intravenous dose of ondansetron, a serotonin type 3 (5-HT$_3$) antagonist, was reported to reduce agitation in delirium patients when a 4-point rating scale was applied prospectively in 35 postcardiotomy patients (mean age = 51 years) (Bayindir et al. 2000). Further research is needed to more carefully assess cognitive and other behavioral effects of this agent.

Haloperidol is the neuroleptic agent most often chosen for the treatment of delirium. It can be administered orally, intramuscularly, or intravenously (Adams 1984, 1988; Dudley et al. 1979; Gelfand et al. 1992; Moulaert 1989; Sanders and Stern 1993; Tesar et al. 1985), although the intravenous route has not been approved by the FDA. Intravenously administered haloperidol is twice as potent as that taken orally (Gelfand et al. 1992). Bolus intravenous doses usually range from 0.5 to 20 mg, although larger doses are sometimes given. In severe, refractory cases, continuous intravenous infusions of 15–25 mg/hr (up to 1,000 mg/day) can be given (Fernandez et al. 1988; J.L. Levenson 1995; Riker et al. 1994; Stern 1994).

The specific brain effects of haloperidol in alleviating delirium are not known, but positron emission tomographic scans show reduced glucose utilization in the limbic cortex, thalamus, caudate nucleus, and frontal and anterior cingulate cortices (Bartlett et al. 1994). These regions are important for behavior and cognition and have been implicated in the neuropathogenesis of delirium.

Based on clinical usage, haloperidol has been considered to be relatively safe in the seriously medically ill and does not cause as much hypotension as droperidol (Gelfand et al. 1992; Moulaert 1989; Tesar et al. 1985). Haloperidol does not antagonize dopamine-induced increases in renal blood flow (Armstrong et al. 1986).

When haloperidol is given intravenously, extrapyramidal symptoms have been considered unusual (Menza et al. 1987; Tesar et al. 1986), except in human immunodeficiency virus (HIV) and Lewy body dementia (Fernandez et al. 1989; McKeith et al. 1992; Swenson et al. 1989). In a case series of five ICU patients receiving 250–500 mg/day of continuous or intermittent intravenous haloperidol, patients had self-limited withdrawal dyskinesia after receiving high-dose haloperidol (Riker et al. 1997). Intravenous lorazepam is sometimes combined with intravenous haloperidol in critically ill cancer patients to lessen extrapyramidal symptoms and produces a deeply sedated state for several days (Menza et al. 1988).

Cases of prolonged QT$_c$ interval on electrocardiogram (ECG) and torsades de pointes tachyarrhythmia (multifocal ventricular tachycardia) have been attributed to intravenously administered haloperidol (Hatta et al. 2001; Huyse 1988; Kriwisky et al. 1990; Metzger and Friedman 1993; O'Brien et al. 1999; Perrault et al. 2000; Wilt et al. 1993; Zee-Cheng et al. 1985). This is a potentially life-threatening event. Risk factors for this arrhythmia are not clearly identified, but prolonged QT$_c$ increases its risk (Sanders et al. 1991). The APA Treatment Guidelines for Delirium (American Psychiatric Association 1999) recommend that QT$_c$ prolongation greater than 450 msec or to greater than 25% over a previous ECG may warrant telemetry, cardiological consultation, dose reduction, or discontinuation. They also recommend monitoring serum magnesium and potassium in critically ill delirious patients whose QT$_c$ is ≥450 msec because of the common use of concomittant drugs and/or electrolyte disturbances that also can prolong the QT$_c$ interval. Wilt et al. (1993) found only 4 cases of torsades de pointes in 1,100 consecutive cases of haloperidol-treated patients admitted to an ICU, and cases who have severe cardiac disease have been reported to tolerate intravenous haloperidol without complication (Tesar et al. 1985), even at daily doses exceeding 1,000 mg (Sanders et al. 1991). In pigs, intravenous haloperidol (50-mg boluses) does not alter mean heart rate, QRS duration, or QT_c interval; in fact, it raises the ventricular fibrillation threshold (Tisdale et al. 1991). However, large intravenous doses of haloperidol were implicated in causing torsades de pointes tachycardia in a delirious post–coronary artery bypass graft patient in the absence of QT_c prolongation (Perrault et al. 2000). High-dose intravenous haloperidol (80 mg) was reported to cause torsades de pointes in an agitated 41-year-old woman without predisposing factors at the first hour of treatment when her QT_c was noted to be 610 msec (O'Brien et al. 1999). A cross-sectional cohort study compared 34 patients receiving intravenous haloperidol plus flunitrazepam to 13 receiving intravenous flunitrazepam for emergency treatment of agitation alone while the ECG was continuously monitored (Hatta et al. 2001). They found mean QT_c was significantly prolonged at 8 hours in the haloperidol group ($P<0.001$), including 4 patients with $QT_c > 500$ msec, and there was a modest correlation between QT_c prolongation and haloperidol dose. These authors note that during agitation the myocardium receives adrenergic stimulation that can trigger automatic ventricular activity and facilitate the onset of reentrant arrhythmias.

Empirical evidence for neuroleptic benefits in treating delirium is substantial, but treatment studies are rare. Itil and Fink (1966) found that chlorpromazine reversed anticholinergic delirium. Using standardized assessment methods and a double-blind, randomized controlled design, Breitbart et al. (1996) found that delirium in acquired immunodeficiency syndrome (AIDS) patients significantly improved with haloperidol or chlorpromazine, but not with lorazepam. In addition, both hypoactive and hyperactive subtypes responded to treatment with haloperidol or chlorpromazine (Platt et al. 1994a). Improvement was noted within hours of treatment, even before the underlying medical causes were addressed (Platt et al. 1994a). Thus, delirium irrespective of motoric presentation should be treated in parallel to identifying and managing comorbid medical conditions.

Haloperidol use in pediatric patients with delirium is not well documented, despite its use in adult delirium and in many other childhood psychiatric disorders (Teicher and Gold 1990). Its efficacy in children for delusions, hallucinations, thought disorder, aggressivity, stereotypies, hyperactivity, social withdrawal, and learning ability (Teicher and Gold 1990) suggests that it may have a potentially beneficial role in pediatric delirium. Clinical experience with haloperidol in pediatric delirium supports its beneficial effects, although there are no controlled studies. A retrospective report of 30 children (mean age, 7 ± 1.0 years; range 8 months to 18 years) with burn injuries supports the use of haloperidol for agitation, disorientation, hallucinations, delusions, and insomnia (Brown et al. 1996). The mean dose of haloperidol was 0.47 ± 0.002 mg/kg, with a mean maximum dose in 24 hours of 0.455 mg/kg, administered intravenously, orally, and intramuscularly. Mean efficacy, as scored on a 0–3 point scale (3 = excellent), was 2.3 ± 0.21, but the drug was not efficacious in 17% of cases (4 of 5 of these failures were via the oral route). Extrapyramidal symptoms were not observed, and there was one episode of hypotension with the intravenous route.

In other psychiatric disorders, pediatric haloperidol doses range from 0.25 to 10 mg/day or from 0.04 to 0.06 mg/kg per day (Locasio et al. 1991; Malone et al. 1991; Spencer et al. 1992). Side effects are similar to those in adults. Sedation and extrapyramidal symptoms occur frequently (Spencer et al. 1992), except in preschool-age children (Teicher and Gold 1990). Dystonias occur more often in adolescents than in children (Teicher and Gold 1990).

Droperidol is sometimes used to treat patients with acute agitation and confusion from a variety of causes, including mania and delirium (Hooper and Minter 1983; Resnick and Burton 1984; H. Thomas et al. 1992), and is superior to placebo (van Leeuwen et al. 1977). After initial use in patients with severe agitated delirium, droperidol can be replaced by haloperidol for continued treatment. Compared with haloperidol, droperidol is more sedating, has a faster onset of action, can only be used parenterally, and is very hypotensive due to potent α-adrenergic antagonism, although continuous intravenous to infusion of 1–10 mg/hr causes less hypotension than do intravenous boluses (Moulaert 1989). Having the patient lie supine is helpful. Dosing is similar to haloperidol, although it may have less antipsychotic activity and fewer extrapyramidal symptoms (Frye et al. 1995). Prolonged QT_c intervals can occur with droperidol (Lawrence and Nasraway 1997; Lischke et al. 1994), although there were no associated ventricular arrhythmias noted in a small series of patients with cardiac conditions (Frye et al. 1995). However, oral droperidol (and thioridazine) was recently reported in Europe to significantly prolong the QT_c interval in a dose-related manner in a study of 495 patients and 101 healthy volunteers (Reilly et al. 2000). Droperidol has been recently withdrawn from the market in several European countries because of risk-benefit issues.

So-called atypical antipsychotic agents—more novel neuroleptic drugs—differ from haloperidol and other conventional neuroleptics in a variety of neurotransmitter activities, in particular serotonin. Some are being used to treat delirium, also mentioned in a few case reports. Receptor activities and adverse event profiles differ among the atypical agents, and extrapyramidal symptoms, QT_c prolongation, and effects on cognition are particularly relevant to any use in delirium.

Clozapine, the first atypical antipsychotic agent, is clinically distinct from the others. It is very sedating, has significant anticholinergic side effects, causes sinus tachycardia, lowers seizure threshold, and is associated with causing agranulocytosis. Clozapine has been reported to cause delirium in 8% of 315 psychiatric inpatients, and in 7 of these 33 delirium cases it was the only drug used (Gaertner et al. 1989). Cholinergic agents were reported to reverse treatment-emergent delirium during clozapine therapy (Schuster et al. 1977).

Risperidone (mean dose, 1.59 ± 0.8 mg/day) has been reported to reduce delirium severity in 8 of 11 patients as measured on the Clinical Global Impression Scale in an open-label case series, with the maximum response on the 5th day (Sipahimalani and Masand 1997). However, in four cases, risperidone use was reported to cause delirium (Chen and Cardasis 1996; Ravona-Springer et al. 1998). Risperidone has dose-related extrapyramidal symptoms beginning at about 2 mg/day based on double-blind placebo-controlled studies (I. R. Katz et al. 1999).

Eleven delirious patients treated with olanzapine (mean dose, 8.2 ± 3.4 mg at bedtime) were compared with 11 delirious patients treated with haloperidol (mean dose, 5.1 ± 3.5 mg at bedtime) in an open-label nonrandomized case series (Masand and Sipahimalani 1998). Drug efficacy was comparable when measured as a greater than 50% reduction on the DRS, although 5 haloperidol patients had extrapyramidal symptoms or excessive sedation versus none in the olanzapine group. Delirium in a medically ill cancer patient responded to olanzapine 10 mg without adverse effects (Passik and Cooper 1999). Breitbart et al. (2002) described 79 consecutive delirious cancer inpatients (mean age = 60 years)—80% of whom had metastases (20% in the brain)—who were treated with olanzapine (dose range = 2.5–20 mg) for delirium. Using standardized measures, the researchers found olanzapine to have a high degree of efficacy (resolution in 76% of patients) and tolerability, without extrapyramidal symptoms. Olanzapine has a favorable extrapyramidal symptom profile and does not appear to have a clinically significant effect on the QT_c interval at therapeutic doses in schizophrenia patients (Czekalla et al. 2001). Olanzapine significantly improved cognitive function to a greater extent than either risperidone or haloperidol, which did not significantly differ from each other, in a head-to-head trial in early-phase schizophrenic patients as measured by sensitive neuropsychological tests (Purdon et al. 2000). Olanzapine increases acetylcholine release measured by in vivo microdialysis in both rat prefrontal cortex (Meltzer 1999) and hippocampus (Schirazi et al. 2000), consistent with procholinergic activity that may improve cognition. Kennedy and colleagues (2001) theorized that presynaptic effects of olanzapine at 5-HT_3, serotonin type 6 (5-HT_6), and m2 receptors may account for this increased acetylcholine release.

A retrospective study of remoxipride (median dose, 75 mg; range, 50–300 mg) in 103 elderly persons, 73 of whom had

delirium (comorbid with dementia in 70 of 73) using DSM-III-R criteria, reported efficacy for 65% of patients with side effects in 25% (tiredness, extrapyramidal symptoms, aggressiveness) (Robertsson et al. 1996). Although it may have had some efficacy for delirium, remoxipride was withdrawn from the market due to an association with aplastic anemia.

There are no reports for ziprasidone or quetiapine use for delirium at this time. However, quetiapine 300 mg bid has been reported to cause delirium in a 62-year-old man, which was associated with a change on his EEG (slowing) compared with a prior normal EEG (Sim et al. 2000). A previous right thalamic lacunar infarct may have increased his risk for delirium. The delirium cleared when quetiapine was discontinued.

Further delirium treatment research is needed, especially randomized, double-blind, placebo-controlled trials. Unlike haloperidol and droperidol, atypical agents have not been available in parenteral forms in the United States, which are often useful in confused patients. Intramuscular forms of olanzapine and ziprasidone are under FDA consideration for agitation in psychiatric patients. Olanzapine has a rapidly dissolving oral formulation that is placed on the tongue, although it has not yet been reported for use in delirium.

Neuropathophysiology

The Final Common Neural Pathway in Delirium

Delirium is considered to result from a generalized disturbance of higher cerebral cortical processes, as reflected by diffuse slowing on the EEG and a breadth of symptoms (cognition, perception, sleep, motor, language, and thought). However, it is not accompanied by primary motor or sensory deficits except when related to a specific etiology (e.g., asterixis). Thus, not all brain regions are equally affected in delirium. Certain regions, circuits, and neurochemistry may be integral in the neuropathogenesis of delirium (Trzepacz 1994a, 1999b, 2000). Henon et al. (1999) found that laterality of lesion location and not metabolic factors accounted for the differences in delirium incidence for superficial cortical lesions.

Even though delirium has many different etiologies, each with its own physiological effects on the body, its constellation of symptoms is largely stereotyped, with some considered "core" symptoms. Somehow this diversity of physiological perturbations translates into a common clinical expression that may well relate to dysfunction of certain neural circuits (as well as neurotransmitters)—that is, a final common neural pathway (Trzepacz 1999b, 2000). An analogy of a funnel (see Figure 5–4) can be used to represent this common neural circuitry. Studies support certain pathways being involved. Specifically, bilateral or right prefrontal cortex, superficial right posterior parietal cortex, basal ganglia, either fusiform cortex (ventromesial temporoparietal) and lingual gyrus, and right anterior thalamus appear to be particularly associated with delirium (Trzepacz 2000). In addition, the pathways linking them (thalamic-frontal-subcortical and temporolimbic-frontal/subcortical) are likely involved. This hypothesis is largely based on structural neuroimaging reports (Table 5–9), only a few of which are consecutive and prospective in design, and a limited number of functional neuroimaging studies.

Lateralization to more right-sided circuitry involvement in delirium is also supported by evidence besides lesion studies. The right prefrontal cortex cognitively processes novel situations, in contrast to the left (which processes familiar situations), and this may account for delirium patients' difficulties with comprehending new environments (E.L. Goldberg 1998). The right posterior parietal cortex subserves sustained attention and attention to the environment (Posner and Boies 1971), and both are often impaired in delirium. Bipolar patients had the highest incidence of delirium (35.5%) among 199 psychiatric inpatients (Ritchie et al. 1996), and because right-sided anterior and subcortical pathways have been implicated in mania (Blumberg et al. 1999), this suggests a predisposition to delirium possibly based on neuroanatomy. Bell's mania is a severe form of mania that causes pseudodelirium. Visual attention and visual memory tests—assessing nondominant hemisphere cognitive functions—distinguished delirious from nondelirious patients (Hart et al. 1997). Dopamine neurotransmission is lateralized such that activity is normally higher in the left prefrontal cortex (Glick et al. 1982), and this difference may become more extreme if right-sided pathways are affected in delirium.

Lesions of the right posterior parietal cortex may be present with severe delirium that overshadows sensory deficits (Boiten and Lodder 1989; Koponen et al. 1989a; Mesulam et al. 1976; Price and Mesulam 1985). Infarctions distributed in the right middle cerebral artery produce fewer localizing neurologic signs when they are accompanied by agitated delirium (Schmidley and Messing 1984). Lesions of the fusiform region may be associated with an acute, agitated delirium accompanied by visual impairment (Horenstein et al. 1967; Medina et al. 1974, 1977). Despite their posterior location, lesions in this basal temporal region also may affect functions of the prefrontal cortex via temporolimbic-frontal pathways.

TABLE 5–9.   Lesions associated with delirium in structural neuroimaging studies

Authors	Lesions associated with delirium
Mesulam et al. 1976; Price and Mesulam 1985	CVA in R posterior parietal, R prefrontal, ventromedial temporal, or occipital cortex
Horenstein et al. 1967	CVAs in fusiform and calcarine cortices
Medina et al. 1977	L or bilateral mesial temporal-occipital CVA
Medina et al. 1974	L hippocampal or fusiform CVA
Vaphiades et al. 1996	R mesial occipital, parahippocampal, and hippocampus (with visual hallucinations)
Nighoghossian et al. 1992	R subcortical CVA (with frontal deactivation)
Bogousslavsky et al. 1988	R anterior thalamus CVA on preexisting L caudate lesion (with ↓ frontal perfusion on SPECT)
Figiel et al. 1989; Martin et al. 1992	Lesions in caudate nucleus (in depressed patients treated with ECT or medications)
Figiel et al. 1991	Parkinson's disease patients (depressed and treated with ECT or medications)
Koponen et al. 1989a	R prefrontal or posterior parietal cortex CVA (many with comorbid dementia)
Dunne et al. 1986	R temporoparietal CVA
Mullaly et al. 1982	R temporal or parietal CVA
Boiten and Lodder 1989	R inferior parietal lobule CVA
Santamaria et al. 1984; Friedman 1985	R anteromedial thalamus CVA
Henon et al. 1999	R superficial CVA (prospective sample)

Note.   ECT = electroconvulsive therapy; CVA = cerebrovascular accident (stroke); L = left; R = right; SPECT = single photon emission computed tomography.
Source.   Reprinted from Trzepacz PT: "Is There a Final Common Neural Pathway in Delirium? Focus on Acetylcholine and Dopamine." *Seminars in Clinical Neuropsychiatry* 5:132-148, 2000. Copyright 2000, with permission from Elsevier.

The thalamus is uniquely positioned to filter, integrate, and regulate information among the brain stem, cortex, and subcortex. The anterior, medial, and dorsal thalamic nuclei have important interconnections with prefrontal, subcortical, and limbic areas that are involved in cognitive and behavioral functions. Because the thalamus is extensively and reciprocally interconnected with all areas of the cerebral cortex, a relatively small thalamic lesion can cause delirium. The thalamus is rich in GABAergic interneurons and glutamatergic neurons (Sherman and Kock 1990) and receives cholinergic, noradrenergic, and serotonergic afferents from brain stem nuclei. Muscarinic influences at the thalamus affect baseline elec-

troencephalographic rhythm. Strokes in the right paramedian and anteromedial thalamus (Bogousslavsky et al. 1988; Friedman 1985; Santamaria et al. 1984) can cause delirium.

Basal ganglia lesions are also associated with delirium. Preexisting lesions of the caudate nucleus (Figiel et al. 1989; Martin et al. 1992) and Parkinson's disease (Figiel et al. 1991) increase the risk of delirium during electroconvulsive therapy and with the use of tricyclic antidepressants. From a study of delirium incidence among 175 consecutive dementia patients, Robertsson et al. (1998) concluded that subcortical damage increased delirium risk and that patients with vascular dementia were more at risk than were those with early

Alzheimer's or frontotemporal dementia.

A retrospective study of 661 stroke patients found 33% to be acutely confused on presentation (Dunne et al. 1986). The 19 patients diagnosed as having delirium almost exclusively had right-sided temporoparietal cortex lesions, although another 26 patients with similar lesions were not classified as having delirium because they lacked "clouded consciousness," which likely underdiagnosed the frequency of delirium associated with such lesions. A retrospective study of 309 neurology consultations found 60 patients with acute confusional state; those with focal lesions had mostly right temporal or parietal locations (Mullaly et al. 1982).

There are a few prospective studies of stroke location and delirium incidence. Using DSM-IV criteria and a DRS score of 10 or more points to define cases, 202 consecutive stroke patients had a 25% incidence of delirium (Henon et al. 1999). Right-sided superficial cortical lesions were more associated with delirium than were left-sided lesions ($P = 0.009$), whereas deep lesions did not show laterality. Computed tomographic scans for 69 consecutively admitted delirious (DSM-III diagnosis) elderly patients, many of whom had comorbid dementia, were compared with 31 age-matched control subjects with other neurological disorders (Koponen et al. 1989a). Delirious patients had more generalized atrophy and focal changes, in particular right hemisphere lesions in the parieto-occipital association area. Using DSM-III-R criteria, 48% of 155 consecutive stroke patients were acutely confused (Gustafson et al. 1991). Among these, more patients with left-sided lesions were confused (58%) than those with right-sided lesions (38%), although the study was not designed to assess effects of laterality. Thus, many patients with strokes can become delirious, through a variety of chemical or structural mechanisms—for example, glutamatergic surges and cholinergic deficiency—but the majority of evidence supports laterality for cortical and thalamic lesions.

Findings from single photon emission computed tomography (SPECT) and positron emission tomography (PET) scans also support the relevance of the prefrontal cortex and subcortical regions in patients with delirium (Trzepacz 1994a). These tests usually show reduced flow or metabolism in the frontal cortex and either increased or decreased flow in subcortical regions. Dysfunction in both cortical and subcortical regions in delirium is also supported by slowing on EEG and evoked potentials (see discussion in "Electroencephalography" section earlier in this chapter).

Neurotransmission

A final common neural pathway for delirium could have neuroanatomical and neurochemical components. The predominance of evidence in the literature supports a low cholinergic excess dopaminergic state in this final common neural theory (Trzepacz 1996, 2000). Although other neurotransmitter systems are known to be involved for certain etiologies (e.g., hepatic insufficiency or alcohol withdrawal deliria), the activity of cholinergic and dopaminergic pathways can be regulated and affected by these neurotransmitters, including serotonergic, opiatergic, GABAergic, and glutamatergic systems. Thus, alterations of these other neurotransmitters may interact with the final common pathway to produce delirium.

Neurotransmission may be altered in many ways, including through widespread effects on oxidative metabolism. Metabolic pathways for the oxidation of glucose involve oxygen, vitamins (cofactors for enzymes), and substrates related to neurotransmission (e.g., amino acids and acetyl coenzyme A). During severe illness, surgery, and trauma, ratios of plasma amino acids may affect synthesis in the brain of neurotransmitters that are associated with immune activation and adaptive metabolic changes that redirect energy consumption (van der Mast and Fekkes 2000).

Whereas some etiologies of delirium alter neurotransmission via general metabolism, others may antagonize or interfere with specific receptors and transmitters. There is evidence for both specific and widespread effects on neurotransmission in delirium. In addition to changes in major neurotransmitter systems, neurotoxic metabolites, such as quinolinic acid from tryptophan metabolism (Basile et al. 1995), and false transmitters, such as octopamine in patients with liver failure, can alter neurotransmission and also have been implicated in the neuropathogenesis of delirium. Because glia regulate neurotransmitter amounts in the synapse, glial dysfunction may also be involved.

A wide variety of medications and their metabolites have anticholinergic activity and cause delirium. Some act postsynaptically; others act presynaptically; and still others, such as norfentanyl and normeperidine, have anticholinergic metabolites (Coffman and Dilsaver 1988). Tune et al. (1992) studied and measured the anticholinergic activity of many medications in "atropine equivalents." They identified medications usually not recognized as being anticholinergic (e.g., digoxin, nifedipine, cimetidine, and codeine). However, the assay used did not discriminate among the muscarinic receptor subtypes, activity at which can result in opposite effects in the brain depending on location in the synapse. Delirium induced by anticholinergic drugs is associated with generalized electroencephalographic slowing and is reversed by treatment with physostigmine or neuroleptics (Itil and Fink 1966; Stern 1983). Centrally active anticholinergic agents can cause electroencephalographic slowing and reduced verbal memory (Sloan et al. 1992).

A rat model of delirium using a range of atropine doses demonstrated similar features as human delirium: cognitive impairment, electroencephalographic slowing, and hyperactivity during objective motor monitoring (Leavitt et al. 1994; Trzepacz et al. 1992). A different rat model using lower atropine doses showed cognitive impairment, but because EEGs were not recorded, intoxication but not delirium per se was shown (O'Hare et al. 1997).

In addition, several medical conditions have anticholinergic effects, including thiamine deficiency, hypoxia, and hypoglycemia, all of which may reduce acetylcholine by affecting the oxidative metabolism of glucose and the production of acetyl coenzyme A, the rate-limiting step for acetylcholine synthesis (Trzepacz 1994a, 1996). Consistent with these findings, glucose has been shown to enhance memory performance via a CNS muscarinic mechanism (Kopf and Baratti 1994). Parietal cortex levels of choline are reduced in chronic hepatic encephalopathy, as measured by magnetic resonance imaging (MRI) spectroscopy (Kreis et al. 1991).

Serum levels of anticholinergic activity are elevated in patients with postoperative delirium and correlate with severity of cognitive impairment (Tune et al. 1981), improving with resolution of the delirium (Mach et al. 1995). Post–electroconvulsive therapy delirium is also associated with higher serum anticholinergic levels (Mondimore et al. 1983). High serum anticholinergic activity levels were associated with reduced self-care ability among nursing home patients (Rovner et al. 1988). A double-blind intervention study in a nursing home showed that reduction of anticholinergic drugs improved cognitive status in those who had had elevated serum anticholinergic levels (Tollefson et al. 1991).

Alzheimer's and vascular dementias reduce cholinergic activity and are associated with increased risk for delirium. Lewy body dementia mimics delirium with its fluctuating symptom severity, confusion, hallucinations (especially visual), delusions, and electroencephalographic slowing and is associated with significant loss of cholinergic nucleus basalis neurons. Its delirium symptoms respond to donepezil (Kaufer et al. 1998). Age-associated changes in cholinergic function also increase delirium propensity.

Stroke and traumatic brain injury are associated with decreased cholinergic activity—especially in the thalamus, amygdala, frontal cortex, hippocampus, and basal forebrain (Yamamoto et al. 1988)—and with increased vulnerability to antimuscarinic drugs (Dixon et al. 1994). The low cholinergic state seems to correlate temporally with delirium following the acute event. Thus, there is broad support for an anticholinergic mechanism for many seemingly diverse mechanisms of delirium.

On the other hand, cholinergic toxicity from organophosphate insecticides, nerve poisons, and tacrine (Trzepacz et al. 1996) can also cause delirium, although this is not as well described as anticholinergic delirium. Perhaps delirium results from extreme imbalances of cholinergic neurotransmitter activity levels.

Increased dopamine activity may occur as a result of reduced cholinergic activity, conceptualized as an imbalance of the activities of dopamine and acetylcholine relative to each other. Hypoxia is associated with increased release of dopamine while decreasing the release of acetylcholine (Broderick and Gibson 1989). In striatum, D_2 receptor stimulation reduces

acetylcholine release, whereas D_1 stimulation increases it (Ikarashi et al. 1997).

Delirium can occur from intoxication with dopaminergic drugs, including levodopa, dopamine, and bupropion (Ames et al. 1992), and from cocaine binges (Wetli et al. 1996). Patients with alcohol withdrawal delirium are more likely to have the A-9 allele of the dopamine transporter gene compared with matched control subjects without delirium (Sander et al. 1997), suggesting a role for dopamine in delirium propensity. Delirium from opiates may be mediated by increased dopamine and glutamate activity in addition to decreased acetylcholine. Hypoxia increases the release of dopamine (Broderick and Gibson 1989), in addition to decreasing acetylcholine (Gibson et al. 1975). Excess dopamine levels occur during hepatic encephalopathy, presumably owing to increased levels of tyrosine and phenylalanine in CSF (Knell et al. 1974) or to changes in dopamine regulation by altered serotonin activity. Dopamine agonists (active at D_1 and D_2 receptors) have been shown to cause electroencephalographic slowing and behavioral arousal in rats (Ongini et al. 1985), findings similar to those seen in rats treated with atropine (Leavitt et al. 1994; Trzepacz et al. 1992). A rat model for delirium using apomorphine (a direct D_1 and D_2 agonist) in a choice reaction task showed reversal of performance deficits by administration of haloperidol and aniracetam, a cholinomimetic, but not by administration of tacrine, which worsened them (K. Nakamura et al. 1998). The investigators concluded that cognitive deficits were mediated by a D_2 mechanism, but because EEGs were not recorded, it is not clear if this could be a delirium animal model.

Little is known about which dopamine receptor subtypes are involved in the neuropathogenesis of delirium, although those related to mesolimbic and mesofrontal dopaminergic pathways are probably involved. Antidopaminergic agents, particularly neuroleptics, can be successfully used to treat delirium, including that arising from anticholinergic causes (Itil and Fink 1966; Platt et al. 1994a). Traditional neuroleptics that are effective in treating delirium are not subtype specific; haloperidol predominantly affects D_2 receptors, although it also affects D_1, D_3, and D_4 receptors (Piercey et al. 1995). Use of selective dopamine antagonists might shed light on the mechanism underlying delirium. For example, differential effects on D_1, D_2, and D_3 receptors might underlie different motoric presentations during an individual delirium episode (Trzepacz 2000).

Both increased and decreased GABA have been implicated in causing delirium. Increased GABAergic activity, in addition to reduced glutamate and increased serotonin activity, is one of several putative mechanisms implicated in hepatic encephalopathy (Mousseau and Butterworth 1994). Increased GABA activity may result from elevated ammonia levels, which increase levels of glutamate and glutamine, which are then converted into GABA (B. Anderson 1984; Schafer and Jones 1982). Consistent with this hypothesis is the improvement observed in some patients with hepatic encephalopathy using flumazenil, which blocks $GABA_A$-benzodiazepine receptors. Glutamine levels have been shown to be elevated in hepatic encephalopathy as measured by MRI spectroscopy, although the chemical relationships among glutamine, GABA, and glutamate confound the meaning of this measurement (Kreis et al. 1991). Reduced GABA activity occurs during delirium due to withdrawal from ethanol and sedative-hypnotic drugs. Decreased GABA activity is also implicated in the mechanism of antibiotic delirium caused by penicillins, cephalosporins, and quinolones (Akaike et al. 1991; Mathers 1987).

Both low and excessive levels of serotonin are associated with delirium (van der Mast and Fekkes 2000). Serotonin activity may be increased in patients with hepatic encephalopathy—related to increased tryptophan uptake in the brain (Mousseau and Butterworth 1994; van der Mast and Fekkes 2000)—as well as in sepsis (Mizock et al. 1990) and serotonergic syndromes (Goldberg and Huk 1992). The precursor of serotonin, tryptophan, is also implicated in delirium. Increases in free tryptophan levels in plasma correlate with reductions in cerebral blood flow on xenon computed tomographic scans in patients with subclinical hepatic encephalopathy (Rodriguez et al. 1987), and l-5-hydroxytryptophan induces delirium (Irwin et al. 1986). In contrast, tryptophan is decreased in patients with postcardiotomy delirium (van der Mast et al. 1994). Serotonin regulates dopamine activity in some brain regions, including the striatum and limbic system (Meltzer 1993), which may explain why neuroleptics are useful in treating serotonergic deliria.

Histamine may play a role in delirium through its effects on arousal and hypothalamic regulation of sleep-wake circadian rhythms. H_1 agonists and H_3 antagonists increase wakefulness (Monti 1993), whereas antihistamines (H_1 antagonists) reduce arousal and are associated with rapid eye movement (REM) sleep (Marzanatti et al. 1989) and delirium (Tejera et al. 1994). H_1 antagonists increase catechols and serotonin levels and have anticholinergic properties (Jones et al. 1986), possibly mediating delirium. H_2 antagonists also cause delirium, possibly related to their anticholinergic properties (Picotte-Prillmayer et al. 1995), although they do not affect brain sleep centers.

Glutamate release is increased during

hypoxia, and glutamatergic receptors may be activated by quinolone antibiotics (Williams and Helton 1991). Activation of glutamatergic receptors is a possible mechanism for quinolones causing delirium. Dopamine and glutamate are both neurotransmitters at the thalamus, a region potentially important in the neuropathogenesis of delirium.

Cytokines have been implicated as causes of inflammatory or infectious-induced delirium, and they also may have a role in sleep (Moldofsky et al. 1986). They are polypeptide hormones secreted in the CNS by glia and macrophages, whose normally low extracellular levels are increased during stress, rapid growth, inflammation, tumor, trauma, and infection (Hopkins and Rothwell 1995; Rothwell and Hopkins 1995; Stefano et al. 1994). Although cytokines are not yet identified as neurotransmitters per se, they may influence the activities of catecholamines, indolamines, GABA, and acetylcholine (Rothwell and Hopkins 1995) and cause increased release and turnover of dopamine and norepinephrine (Stefano et al. 1994), thereby causing delirium. Cytokines acting as neurotoxins, as in HIV dementia, is another mechanism for causing brain dysfunction (Lipton and Gendelman 1995).

Conclusions

Delirium is a common neuropsychiatric disorder affecting cognition, thinking, perception, sleep, language, and other behaviors. It is associated with an increased mortality rate, the attribution of which to delirium itself or underlying medical problems is unclear. It affects persons of any age, although elderly patients may be particularly vulnerable, especially if demented. Research on delirium in children is sorely needed. The assessment of delirium can be aided through the use of diagnostic criteria and rating scales, as well as knowledge of which populations are at risk.

Certain symptoms of delirium may represent "core" symptoms, whereas others may be associated symptoms that occur under certain conditions. Core symptoms may reflect dysfunction of certain brain regions and neurotransmitter systems that constitute a "final common neural pathway" that is responsible for the presentation of the syndrome of delirium. Regions implicated include prefrontal cortex, thalamus, basal ganglia, right temporoparietal cortex, and fusiform and lingual gyri. A diversity of physiologies related to the wide variety of etiologies may funnel into a common neurofunctional expression for delirium via elevated brain dopaminergic and reduced cholinergic activity, or a relative imbalance of these. Other neurochemical candidates include serotonin, GABA, and glutamate, although these may interact to regulate and alter activity of acetylcholine and dopamine.

The clinical standard of treatment involves a dopamine antagonist medication—usually haloperidol—although, theoretically, procholinergic drugs should help. There is a dearth of drug treatment studies for delirium, in particular double-blind, and there are none with placebo controls. Newer agents deserve more study as well. It is important to initiate treatment even before medical causes have been rectified, for both hypoactive and hyperactive psychomotoric subtypes.

References

Adams F: Neuropsychiatric evaluation and treatment of delirium in the critically ill cancer patient. Cancer Bull 36:156–160, 1984

Adams F: Emergency intravenous sedation of the delirious medically ill patient. J Clin Psychiatry 49 (suppl):22–26, 1988

Akaike N, Shirasaki T, Yakushiji T: Quinolone and fenbufen interact with GABA-A receptors in dissociated hippocampal cells of rats. J Neurophysiol 66:497–504, 1991

American Psychiatric Association: Diagnostic and Statistical Manual of Mental Disorders, 3rd Edition. Washington, DC, American Psychiatric Association, 1980

American Psychiatric Association: Diagnostic and Statistical Manual of Mental Disorders, 3rd Edition, Revised. Washington, DC, American Psychiatric Association, 1987

American Psychiatric Association: Diagnostic and Statistical Manual of Mental Disorders, 4th Edition. Washington, DC, American Psychiatric Association, 1994

American Psychiatric Association: Practice guidelines for the treatment of patients with delirium. Am J Psychiatry 156 (suppl):1–20, 1999

American Psychiatric Association: Diagnostic and Statistical Manual of Mental Disorders, 4th Edition, Text Revision. Washington, DC, American Psychiatric Association, 2000

Ames D, Wirshing WC, Szuba MP: Organic mental disorders associated with bupropion in three patients. J Clin Psychiatry 53:53–55, 1992

Anderson B: A proposed theory for the encephalopathies of Reye's syndrome and hepatic encephalopathy. Med Hypotheses 15:415–420, 1984

Anderson SD: Treatment of elderly patients with delirium. CMAJ 152:323–324, 1995

Andreasen NJC, Hartford CE, Knott JR, et al: EEG changes associated with burn delirium. Dis Nerv Syst 38:27–31, 1977

Armstrong DH, Dasts JF, Reilly TE, et al: Effect of haloperidol on dopamine-induced increase in renal blood flow. Drug Intell Clin Pharm 20:543–546, 1986

Bartlett EJ, Brodie JD, Simkowitz P, et al: Effects of haloperidol challenge on regional cerebral glucose utilization in normal human subjects. Am J Psychiatry 151:681–686, 1994

Basile AS, Saito K, Li Y, et al: The relationship between plasma and brain quinolinic acid levels and the severity of hepatic encephalopathy in animal models of fulminant hepatic failure. J Neurochem 64:2607–2614, 1995

Bayindir O, Akpinar B, Can E, et al: The use of the 5-HT_3-receptor antagonist ondansetron for the treatment of postcardiotomy delirium. J Cardiothorac Vasc Anesth 14:288–292, 2000

Bedford PD: General medical aspects of confusional states in elderly people. Br Med J 2: 185–188, 1957

Blumberg HP, Stern E, Ricketts S, et al: Rostral orbitofrontal prefrontal cortex dysfunction in the manic state of bipolar disorder. Am J Psychiatry 156:1986–1988, 1999

Bogousslavsky J, Ferranzzini M, Regli F, et al: Manic delirium and frontal-like syndrome with paramedian infarction of the right thalamus. J Neurol Neurosurg Psychiatry 51:116–119, 1988

Boiten J, Lodder J: An unusual sequela of a frequently occurring neurologic disorder: delirium caused by brain infarct. Ned Tijdschr Geneeskd 133:617–620, 1989

Brauer C, Morrison S, Silberzweig SB, et al: The cause of delirium in patients with hip fracture. Arch Intern Med 160: 1856–1860, 2000

Breitbart W, Marotta R, Platt MM, et al: A double-blind trial of haloperidol, chlorpromazine, and lorazepam in the treatment of delirium in hospitalized AIDS patients. Am J Psychiatry 153:231–237, 1996

Breitbart W, Rosenfeld B, Roth A, et al: The Memorial Delirium Assessment Scale. J Pain Symptom Manage 13:128–137, 1997

Breitbart W, Tremblay A, Gibson C: An open trial of olanzapine for the treatment of delirium in hospitalized cancer patients. Psychosomatics 43:175–182, 2002

Broderick PA, Gibson GE: Dopamine and serotonin in rat striatum during in vivo hypoxic-hypoxia. Metab Brain Dis 4:143–153, 1989

Brown RL, Henke A, Greenhalgh DG, et al: The use of haloperidol in the agitated, critically ill pediatric patient with burns. J Burn Care Rehabil 17:34–38, 1996

Brown TM: Drug-induced delirium. Semin Clin Neuropsychiatry 5:113–125, 2000

Burke WJ, Roccaforte WH, Wengel SP: Treating visual hallucinations with donepezil. Am J Psychiatry 156:1117–1118, 1999

Cameron DJ, Thomas RI, Mulvihill M, et al: Delirium: a test of DSM-III criteria on medical inpatients. J Am Geriatr Soc 35:1007–1010, 1987

Camus V, Gonthier R, Dubos G, et al: Etiologic and outcome profiles in hypoactive and hyperactive subtypes of delirium. J Geriatr Psychiatry Neurol 13:38–42, 2000

Chedru F, Geschwind N: Writing disturbances in acute confusional states. Neuropsychologia 10:343–353, 1972

Chen B, Cardasis W: Delirium induced by lithium and risperidone combination. Am J Psychiatry 153:1233–1234, 1996

Coffman JA, Dilsaver SC: Cholinergic mechanisms in delirium. Am J Psychiatry 145:382–383, 1988

Cole MG, Primeau FJ: Prognosis of delirium in elderly hospital patients. CMAJ 149:41–46, 1993

Cole MG, Primeau FJ, Bailey RF, et al: Systematic intervention for elderly inpatients with delirium: a randomized trial. CMAJ 151:965–970, 1994

Cutting J: The phenomenology of acute organic psychosis: comparison with acute schizophrenia. Br J Psychiatry 151:324–332, 1987

Czekalla J, Beasley CM Jr, Dellva MA, et al: Analysis of the QTc interval during olanzapine treatment of patients with schizophrenia and related psychoses. J Clin Psychiatry 62:191–198, 2001

Dickson LR: Hypoalbuminemia in delirium. Psychosomatics 32:317–323, 1991

Dixon CE, Hamm RJ, Taft WC, et al: Increased anticholinergic sensitivity following closed skull impact and controlled cortical impact traumatic brain injury in the rat. J Neurotrauma 11:275–287, 1994

Drake ME, Coffey CE: Complex partial status epilepticus simulating psychogenic unresponsiveness. Am J Psychiatry 140:800–801, 1983

Dudley DL, Rowlett DB, Loebel PJ: Emergency use of intravenous haloperidol. Gen Hosp Psychiatry 1:240–246, 1979

Dunne JW, Leedman PJ, Edis RH: Inobvious stroke: a cause of delirium and dementia. Aust N Z J Med 16:771–778, 1986

Ely EW, Gordan S, Francis J, et al: Evaluation of delirium in critically ill patients: validation of the Confusion Assessment Method for the intensive care unit (CAM-ICU). Crit Care Med 29:1370–1379, 2001

Engel GL, Romano J: Delirium, II: reversibility of electroencephalogram with experimental procedures. Archives of Neurology and Psychiatry 51:378–392, 1944

Engel GL, Romano J: Delirium, a syndrome of cerebral insufficiency. J Chronic Dis 9:260–277, 1959

Erkinjuntti T, Wikstrom J, Parlo J, et al: Dementia among medical inpatients: evaluation of 2000 consecutive admissions. Arch Intern Med 146:1923–1926, 1986

Ewert J, Levin HS, Watson MG, et al: Procedural memory during posttraumatic amnesia in survivors of severe closed head injury: implications for rehabilitation. Arch Neurol 46:911–916, 1985

Fann JR: The epidemiology of delirium: a review of studies and methodological issues. Semin Clin Neuropsychiatry 5:86–92, 2000

Fernandez F, Holmes VF, Adams F, et al: Treatment of severe, refractory agitation with a haloperidol drip. J Clin Psychiatry 49:239–241, 1988

Fernandez F, Levy JK, Mansell PWA: Management of delirium in terminally ill AIDS patients. Int J Psychiatry Med 19:165–172, 1989

Figiel GS, Krishman KR, Breitner JC, et al: Radiologic correlates of antidepressant-induced delirium: the possible significance of basal ganglia lesions. J Neuropsychiatry Clin Neurosci 1:188–190, 1989

Figiel GS, Hassen MA, Zorumski C, et al: ECT-induced delirium in depressed patients with Parkinson's disease. J Neuropsychiatry Clin Neurosci 3:405–411, 1991

Foley CM, Polinsky MS, Gruskin AB, et al: Encephalopathy in infants and children with chronic renal disease. Arch Neurol 38:656–658, 1981

Forman LJ, Cavalieri TA, Galski T, et al: Occurrence and impact of suspected delirium in hospitalized elderly patients. J Am Osteopath Assoc 95:588–591, 1995

Frances J: Sensory and environmental factors in delirium. Paper presented at Delirium: Current Advancements in Diagnosis, Treatment and Research, Geriatric Research, Education, and Clinical Center (GRECC), Veterans Administration Medical Center, Minneapolis, MN, September 13–14, 1993

Francis J, Kapoor WN: Prognosis after hospital discharge of older medical patients with delirium. J Am Geriatr Soc 40:601–606, 1992

Francis J, Martin D, Kapoor WN: A prospective study of delirium in hospitalized elderly. JAMA 263:1097–1101, 1990

Friedman JH: Syndrome of diffuse encephalopathy due to nondominant thalamic infarction. Neurology 35:1524–1526, 1985

Frye MA, Coudreaut MF, Hakeman SM, et al: Continuous droperidol infusion for management of agitated delirium in an ICU. Psychosomatics 36:301–305, 1995

Gaertner HJ, Fischer E, Hoss J: Side effects of clozapine. Psychopharmacology 99:S97–S100, 1989

Gelfand SB, Indelicato J, Benjamin J: Using intravenous haloperidol to control delirium (abstract). Hosp Community Psychiatry 43:215, 1992

George J, Bleasdale S, Singleton SJ: Causes and prognosis of delirium in elderly patients admitted to a district general hospital. Age Ageing 26:423–427, 1997

Gibson GE, Jope R, Blass JP: Decreased synthesis of acetylcholine accompanying impaired oxidation of pyruvate in rat brain slices. Biochem J 26:17–23, 1975

Glick SD, Ross DA, Hough LB: Lateral asymmetry of neurotransmitters in human brain. Brain Res 234:53–63, 1982

Goldberg EL: Lateralization of frontal lobe functions and cognitive novelty. J Neuropsychiatry Clin Neurosci 6:371–378, 1998

Goldberg RJ, Huk M: Serotonergic syndrome from trazodone and buspirone (letter). Psychosomatics 33:235–236, 1992

Gustafson Y, Berggren D, Brahnstrom B, et al: Acute confusional states in elderly patients treated for femoral neck fracture. J Am Geriatr Soc 36:525–530, 1988

Gustafson Y, Olsson T, Eriksson S, et al: Acute confusional state (delirium) in stroke patients. Cerebrovasc Dis 1:257–264, 1991

Hales RE, Polly S, Orman D: An evaluation of patients who received an organic mental disorder diagnosis on a psychiatric consultation-liaison service. Gen Hosp Psychiatry 11:88–94, 1988

Hart RP, Levenson JL, Sessler CN, et al: Validation of a cognitive test for delirium in medical ICU patients. Psychosomatics 37:533–546, 1996

Hart RP, Best AM, Sessler CN, et al: Abbreviated Cognitive Test for Delirium. J Psychosom Res 43:417–423, 1997

Hatta K, Takahashi T, Nakamura H, et al: The association between intravenous haloperidol and prolonged QT interval. J Clin Psychopharmacol 21:257–261, 2001

Hemmingsen R, Vorstrup S, Clemmesen L, et al: Cerebral blood flow during delirium tremens and related clinical states studied with xenon-133 inhalation tomography. Am J Psychiatry 145:1384–1390, 1988

Henon H, Lebert F, Durieu I, et al: Confusional state in stroke. Relation to preexisting dementia, patient characteristics and outcome. Stroke 30:773–779, 1999

Henry WD, Mann AM: Diagnosis and treatment of delirium. Can Med Assoc J 93:1156–1166, 1965

Hooper JF, Minter G: Droperidol in the management of psychiatric emergencies. J Clin Psychopharmacol 3:262–263, 1983

Hopkins SJ, Rothwell NJ: Cytokines and the nervous system, I: expression and recognition. Trends Neurosci 18:83–88, 1995

Horenstein S, Chamberlin W, Conomy J: Infarction of the fusiform and calcarine regions: agitated delirium and hemianopia, in Translations of the American Neurological Association 1967, Vol 92. Edited by Yahr MD. New York, Springer, 1967, pp 85–89

Huang S-C, Tsai S-J, Chan C-H, et al: Characteristics and outcome of delirium in psychiatric inpatients. Psychiatry Clin Neurosci 52:47–50, 1998

Huyse F: Haloperidol and cardiac arrest. Lancet 2:568–569, 1988

Ikarashi Y, Takahashi A, Ishimaru H, et al: Regulation of dopamine D1 and D2 receptors on striatal acetylcholine release in rats. Brain Res Bull 43:107–115, 1997

Inouye SK, Charpentier PA: Precipitating factors for delirium in hospitalized elderly patients: predictive model and interrelationships with baseline vulnerability. JAMA 275:852–857, 1996

Inouye SK, van Dyke CH, Alessi CA, et al: Clarifying confusion: the Confusion Assessment Method. Ann Intern Med 113:941–948, 1990

Inouye SK, Viscoli CM, Horwitz RI, et al: A predictive model for delirium in hospitalized elderly medical patients based on admission characteristics. Arch Intern Med 119:474–481, 1993

Inouye SK, Rushing JT, Foreman MD, et al: Does delirium contribute to poor hospital outcome? J Gen Intern Med 13:234–242, 1998

Inouye SK, Bogardus ST, Charpentier PA, et al: A multicomponent intervention to prevent delirium in hospitalized older patients. N Engl J Med 340:669–676, 1999

Irwin M, Fuentenebro F, Marder SR, et al: L-5-Hydroxytryptophan-induced delirium. Biol Psychiatry 21:673–676, 1986

Itil T, Fink M: Anticholinergic drug-induced delirium: experimental modification, quantitative EEG, and behavioral correlations. J Nerv Ment Dis 143:492–507, 1966

Jacobson SA, Jerrier S: EEG in delirium. Semin Clin Neuropsychiatry 5:86–93, 2000

Jacobson SA, Leuchter AF, Walter DO: Conventional and quantitative EEG diagnosis of delirium among the elderly. J Neurol Neurosurg Psychiatry 56:153–158, 1993a

Jacobson SA, Leuchter AF, Walter DO, et al: Serial quantitative EEG among elderly subjects with delirium. Biol Psychiatry 34:135–140, 1993b

Jitapunkul S, Pillay I, Ebrahim S: Delirium in newly admitted elderly patients: a prospective study. Q Med 83:307–314, 1992

Johnson JC, Gottlieb GL, Sullivan E, et al: Using DSM-III criteria to diagnose delirium in elderly general medical patients. J Gerontol 45:M113–M119, 1990

Johnson JC, Kerse NM, Gottlieb G, et al: Prospective versus retrospective methods of identifying patients with delirium. J Am Geriatr Soc 40:316–319, 1992

Jones J, Dougherty J, Cannon L: Diphenhydramine-induced toxic psychosis. Am J Emerg Med 4:369–371, 1986

Katz IR, Jeste DV, Mintzer JE, et al: Comparison of risperidone and placebo for psychosis and behavioral disturbances associated with dementia: a randomized double-blind trial. J Clin Psychiatry 60:107–115, 1999

Katz JA, Mahoney DH, Fernbach DJ: Human leukocyte alpha-interferon induced transient neurotoxicity in children. Invest New Drugs 6:115–120, 1988

Kaufer DI, Catt KE, Lopez OL, et al: Dementia with Lewy bodies: response of delirium-like features to donepezil. Neurology 51:1512–1513, 1998

Kennard MA, Bueding E, Wortis WB: Some biochemical and electroencephalographic changes in delirium tremens. Q Stud Alcohol 6:4–14, 1945

Kennedy JS, Zagar A, Bymaster F, et al: The central cholinergic system profile of olanzapine compared with placebo in Alzheimer's disease. Int J Geriatr Psychiatry 16(suppl 1):S24–S32, 2001

Kishi Y, Iwasaki Y, Takezawa K, et al: Delirium in critical care unit patients admitted through an emergency room. Gen Hosp Psychiatry 17:371–379, 1995

Knaus WA, Draper EA, Wagner DP, et al: APACHE II: a severity of disease classification system. Crit Care Med 13:818–829, 1985

Knell AJ, Davidson AR, Williams R, et al: Dopamine and serotonin metabolism in hepatic encephalopathy. Br Med J 1:549–551, 1974

Kobayashi K, Takeuchi O, Suzuki M, et al: A retrospective study on delirium type. Jpn J Psychiatry Neurol 46:911–917, 1992

Kolbeinsson H, Jonsson A: Delirium and dementia in acute medical admissions of elderly patients in Iceland. Acta Psychiatr Scand 87:123–127, 1993

Kopf SR, Baratti CM: Memory-improving actions of glucose: involvement of a central cholinergic muscarinic mechanism. Behav Neural Biol 62:237–243, 1994

Koponen H, Hurri L, Stenback U, et al: Computed tomography findings in delirium. J Nerv Ment Dis 177:226–231, 1989a

Koponen H, Partanen J, Paakkonen A, et al: EEG spectral analysis in delirium. J Neurol Neurosurg Psychiatry 52:980–985, 1989b

Koponen H, Sirvio J, Lepola U, et al: A long-term follow-up study of cerebrospinal fluid acetylcholinesterase in delirium. Eur Arch Psychiatry Clin Neurosci 243:347–351, 1994

Kreis R, Farrow N, Ross BN: Localized NMR spectroscopy in patients with chronic hepatic encephalopathy: analysis of changes in cerebral glutamine, choline, and inositols. NMR Biomed 4:109–116, 1991

Kriwisky M, Perry GY, Tarchitsky, et al: Haloperidol-induced torsades de pointes. Chest 98:482–484, 1990

Kullmann F, Hollerbach S, Holstege A, et al: Subclinical hepatic encephalopathy: the diagnostic value of evoked potentials. J Hepatol 22:101–110, 1995

Lawlor PG, Gagnon B, Mancini IL, et al: Occurrence, causes and outcome of delirium in patients with advanced cancer. Arch Intern Med 160:786–794, 2000

Lawrence KR, Nasraway SA: Conduction disturbances associated with administration of butyrophenone antipsychotics in the critically ill: a review of the literature. Pharmacotherapy 17:531–537, 1997

Leavitt M, Trzepacz PT, Ciongoli K: Rat model of delirium: atropine dose-response relationships. J Neuropsychiatry Clin Neurosci 6:279–284, 1994

Levenson JA: Should psychostimulants be used to treat delirious patients with depressed mood? (letter). J Clin Psychiatry 53:69, 1992

Levenson JL: High-dose intravenous haloperidol for agitated delirium following lung transplantation. Psychosomatics 36:66–68, 1995

Levkoff SE, Evans DA, Liptzin B, et al: Delirium: the occurrence and persistence of symptoms among elderly hospitalized patients. Arch Intern Med 152:334–340, 1992

Levkoff SE, Liptzin B, Evans D, et al: Progression and resolution of delirium in elderly patients hospitalized for acute care. Am J Geriatr Psychiatry 2:230–238, 1994

Lipowski ZJ: Delirium: Acute Confusional States. New York, Oxford University Press, 1990

Lipton SA, Gendelman HE: Dementia associated with the acquired immunodeficiency syndrome. N Engl J Med 332:934–940, 1995

Liptzin B, Levkoff SE: An empirical study of delirium subtypes. Br J Psychiatry 161:843–845, 1992

Lischke V, Behne M, Doelken P, et al: Droperidol causes a dose-dependent prolongation of the QT interval. Anesth Analg 79:983–986, 1994

Locasio JJ, Malone RP, Small AM, et al: Factors related to haloperidol response and dyskinesias in autistic children. Psychopharmacol Bull 27:119–125, 1991

Mach J, Dysken M, Kuskowski M, et al: Serum anticholinergic activity in hospitalized older persons with delirium: a preliminary study. J Am Geriatr Soc 43:491–495, 1995

Magaziner J, Simonsick EM, Kashner M, et al: Survival experience of aged hip fracture patients. Am J Public Health 79: 274–278, 1989

Malone RP, Ernst M, Godfrey KA, et al: Repeated episodes of neuroleptic-related dyskinesias in autistic children. Psychopharmacol Bull 27:113–117, 1991

Manos PJ: The utility of the ten-point clock test as a screen for cognitive impairment in general hospital patients. Gen Hosp Psychiatry 19:439–444, 1997

Manos PJ, Wu R: The duration of delirium in medical and postoperative patients referred for psychiatric consultation. Ann Clin Psychiatry 9:219–225, 1997

Marcantonio ER, Goldman L, Mangione CM, et al: A clinical prediction rule for delirium after elective noncardiac surgery. JAMA 271:134–139, 1994a

Marcantonio ER, Juarez G, Goldman L, et al: The relationship of postoperative delirium with psychoactive medications. JAMA 272:1518–1522, 1994b

Martin M, Figiel G, Mattingly G, et al: ECT-induced interictal delirium in patients with a history of a CVA. J Geriatr Psychiatry Neurol 5:149–155, 1992

Marzanatti M, Monopoli A, Trampus M, et al: Effects of nonsedating histamine H-1 antagonists on EEG activity and behavior in the cat. Pharmacol Biochem Behav 32: 861–866, 1989

Masand PS, Sipahimalani A: Olanzapine in the treatment of delirium. Psychosomatics 39:422–430, 1998

Mathers DA: The GABA-A receptor: new insights from single channel recording. Synapse 1:96–101, 1987

Matsuoka Y, Miyake Y, Arakaki H, et al: Clinical utility and validation of the Japanese version of the Memorial Delirium Assessment Scale in a psychogeriatric inpatient setting. Gen Hosp Psychiatry 23:36–40, 2001

McKeith I, Fairbairn A, Perry R, et al: Neuroleptic sensitivity in patients with senile dementia of Lewy body type. BMJ 305:673–678, 1992

Meagher DJ, Trzepacz PT: Motoric subtypes of delirium. Semin Clin Neuropsychiatry 5:76–86, 2000

Meagher DJ, O'Hanlon D, O'Mahony E, et al: Use of environmental strategies and psychotropic medication in the management of delirium. Br J Psychiatry 168:512–515, 1996

Medina JL, Rubino FA, Ross E: Agitated delirium caused by infarctions of the hippocampal formation and fusiform and lingual gyri. Neurology 24:1181–1183, 1974

Medina JL, Sudhansu C, Rubino FA: Syndrome of agitated delirium and visual impairment: a manifestation of medial temporo-occipital infarction. J Neurol Neurosurg Psychiatry 40:861–864, 1977

Meltzer HY: Serotonin-dopamine interactions and atypical antipsychotic drugs. Psychiatr Ann 23:193–200, 1993

Meltzer HY, O'Laughlin IA, Dai J, et al: Atypical antipsychotic drugs but not typical increased extracellular acetylcholine levels in rat medial prefrontal cortex in the absence of acetylcholinesterase inhibition. Abstr Soc Neurosci 25:452, 1999

Mendelson G: Pheniramine aminosalicylate overdose. Reversal of delirium and choreiform movements with tacrine treatment. Arch Neurol 34:313, 1977

Menza MA, Murray GB, Holmes VF, et al: Decreased extrapyramidal symptoms with intravenous haloperidol. J Clin Psychiatry 48:278–280, 1987

Menza MA, Murray GB, Holmes VF, et al: Controlled study of extrapyramidal reactions in the management of delirious, medically ill patients: intravenous haloperidol versus intravenous haloperidol plus benzodiazepines. Heart Lung 17: 238–241, 1988

Mesulam M-M, Waxman SG, Geschwind N, et al: Acute confusional states with right middle cerebral artery infarction. J Neurol Neurosurg Psychiatry 39:84–89, 1976

Metzger E, Friedman R: Prolongation of the corrected QT and torsades de pointes cardiac arrhythmia associated with intravenous haloperidol in the medically ill. J Clin Psychopharmacol 13:128–132, 1993

Minagawa H, Uchitomi Y, Yamawaki S, et al: Psychiatric morbidity in terminally ill cancer patients: a prospective study. Cancer 78:1131–1137, 1996

Mizock BA, Sabelli HC, Dubin A, et al: Septic encephalopathy: evidence for altered phenylalanine metabolism and comparison with hepatic encephalopathy. Arch Intern Med 150:443–449, 1990

Moldofsky H, Lue FA, Eisen J, et al: The relationship of interleukin-1 and immune functions to sleep in humans. Psychosom Med 48:309–318, 1986

Moller JT, Cluitmans P, Rasmussen LS, et al: Long-term postoperative cognitive dysfunction in the elderly ISPOCD1 study. ISPOCD investigators. International Study of Post-Operative Cognitive Dysfunction. Lancet 351:857–861, 1998

Mondimore FM, Damlouji N, Folstein MF, et al: Post-ECT confusional states associated with elevated serum anticholinergic levels. Am J Psychiatry 140:930–931, 1983

Monette J, Galbaud du Fort G, Fung SH, et al: Evaluation of the Confusion Assessment Method (CAM) as a screening tool for delirium in the emergency room. Gen Hosp Psychiatry 23:20–25, 2001

Montgomery EA, Fenton GW, McClelland RJ, et al: Psychobiology of minor head injury. Psychosom Med 21:375–384, 1991

Monti JM: Involvement of histamine in the control of the waking state. Life Sci 53:1331–1338, 1993

Moulaert P: Treatment of acute nonspecific delirium with IV haloperidol in surgical intensive care patients. Acta Anaesthesiol Belg 40:183–186, 1989

Mousseau DD, Butterworth RF: Current theories on the pathogenesis of hepatic encephalopathy. Proc Soc Exp Biol Med 206:329–344, 1994

Mullaly W, Huff K, Ronthal M, et al: Frequency of acute confusional states with lesions of the right hemisphere (abstract). Ann Neurol 12:113, 1982

Murphy KM: The baseline predictors and 6-month outcomes of incident delirium in nursing home residents: a study using the minimum data set. Psychosomatics 40:164–165, 1999

Murray AM, Levkoff SE, Wetle TT, et al: Acute delirium and functional decline in the hospitalized elderly patient. J Gerontol 48:M181–M186, 1993

Nakamura J, Uchimura N, Yamada S, et al: The effect of mianserin hydrochloride on delirium. Hum Psychopharmacol 10:289–297, 1995

Nakamura J, Uchimura N, Yamada S, et al: Does plasma free-3-methoxy-4-hydroxyphenyl(ethylene)glycol increase the delirious state? A comparison of the effects of mianserin and haloperidol on delirium. Int Clin Psychopharmacol 12: 147–152, 1997a

Nakamura J, Uchimura N, Yamada S, et al: Mianersin suppositories in the treatment of post-operative delirium. Hum Psychopharmacol 12:595–599, 1997b

Nakamura K, Kurasawa M, Tanaka Y: Apomorphine-induced hypoattention in rat and reversal of the choice performance impairment by aniracetam. Eur J Pharmacol 342: 127–138, 1998

Nicholas LM, Lindsey BA: Delirium presenting with symptoms of depression. Psychosomatics 36:471–479, 1995

Nighoghossian N, Trouillas P, Vighetto A, et al: Spatial delirium following a right subcortical infarct with frontal deactivation. J Neurol Neurosurg Psychiatry 55:334–335, 1992

O'Brien JM, Rockwood RP, Suh KI: Haloperidol-induced torsades de pointes. Ann Pharmacother 33:1046–1050, 1999

O'Hare E, Weldon DT, Bettin K, et al: Serum anticholinergic activity and behavior following atropine sulfate administration in the rat. Pharmacol Biochem Behavior 56:151–154, 1997

Okamoto Y, Matsuoka Y, Sasaki T, et al: Trazodone in the treatment of delirium. J Clin Psychopharmacol 19:280–282, 1999

O'Keeffe ST: Clinical subtypes of delirium in the elderly. Dement Geriatr Cogn Disord 10:380–385, 1999

O'Keeffe ST, Lavan JN: Predicting delirium in elderly patients: development and validation of a risk-stratification model. Age Ageing 25:317–321, 1996

O'Keeffe S, Lavan J: The prognostic significance of delirium in older hospital patients. J Am Geriatr Soc 45:174–178, 1997

O'Keeffe ST, Lavan JN: Clinical significance of delirium subtypes in older people. Age Ageing 28:115–119, 1999

O'Keeffe ST, Tormey WP, Glasgow R, et al: Thiamine deficiency in hospitalized elderly patients. Gerontology 40:18–24, 1994

Olofsson SM, Weitzner MA, Valentine AD, et al: A retrospective study of the psychiatric management and outcome of delirium in the cancer patient. Support Care Cancer 4:351–357, 1996

Ongini E, Caporali MG, Massotti M: Stimulation of dopamine D-1 receptors by SKF 38393 induces EEG desynchronization and behavioral arousal. Life Sci 37:2327–2333, 1985

Onofrj M, Curatola L, Malatesta G, et al: Reduction of P3 latency during outcome from post-traumatic amnesia. Acta Neurol Scand 83:273–279, 1991

Passik SD, Cooper M: Complicated delirium in a cancer patient successfully treated with olanzapine. J Pain Symptom Manage 17:219–223, 1999

Patten SB, Lamarre CJ: Dysgraphia (letter). Can J Psychiatry 34:746, 1989

Perrault LP, Denault AY, Carrier M, et al: Torsades de pointes secondary to intravenous haloperidol after coronary artery bypass graft surgery. Can J Anesth 47:251–254, 2000

Picotte-Prillmayer D, DiMaggio JR, Baile WF: H-2 blocker delirium. Psychosomatics 36:74–77, 1995

Piercey MF, Camacho-Ochoa M, Smith MW: Functional roles for dopamine-receptor subtypes. Clin Neuropharmacol 18:S34–S42, 1995

Platt MM, Breitbart W, Smith M, et al: Efficacy of neuroleptics for hypoactive delirium. J Neuropsychiatry Clin Neurosci 6:66–67, 1994a

Platt MM, Trautman P, Frager G, et al: Pediatric delirium: research update. Paper presented at the annual meeting of the Academy of Psychosomatic Medicine, Phoenix, AZ, November 1994b

Pompeii P, Foreman M, Rudberg MA, et al: Delirium in hospitalized older persons: outcomes and predictors. J Am Geriatr Soc 42:809–815, 1994

Posner ML, Boies SJ: Components of attention. Psychol Rev 78:391–408, 1971

Price BH, Mesulam M: Psychiatric manifestations of right hemisphere infarctions. J Nerv Ment Dis 173:610–614, 1985

Prugh DG, Wagonfeld S, Metcalf D, et al: A clinical study of delirium in children and adolescents. Psychosom Med 42:177–195, 1980

Purdon SE, Jones BDW, Stip E, et al: Neuropsychological change in early phase schizophrenia during 12 months of treatment with olanzapine, risperidone, or haloperidol. Arch Gen Psychiatry 57:249–258, 2000

Rabins PV, Folstein MF: Delirium and dementia; diagnostic criteria and fatality rates. Br J Psychiatry 140:149–153, 1982

Ravona-Springer R, Dohlberg OT, Hirschman S, et al: Delirium in elderly patients treated with risperidone: a report of three cases. J Clin Psychopharmacol 18:171–172, 1998

Reilly JG, Ayis AS, Ferrier IN, et al: QT_c-interval abnormalities and psychotropic drug therapy in psychiatric patients. Lancet 355:1048–1052, 2000

Resnick M, Burton BT: Droperidol versus haloperidol in the initial management of acutely agitated patients. J Clin Psychiatry 45:298–299, 1984

Reyes RL, Bhattacharyya AK, Heller D: Traumatic head injury: restlessness and agitation as prognosticators of physical and psychological improvement in patients. Arch Phys Med Rehabil 62:20–23, 1981

Riker RR, Fraser GL, Cox PM: Continuous infusion of haloperidol controls agitation in critically ill patients. Crit Care Med 22:433–440, 1994

Riker RR, Fraser GL, Richen P: Movement disorders associated with withdrawal from high-dose intravenous haloperidol therapy in delirious ICU patients. Chest 111: 1778–1781, 1997

Ritchie J, Steiner W, Abrahamowicz M: Incidence of and risk factors for delirium among psychiatric patients. Psychiatr Serv 47:727–730, 1996

Robertsson B, Karlsson I, Eriksson L, et al: An atypical neuroleptic drug in the treatment of behavioral disturbances and psychotic symptoms in elderly people. Dementia 7:142–146, 1996

Robertsson B, Blennow K, Gottfries CG, et al: Delirium in dementia. Int J Geriatr Psychiatry 13:49–56, 1998

Rockwood K: Acute confusion in elderly medical patients. J Am Geriatr Soc 37:150–154, 1989

Rockwood K: The occurrence and duration of symptoms in elderly patients with delirium. Journal of Gerontological Medical Science 48:M162–M166, 1993

Rockwood K, Cosway S, Stolee P, et al: Increasing the recognition of delirium in elderly patients. J Am Geriatr Soc 42:252–256, 1994

Rockwood K, Cosway S, Carver D, et al: The risk of dementia and death after delirium. Age Ageing 28:551–556, 1999

Rodriguez G, Testa R, Celle G, et al: Reduction of cerebral blood flow in subclinical hepatic encephalopathy and its correlation with plasma-free tryptophan. J Cereb Blood Flow Metab 7:768–772, 1987

Rolfson DB, McElhaney JE, Jhangri GS, et al: Validity of the Confusion Assessment Method in detecting post-operative delirium in the elderly. Int Psychogeriatr 11:431–438, 1999

Romano J, Engel GL: Delirium, I: electroencephalographic data. Archives of Neurology and Psychiatry 51:356–377, 1944

Rosenberg PB, Ahmed I, Hurwitz S: Methylphenidate in depressed medically ill patients. J Clin Psychiatry 52:263–267, 1991

Ross CA, Peyser CE, Shapiro I, et al: Delirium: phenomenologic and etiologic subtypes. Int Psychogeriatr 3:135–147, 1991

Rothwell NJ, Hopkins SJ: Cytokines and the nervous system, II: actions and mechanisms of action. Trends Neurosci 18:130–136, 1995

Rovner BW, David A, Lucas-Blaustein MJ, et al: Self-care capacity and anticholinergic drug levels in nursing home patients. Am J Psychiatry 145:107–109, 1988

Ruijs MB, Keyser A, Gabreels FJ, et al: Somatosensory evoked potentials and cognitive sequelae in children with closed head injury. Neuropediatrics 24:307–312, 1993

Ruijs MB, Gabreels FJ, Thijssen HM: The utility of electroencephalography and cerebral CT in children with mild and moderately severe closed head injuries. Neuropediatrics 25:73–77, 1994

Sandberg O, Gustafson Y, Brannstrom B, et al: Prevalence of dementia, delirium and psychiatric symptoms in various care settings for the elderly. Scan J Soc Med 26:56–62, 1998

Sander T, Harms H, Podschus J, et al: Alleleic association of a dopamine transporter gene polymorphism in alcohol dependence with withdrawal seizures or delirium. Biol Psychiatry 41:299–304, 1997

Sanders KM, Stern TA: Management of delirium associated with use of the intra-aortic balloon pump. Am J Crit Care 2:371–377, 1993

Sanders KM, Murray GB, Cassem NH: High-dose intravenous haloperidol for agitated delirium in a cardiac patient on intra-aortic balloon pump. J Clin Psychopharmacol 11:146–147, 1991

Santamaria J, Blesa R, Tolosa ES: Confusional syndrome in thalamic stroke. Neurology 34:1618–1619, 1984

Schafer DF, Jones EA: Hepatic encephalopathy and the gamma-aminobutyric acid neurotransmitter system. Lancet 1:18–20, 1982

Schirazi S, Rodriguez D, Nomikos GG: Effects of typical and atypical antipsychotic drugs on acetylcholine release in the hippocampus. Abstr Soc Neurosci 26:2144, 2000

Schmidley JW, Messing RO: Agitated confusional states with right hemisphere infarctions. Stroke 5:883–885, 1984

Schor JD, Levkoff SE, Lipsitz LA, et al: Risk factors for delirium in hospitalized elderly. JAMA 267:827–831, 1992

Schuster P, Gabriel E, Kufferle B, et al: Reversal by physostigmine of clozapine-induced delirium. Clin Toxicol 10:437–441, 1977

Seear M, Lockitch G, Jacobson B, et al: Thiamine, riboflavin and pyridoxine deficiency in a population of critically ill children. J Pediatr 121:533–538, 1992

Sherman SM, Kock C: Thalamus, in The Synaptic Organization of the Brain, 3rd Edition. Edited by Shepherd GM. New York, Oxford University Press, 1990, pp 246–278

Sim FH, Brunet DG, Conacher GN: Quetiapine associated with acute mental status changes (letter). Can J Psychiatry 3:299, 2000

Sipahimalani A, Masand PS: Use of risperidone in delirium: case reports. Ann Clin Psychiatry 9:105–107, 1997

Sloan EP, Fenton GW, Standage KP: Anticholinergic drug effects on quantitative EEG, visual evoked potentials, and verbal memory. Biol Psychiatry 31:600–606, 1992

Spencer EK, Kafantaris V, Padron-Gayol MV, et al: Haloperidol in schizophrenic children: early findings from a study in progress. Psychopharmacol Bull 28:183–186, 1992

Stefano GB, Bilfinger TV, Fricchione GL: The immune-neuro-link and the macrophage: post-cardiotomy delirium, HIV-associated dementia and psychiatry. Prog Neurobiol 42:475–488, 1994

Stern TA: Continuous infusion of physostigmine in anticholinergic delirium: a case report. J Clin Psychiatry 44:463–464, 1983

Stern TA: Continuous infusion of haloperidol in agitated critically ill patients. Crit Care Med 22:378–379, 1994

Sundaram M, Dostrow V: Epilepsy in the elderly. Neurolog 1:232–239, 1995

Swenson JR, Erman M, Labelle J, et al: Extrapyramidal reactions: neuropsychiatric mimics in patients with AIDS. Gen Hosp Psychiatry 11:248–253, 1989

Tarter RE, van Thiel DH, Arria AM, et al: Impact of cirrhosis on the neuropsychological test performance of alcoholics. Alcohol Clin Exp Res 12:619–621, 1988

Teicher MH, Gold CA: Neuroleptic drugs: indications and guidelines for their rational use in children and adolescents. J Child Adolesc Psychopharmacol 1:33–56, 1990

Tejera CA, Saravay SM, Goldman E, et al: Diphenhydramine-induced delirium in elderly hospitalized patients with mild dementia. Psychosomatics 35:399–402, 1994

Tesar GE, Murray GB, Cassem NH: Use of high-dose intravenous haloperidol in the treatment of agitated cardiac patients. J Clin Psychopharmacol 5:344–347, 1985

Tesar GE, Murray GB, Cassem NH: Response to Dr. Weiden (letter). J Clin Psychopharmacol 6:375, 1986

Thomas H, Schwartz E, Petrilli R: Droperidol versus haloperidol for chemical restraint of agitated and combative patients. Ann Emerg Med 21:407–413, 1992

Thomas RI, Cameron DJ, Fahs MC: A prospective study of delirium and prolonged hospital stay. Arch Gen Psychiatry 45:937–946, 1988

Tisdale JE, Kambe JC, Chow MSS, et al: The effect of haloperidol on ventricular fibrillation threshold in pigs. Pharmacol Toxicol 69:327–329, 1991

Tollefson GD, Montagne-Clouse J, Lancaster SP: The relationship of serum anticholinergic activity to mental status performance in an elderly nursing home population. J Neuropsychiatry Clin Neurosci 3:314–319, 1991

Treloar AJ, MacDonald AJ: Outcome of delirium, I: outcome of delirium diagnosed by DSM III-R, ICD-10 and CAMDEX and derivation of the Reversible Cognitive Dysfunction Scale among acute geriatric inpatients. Int J Geriatr Psychiatry 12:609–613, 1997

Trzepacz PT: Neuropathogenesis of delirium: a need to focus our research. Psychosomatics 35:374–391, 1994a

Trzepacz PT: A review of delirium assessment instruments. Gen Hosp Psychiatry 16:397–405, 1994b

Trzepacz PT: Anticholinergic model for delirium. Semin Clin Neuropsychiatry 1:294–303, 1996

Trzepacz PT: The Delirium Rating Scale: its use in consultation/liaison research. Psychosomatics 40:193–204, 1999a

Trzepacz PT: Update on the neuropathogenesis of delirium. Dement Geriatr Cogn Disord 10:330–334, 1999b

Trzepacz PT: Is there a final common neural pathway in delirium? focus on acetylcholine and dopamine. Semin Clin Neuropsychiatry 5:132–148, 2000

Trzepacz PT, Dew MA: Further analyses of the Delirium Rating Scale. Gen Hosp Psychiatry 17:75–79, 1995

Trzepacz PT, Francis J: Low serum albumin and risk of delirium (letter). Am J Psychiatry 147:675, 1990

Trzepacz PT, Teague GB, Lipowski ZJ: Delirium and other organic mental disorders in a general hospital. Gen Hosp Psychiatry 7:101–106, 1985

Trzepacz PT, Baker RW, Greenhouse J: A symptom rating scale for delirium. Psychiatry Res 23:89–97, 1988a

Trzepacz PT, Brenner R, Coffman G, et al: Delirium in liver transplantation candidates: discriminant analysis of multiple test variables. Biol Psychiatry 24:3–14, 1988b

Trzepacz PT, Leavitt M, Ciongoli K: An animal model for delirium. Psychosomatics 33:404–415, 1992

Trzepacz PT, Ho V, Mallavarapu H: Cholinergic delirium and neurotoxicity associated with tacrine for Alzheimer's dementia. Psychosomatics 37:299–301, 1996

Trzepacz PT, Mulsant BH, Dew MA, et al: Is delirium different when it occurs in dementia? A study using the Delirium Rating Scale. J Neuropsychiatry Clin Neurosci 10:199–204, 1998

Trzepacz PT, Mittal D, Torres R, et al: Validation of the Delirium Rating Scale–Revised-98: comparison to the Delirium Rating Scale and Cognitive Test for Delirium. J Neuropsychiatry Clin Neurosci 13:229–242, 2001

Tsutsui S, Kitamura M, Higachi H, et al: Development of postoperative delirium in relation to a room change in the general surgical unit. Surg Today 26:292–294, 1996

Tune LE, Dainloth NF, Holland A, et al: Association of postoperative delirium with raised serum levels of anticholinergic drugs. Lancet 2:651–653, 1981

Tune L, Carr S, Hoag E, et al: Anticholinergic effects of drugs commonly prescribed for the elderly: potential means for assessing risk of delirium. Am J Psychiatry 149:1393–1394, 1992

Uchiyama M, Tanaka K, Isse K, et al: Efficacy of mianserin on symptoms of delirium in the aged: an open trial study. Prog Neuropsychopharmacol Biol Psychiatry 20:651–656, 1996

van der Mast RC: Detecting and measuring the severity of delirium with the symptom rating scale for delirium, in Delirium After Cardiac Surgery. Thesis, Erasmus University Rotterdam, Benecke Consultants, Amsterdam, The Netherlands, 1994, pp 78–89 van der Mast RC, Fekkes D: Serotonin and amino acids: partners in delirium pathophysiology? Semin Clin Neuropsychiatry 5:125–131, 2000

van der Mast RC, Fekkes D, van den Broek WW, et al: Reduced cerebral tryptophan availability as a possible cause for postcardiotomy delirium. Psychosomatics 35:195, 1994

van Hemert AM, van der Mast RC, Hengeveld MW, et al: Excess mortality in general hospital patients with delirium: a 5-year follow-up study of 519 patients seen in psychiatric consultation. J Psychosom Res 38:339–346, 1994

van Leeuwen AMH, Molders J, Sterkmans P, et al: Droperidol in acutely agitated patients: a double-blind placebo-controlled study. J Nerv Ment Dis 164:280–283, 1977

Vaphiades MS, Celesia GG, Brigell MG: Positive spontaneous visual phenomena limited to the hemianopic field in lesions of central visual pathways. Neurology 47:408–417, 1996

Wahlund LA, Bjorlin GA: Delirium in clinical practice: experiences from a specialized delirium ward. Dement Geriatr Cogn Disord 10:389–392, 1999

Weddington WW: The mortality of delirium: an underappreciated problem? Psychosomatics 23:1232–1235, 1982

Wengel SP, Roccaforte WH, Burke WJ: Donepezil improves symptoms of delirium in dementia. J Geriatr Psychiatry Neurol 11:159–161, 1998

Wengel SP, Burke WJ, Roccaforte WH: Donepezil for postoperative delirium associated with Alzheimer's disease. J Am Geriatr Soc 47:379–380, 1999

Wetli CV, Mash D, Karch SB: Cocaine-associated agitated delirium and the neuroleptic malignant syndrome. Am J Emerg Med 14:425–428, 1996

Williams PD, Helton DR: The proconvulsive activity of quinolone antibiotics in an animal model. Toxicol Lett 58:23–28, 1991

Wilson LM: Intensive care delirium: the effect of outside deprivation in a windowless unit. Arch Intern Med 130:225–226, 1972

Wilt JL, Minnema AM, Johnson RF, et al: Torsades de pointes associated with the use of intravenous haloperidol. Ann Intern Med 119:391–394, 1993

Wolff HG, Curran D: Nature of delirium and allied states: the dysergastic reaction. Archives of Neurology and Psychiatry 33:1175–1215, 1935

World Health Organization: International Statistical Classification of Diseases and Related Health Problems, 10th Revision. Geneva, World Health Organization, 1992

Yamamoto T, Lyeth BG, Dixon CE, et al: Changes in regional brain acetylcholine content in rats following unilateral and bilateral brainstem lesions. J Neurotrauma 5:69–79, 1988

Zee-Cheng C-S, Mueller CE, Siefert CF, et al: Haloperidol and torsades de pointes (letter). Ann Intern Med 102:418, 1985

Neuropsychiatric Aspects of Aphasia

Mario F. Mendez, M.D., Ph.D.

Jeffrey L. Cummings, M.D.

Aphasia is the loss or impairment of language caused by brain dysfunction. Language is the unique human ability to communicate through symbols, whether these are in the form of spoken or written language, braille, musical notation, or sign language. Normal language requires the ability to decode, encode, and interrupt these symbols for the exchange of information. In aphasic patients, some or all of these language functions become disturbed, usually as a consequence of acquired brain damage in the language structures of the left hemisphere.

The aphasic syndromes disturb communication and can be severely disabling. In addition to disturbances in linguistic processing, the aphasic syndromes are associated with other neuropsychiatric manifestations. Aphasic patients are prone to psychiatric problems, including depression or paranoid ideation, cognitive abnormalities, and psychosocial challenges in adjusting to the impact of their disorder. These complications may cause more disability than the aphasia itself.

Classification and Diagnosis of Aphasia

The Language Examination

The syndrome classification based on the Wernicke-Geschwind model remains the core of both clinical and academic studies of aphasia (Figure 6–1). Classification of aphasia syndromes by this model requires the examination of six major language areas: 1) fluency, 2) auditory comprehension, 3) confrontational naming, 4) repetition, 5) reading (aloud and for comprehension), and 6) writing. Six additional and helpful areas of examination are 1) word list generation, 2) automatic speech, 3) content of speech, 4) presence of language errors (paraphasias and neologisms), 5) prosody, and 6) speech mechanics. Table 6–1 presents an abridged version of this classification with the major language abnormalities associated with each syndrome (Benson and Ardila 1996; Damasio 1992; Kertesz 1979; Kirshner 1995).

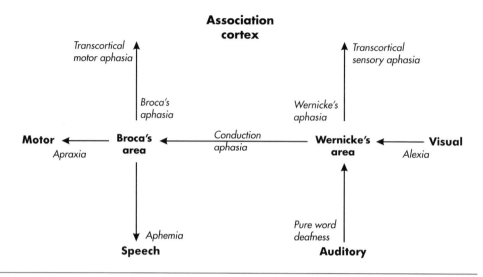

FIGURE 6–1. Wernicke-Geschwind model.

The diagram illustrates the organization of language and corresponding aphasia syndromes in the left hemisphere. The perisylvian language region receives auditory and visual input and produces speech and motor output. Disturbances in the corresponding regions are indicated in italics. Aphemia and pure word deafness are disturbances at the prelanguage and postlanguage levels, respectively. Alexia and apraxia reflect disorders of visual language input and nonspeech motor output, respectively. Language symbols must be interpreted by relating to other associations in higher association cortex. Lesions outside the perisylvian language region may result in the transcortical aphasias, sparing the direct perisylvian pathway mediating repetition.

Fluency evaluation requires an assessment of the generation and ease of production of language. The examiner elicits language in spontaneous conversation, listening for several elements of potential dysfluency. These include a decrease in the number of words generated per minute (usually fewer than 50 in English), shortened phrase length (no more than a few words per phrase), a drop-out of grammatic words such as prepositions or conjunctions (agrammatic or "telegraphic" speech), and effort or struggle in speech production. In addition, aphasic patients often have a dysarthric or poorly articulated verbal output with loss of the normal components of prosody or intonation. Often, their verbal output is brief and strained, but succinct and informative. In the assessment of fluency, it is also valuable to have the patient generate a list of words, such as animal names, in a 1-minute timed sample (normal is 12 or more). The patient's ability to produce automatic speech, such as counting numbers or reciting the days of the week, also reflects his or her ability to generate and produce language.

A second step in the language examination is an assessment of auditory comprehension. This is achieved by giving the patient simple commands or asking yes/no questions. Commands such as "close your eyes" or "open your mouth" can be escalated to more complex pointing commands such as "first touch your chin and then touch your right shoulder." The patient should be able to comprehend and follow these instructions. Additional bedside tasks include syntactically difficult questions, for example, "If a lion was killed by a tiger, which animal is dead?"

The ability to produce names is probably the most commonly impaired language

TABLE 6–1. Principal aphasia syndromes

Aphasia syndrome	Fluency	Auditory comprehension	Repetition	Naming	Reading	Writing comprehension
Broca's	Abnormal	Relatively normal	Abnormal	Abnormal	Normal or abnormal	Abnormal
Wernicke's	Normal, paraphasic	Abnormal	Abnormal	Abnormal	Abnormal	Abnormal
Global	Abnormal	Abnormal	Abnormal	Abnormal	Abnormal	Abnormal
Conduction	Normal, paraphasic	Relatively normal	Abnormal	Usually abnormal	Relatively normal	Abnormal
Transcortical motor	Abnormal	Relatively normal	Relatively normal	Abnormal	Relatively normal	Abnormal
Transcortical sensory	Normal, echolalic	Abnormal	Relatively normal	Abnormal	Abnormal	Abnormal
Anomic	Normal	Relatively normal	Normal	Abnormal	Normal or abnormal	Normal or abnormal

function in aphasia. The evaluation of confrontational naming requires the patient to name objects or pictures. The examiner initially asks the patient to name common items present in his or her environment, such as pen, watch, ring, tie, keys. Subsequently, the examiner asks the patient to name less common items and parts of objects, such as face of a watch, heels of shoes, cuff of sleeve.

In addition to fluency, auditory comprehension, and confrontational naming, the examiner must evaluate repetition, reading, writing, and the presence or absence of paraphasic errors. The examiner asks the patient to repeat sentences or phrases such as "no ifs, ands, or buts" and listens for the presence of literal paraphasias (language errors involving the substitution of incorrect syllables in a word). The patient must read a brief written passage aloud and is then queried for his or her comprehension of the passage. A brief written sample, preferably a sentence of their own composition and a dictated sentence, screens for agraphias or acquired writing disturbances. Finally, the examiner carefully assesses the patient's language output for paraphasic errors, not only literal but also semantic paraphasias (the substitution of an incorrect word) and neologisms (the production of "new" or made-up–sounding words).

Syndromes of Abnormal Verbal Output

Broca's Aphasia

Nonfluent verbal output characterizes Broca's aphasia. Spontaneous speech is sparse, effortful, dysarthric, dysprosodic, short in phrase length, and agrammatic. Decreased fluency occurs in the presence of relatively preserved comprehension (although relational words such as "above" and "behind" may be poorly understood), abnormal repetition and naming, a distur-

bance in reading (particularly for relational and syntactic words), and disturbed writing. Most patients with Broca's aphasia have right-sided weakness varying from mild paresis to total hemiplegia, and some have sensory loss as well. Apraxia of the left limb and buccal-lingual apraxia are common. The neuropathology involves the left hemisphere frontal operculum containing Broca's area. If the lesion is superficial and involves only the cortex, the prognosis for improvement is good. However, if the lesion extends sufficiently deep to involve the basal ganglia and internal capsule, the language defect tends to be permanent.

Wernicke's Aphasia

The most striking abnormality of Wernicke's aphasia is a disturbance of comprehension, which may range from a total inability to understand spoken language to a partial difficulty in decoding the spoken word. The characteristics of Wernicke's aphasia include fluent verbal output with normal word count and phrase length; no abnormal effort, articulatory problems, or prosodic difficulties; and difficulty in repetition and in word finding. The verbal output is often empty of content words and full of paraphasic substitutions and neologisms. *Jargon aphasia* refers to this output when it is extreme and unintelligible, and it must be distinguished from the "word salad" of schizophrenia (Table 6–2). Often there are no basic neurologic defects, but a superior quadrantanopsia may be present. The neuropathology involves the posterior superior temporal lobe of the left hemisphere (the auditory association cortex) and, in some cases, the primary auditory sensory area as well.

Conduction Aphasia

Conduction aphasia features a prominent disturbance in repetition out of proportion to any other language disturbance.

TABLE 6–2. Comparison of language characteristics for Wernicke's aphasia, delirium, schizophrenia, and mania

	Wernicke's aphasia	Delirium	Schizophrenia	Mania
Basic language				
Fluency	Normal	Mildly abnormal	Extended	Logorrheic
Comprehension	Abnormal	Variable	Intact	Normal
Repetition	Abnormal	Mildly abnormal	Intact	Normal
Naming	Abnormal	Nonaphasic	Intact	Normal
Reading comprehension	Abnormal		Intact	Normal
Writing	Abnormal	Abnormal	Resembles spoken output	Normal
Other examination				
Word list generation	Diminished	Abnormal	Diminished on average, bizarre	Increased
Automatic speech	Paraphasic	Normal	Normal, bizarre	Normal
Content	Empty	Incoherent	Impoverished, bizarre, restricted	Grandiose
Neologisms and paraphasias	Common	Absent	Rare (stable meaning)	
Prosody	Normal	Mildly abnormal	Mildly abnormal	Mildly abnormal
Motor speech	Normal	Dysarthric and incoherent	Possible clanging	Press of speech
Associated features				
Thinking	Present	Confused	Special productions	Rapid, flight of ideas
Awareness of deficit	Possibly abnormal	Partial	Absent	Absent
Neurologic examination		Possibly abnormal	Normal	Normal

Patients with conduction aphasia have fluent verbal output and a preserved ability to comprehend. Paraphasias are common, particularly substitutions of phonemes, and confrontational naming is often limited by these paraphasic intrusions. Reading aloud and writing are disturbed, but reading comprehension can be entirely normal. Apraxia of both the right and the left limb is often present, and cortical sensory loss of the left hand or the left side of the face is common. Most cases of conduction aphasia have neuropathology involving the anterior inferior parietal lobe, including the supramarginal gyrus and the arcuate fasciculus (Damasio and Damasio 1980), but exceptions are recognized (Mendez and Benson 1985).

Global Aphasia

A severe language impairment in which all modalities—verbal fluency, comprehension, repetition, naming, reading, and writing—are impaired is known as *global aphasia* or *total aphasia*. Most patients have a right hemiparesis or hemiplegia, a right hemisensory deficit, and a right homonymous hemianopsia. Global aphasia is usually caused by a complete infarction in the territory of the middle cerebral artery. Exceptions are noted, however, including some in which there is global aphasia without hemiparesis due to multiple cerebral emboli to the left hemisphere.

Transcortical Aphasias

The major factor underlying transcortical aphasias is the relative preservation of the ability to repeat spoken language in the presence of other language impairments. Transcortical motor aphasia resembles Broca's aphasia in its decreased verbal fluency but differs in the normal or nearly normal ability to repeat. Patients with this disorder present the strange picture of struggling to utter words in spontaneous conversation but of easily saying the same words on repetition.

The neuropathologic lesions underlying transcortical aphasias are most often located in the supplementary motor area of the left hemisphere or between that area and the frontal operculum. Transcortical sensory aphasia resembles Wernicke's aphasia in its fluent paraphasic output and decreased comprehension but differs in the preserved ability to repeat. When extreme, there is a tendency to exhibit echolalia. Patients with this disorder may manifest the peculiar tendency to repeat everything that the examiner says, as if mimicking them. This tendency to echolalia can lead to the misdiagnosis of the aphasia as a factitious or primary psychiatric condition.

The most common site of neuropathology in transcortical sensory aphasia is in the angular gyrus in the left parietal region. Mixed transcortical aphasia, also known as isolation of the speech area, is the transcortical equivalent of global aphasia. Patients with this disorder may be entirely unable to speak or to comprehend language, but they are able to repeat spoken words. The neuropathology in the mixed transcortical syndrome involves the vascular border zone or watershed areas in both the frontal and parietal lobes. Some patients with transcortical aphasia have widespread pathology with involvement of the frontal lobes. In these cases, the echolalia is a manifestation of environmental dependency.

Anomic Aphasia

Anomic aphasia is a common residual effect following improvement from other types of aphasia. Although verbal output is fluent and repetition and comprehension are intact, naming to confrontation is significantly disturbed. There are multiple word-finding pauses, a tendency to circumlocution, and a somewhat stumbling verbal output. Many individuals with anomic aphasia also have reading and writing disturbances (alexia and agraphia). There is no specific causative location, although neuropathology often involves the left hemisphere angular gyrus. Anomic aphasia has also been reported with lesions of the left temporal pole.

Subcortical Aphasia

With the advent of brain imaging, it became apparent that predominant subcortical lesions (hemorrhage or infarction) could produce acute aphasia syndromes or variable symptomatology (Nadeau and Crosson 1997). Subcortical aphasias characteristically begin with a period of mutism followed by a period of abnormal motor speech, usually hypophonia and articulatory difficulty. As recovery ensues, patients regain much of their speech but are left with paraphasic errors. Similar to the transcortical aphasias, repetition is near normal, and comprehension, naming, reading, and writing may or may not show abnormality. If the lesion is entirely subcortical, recovery usually ensues; many individuals recover totally from the aphasia but are left with residual speech impairments. Studies suggest that basal ganglia or thalamic lesions alone are insufficient to produce permanent aphasia and that cortical involvement is necessary to produce permanent language changes (Bhatia and Marsden 1994).

Neuropsychiatric Aspects of Aphasia

Patients with aphasias or related disorders often have neuropsychiatric disturbances that may be more debilitating than the language impairment itself. Lack of awareness of these disturbances stems in part from the fact that the language disorder interferes with communication and with the psychiatric assessment of patients. The behavioral assessment of aphasic patients through their language impairment requires a great deal of skill and expertise. In the following sections, we discuss the neuropsychiatric aspects of aphasia by examining the psychiatric and cognitive aspects of the disorder.

Psychiatric Aspects

Two distinct, long-term behavioral syndromes accompany aphasia syndromes. One accompanies nonfluent (anterior) aphasia, and the other appears in cases of fluent (posterior) aphasia (Benson 1973).

Anterior Aphasia Behavioral Syndrome

Persons with Broca's aphasia or transcortical motor aphasia know exactly what they wish to say, but their verbal output is restricted and barely intelligible. This inability to explain their wishes or thoughts in other than telegraphic words can cause intense frustration. These nonfluent aphasic patients may manifest their attempts to communicate with agitated gestures and expletives.

Depression is another aspect of the anterior aphasia behavioral reaction. Nonfluent aphasic patients develop intense feelings of personal worthlessness and hopelessness. Depression is considerably more common and intense in patients with anterior aphasia than in those with posterior aphasia (Robinson 1997). This is due in part to the patient's ability to recognize the disability and the frustration of not being able to express thoughts and desires, but there are neurobiological causes for the depression as well.

The occurrence of depression correlates with acute strokes in the left prefrontal region and surrounding areas (Robinson and Szetela 1981). The depressive reaction typically starts with feelings of futility that lead to an unwillingness to participate in self-care or in rehabilitation activities. During the depressed period, aphasic patients may sink deep within themselves; stop eating; refuse social interaction with therapists, other patients, or even family members; and manifest a strong but passive noncooperation. In rare instances, the negative reaction may become intense and explosive, a catastrophic reaction (Goldstein 1948). Although the depression, frustration, and catastrophic reaction of the patient with anterior aphasia suggest a strong potential for suicide, it is rarely reported in this group.

Posterior Aphasia Behavioral Syndrome

Most patients with posterior aphasia have difficulty comprehending spoken language and remain unaware of their deficit, producing a persistent unconcern that is pathologic. Because they are unable to monitor their own verbal output, they often fail to realize that they are producing an incomprehensible jargon. In fact, when tape recordings of such jargon have been made and then replayed immediately, many patients with posterior aphasia deny that it is their own speech. The persistent unawareness and unconcern in patients with posterior aphasia stands in sharp contrast to the frustrated, depressed condition in individuals with anterior aphasia.

Paranoia with agitation, another aspect of posterior aphasia behavioral syndrome, occurs when damage is limited to the posterior temporal lobe (Wernicke's aphasia). This feature is much less common in patients with transcortical sensory aphasia and is virtually unknown in those with anterior aphasia. Paranoid behavior is also universally present in the prelanguage disorder of pure word deafness. Unaware of their own comprehension disturbance, individuals with posterior aphasia or pure word deafness tend to blame their communication difficulties on others. They suggest that the person they are talking to is not speaking clearly or is not paying sufficient attention. Some of these patients come to believe that persons they observe talking together must be using a special code because their conversation cannot be understood. This reaction is similar to the paranoid reaction of acquired deafness, but there are also neurobiological causes for the paranoia. A paranoid reaction correlates with lesions in the left temporal lobe, suggesting that damage to this anatomic region facilitates the perception of threat.

In addition, some patients with posterior aphasia display impulsive behavior. The combination of unawareness, paranoia, and impulsiveness makes them potentially dangerous to others. Physical attacks against medical personnel, family members, or other patients can occur, particularly when the patients misinterpret the behaviors of others. Almost all aphasic patients who need custodial management because of dangerous behavior have a posterior, fluent aphasia (Benson and Geschwind 1985). Moreover, compared with patients having anterior aphasia with depression, those having posterior aphasia with both paranoia and impulsiveness tend to commit suicide more often, particularly as self-awareness of their deficit occurs.

Cognitive Aspects

Aphasic patients often present initially with delirium followed by a period of decreased insight into the existence of their language deficit. If the brain insult is sufficiently large, the patient with aphasia is lethargic or has a clouding of consciousness from the cerebral edema, diaschisis, and other acute neuropathologic changes. After resolution of the initial delirium, in days to weeks, a more prolonged period ensues in which the aphasic patient fails to fully realize the alterations that have occurred. Although alert and responsive, the patient does not yet grasp the significance of the language defect. At this stage, the patient cannot participate rationally in plans for the future because of a decreased appreciation of reality. As previously discussed, some patients with posterior aphasia have a permanent impairment in awareness and concern, but for most, the insight that they are language impaired eventually dawns on them, sometimes rather acutely, and can lead directly to reactive depression.

Language facilitates thought. Among aphasic individuals, thinking processes are less efficient, due to language deficits. Following Bastian (1898), who declared that humans think in words, many experts have emphasized the symbolic nature of cognition and have concluded that defective use of language symbols produces defective thinking. Both Goldstein (1948) and Bay (1964) accepted aphasia as proof that thinking was abnormal, either regressed or concrete. Furthermore, pathology of the posterior language area may be more likely than anterior damage to interfere with intellectual competency (Benson 1979).

Despite these observations, the studies of intelligence in aphasic patients have provided somewhat nebulous results (Basso et al. 1981; Hamsher 1981; Lebrun 1974; Zangwill 1964). Most aphasic patients perform poorly on standard tests of intellectual competency, sometimes in both verbal and nonverbal portions, but many retain considerable nonverbal capability. Standard IQ tests, however, emphasize language skills and thus exaggerate intellectual deficits among aphasic patients. Moreover, most intelligence studies treat aphasia as a single, unitary disturbance, failing to note that intellectual dysfunction varies considerably with the specific aphasia syndrome and the locus of neuropathology. In real life, the examiner must base a decision about the intellectual competence of an aphasic patient on observations; test results alone are not sufficient. Important information, such as the retention of social graces; counting; making change; exhibiting appropriate concern about family, business, and personal activities; finding their way about; socializing; and showing self-concern, may provide valuable indications of residual intelligence in individuals with aphasia.

Prognosis and Treatment

Most poststroke aphasia patients recover significant language function (Basso 1992; Benson and Ardila 1996; Robey 1998). Patients with anomic or conduction aphasia have an excellent recovery and are often left with some more minor degree of language impairment. Many patients with initial Broca's or Wernicke's aphasia recover to anomic or conduction aphasia. The exception is patients with initial global aphasia. In general, these patients have a poor prognosis for recovery of functional language. In addition, patients with aphasia due to dementia or primary progressive aphasia continue to have a slowly progressive deterioration in their language ability, eventually complicated by deficits in other areas of cognition.

The treatment for aphasia requires a careful assessment, usually performed by a speech-language pathologist. The assessment includes evaluation with one of the commonly used aphasia tests, such as the Boston Diagnostic Aphasia Examination, the Psycholinguistic Assessment of Language Processing in Aphasia, or the Communicative Abilities of Daily Living (Lezak 1994). The therapist then formulates a therapy program based on specific goals. In addition to traditional rote repetition and rehearsal, a range of other language therapy techniques are available. These include stimulation-facilitation techniques such as melodic intonation therapy and emotional speech techniques (Benson and Ardila 1996; Reuterskiold 1991). Some techniques focus on modular treatments aimed at specific deficits, such as verbal fluency. Other techniques focus on functional improvement, caregiver interventions, manual or visual symbol systems, use of communication aids, or more recent neurocognitive and psycholinguistic approaches. Whatever the program, a significant emphasis is directed toward positive language competency, allowing few failures and rewarding all successes.

Drug treatments for language disturbances have had little success. Although bromocriptine, bupropion, and methylamphetamine have improved fluency in some nonfluent patients, more rigorous studies have failed to show significant benefits (Gupta et al. 1995). In addition, some aphasic patients need extensive rehabilitation measures other than speech and language therapy. These measures include physical therapy, gait training, mechanical aids such as crutches and leg braces, recreational therapy, and occupational therapy, including instruction and training in activities of daily living.

Despite the language disturbance, many forms of psychotherapy may be useful for aphasic patients, not the least of which is the support provided by family members, nursing staff, therapists, physicians, and others in contact with the patient. There is almost always a positive transference between the patient with aphasia and the speech-language pathologist, a phenomenon that can be used therapeutically. Most language therapists, however, are not formally trained in psychotherapy, and they may become discouraged, for example, if the patient's psychiatric manifestations obviate good

language rehabilitation. Moreover, the comprehension deficit of patients with posterior aphasia precludes more traditional insight-oriented psychotherapy. These barriers need to be considered and overcome. Group psychotherapy, when possible, can decrease feelings of isolation and provide encouragement as patients observe improvements in others. Finally, family counseling often represents a crucial factor in the successful management of an aphasic patient's neuropsychiatric problems.

Among patients with an aphasia syndrome, the early recognition of a mood disorder is critical to the treatment of depression. Awareness of the onset of depression in an aphasic patient should be immediately followed by supportive measures. Challenging therapies (e.g., language, occupational, and physical) should be halted and replaced with activities that the patient can perform successfully. The patient should not be allowed to fail, particularly at tasks that would be considered simple and mundane in normal life. Careful monitoring is needed, and suicide precautions may become necessary, particularly for patients with posterior aphasia. Physicians often use antidepressant medications, particularly for the depression of patients with anterior aphasia. Because aphasic patients are often elderly and have cardiovascular disease, selective serotonin reuptake inhibitors are usually the medications of choice. Drugs such as sertraline and paroxetine have been beneficial in relieving symptoms of depression in these patients.

In addition to antidepressants, a range of psychoactive medications can be useful in the management of aphasic patients. Benzodiazepines can help alleviate anxiety and hyperactivity, but their potential suppression of learning and memory may impede rehabilitation. Atypical antipsychotics, such as quetiapine, olanzapine, or risperidone, are useful in selected aphasic patients, especially those with posterior aphasia who have impulsive, paranoid behavior. Patients with Wernicke's aphasia and pure word deafness who are treated with these psychotropic medications appear to have less agitation and are more compliant with rehabilitation measures. Doses should be kept low to avoid interference with residual mental functions. When brain damage causes apathy, lethargy, and decreased drive, judicious use of a stimulant such as methylphenidate could be beneficial. Again, these drugs need to be monitored carefully because of the increased susceptibility of brain-damaged patients to potential complications.

Conclusions

Patients with aphasia and related disorders often suffer significant psychiatric, cognitive, and psychosocial complications. These changes result from their altered ability to communicate, from their compromised personal and social status, and directly from the brain lesion itself. The neuropsychiatric aspects of aphasia hamper language rehabilitation and may produce serious dysfunction. The optimal management of aphasic patients does not stop with language therapy but also requires competence in the management of the neuropsychiatric aspects of these syndromes.

References

Basso A: Prognostic factors in aphasia. Aphasiology 6:337–348, 1992

Basso A, Capitani E, Luzzatti C, et al: Intelligence and left hemisphere disease: role of aphasia, apraxia and size of lesion. Brain 104:721–734, 1981

Bastian HC: Aphasia and Other Speech Defects. London, HK Lewis, 1898

Bay E: Principles of classification and their influence on our concepts of aphasia, in Disorders of Language. Edited by De Renck AV, O'Connor M. Boston, MA, Little, Brown, 1964, pp 122–139

Benson DF: Psychiatric aspects of aphasia. Br J Psychiatry 123:555–566, 1973

Benson DF: Aphasia, Alexia, and Agraphia. New York, Churchill Livingstone, 1979

Benson DF, Ardila A: Aphasia: A Clinical Approach. New York, Oxford University Press, 1996

Benson DF, Geschwind N: The aphasias and related disturbances, in Clinical Neurology, Vol 1. Edited by Baker AB, Joynt R. Philadelphia, PA, Harper & Row, 1985, pp 1–34

Bhatia KP, Marsden CD: The behavioural and motor consequences of focal lesions of the basal ganglia in man. Brain 117:859–876, 1994

Damasio AR: Aphasia. N Engl J Med 326:531–539, 1992

Damasio H, Damasio A: The anatomical basis of conduction aphasia. Brain 103:337–350, 1980

Goldstein K: Language and Language Disturbances: Aphasic Symptom Complexes and Their Significance for Medicine and Theory of Language. New York, Grune & Stratton, 1948

Gupta SR, Mlcoch G, Scolaro C, et al: Bromocriptine treatment of nonfluent aphasia. Neurology 45:2170–2173, 1995

Hamsher K: Intelligence and aphasia, in Acquired Aphasia. Edited by Sarno MT. New York, Academic Press, 1981, pp 327–359

Kertesz A: Aphasia and Associated Disorders. New York, Grune & Stratton, 1979

Kirschner HS (ed): Handbook of Neurological Speech and Language Disorders. New York, Marcel Dekker, 1995

Lebrun Y: Intelligence and Aphasia. Amsterdam, The Netherlands, Swets & Zeitlinger, 1974

Lezak M: Neuropsychological Assessment, 3rd Edition. New York, Oxford University Press, 1994

Mendez MF, Benson DE: Atypical conduction aphasia: a disconnection syndrome. Arch Neurol 42:886–891, 1985

Nadeau SE, Crosson B: Subcortical aphasia. Brain Lang 58:355–402, 1997

Reuterskiold C: The effects of emotionality on auditory comprehension in aphasia. Cortex 27:595–604, 1991

Robey RR: A meta-analysis of clinical outcomes in the treatment of aphasia. J Speech Lang Hear Res 41:172–187, 1998

Robinson RG: Neuropsychiatric consequences of stroke. Annu Rev Med 48:217–229, 1997

Robinson R, Szetela B: Mood change following left hemisphere brain injury. Ann Neurol 9:447–453, 1981

Zangwill OL: Intelligence in aphasia, in Disorders of Language. Edited by De Renck AV, O'Connor M. Boston, MA, Little, Brown, 1964, pp 261–274

Neuropsychiatric Aspects of Memory and Amnesia

Yaakov Stern, Ph.D.

Harold A. Sackeim, Ph.D.

Memory Systems

Our understanding of memory has increased dramatically during the past decade. Three related lines of research have demonstrated that memory is not a unitary entity and have outlined the nature of different memory "systems." First, in experimental cognitive research with healthy individuals, comparisons of different types of tasks have dissected memory into interrelated, but discriminable, processes. Second, studies of abilities that are differentially affected and retained in patients with discrete brain lesions have also supported the concept of distinct memory systems. Third, functional brain imaging studies, using cognitive challenge procedures with positron emission tomography (PET) or functional magnetic resonance imaging (fMRI), have contributed to the separation of memory processes and to our understanding of the neural network mediating memory per-

formance. For some memory systems, there is relatively good evidence that they are subserved by specific areas of the brain or by specific neural networks. Other systems without clear-cut anatomical correlates have been identified experimentally on the basis of the type of information they process or how they operate. Thus, whether some distinct memory systems actually represent different brain systems remains to be seen. In this section, we review the different aspects of memory that have been identified. The various systems are summarized in Figure 7–1.

Most memory researchers make an initial separation of memory into two categories: *declarative* and *nondeclarative* (Cohen and Squire 1980; Squire 1992). Declarative memory describes the conscious recollection of words, scenes, faces, stories, and events. It is the type of memory assessed by traditional tests of recall and recognition, which rely on what has been called the *explicit* retrieval of information (Graf and Schacter 1985). Non-

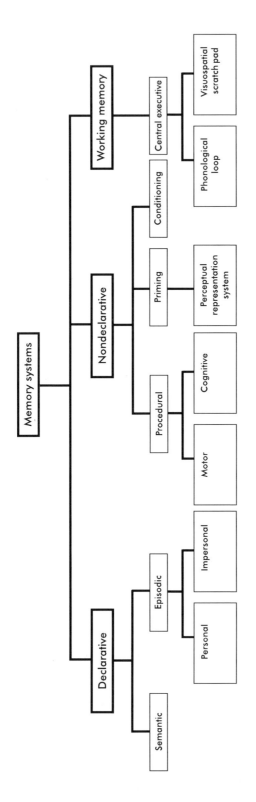

FIGURE 7–1.   An outline of the components of memory.
Source.   Adapted from Squire 1992.

declarative memory is best described in the negative—as a collection of memory processes that are not declarative. The hallmark of nondeclarative memory is evidence that some types of life experience can result in behavioral change without requiring conscious access to the experience—that is, without explicit recall. Tests of nondeclarative memory typically rely on what has been called *implicit* retrieval, and they attempt to demonstrate that a particular type of experience has resulted in a later change in behavior. Several types of memory are subsumed under the heading of nondeclarative memory. These include procedural memory, classical conditioning, simple associative learning, and priming. Separate from the declarative-nondeclarative distinction is working memory, which is viewed as an active memory buffer that can serve either as a scratch pad for newly acquired information or as a locus/mechanism for retrieving and operating on already stored information.

Declarative Memory

Declarative memory is the aspect of memory that is most often assessed clinically with tests of recall or recognition. It is usually subdivided into two components: *semantic* and *episodic* memory (Tulving 1972, 1983). Semantic memory refers to the acquisition of factual information about the world. Typically, semantic memories cannot be fixed as having been acquired at a specific time. For example, although most people know that Shakespeare is the author of *Hamlet*, few can recall when they first acquired this information. Episodic memory refers to the recording and conscious recollection of personal experiences. Semantic memory is required for episodic memory. However, our typical recollections are more than simple facts. They include the spatial and temporal context of events as well as other associated features, such as the emotions associated with life events and the specific details that encompass life events. Episodic memory encompasses personal or autobiographical memories as well as memories for public events. Most standard clinical assessments of memory evaluate episodic memory. It is important to recognize that personal or autobiographical events may become episodic memories, losing any associated recall of spatial or temporal context. As a fact, we may remember that we graduated from college in a particular year but have no recall of the events surrounding the graduation.

A key observation underlying the current memory taxonomy is the view that declarative memory is dependent on the integrity of the hippocampus and its related structures. This was demonstrated most dramatically by the famous case of H.M., who underwent surgery for severe epilepsy (Milner 1959). The medial temporal region of this individual's brain was removed bilaterally, including the uncus, amygdala, anterior two-thirds of the hippocampus, and hippocampal gyrus. After the operation, H.M. was unable to retain new information if he was distracted for more than a few seconds from rehearsing the material. Thus, his performance on standard tests of recall was impaired, and he could not learn new vocabulary words. On the other hand, his recall of events remote from the operation was close to normal (Corkin 1984; Marslen-Wilson and Teuber 1975). Other intellectual functions, including IQ, were spared. H.M. remains densely amnesic to this day. H.M.'s case provided compelling evidence for the importance of the hippocampus and related structures to the process of memory formation and storage that underlies the laying down of new declarative memories. Indeed, the strongest argument for the existence of a memory system can be made for declarative memory, which can be convincingly demonstrated to rely, at least in part, on a specific set of brain structures.

Nondeclarative Memory

The concept of nondeclarative memory stems from the observation that several types of memory tasks can be performed successfully even by patients who have sustained damage to the hippocampus and its associated structures (Cohen and Squire 1980) with marked deficits in declarative memory. The fact that studies of healthy control subjects have also demonstrated dissociations in task performance suggests that some tasks do not require declarative memory. Unlike declarative memory, nondeclarative memory cannot be considered a system. Rather, the term is simply a general classification for a disparate group of tasks (and presumably memory processes) whose performance is not mediated by conscious recall. Some of these tasks have been grouped into hypothetical systems, and these are described in the following sections. One unifying feature of nondeclarative memory tasks is that they demand implicit recall, in which there is no need for conscious storage or recall of material.

Procedural Memory

The term *procedural memory* is typically applied to tasks that assess the acquisition of motor or cognitive skills. One can describe procedural memory as "knowing how," as opposed to declarative memory's "knowing that" (Cohen and Squire 1980).

A well-investigated test of procedural memory is the Tower of Hanoi task. In this task, which is based on an old puzzle, the subject is given a board with three posts. On one of the posts is a pile of disks of graduated sizes, so that each disk is smaller than the one below it. The subject's task is to move all of the disks from one post to another, following two rules:

only one disk can be moved at a time, and a larger disk can never be put on top of a smaller disk. The key to solving this puzzle is to develop the optimal sequence of moves needed to move the disks. With practice, an amnesic patient can improve his or her performance on this task to the optimal level (Cohen 1984; Cohen and Corkin 1981). When given the task again at a later date, the amnesic patient does not remember ever having performed it and needs to be taught the rules as if this were his or her first exposure. However, once the patient begins to perform the task, it is clear that the performance level is far better than at the first exposure to the task. Thus, although the individual has no episodic memory for the task or its rules, the procedures or strategies that contribute to task performance have been retained. This procedural memory is thought to be not dependent on the parahippocampal structures and is *implicit*.

Procedural memory has also been demonstrated for motor tasks. One example is the pursuit rotor task, in which the subject must learn to keep a stylus touching a spot on a revolving turntable. As with the more cognitively based Tower of Hanoi task, amnesic patients can learn and retain this skill (Corkin 1968). Other tests of procedural learning include mirror reading and jigsaw puzzle assembly.

The brain areas that mediate procedural memory have not been identified. However, because several studies have suggested that learning the pursuit rotor task depends on the integrity of the basal ganglia, the possibility exists that procedural memory for motor tasks depends on areas of the brain associated with initial task acquisition and performance (Butters et al. 1990). Similarly, it has been suggested that the brain structures that mediate the acquisition and initial performance of nonmotor tasks also mediate procedural memory for these cognitive skills.

Simple Conditioning and Simple Associative Learning

Amnesic patients can acquire new conditioned responses. In one early study, Weiskrantz and Warrington (1979) assessed classical conditioning of the blink response in two amnesic patients. These patients retained conditioned responses for as long as 24 hours even though they did not recognize the conditioning apparatus. Other simple associative learning is also intact in amnesic patients.

Priming

Priming is another type of nondeclarative memory that requires implicit recall. Some investigators have suggested that distinct memory systems may underlie performance on priming tasks. *Priming* can be defined as the facilitated identification of perceptual objects from reduced cues as a consequence of prior exposure to those objects (Tulving and Schacter 1990).

In a typical priming task, the subject studies some material but is not told that he or she will be expected to recall it. For example, the subject may be given a list of words and asked to identify those that contain a particular letter or to make some judgment about the words (e.g., degree of pleasantness). A key feature of the subsequent retrieval task is that it is also implicit. For example, in one typical retrieval task, the subject is given the first three letters of words (i.e., word stems) and is asked to generate words that begin with those stems as quickly as possible. Half of the word stems are the beginnings of words to which the subject was previously exposed, whereas the other half correspond to new words. In this experiment, the subject will generate words more rapidly for stems of previously studied words. This priming effect is not dependent on explicit recall and is present in amnesic patients (Graf and Schacter

1985). In addition, this priming experiment includes an explicit-recall component, usually a recognition task in which the subject is given a list of words containing both previously studied and new words. Typically, the subject's ability to discriminate the "old" from the "new" words is quite poor, thus demonstrating that exposure to the words was not sufficient for retrieval in a standard explicit recall task.

A wide range of priming paradigms have been used. The studied material has included words, shapes, and sounds. The mode of exposure of the studied list has also been extensively varied, and these studies have provided insight into the memory processes underlying priming. An important feature of the subject's initial exposure to the list is the "level of processing." A distinction can be made between instructions that call attention to the perceptual features of items (e.g., their shape, constituent letters) and those that require a deeper or more conceptual level of processing (e.g., making judgments about whether words belong to specific categories). In general, the more the mode of study is perceptual in nature (a quality some call "data driven"), the better the priming performance. In contrast, deeper conceptual study is more beneficial to declarative modes of recall (Blaxton 1995).

Some priming tasks benefit from deeper levels of processing. These tasks, known as conceptual priming tasks, require semantic processing of the task stimuli and often require responses that are conceptually or semantically related to a stimulus. For example, subjects are given the name of a category (e.g., animal) and asked to produce the first instance that comes to mind (e.g., bear). It has been argued that these conceptual priming tasks differ from standard perceptual priming and rely on semantic learning

(Tulving and Schacter 1990).

The sensitivity of priming performance to perceptual manipulation, as well as its lack of reliance on hippocampal systems, has led some theorists to suggest that priming is an expression of *perceptual representation systems* (PRSs)—a group of domain-specific subsystems that process and represent information about the form and structure, but not the meaning or other associative properties, of words and objects (Tulving and Schacter 1990). PRSs are thought to involve the brain areas responsible for the initial perception and processing of material. Schacter and colleagues have proposed three such systems: *visual word form* (Schacter 1990), *auditory word form* (Schacter and Church 1992), and *structural description* (Schacter et al. 1990). The most carefully worked out of these hypothesized systems is the visual word form PRS, which presumably mediates most of the visually presented verbal priming tasks. This system would include areas in the occipital cortex and elsewhere that are important for visual processing, but would exclude both those areas involved in the semantic processing of words and those implicated in explicit recall.

Working Memory

Working memory is typically viewed as distinct from the declarative and non-declarative memory systems. In one sense, working memory is similar to what in the past has been called short-term memory. It provides a repository for briefly holding on to information such as a telephone number or the name of a newly met person. It is also important in tasks that require mental manipulation of information, such as multistep arithmetic problems. However, for many theorists (e.g., Goldman-Rakic 1992), working memory also has a more important role as the work space where recalled informa-

tion is actually used, manipulated, and related to other information, thus allowing complex cognitive processes such as comprehension, learning, and reasoning to take place.

A detailed model of working memory was proposed by Baddeley and colleagues (Baddeley 1986). In this model, working memory is viewed not as a single memory buffer, but instead as three interrelated components: an attentional controller termed the *central executive*, which is aided by two active slave subsystems, the articulatory or phonological loop and the visuospatial scratch pad or sketch pad.

The phonological loop maintains speech-based information. Without any intervention, this information would fade rapidly. However, the information can be maintained for longer periods in the loop by an articulatory control process, which in effect recycles or rehearses the information. Thus, one way to hold on to a telephone number until it is dialed is to mentally repeat it continuously. Similar to the phonological loop, the visuospatial scratch pad briefly stores and rehearses visuospatial information.

Although the central executive is presumably the most important component of working memory, its role is the least well defined. One function of the central executive is to coordinate information from the separate subsystems. In one study of this function, subjects were asked to simultaneously perform pursuit-tracking and digit-span tasks, the latter of which involves remembering a newly presented string of numbers. Because these two tasks rely on the phonological loop and the visuospatial scratch pad, a subject's relative ability or inability to perform them simultaneously may reflect the capacity of the central executive. Another function attributed to the central executive is the organization and generation of new strategies for the retrieval or processing of information.

Memory Consolidation

Studies of amnesic patients, as well as of nonamnesic humans and animals treated with electroconvulsive shock or specific medications, suggest that there is a difference between how memory is stored for short and for longer periods of time. The short-term memory store has limited capacity and persists for just a few minutes without rehearsal. This level of storage is probably comparable to that described in the working memory system. The short-term memory store is thought to be based on either short-term changes in synaptic transmission or on some form of ongoing neural activity that maintains the information. Manipulations that silence neuronal activity, such as cooling or anoxia, can disrupt short-term memory but not long-term memory.

If memory is to persist longer, it must be transferred into a long-term memory store. However, the long-term memory store can also be subdivided into an earlier phase that is relatively sensitive to disruption and a later phase that is more insensitive to disruption. As reviewed below, immediately following a treatment course with electroconvulsive therapy (ECT), deficits in the recall or recognition of both personal and public information learned before treatment are common; that is, retrograde amnesia (Lisanby et al. 2000; Sackeim 1992; Sackeim et al. 1993, 2000). These deficits are greatest for events that occurred temporally closest to the treatment (i.e., typically within weeks or months) (Lisanby et al. 2000; McElhiney et al. 1995; Squire 1986). Thus, whereas memory for more remote events is intact, patients may have difficulty recalling events that occurred during and several months—or, in some cases, a few years—before the ECT course. This observation is consistent with the idea that the more recent memories are more easily disrupted because they have not yet been stored in their final long-term memory form. In classic amnesia, the retrograde amnesia can also have a temporal gradient, with poorer recall for more recent information (Russell and Nathan 1946). The observation that ECT-caused retrograde amnesia is mostly transitory argues that the memory stores themselves are not affected by ECT, but rather the ability to retrieve these memories (Sackeim 1992).

Animal studies using agents designed to block protein or mRNA synthesis have shown that long-term memory is selectively impaired and short-term memory is unaffected (Davis and Squire 1984). In this case, the actual long-term storage of the material may be affected, rather than the retrieval from long-term storage. Thus, memories in the later phase of long-term storage are probably in the form of actual protein changes that alter the connections between neurons.

System Versus Process Concepts

Some investigators have preferred to categorize memory tasks in a way that does not rely on the concept of systems. Thus, for example, the dissociations between performance on a task that requires implicit retrieval (such as priming) and one that requires explicit retrieval (such as a word recognition test) might not be a function of the use of separate memory systems. Rather, a *process-based* view of memory would posit that these dissociations are a function of the type of processing performed on the test material at study and test. In general, to the degree that the type of processing at study is recapitulated at test, memory performance will improve (Blaxton 1995; Gabrieli 1995). Two types of processing are typically considered: conceptually driven, which is based on the semantic meaning of stimuli, and data driven, which is based on perceptual features of stimuli. Often, the study phase of priming tests is data driven, with the subject instructed to attend to some perceptual feature of the studied material. This procedure creates an advantage in a data-driven test such as the word-stem technique sometimes used in priming tasks (as described earlier) and a disadvantage in a more conceptually driven task such as word recognition. Alternatively, when material is studied at a conceptually driven level—for example, by generating synonyms to the studied words—an advantage is created in tests that also require this type of processing. Thus, the process-based approach argues that it is not necessary to posit that implicit and explicit retrieval reflect two distinct memory systems. Rather, processing matches or mismatches can be introduced into tasks requiring either type of retrieval with predictable results.

Proponents of the process-based approach most often study healthy subjects, although predictions from this approach have been supported in some studies of populations with brain damage, including left temporal lobe epilepsy and Alzheimer's disease (Blaxton 1992). The process-based predictions are not completely upheld, however, in individuals with diencephalic/bilateral medial temporal amnesia (Keane et al. 1993). These patients appear to have normal priming on implicit conceptual memory tasks but are impaired on explicit conceptual tasks. This pattern supports the argument that these patients have a deficit in explicit recall, as systems theorists would predict. Most theorists now agree that systems-based and process-based approaches are not mutually exclusive and that manipulations of processing type can enrich insights about the nature of memory systems.

Coordinating Memory Systems

Although experimental manipulations and careful observation of patients with brain lesions support the concept of dissociable memory systems, it should be emphasized that these systems do not usually operate independently. For example, in a healthy subject, a priming task probably does not measure implicit recall only, because performance might also be aided by explicit recall. Consequently, most experimenters design priming studies to minimize the influence of explicit recall. Others, however, have developed techniques that attempt to evaluate the relative contribution of explicit (or conscious) and implicit (or unconscious) recall during the performance of a memory task (Jacoby et al. 1992).

More importantly, memory theorists have proposed models of memory that suggest how the different memory systems are normally integrated. Presented here is a simplification of one such model, proposed by Moscovitch (1994). Modules similar to the PRS previously described are responsible for the perception and encoding of information. Other associated central systems semantically encode the perceptual information. These systems operate automatically (without awareness) and may subserve implicit recall. The information from these systems can be delivered to working memory, where it can be briefly stored or processed. According to Moscovitch, information in working memory that receives full conscious attention is automatically processed by the hippocampus and related structures. Storage in these structures is in the form of simple association, in which a cue in working memory will produce the associated memories from the hippocampal structures regardless of whether they are relevant. Input to the hippocampus from working memory and output from the hippocampus to working memory can be guided, organized, and evaluated by executive systems, most likely located in prefrontal cortex. In this model, "the frontal lobes are necessary for converting remembering from a stupid reflexive act triggered by a cue to an intelligent, reflective, goal-directed activity under voluntary control" (Moscovitch 1994, pp. 278–279). Acquisition and retention of skills in procedural memory tasks may be mediated by modification of the same structures that are involved in task performance, similar to the operation of PRSs in priming tasks. This model integrates the reviewed declarative and nondeclarative memory systems, as well as the components of working memory, into a coordinated system and provides a framework for how these systems interact. Clearly, in the course of day-to-day activities, all of these systems must work together to allow us to store, recall, and use memories.

Amnesia

Amnesia is the generic term for severe memory deficit, regardless of cause. Table 7–1 summarizes the DSM-IV-TR (American Psychiatric Association 2000) criteria for amnesia.

Four clinical characteristics are typical of most amnesic patients: anterograde amnesia, retrograde amnesia, confabulation, and intact intellectual function. Anterograde amnesia is the hallmark of an amnestic disorder; it refers to the inability after the onset of the disorder to acquire new information for explicit retrieval. Retrograde amnesia refers to difficulty in retrieving events that occurred before the onset of the amnestic disorder, often demarcated as the time of head trauma, stroke, or other injury. It is more variably present in different amnesias. When amnesic patients are asked to recall information and cannot, they may confabulate, providing made-up or inaccurate information without having any apparent awareness that their responses are incorrect.

TABLE 7–1. DSM-IV-TR criteria for amnestic disorder

A. The development of memory impairment as manifested by impairment in the ability to learn new information or the inability to recall previously learned information.
B. The memory disturbance causes significant impairment in social or occupational functioning and represents a significant decline from a previous level of functioning.
C. The memory disturbance does not occur exclusively during the course of a delirium or a dementia.

Source. Reprinted from the *Diagnostic and Statistical Manual of Mental Disorders*, 4th Edition, Text Revision. Washington, DC, American Psychiatric Association, 2000. Copyright 2000, American Psychiatric Association. Used with permission.

Again, confabulation does not occur in all amnesias, and it is often more common in the acute stage of the neuropsychiatric illness. Finally, in the classic amnestic disorders, the patients' intellectual function remains relatively intact even though some specific secondary cognitive defects may be noted on careful neuropsychological testing.

Lesions of the Mesial Regions of the Temporal Lobes

The classic case of bilateral mesial temporal lobe (MTL) ablation is the patient H.M., who was described earlier in this chapter. Since his surgery, H.M. has had severe anterograde amnesia and essentially cannot recall or recognize virtually any newly learned information. He can remember events from his early childhood but has difficulty with events that occurred just before his operation, indicating a restricted retrograde amnesia. His IQ is in the normal range.

Although bilateral temporal lobectomies are rare, unilateral temporal lobectomies are commonly performed to treat intractable seizure disorders. This operation is usually effective in treating the seizure disorder, and patients may have no obvious memory deficits. However, careful testing often demonstrates subtle memory impairments, with removal of the left temporal lobe commonly producing relative deficits in verbal memory and removal of the right temporal lobe producing relative deficits in remembering nonverbal information, indicating material-specific amnesia. A similar pattern has often been demonstrated in the acute postictal state following ECT, where unilateral treatment with electrodes on the left side produces greater persistence of postictal confusion and verbal anterograde and retrograde memory deficits, whereas stimulation over the right hemisphere produces greater anterograde and retrograde memory deficits for nonverbal material (Sackeim 1992). Likewise, left and right medial temporal lobe sclerosis due to epilepsy has been associated with material-specific amnesia.

Wernicke-Korsakoff Syndrome

Wernicke-Korsakoff syndrome is the prototypical example of diencephalic amnesia, given that the memory disorders seen in this condition are attributed to lesions of mesial diencephalic brain structures, including the dorsomedial nucleus of the thalamus and/or the mamillary bodies (Victor et al. 1989). The syndrome is typically observed in nutritionally depleted alcoholic patients. When the diet is insufficient, neuronal injury occurs in thiamine-dependent areas of the brain and can lead to the characteristic lesions associated with this condition. In the acute phase, Wernicke's encephalopathy, common presenting complaints include mental confusion, staggering gait, ocular symptoms, and polyneuropathy. The chronic phase of the disease, Korsakoff's psychosis, is characterized by both antero-

grade and retrograde memory deficits. The anterograde amnesia is dense, with the patient unable to recall events that are no longer in working memory. Retrograde amnesia consists of difficulty recalling past personal or public events. Recall is poorest for events that are closest to the onset of the amnesia and improves for events in the more distant past. This pattern of retrograde amnesia is called a temporal gradient (Albert et al. 1979). Performance on IQ tests is comparable to that of chronic alcoholic individuals without amnesia. Deficits can be demonstrated, however, on tests that require speed and visuoperceptual and spatial organization components. The neuropathology of this syndrome consists of lesions to the paraventricular regions of the thalamus, the hypothalamus, the mamillary bodies, the periaqueductal region of the midbrain, the floor of the fourth ventricle, and the superior vermis (Victor et al. 1989).

Frontal Lobe Lesions and the Role of the Frontal Lobes in Memory

Most of the literature investigating frontal lobe lesions has concentrated on cognitive functions other than memory. Although the frontal lobes are complex structures with many differentiated areas and functions, the consensus had long been that lesions to the frontal lobes do not produce the kinds of memory deficits that are seen in amnesia. Memory performance is affected in patients with frontal lobe lesions, but this has been attributed to the role of frontal structures in the placement of information into spatial and temporal contexts and in the execution of complex mnemonic strategies (Baddeley 1986; Milner et al. 1985). Without context, it is difficult to organize information for storage or retrieval. Some patients with frontal lobe lesions have been described as not being able to remember to remember; that is, they do not spontaneously initiate the activity required to retrieve information or to identify a retrieval strategy. This view of the frontal lobes in memory loss is concordant with the model of memory systems set forth above.

However, a recent meta-analysis of studies relating frontal lobe lesions to tests of recognition, cued recall, and free recall suggests that all three types of performance are disrupted in patients with frontal lobe lesions (Wheeler et al. 1995). In many published studies, there was a nonsignificant trend toward better performance in the control groups, and the failure to obtain statistically significant differences was often attributed to a lack of statistical power. This weakness is eliminated with meta-analysis. The review found that these patients performed more poorly on recall than on recognition tests, which again may implicate the processes involved in the organization of information and the initiation of recall as the primary reasons for the memory deficit. However, the patients' performances were also poorer than those of control subjects on recognition tasks, which may suggest that the frontal lobes have a more primary role in episodic memory.

Nonetheless, the role of the frontal lobe in memory processes is undergoing substantial reevaluation. This stems principally from several sources of evidence. First, frontal lobe damage can result in a profound, temporally graded retrograde amnesia (Kopelman 1992; Kopelman et al. 1999; Moscovitch 1994; Shimamura 1994; Stuss and Benson 1986), in some comparisons as great as MTL pathology (Kopelman et al. 1999) and presumably due to the disruption of retrieval processes. In amnesic patients, anterograde and retrograde amnesia are often weakly associated, and there is evidence that tests

of frontal lobe (executive) function covary with the magnitude of retrograde amnesia (Kopelman 1992).

Markowitsch (1995, 2000) conducted a careful analysis of the sites of injury in brain-damaged patients with preserved anterograde memory but marked retrograde amnesia. He proposed that ventrolateral (orbital) prefrontal cortex and temporopolar cortex, interconnected through the ventral branch of the uncinate fasciculus, are essential for the retrieval of declarative information from long-term memory, with the caveat that right-side damage was especially associated with retrograde amnesia. A host of imaging studies in normal samples have shown activation of ventrolateral prefrontal cortex and anterolateral portions of the temporal cortex during episodic memory retrieval (Buckner 1996; Buckner et al. 1995, 1998a, 1998b, 1999, 2000; S. Kapur et al. 1995; Lepage et al. 2000; Shallice et al. 1994; Tulving and Markowitsch 1997; Tulving et al. 1994a, 1994b, 1999). Thus, the evidence from focal retrograde amnesia (N. Kapur 1999) and imaging studies of normal recall or recognition of newly learned information emphasizes a key contribution of the ventrolateral prefrontal cortex and the temporal pole.

More generally and surprisingly, early imaging studies of the retrieval of newly learned information had difficulty in showing MTL activation (Schacter and Wagner 1999). However, recent work has suggested that there may be differential encoding/retrieval activation within the hippocampus along the rostral-caudal axis (Lepage et al. 1998). In addition, the novelty of stimuli may strongly affect the nature of MTL activation. Saykin et al. (1999) and Johnson et al. (2001), using fMRI in healthy participants, found that the processing of novel words led to activation of the left anterior hippocampus, whereas recognition of familiar words activated the left posterior parahippocampal gyrus and right dorsolateral prefrontal cortex. In particular, retrieval success was strongly associated with activation of the right dorsolateral prefrontal cortex (Johnson et al. 2001).

Overall, it is more firmly established from imaging studies that dorsal prefrontal cortical regions participate in retrieval of newly learned information. Tulving and colleagues offered the hemispheric encoding/retrieval asymmetry (HERA) model (S. Kapur et al. 1995; Nyberg et al. 1996a, 1996b, 1996c, 1998, 2000; Tulving and Markowitsch 1997, 1998; Tulving et al. 1994a, 1994b), which posits that the left prefrontal cortex (particularly the dorsolateral prefrontal cortex) is critical to the encoding of novel information in episodic memory and retrieval from semantic memory. In contrast, the right prefrontal cortex (particularly the dorsolateral prefrontal cortex) is critical in episodic memory retrieval. HERA has been carefully critiqued (Buckner 1996; Nyberg et al. 1996a), and regions involved in encoding/retrieval have been refined. For instance, S. Kapur et al. (1995) distinguished between general retrieval attempt and successful retrieval of stored memories ("ecphory"). Although the former was associated with primarily right prefrontal (Brodmann's area[s] [BA] 9, 10, 46) activation, the latter was characterized by activation of more posterior right-sided regions (right cuneus-precuneus). Subsequently, Lepage et al. (2000) made the distinction between episodic retrieval mode and ecphory. Retrieval mode was associated with right greater than left prefrontal cortical activation, including BA 9 and 10. They concluded that the retrieval asymmetry in HERA is explained by the asymmetry in retrieval mode, but that the new findings did not necessitate reformulation of the encoding asymmetry aspect of HERA (left greater than right). In other

work, this group used partial least squares analyses of imaging data and identified a functional network involving the right prefrontal cortex, left MTL, and left parietal regions (cuneus-precuneus) in episodic retrieval (Nyberg et al. 2000). Thus, beyond the MTL, recent work on memory retrieval of newly learned information in normal subjects has generally emphasized right-sided dorsal prefrontal (typically dorsolateral) structures, as well as ventromedial and temporopolar regions. Of note, the left dorsolateral prefrontal cortex is thought to be critical in the retrieval of semantic memories (facts about the world).

This imaging work with normal participants has focused on retrieval of (impersonal) newly learned information (e.g., word lists). Relevance to our understanding of retrograde amnesia in patients with lesions (or who have received ECT) or for the processes mediating memories of our own past may be questionable. Only a small set of studies has examined activation patterns during recall of autobiographical memories in healthy subjects (with only case studies of patients with retrograde amnesia), and, in general, this literature is methodologically compromised (e.g., no control over the age of events recalled, no verification of accuracy of recall, etc.). Andreasen et al. (1995) found left dorsolateral prefrontal activation during recall of autobiographical or personal memories. Because their procedure involved verbalization during scanning, the researchers repeated the experiment with silent recall (Andreasen et al. 1999), finding activation of medial and orbital frontal cortex, anterior cingulate gyrus, left parietal regions, and left thalamus. In line with HERA, Fink et al. (1996) found that retrieval of autobiographical memories activated multiple right hemisphere regions, including dorsal prefrontal cortex (BA 6), temporomedial, temporoparietal, and temporolateral cortex, and posterior cingulate gyrus. There was also activation of MTL structures, including amygdala, hippocampus, and parahippocampus. In contrast, Conway et al. (1999) found activation predominantly of the left side (frontal BA 6, 44, 45) and the inferior temporal lobe (BA 20) in response to recall of both recent and remote autobiographical memories. These researchers also detected hippocampal activation under both conditions, implying that even if remote memory storage extends beyond MTL regions, intact hippocampal function may be necessary for successful retrieval. Finally, Maguire and Mummery (1999) found evidence of activation of the left temporal pole, left medial frontal cortex (BA 10), and the left hippocampus during retrieval of autobiographical memories. Taken together, these studies indicate that there is great uncertainty about the exact region(s) necessary for retrieval of autobiographical memories in normal participants. Furthermore, unlike the larger literature on retrieval of newly learned information, this handful of imaging studies of autobiographical memory has not explicitly examined the consequences of unsuccessful ecphory of events, that is, amnesia. Finally, aside from Conway et al. (1999), no study has examined differential activation of recent versus remote autobiographical memories, despite the fact that most theories suggest a time-limited role for events to be stored in the MTL before being permanently transferred to cortical representations (e.g., Moscovitch 1994).

Alzheimer's Disease

Alzheimer's disease is a progressive dementing disorder that affects a wide range of intellectual functions. The hallmark of all dementias is acquired amnesia, along with deficits in other cognitive functions. Patients with Alzheimer's disease

have difficulty learning new material. In addition, their memory deficit is characterized by rapid forgetting of newly acquired material (Welsh et al. 1992). In addition, as the disease progresses, there is a growing retrograde amnesia, typically manifesting a classic temporal gradient, with greatest preservation of remote memories. Studies suggest that the memory deficit of Alzheimer's disease is actually present years before the clinical diagnosis becomes apparent (Jacobs et al. 1995). The histopathologic manifestations of Alzheimer's disease—cell loss, senile plaques, and neurofibrillary tangles—are relatively widespread but early in the disease are primarily present in the hippocampus and surrounding entorhinal cortex (Ball et al. 1985).

Twelve elderly persons who had documented isolated memory decline over 3 years but no dementia were studied with an fMRI paradigm in which they studied pictured faces for later recall (Small et al. 1999). The subjects were dichotomized into two subgroups: four with diminished entorhinal activation (i.e., entorhinal activation at least 2 standard deviations below that of the normal elderly) and eight with normal entorhinal activation. The diminished entorhinal activation subgroup had diminished activation in the hippocampus proper and the subiculum compared with healthy elderly persons. This group may have preclinical Alzheimer's disease. The normal-activation subgroup had diminished activation restricted to the subiculum. This subgroup of subjects is unlikely to have early Alzheimer's disease, but may have memory decline for some other reason. Thus, dimished activation of the entorhinal cortex and hippocampus may be an early marker of Alzheimer's disease. This is compatible with the evidence that atropy of the hippocampus and surrounding entorhinal cortex is an early marker of Alzheimer's disease.

Recent imaging work suggests that some patients with early Alzheimer's disease utilize the same neural networks as matched elderly control subjects when performing memory tasks (Stern et al. 2000). In contrast, other patients appear to utilize different and apparently compensatory networks. The use of compensatory networks is associated with poorer memory performance and may mark a stage of disease progression in which pharmacologic attempts to arrest the disease process may be less successful.

Psychiatric Disorders and Normal Aging

The major psychiatric disorders—schizophrenia, mania, and major depression—almost invariably compromise aspects of attention and concentration (Goldberg and Gold 1995; Sackeim and Steif 1988). Because the ability to focus and sustain attention is central to the acquisition of new information in general and declarative memory in particular, deficits in acquiring new information are common among these patients.

Mood Disorders

Since the classic work of Cronholm and Ottosson (1961), it has been repeatedly demonstrated that although patients experiencing an episode of major depression or mania have a reduced capacity to learn new, unstructured information, they are usually less impaired in retaining whatever information they do learn. For example, in verbal and nonverbal paired-associate tasks, depressed patients will typically recall fewer items than will matched control subjects when tested immediately after stimulus presentation, with the extent of this deficit often associated with measures of depression severity and reversing with successful

treatment (Bornstein et al. 1991; Steif et al. 1986; Sternberg and Jarvik 1976). In contrast, after controlling for the amount of information learned, researchers have found that depressed patients and control subjects typically do not differ in the percentage of the material recalled after a delay. Thus, in general, depression appears to have a greater influence on the acquisition than the retention of information (D.B. Burt et al. 1995). This is not to say that memory impairments cannot be identified in mood disorder samples. In a meta-analysis, Zakzanis et al. (1998) found that anterograde memory tests were among the most discriminative neuropsychological measures in distinguishing patients with major depression and matched control subjects. In part, this may be due to the contribution of attentional deficits to memory performance.

This acquisition impairment is most marked for material that is unstructured and that exceeds the capacity of working memory. Healthy individuals are capable of recalling or recognizing 7 ± 2 items immediately after presentation, and this aspect of short-term memory is often assessed with digit-span tests. The evidence is mixed that digit-span performance is impaired in the major mood disorders (Breslow et al. 1980; Gass and Russell 1986; Whitehead 1973). When deficits on this measure are observed in mood disorder patients, it is generally thought that the deficits reflect not an inherent limitation in the capacity of working memory, but rather an attentional dysfunction, with difficulties in concentration leading to greater distractibility and interference effects.

Other sources support the notion that attentional dysfunction and, more generally, impaired executive skills commonly form the basis for memory deficits in mood disorders (Sackeim and Steif 1988). Calev and Erwin (1985) compared depressed patients and healthy control subjects on a verbal memory task in which the difficulty of recall and recognition was matched. Depressed patients demonstrated deficits in recall but not in recognition. This finding suggested that there were no deficits in the consolidation and storage of information, but that depressed patients had a reduced ability to organize effective retrieval strategies. Furthermore, the deficits in episodic memory seen in depressed patients are most pronounced when the material to be learned is unstructured. For example, when given a list of words to remember that are drawn from semantic categories (e.g., pants, shirt, shoe) in which the order of words is clustered by category, depressed patients are typically equivalent to healthy control subjects in recall. However, when overt clustering is not provided, patients manifest a recall deficit (Backman and Forsell 1994; Channon et al. 1993; Weingartner et al. 1981). This finding suggests that depressed patients are less likely both to spontaneously impose organization on new information and to link that information to preexisting knowledge. Consequently, the depth of encoding is more shallow, resulting in impaired learning and retrieval.

Cognitive psychologists have distinguished between *automatic* and *effortful* processing (Hasher and Zacks 1979). Similar to the notion of nondeclarative memory, automatic operations place limited demands on attentional capacity and occur without intention or awareness. Our learning and retaining what we had for breakfast—that is, *incidental* learning—is an example of automatic processing. In contrast, effortful processing requires the use of limited attentional capacity, is initiated intentionally, and benefits from rehearsal. Committing to memory a long shopping list is an example of effortful processing. In general,

depressed patients are more likely to manifest deficits on tasks that require effort or greater depth of processing but not on tasks that can be completed automatically (Roy-Byrne et al. 1986; Weingartner et al. 1981). Similarly, most studies that have compared implicit and explicit memory in major depression have noted deficits in the declarative, explicit domain but not in the nondeclarative, implicit domain (Bazin et al. 1994; Watkins et al. 1996). This overall pattern may be useful clinically in distinguishing depressed patients from those with Alzheimer's disease. Anterograde memory deficits in Alzheimer's disease are expected even when tasks call for shallow processing and minimal effort. Furthermore, a conservative response bias is commonly observed in major depression, where recognition errors tend to be of the sort in which patients fail to recognize a previously learned stimulus (false-negative errors) (Corwin et al. 1990). In contrast, patients with Alzheimer's disease are often more prone to false-positive errors, misidentifying a novel stimulus as part of a learning set (Gainotti and Marra 1994; Lachner and Engel 1994).

Often, depressed patients not only are impaired in their capacity for effortful learning but also manifest changes in the content of memory. In clinical interviews, it is evident that much of the recollection of depressed patients involves autobiographical events with negative emotional valence. The concept of the effects of *mood congruence* on memory stipulates that the efficiency of mnemonic processing is influenced by the match between an existing mood state and the affective tone of the material to be remembered (Blaney 1986; Singer and Salovey 1988). There will be greater access to memories whose affective valence is congruent with the current mood state. For example, some evidence exists that depressed psychiatric patients are more likely to recall experiences of failure relative to experiences of success (DeMonbreun and Craighead 1977). Furthermore, this biasing of memory may extend beyond explicit, conscious recall. Watkins et al. (1996) recently found that whereas healthy control subjects showed greater implicit priming effects for positively emotionally toned words than for negative words, the opposite characterized depressed patients. The concept of mood congruence is attractive in helping to account for the apparent bias in accessibility of personal memories among depressed patients. However, in clinical samples, such mood-congruence effects have been observed mostly in memory tests for experimenter-presented material (Breslow et al. 1981). When effects have been obtained for "real life" autobiographical memories, they have often pertained to the latency of recall (e.g., Lloyd and Lishman 1975) or to the extent of detail in the reported memories (Brittlebank et al. 1993). In addition, there is evidence that mood-congruence effects are most readily obtained when the recall of autobiographical memories is relatively unstructured (Eich et al. 1994). Typical procedures involve presentation of cue words as free-association stimuli for recalling autobiographical events. In contrast, when using procedures that required a deliberate memory search for specific classes of events, McElhiney et al. (1995) found no difference between severely depressed patients and healthy control subjects in capacity to recall negatively versus positively charged autobiographical memories. If this formulation is correct, it suggests that the spontaneous trains of thought of depressed patients are biased to retrieve negative affective memories, but that no abnormalities are seen when retrieval is guided or structured.

There is increasing evidence that the neuropsychological impairments—and, in particular, memory disturbance—in mood disorder patients may not fully reverse with resolution of the depressive or manic episode and may intensify with repeated episodes. T. Burt et al. (2000) compared young and elderly unipolar and bipolar patients in an episode of major depression on a variety of anterograde memory tasks. Elderly bipolar patients, even though free of psychotropic medication, had the poorest performance of all groups, suggesting a particular iatrogenic effect of a long-term history of bipolar disorder. This is all the more impressive because in evaluations of neuropsychological differences between young adults with unipolar and bipolar illness, those with bipolar illness have generally fared better (Donnelly et al. 1982; Mason 1956; McKay et al. 1995; Overall et al. 1978). In a meta-analysis of 40 studies, Kindermann and Brown (1997) reported that studies that examined both bipolar and unipolar patients found greater dysfunction of moderate effect size compared with studies examining only unipolar depressed patients. The larger differences were found for 1) figural (vs. verbal) memory, 2) delayed (vs. immediate) memory, and 3) recognition (vs. free and cued recall). Similarly, D.B. Burt et al. (1995) in another meta-analysis noted that recall deficits were of greater magnitude in samples that contained both bipolar and unipolar depressed patients compared with samples restricted only to unipolar major depression.

Several studies have shown that bipolar patients in the euthymic state manifest neuropsychological deficits relative to matched control subjects, but the characterization of these deficits is still unclear, with the exception possibly of impairments in verbal learning and executive functions (Coffman et al. 1990; Kessing 1998; van Gorp et al. 1998) and the suggestion that greater frequency of episodes or duration of illness may be related to greater impairment. Of particular note, Shelline and colleagues (1999) examined euthymic women with a history of unipolar major depression and reported that the number of days lifetime in a depressive episode was inversely related to hippocampal volume. The interpretation offered is that excessive glucocorticoids (e.g., hypercortisolemia) during the episode have an atrophic effect on hippocampal volume. Of note, reduced hippocampal size was associated with inferior performance on a verbal memory test. Thus, in the last several years, there has been a major change in perspective. Memory deficits in mood disorders were largely seen as a state-dependent phenomenon, mainly attributable to attentional disturbance and difficulties with effortful processing. There is incomplete, but increasing, evidence that learning and memory abnormalities may persist during euthymia and may reflect structural brain abnormalities induced by the mood disorder episodes.

Schizophrenia

Schizophrenia is associated with disturbance in attention, motor behavior, speed of processing, abstraction, learning, and memory. Indeed, patients with schizophrenia perform poorly on a wide variety of cognitive and behavioral tasks. This generalized intellectual decline seems to be present early in the illness and, in most cases, does not appear to be subsequently progressive (Hyde et al. 1994; Nopoulos et al. 1994). Given the multiple dimensions of deficit, one goal of neuropsychological investigation has been to determine whether certain cognitive domains are especially impaired in schizophrenia. The belief has been that identifying such differential deficits may provide leads regarding the cognitive dysfunction that plays a more primary role in the disorder's

pathoetiology (Blanchard and Neale 1994; Chapman and Chapman 1973). Related goals have been to determine whether subgroups of patients differ in their profiles of cognitive disability and to relate findings of cognitive impairment to functional and structural brain abnormalities (Goldberg and Gold 1995).

In recent years, the focus of research on memory impairment in schizophrenia has been to improve characterization of the deficits in working and declarative memory. In line with imaging studies of function and structure, the most characteristic neuropsychological profile in schizophrenia is compatible with deficits in systems mediated by the prefrontal and temporohippocampal cortices (M.A. Taylor and Abrams 1984), with relative sparing of language and visuospatial processing mediated by the posterior cortex.

There is debate concerning whether the deficits in working memory and associated executive functions in schizophrenia are less or more profound than those in verbal, declarative memory (Goldberg and Gold 1995; Saykin et al. 1994). In a large study of first-episode, never-medicated patients; medication-free, previously treated patients; and healthy control subjects, Saykin et al. (1994) reported that verbal memory impairment was the most profound deficit and was present early in the course of the illness. The magnitude of impairment in this domain was extensive even after the investigators controlled for impairments in executive functions (i.e., attention-vigilance, abstraction-flexibility). Similarly, in a recent community-based study of 138 patients with schizophrenia, Kelly et al. (2000) found that 15% had significant global cognitive impairment, 81% had impaired memory, 25% had executive dyscontrol, and 49% had impaired verbal fluency. Elvevag et al. (2000) attempted to examine how various manipulations of paired-associate learning would interfere with the memory performance of schizophrenic patients in a manner akin to the interference seen with patients with frontal lobe damage. They concluded that that susceptibility to interference effects was not a specific problem in patients with schizophrenia but reflected a more general disturbance in memory. Verdoux and Liraud (2000) compared the memory and executive abilities of patients with schizophrenia, other nonschizophrenic psychoses, bipolar disorder, and major depression. Memory deficits were most discriminatory between patients with schizophrenia and those with other psychotic or mood disorders.

The verbal memory deficit seen in patients with schizophrenia is compatible with left temporohippocampal dysfunction and has been observed in patients with schizotypal personality disorder (Voglmaier et al. 2000). Related imaging research with fluorodeoxyglucose PET in the resting state revealed that increased metabolic activity in the left inferior frontal and left midtemporal regions was associated with increased verbal memory deficits (Mozley et al. 1996). This finding was interpreted as indicating dysfunction in the circuitry subserving declarative verbal memory and, in particular, excessive activation in these regions. Compatible with these findings are a highly consistent set of observations of volume reduction in the left temporal lobe of patients with schizotypal personality disorder, first-episode schizophrenia, and chronic schizophrenia (Gur et al. 2000; McCarley et al. 1999) and reduced P300 evoked potential amplitudes over the left temporal lobe in patients with schizophrenia (O'Donnell et al. 1999; Salisbury et al. 1999). Compared with control subjects and patients with manic psychosis, patients with first-episode schizophrenia have smaller gray matter left planum temporale and Heschl

gyrus volume (Hirayasu et al. 2000). Patients with chronic schizophrenia may be more likely to show volume reductions in MTL structures, particularly the hippocampus (Dickey et al. 1999).

However, Gold et al. (1995) compared neuropsychological profiles in patients with schizophrenia and patients with left or right temporal lobe epilepsy. Among the epileptic patients, particularly those with left temporal lobe epilepsy, memory was selectively impaired relative to other domains, particularly attention. Among schizophrenic patients, the magnitude of attentional and memory impairments was relatively equal. Other research has suggested that individual patients may differ in the extent to which they manifest neuropsychological impairments characteristic of frontal lobe (executive function) or temporal lobe (episodic memory) dysfunction (Harvey et al. 1995) and that impairments in each domain may have distinct clinical correlates (Sullivan et al. 1994). Indeed, in a recent study, Weickert et al. (2000) examined neuropsychological profiles in a large group of patients with chronic schizophrenia in relation to estimates of current and premorbid intellectual level. Across the subgroups, they concluded that executive function and attention deficits may be core cognitive features of the disorder, independent of variations in intelligence. In examining patients with schizophrenia, healthy siblings, and control subjects, Staal et al. (2000) found that executive function deficits and, to some extent, sensorimotor impairments characterized both the patients and siblings, suggesting that these cognitive abnormalities may be related to the schizophrenia genotype.

The focus on executive function and working memory impairments suggests disruption of prefrontal cortical function. Compatible physiological and biochemical data have been obtained. Callicott et al.

(2000) reported that during the performance of a working memory task (N-Back), patients with schizophrenia manifested abnormal activation in the dorsolateral prefrontal cortex, with the correlation between the degree of activation response and performance opposite in direction in patients and control subjects. Furthermore, N-acetylaspartate (NAA) concentrations, measured by proton magnetic resonance spectroscopy, were lower in this region (BA 9 and 46) in patients compared with control subjects, suggesting prefrontal neuronal pathology, and the NAA levels predicted the fMRI response to the working memory challenge. Thus, in addition to the substantial evidence for a (verbal) declarative memory deficit in schizophrenia, it is evident that many patients also manifest deficits in working memory and other executive functions.

The nature of the declarative memory deficits in schizophrenia has been further specified. Deficits are usually more pronounced in tests of recall than in tests of recognition (Beatty et al. 1993; Calev 1984). The deficits in explicit recall have often been attributed to shallow or inefficient encoding of information, disorganized or inefficient retrieval strategies, and rapid forgetting (Goldberg and Gold 1995; McKenna et al. 1990). Of note, a growing number of studies report that schizophrenic patients evidence little or no deficits in nondeclarative memory tasks, including procedural memory (as reflected in motor skill learning) and implicit memory (as reflected in various tests of perceptual and conceptual priming) (Clare et al. 1993; Gras-Vincendon et al. 1994; Perry et al. 2000).

As indicated, schizophrenia is also associated with often profound impairments in aspects of working memory. Primate and human research has indicated that various prefrontal areas are critical to the capacity to hold information in consciousness, update past and current information based on a changing environment, and guide behavior on the basis of these representations (Goldman-Rakic 1994). Lesions in selective prefrontal areas in primates result in characteristic deficits in modality-specific aspects of working memory. Neuropsychological tests designed to sample analogous functions in humans have repeatedly shown marked deficits in patients with schizophrenia (Keefe et al. 1995; Park and Holzman 1993). Indeed, a diverse number of deficits are subsumed under the concept of "working memory" or "executive function." The central executive is responsible for selecting stimuli for further processing (i.e., allocating attention). Deficits in this function will be reflected in increased distractibility and inability to maintain vigilance. In line with decades of research suggesting increased distractibility, Fleming et al. (1995) demonstrated that even a simple concurrent task will interfere with short-term memory performance in patients with schizophrenia. Furthermore, the central executive is responsible for shifting sets (i.e., changing strategies and behavior when they no longer meet environmental demands). A deficit in this domain would be expressed as perseveration and as difficulty with rule learning and concept formation. Impairments in these domains are characteristic, as reflected in performance deficits on the Wisconsin Card Sorting Test (Heaton et al. 1993) or the Category Test from the Halstead-Reitan Battery (Reitan and Wolfson 1985). Nonetheless, it has still not been established that dysfunction of specific prefrontal areas is responsible for the working memory deficits seen in schizophrenia. Indeed, there is preliminary evidence that schizophrenic patients may have marked deficits in aspects of working memory that are less reliant on the prefrontal cortex. Using a remarkably simple task, Strous et al. (1995) demonstrated that schizophrenic patients were impaired in matching two tones after a brief delay of only 300 milliseconds but were unimpaired when there was no intertone interval. This aspect of auditory sensory (echoic) memory is thought to be subserved by nonassociation cortex outside the frontal lobes (superior temporal plane). Thus, both prefrontal and nonprefrontal components of working memory may be preferentially disturbed in schizophrenia.

Dissociative Amnesia

Table 7–2 provides the DSM-IV-TR diagnostic criteria for dissociative amnesia (formerly called psychogenic amnesia). Dissociative amnesia is a disorder in which memory loss is attributed to functional factors. The memory loss may be localized in time, may be selective for elements of history, and, most rarely, may be generalized and continuous. In the generalized form, patients may have amnesia for their own identity and history.

Dissociative amnesia is rarely diagnosed. Several factors may account for its low incidence. First, even among patients who at one time received diagnoses of hysteric disorders, amnesia was a relatively uncommon symptom. Perley and Guze (1962) examined the frequency of a wide range of symptoms in a sample of patients with "hysterical neurosis." (At that time, dissociative disorders were included in this grouping.) First, whereas symptoms such as dizziness, headache, fatigue, and abdominal pain occurred at high rates (all in more than 70% of patients), amnesia was found in only 8% of cases. Second, patients presenting with forms of functional amnesia typically have a number of other psychiatric disorders or manifest the amnesia after trauma—as may occur, for instance, in combat situa-

TABLE 7–2. DSM-IV-TR criteria for dissociative amnesia

A. The predominant disturbance is one or more episodes of inability to recall important personal information, usually of a traumatic or stressful nature, that is too extensive to be explained by ordinary forgetfulness.

B. The disturbance does not occur exclusively during the course of dissociative identity disorder, dissociative fugue, posttraumatic stress disorder, acute stress disorder, or somatization disorder and is not due to the direct physiological effects of a substance (e.g., a drug of abuse, a medication) or a neurological or other general medical condition (e.g., amnestic disorder due to head trauma).

C. The symptoms cause clinically significant distress or impairment in social, occupational, or other important areas of functioning.

Source. Reprinted from the *Diagnostic and Statistical Manual of Mental Disorders*, 4th Edition, Text Revision. Washington, DC, American Psychiatric Association, 2000. Copyright 2000, American Psychiatric Association. Used with permission.

tions. Current nosology excludes diagnosis of dissociative amnesia in many such instances. Third, functional amnesia does not necessarily interfere with social or occupational functioning. The most common varieties involve forgetting of isolated events. Furthermore, patients with dissociative amnesia may display indifference to their symptoms and thus may be unlikely to present for treatment.

Dissociative amnesia may be more common among females, and it is thought to occur more often in adolescents and young adults than in elderly persons. Most patients demonstrate rapid recovery of memory, and therefore the disorder is usually transient. Abeles and Schilder (1935) and Herman (1938) reported on 63 cases of dissociative amnesia (they also included fugue states in this categorization). Of these individuals, 27 recovered within 24 hours; 21, within 5 days; 7, within a week; and 4, within 3 weeks or more.

Problems of differential diagnosis usually involve distinguishing dissociative amnesia from two other types of conditions: trauma to the brain, which may produce similar syndromes, and malingering.

The DSM-IV-TR grouping of dissociative disorders is an attempt to categorize disturbances of higher cognitive functions that resemble effects of neurologic dysfunction but that are believed to be functional in origin. If a patient's amnesia can be related to a neurologic disorder, the diagnosis of dissociative disorder is inappropriate. To date, no studies have examined the frequency with which patients with dissociative disorder diagnoses concurrently or ultimately show signs of neurologic disease. However, such work in the case of hysterical conversion reactions indicates that a disturbingly large number of patients thus diagnosed manifested neurologic disorders (at the time or shortly thereafter) that in some proved fatal (Slater and Glithero 1965; Whitlock 1967).

The difficulties of differential diagnosis in this area can be illustrated with the syndrome of transient global amnesia (Fisher and Adams 1964; Pantoni et al. 2000). Without warning, individuals, usually middle-aged, display retrograde amnesia for events that occurred in the previous days, weeks, or years and a dense anterograde amnesia. The amnesia is typically transient, lasting from minutes to several hours. When memory returns, there is typically a progressive recall of distant events, with memory of the most recent past returning last. Retrograde amnesia may resolve before the anterograde component (N. Kapur et al. 1998). During the amnesia, the individual is usually well oriented, with perception, sense of identity, and other higher cognitive functions intact. There is typically considerable concern and upset on the part of the individual about the memory loss. The attacks may strike only once or may be recurrent (Heathfield et al. 1973).

The transient nature of the amnesia and its occurrence in individuals who appear medically healthy might suggest a dissociative reaction. Heathfield et al. (1973) reported on 31 patients who were referred for transient loss of memory. Of the 31 patients, memory loss was associated with epilepsy in 6 patients (19%), with migraine in 1 patient (3%), and with temporal lobe encephalitis in 2 patients (6%). Three patients (10%) received the diagnosis of dissociative (psychogenic) amnesia. The remaining 19 patients (61%) were considered as presenting the syndrome of transient global amnesia. The ages of these 19 patients (13 men, 6 women) ranged from 46 to 68 years; amnesic episodes lasted from 30 minutes to 5 days; 11 had only one attack during the period of study. Cerebrovascular dysfunction was suggested in 9 of the 19 patients. Heathfield et al. (1973) concluded, "It is probable that most episodes of transient global amnesia result from bilateral temporal lobe or thalamic lesions. In some of our patients there was clear evidence of ischemia in the territory of the posterior cerebral circulation, and we consider that such ischemia is the cause of this syndrome" (p. 735). However, recent investigations have suggested that etiologies based on migraine, seizures, transient cerebral arterial ischemia, or a thromboembolic pathogenesis are unlikely to account for transient global amnesia (Lauria et al. 1998; Lewis 1998). Receiving greater attention is the possibility that a blockage of venous return (such as in a Valsalva maneuver) results in high venous retrograde pressure to the cerebral venous system and produces venous ischemia in the diencephalon and MTL (Lewis 1998; Sander et al. 2000). Regardless, several imaging studies, using single photon emission computed tomography (SPECT), PET, or diffusion-weighted magnetic resonance imaging have reported decreased activity in MTL structures during transient global amnesia with normalization on recovery (Jovin et al. 2000; Strupp et al. 1998; Tanabe et al. 1999).

Some general guidelines may be useful in distinguishing dissociative amnesia from the memory loss that accompanies neurologic disease. Typically, the memory loss associated with head trauma, Korsakoff's psychosis, temporal lobe dysfunction, and ECT has both retrograde and anterograde components, whereas patients with dissociative amnesia will often show unaltered ability to acquire and retain new information (as also opposed to transient global amnesia). It is rare in the context of neurologic disease for a patient to manifest global amnesia across the life span, and personal identity and early memories are typically preserved. Dissociative amnesia may selectively affect autobiographical memory, whereas both personal and impersonal memory is disturbed in amnesia associated with neurologic insult.

Contributing to differential diagnosis is the collateral behavior of the patient and the nature of the recovery of memory. Patients who present with amnesia accompanied by clouded consciousness, disorientation, and/or mood change are likely manifesting neurologic disturbance. Indifference to amnesia concerning events that would ordinarily be associated with guilt and shame for the patient suggests a dissociative basis. Dissociative amnesia usually pertains to traumatic events, and amnesia for the ordinary events of life would suggest a neurologic disturbance.

Amnesia during or after a stressful experience is not, however, a reliable sign of dissociative origin (it is excluded by DSM-IV-TR). Stress may precipitate a transient ischemic attack (TIA) or epileptic event, resulting in amnesia. Retrograde amnesia associated with known neurologic insult typically also has a standard course of recovery. Events in the most distant past are recovered before more recent events. In dissociative amnesia, there is usually a sudden return of memory (Nemiah 1979). Interviews employing hypnotism and/or sodium amobarbital may be useful to distinguish dissociative amnesia from neurologic disturbance. A number of reports exist of patients who recovered memory with either procedure, and in some cases the recovery was permanent (e.g., Herman 1938). Recovery of memory with the use of hypnosis or amobarbital should not occur in cases of neurologic disturbance.

Malingering refers to deliberate and voluntary simulation of psychological or physical disorder. The assumption in a diagnosis of dissociative amnesia is that the loss of memory and its subsequent recovery are not under voluntary control. It should be noted that some clinicians with considerable exposure to amnesia of psychological origin question whether a distinction between malingering and dissociative amnesia can or should be made. Differentiating between dissociative amnesia and malingering is difficult. The degree to which a malingerer is successful at simulation likely depends on the sophistication of the patient with regard to manifestations of psychological and neurologic disease. In a somewhat similar context, it should be noted that experienced hypnotists cannot reliably distinguish hypnotized subjects from individuals simulating the effects of hypnosis (Orne 1979). It should be noted that in recent years, psychometric instruments have been validated that appear to be successful in distinguishing between the malingering of anterograde amnesia and a true amnestic syndrome. The basis of this approach is to use memory tests that are subjectively experienced as difficult, but in which patients with amnesia show high performance accuracy. In contrast, individuals who are malingering generate low scores (Rees et al. 1998; Tombaugh 1996).

Normal Aging

Complaints about memory loss are common in the elderly, and normal aging is accompanied by characteristic decrements in memory performance (Parkin et al. 1995; West 1996). However, the decline in memory with aging is selective, affecting some cognitive processes more than others. The capacity to deliberately acquire and retain new information (declarative episodic memory) is often impaired by age 50, particularly when the material to be learned is unstructured, such as random lists of words (Albert et al. 1987). This deficit seems to reflect not a more rapid forgetting with aging, but rather the use of less-efficient encoding and retrieval strategies. In part, this deficit, as in major depression, may reflect limited attentional capacity and reduced capacity for "effortful processing." Aging also exerts greater negative effects on memory for the context in which information was learned as opposed to memory for the information itself. For example, age-related changes have been demonstrated in memory for the temporal order (Parkin et al. 1995) and the source (Craik et al. 1990) of information. This pattern of memory deficits, with decrements in source memory and in the acquisition and retention of unstructured, but not highly structured, material is suggestive of an age-related decline in the memory processes supported by prefron-

tal cortex (West 1996). Indeed, the age-related impairment in source memory has been found to covary with other measures of frontal lobe function, the Wisconsin Card Sorting Test, and verbal fluency (Craik et al. 1990; Parkin et al. 1995). There is also evidence that with aging, the frontal lobe undergoes greater reductions in volume and in resting functional activity than do other brain areas (West 1996).

The literature on the effects of aging on nondeclarative memory is inconsistent. Although it appears that many of the cognitive processes that underlie these aspects of learning and memory are unaltered by age (Light and La Voie 1993), age-related deficits have been reported, particularly for priming tasks. Indeed, there is also evidence linking impaired implicit memory to age-related frontal lobe dysfunction (Winokur et al. 1996).

The Subjective Evaluation of Memory: Metamemory

In clinical circumstances, we often obtain individuals' assessments of their own memory functioning, a domain referred to as *metamemory*. The perception of memory decline may be the first indication of valid incipient changes in cognitive function. A large number of studies, conducted in neurologic, psychiatric, and healthy populations, have examined the relationships between self-evaluations of memory and objective test results.

The most consistent finding in this literature is that the strongest predictor of memory self-evaluation is current mood state (Bennett-Levy and Powell 1980; Coleman et al. 1996; Hinkin et al. 1996; Larrabee and Levin 1986). Almost invariably, depressed mood, whether assessed by observers or by self-report, is associated with self-evaluations of impaired cognitive function (Prudic et al. 2000). In contrast, although significant associations between objective neuropsychological and subjective cognitive evaluations have been occasionally reported (Riege 1982), for the most part such associations are either small in magnitude or nonexistent. Furthermore, when associations have been reported, they have not always been in the expected direction. Hinkin et al. (1996) found that men who were seropositive for human immunodeficiency virus type 1 (HIV-1) with a low level of memory complaints performed worse on memory testing than did those with a higher level of complaints.

It is sobering that, independent of neurologic or psychiatric illness, we are generally poor judges of the quality of our memory. To some extent, this lack of association might be attributed to the limited ecological validity of standard memory-assessment batteries, which may fail to capture the type of memory failures experienced in everyday life (e.g., incidental learning and forgetting). Furthermore, it is clear that a variety of neurologic and psychiatric conditions, including but not limited to Alzheimer's disease and schizophrenia, may be associated with distinct deficits in metamemory, such that patients are particularly likely to deny or be unaware of cognitive deficits. However, the fact that current mood state is a consistent predictor of memory functioning strongly implies that factors other than actual memory performance influence self-evaluations. Figure 7–2 illustrates changes on the Squire Subjective Memory Questionnaire (Squire et al. 1979) in patients with major depression who did and did not respond to ECT (Coleman et al. 1996). Both at baseline and shortly after the ECT course, patient scores on this metamemory measure were strongly associated with depression-severity scores. Despite the fact that patients had characteristic anterograde and retrograde

memory disturbances at the time of post-ECT metamemory evaluation, approximately 80% of patients reported improved memory functioning after ECT relative to before ECT. Although the magnitude of these memory deficits was generally equivalent in ECT responders and nonresponders, the improvement in the metamemory measure was particularly pronounced in patients whose depression responded to ECT.

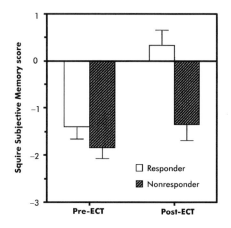

FIGURE 7–2. Scores on the Squire Subjective Memory Questionnaire in depressed patients treated with electroconvulsive therapy (ECT).

A score of 0 indicates that the patient assesses memory function to be the same as it was before the episode of depressive illness, whereas a negative score indicates that the patient considers current memory function to be impaired. Before receiving ECT, patients report marked impairment, the magnitude of which covaries with the severity of depressive symptoms. Patients who respond to ECT report marked improvement even though objective tests indicate memory deficits.

Source. Adapted from Coleman et al. 1996.

Little consensus exists about the theoretical underpinnings of metamemory or subjective memory judgments. The field is largely driven by empirical interest in the relationship of objective memory performance to subjective complaints, and, in particular, the disjunction between the two, that is, why reports of memory performance deviate so markedly from actual performance, a common occurrence. For example, it was hypothesized that there exists an internal memory monitor that reviews memory contents in an unbiased manner and forms judgments about the retrievability of memories (Burke et al. 1991). A later view suggested that judgments about memory are highly inferential, and that evaluations of the objective status of memory must be made based on sources of information other than access to a review of memory content. Other sources of information that affect subjective judgments may include retrieval fluency, the amounts of related and unrelated information activated by attempts to remember (Koriat 1993), and feelings about memory, such as the feeling of familiarity (Schwartz et al. 1997).

As a result, there are likely to be multiple dimensions to assess when evaluating subjective memory. An inclusive conceptual approach offered four dimensions: 1) memory knowledge, which involves factual knowledge about memory and its processes; 2) memory monitoring, which includes awareness of the current state of one's memory and of how one uses memory; 3) memory-related affect; and 4) memory self-efficacy, a set of beliefs about one's memory, including changes in memory status (Hultsch et al. 1988). Evaluations of the psychometric properties of questionnaires developed to examine subjective assessments of memory indicated that assessments of memory capacity and change in memory status were best related to beliefs about memory, which were, in turn, subject to a variety of influences, including mood and locus of control (Cavanaugh and Green 1990). In a meta-analysis of the effects of memory training on subjective memory assessment, Floyd and Scoggin (1997) found that memory training and improve-

ment in performance did not alter subjective memory assessment in normal elderly adults. Instead, techniques such as relaxation training, which may alter affect or mood, and interventions directed at changing participants' beliefs about the effects of aging on memory significantly improved subjective assessment of memory. This suggests that interventions that improve objective memory performance have less impact on subjective evaluations than do interventions targeted either at beliefs about memory or affective state.

Effects of Somatic Treatments on Learning and Memory

Psychotropic Agents

In addition to the deleterious effects of benzodiazepines on psychomotor performance, this class of medications can produce consistent adverse effects on memory. The most characteristic deficit is diminished delayed recall for newly learned information (J.L. Taylor and Tinklenberg 1987). This deficit is most evident acutely after ingestion and is most marked in the first hour or two postingestion for diazepam and the third or fourth hour postingestion for lorazepam. Despite producing this deficit in anterograde declarative memory, benzodiazepines do not appear to impair retrograde memory. Indeed, lists of words learned before benzodiazepine administration may be better recalled in the postingestion period, a phenomenon termed *retrograde facilitation*. This effect may be more pronounced at higher benzodiazepine dosages and has been interpreted as reflecting reduced retroactive interference due to diminished learning after drug ingestion. The capacity of short-term or working memory does not appear to be altered by benzodiazepine use, although the speed at which information is processed may be slowed. Contrary to the case for psychomotor performance, there is evidence that tolerance to adverse acute effects of benzodiazepines on memory functions may not develop with long-term use (Gorenstein et al. 1994) and that elderly individuals are particularly sensitive to the amnesic effects of benzodiazepines.

A wide range of medications have anticholinergic properties, including heterocyclic antidepressants (e.g., amitriptyline, imipramine, and nortriptyline), neuroleptics (e.g., chlorpromazine), antiparkinsonism agents (e.g., benztropine), and sleep and cold preparations that contain antihistamines. Anticholinergics can produce sedation, attentional impairment, memory disturbance, and, in extreme cases, an anticholinergic delirium. There is compelling evidence that psychotropic medications that differ in anticholinergic properties also differ in their effects on learning and memory. For example, despite equivalent clinical improvement, patients with major depression will show superior performance on declarative memory measures when treated with fluoxetine relative to amitriptyline (Richardson et al. 1994). In a double-blind, crossover study in chronic schizophrenic patients, Silver and Geraisy (1995) found that biperiden (an anticholinergic) but not amantadine (a dopamine agonist) produced detectable deficits in both working and declarative memory. As with the benzodiazepines, vulnerability to the adverse cognitive effects of anticholinergic agents may be augmented in the elderly. There is evidence that tolerance develops to the adverse cognitive effects of anticholinergics, but there is no such evidence for benzodiazepines. Nonetheless, all else being equal, avoidance of agents with pronounced anticholinergic effects may be advisable, particularly in patients with preexisting memory impairment.

Aside from the anticholinergic properties of antidepressants or neuroleptics, there is not convincing evidence that standard antidepressants or traditional neuroleptics exert intrinsic detrimental effects on learning and memory. For example, differences among the selective serotonin reuptake inhibitors (SSRIs) in neuropsychological effects are largely attributable to differences among their anticholinergic properties. Although excessive dosages can produce sedation with traditional neuroleptic treatment, most studies comparing patients with schizophrenia with themselves in unmedicated and neuroleptic-treated states have found no change or slight improvement in the medicated state, particularly in measures of attention. This pattern also appears to hold for atypical neuroleptics such as clozapine (Goldberg et al. 1993).

At present, considerable attention is being paid to the possibility that atypical antipsychotic medications have an ameliorative effect on cognitive deficits in schizophrenia (Purdon 1999). Currently, much of the evidence is circumstantial and tentative. At least 12 studies have examined the effects of clozapine on cognitive parameters, with the most general finding being an improvement in measures of attention and verbal fluency, with some additional evidence for improved executive function. However, as reviewed by Meltzer and McGurk (1999), effects of clozapine on working memory and standard measures of verbal and nonverbal learning and memory are inconclusive. Somewhat similarly, risperidone appears to exert positive effects on working memory, executive function, and attention, whereas effects on standard measures of learning and memory are inconsistent. There is preliminary evidence that olanzapine may have a different profile, improving verbal learning and memory, verbal fluency, and executive function, but not attention, working memory, or visual (nonverbal) learning and memory (e.g., Purdon et al. 2000). Thus, the possibility has been raised that atypical antipsychotics differ in their effects on memory, with risperidone having stronger beneficial effects on working (short-term) memory and olanzapine exerting stronger action on verbal learning and memory.

Electroconvulsive Therapy and Other Brain Stimulation Treatments

ECT is a remarkably effective treatment for specific psychiatric disorders (American Psychiatric Association et al. 2001; Sackeim et al. 1995). However, its cognitive side effects are the major factor limiting its use. As with spontaneous seizures, in the immediate postictal period, patients may manifest transient neurologic abnormalities, alterations of consciousness (disorientation, attentional dysfunction), sensorimotor abnormalities, and disturbances in higher cognitive functions, particularly learning and memory (Sackeim 1992). Technical factors in ECT administration, including electrode placement (bilateral versus unilateral), stimulus dosage, and electrical waveform, strongly determine the severity and persistence of these acute effects. Indeed, these factors determine whether patients require on average a few minutes or several hours to achieve full reorientation after seizure termination (Sackeim 1992; Sackeim et al. 1993, 2000; Weiner et al. 1986).

There is rapid recovery of cognitive function after a single treatment. However, with forms of ECT that exert more severe acute cognitive effects, recovery may be incomplete by the time of the next treatment. In such cases, deterioration may occur over the treatment course, particularly when treatments are closely spaced in time. Some patients may develop an organic mental syndrome with marked disorientation during the ECT course. With milder forms of ECT, cumulative deterioration in cognitive functions need not occur. Indeed, with specific alterations of ECT technique, cumulative *improvement* in some acute cognitive measures has been demonstrated (Sackeim 1992).

Associations between the magnitude of cognitive effects and ECT treatment parameters diminish with time after ECT treatment. Differences between bilateral and unilateral electrode placement are difficult to detect after more than a few months have elapsed since the end of the ECT course (Lisanby et al. 2000; Sackeim 1992; Sackeim et al. 1993, 2000; Weiner et al. 1986). Within days of the end of an ECT course, depressed patients manifest superior performance in most cognitive domains relative to their pretreatment baseline. On tests of intelligence, patients' scores shortly after ECT will typically be superior to those produced in the untreated depressed state (Sackeim et al. 1992). Similarly, before treatment, depressed patients usually manifest deficits in the acquisition of information, as revealed by tests of immediate recall or recognition of item lists. Within days after an ECT course, patients are typically unchanged or improved in these measures of learning, with the change in clinical state being the critical predictor of the magnitude of improvement. In contrast, patients often manifest impaired ability to retain information over a delay. This impairment reflects a double dissociation between the effects of depression and ECT on anterograde learning and memory (Steif et al. 1986). ECT introduces a new deficit in consolidation or retention, so that information that is newly learned is rapidly forgotten.

During and shortly after a course of

ECT, patients also display retrograde amnesia. Deficits in the recall or recognition of both personal and public information learned before ECT are common, and there is evidence that these deficits are greatest for events that occurred temporally closest to the treatment (McElhiney et al. 1995; Squire 1986). Thus, whereas memory for more remote events is intact, patients may have difficulty recalling events that occurred during and several months to years before the ECT course. The retrograde amnesia is rarely dense, as patients typically show spottiness in memory for recent events. It has typically been thought that the amnesia is most dense for autobiographical information (Weiner 1984). However, careful analysis of the extent of amnesia for public and personal events, and the details of those events, indicates that information about the world (public events) is subject to greater memory loss (Lisanby et al. 2000). This is in contrast to the pattern often seen with MTL brain damage, in which retrograde amnesia for personal information is greater than that for impersonal or public events (Nadel and Moscovitch 1997).

As time from treatment increases, there is improved retrograde functioning, with a return of more distant memories (Lisanby et al. 2000; McElhiney et al. 1995). This temporally graded pattern is compatible with similar findings of the effects of repeated electroconvulsive shock in animals (Krueger et al. 1992). Both the anterograde and the retrograde amnesia are most marked for explicit or declarative memory, whereas no effects of ECT have been seen on measures of implicit or procedural memory (Squire et al. 1985). In this respect, the effects of ECT on memory are similar to those associated with MTL dysfunction. In general, there is no relation between the magnitude of the adverse effects of ECT on

memory and its therapeutic properties (McElhiney et al. 1995).

Within a few weeks after the end of ECT, objective evidence of persistent cognitive deficits is difficult to document. The anterograde amnesia typically resolves rapidly after ECT termination (Sackeim et al. 1993, 2000). The retrograde amnesia will often show a more gradual reduction, with substantial return of memory for events that were seemingly "forgotten" when assessed immediately after the treatment course. However, ECT can result in persistent deficits (McElhiney et al. 1995; Sackeim 2000a; Weiner et al. 1986), most likely due to a combination of retrograde and anterograde effects. Even when tested at substantial time periods after treatment, patients may manifest persistent amnesia for some events that occurred several months immediately before and after ECT. Some research suggests that the patients most vulnerable to persistent retrograde amnesia are those with preexisting cognitive impairment and those who manifest the most prolonged disorientation immediately after seizure induction (Sobin et al. 1995). In rare patients, the extent of persistent or permanent retrograde amnesia may extend several years into the past (Sackeim 2000a).

In recent years, other brain stimulation treatments have been developed. There have been more than 20 reports on the use of repetitive transcranial magnetic stimulation (rTMS) in the treatment of major depression, as well as application to other neuropsychiatric conditions (George et al. 1999). This noninvasive technique, which involves inducing focal current flow in cortical tissue by imposing a time-varying magnetic field, has shown remarkable promise as a method to map brain function (through transitory disruption of local activity) and brain connectivity, when combined with functional imaging techniques. Although neuropsychological investigation has been limited in the standard treatment trials in neuropsychiatric disorders (usually at least 10 days of stimulation, each for 15–20 periods), initial impressions are that rTMS (either at slow or fast frequencies) is benign in cognitive effects. Of greater uncertainty, at least in the treatment of major depression, is whether nonconvulsive rTMS will have a significant clinical role. Therapeutic properties have been highly variable in effect size, and there is little information on the persistence of clinical benefit (Sackeim 2000b). Using similar technology, an alternative that is being developed is the deliberate induction of seizure activity under general anesthesia with rTMS, termed magnetic seizure therapy (MST). Due to the greater control magnetic stimulation affords over the site of seizure initiation and electrical dosage in the brain, MST may have advantages over ECT in reducing adverse amnestic effects (Lisanby et al. 2001).

Finally, another new brain stimulation approach is the use of vagus nerve stimulation (VNS) in the therapy of treatment-resistant major depressive episodes. VNS is approved for treatment-resistant epilepsy, with approximately 10,000 implants having been performed. The procedure involves inserting a stimulator in the chest wall and running leads to electrodes attached to the left vagus nerve in the neck. Stimulation is continuous, with the 24-hour cycle usually involving 30 seconds of stimulation followed by a 5-minute off period. Intensity of the current administered is the primary variable adjusted, and it is usually varied in relation to tolerability. An initial open-label pilot study suggested that a substantial number of patients with treatment-resistant depression showed marked and sustained clinical improvement (Rush et al. 2000).

Neuropsychological investigation in this sample before and after the acute VNS treatment phase did not reveal any deleterious effects. Indeed, there was improvement in a variety of neurocognitive measures, including memory, but especially executive functions, that tended to covary with the extent of clinical improvement (Sackeim et al. 2001).

References

Abeles M, Schilder P: Psychogenic loss of personal identity. Archives of Neurology and Psychiatry 34:587–604, 1935

Albert MS, Butters N, Levin J: Temporal gradients in the retrograde amnesia of patients with alcoholic Korsakoff's disease. Arch Neurol 36:211–216, 1979

Albert MS, Duffy FH, Naeser MA: Nonlinear changes in cognition and their neurophysiologic correlates. Can J Psychol 41:141–157, 1987

American Psychiatric Association: Diagnostic and Statistical Manual of Mental Disorders, 4th Edition, Text Revision. Washington, DC, American Psychiatric Association, 2000

American Psychiatric Association and Weiner RD, Coffey CE, Fochtmann L, et al: The Practice of ECT: Recommendations for Treatment, Training and Privileging, 2nd Edition. Washington, DC, American Psychiatric Press, 2001

Andreasen NC, O'Leary DS, Cizadlo T, et al: Remembering the past: two facets of episodic memory explored with positron emission tomography. Am J Psychiatry 152:1576–1585, 1995

Andreasen NC, O'Leary DS, Paradiso S, et al: The cerebellum plays a role in conscious episodic memory retrieval. Hum Brain Mapp 8:226–234, 1999

Backman L, Forsell Y: Episodic memory functioning in a community-based sample of old adults with major depression: utilization of cognitive support. J Abnorm Psychol 103:361–370, 1994

Baddeley AD: Working Memory. Oxford, UK, Oxford University Press, 1986

Ball MJ, Fishman M, Hachinski V, et al: A new definition of Alzheimer's disease: a hippocampal dementia. Lancet 1:14–16, 1985

Bazin N, Perruchet P, De Bonis M, et al: The dissociation of explicit and implicit memory in depressed patients. Psychol Med 24:239–245, 1994

Beatty WW, Jocic Z, Monson N, et al: Memory and frontal lobe dysfunction in schizophrenia and schizoaffective disorder. J Nerv Ment Dis 181:448–453, 1993

Bennett-Levy J, Powell GE: The Subjective Memory Questionnaire (SMQ): an investigation into the self-reporting of "real-life" memory skills. Br J Soc Clin Psychol 19:177–188, 1980

Blanchard JJ, Neale JM: The neuropsychological signature of schizophrenia: generalized or differential deficit? Am J Psychiatry 151:40–48, 1994

Blaney PH: Affect and memory: a review. Psychol Bull 99:229–246, 1986

Blaxton TA: Dissociations among memory measures in memory-impaired subjects: evidence for a processing account of memory. Mem Cognit 20:549–562, 1992

Blaxton TA: A process-based view of memory. J Int Neuropsychol Soc 1:112–114, 1995

Bornstein RA, Baker GB, Douglass AB: Depression and memory in major depressive disorder. J Neuropsychiatry Clin Neurosci 3:78–80, 1991

Breslow R, Kocsis J, Belkin B: Memory deficits in depression: evidence utilizing the Wechsler Memory Scale. Percept Mot Skills 51:541–542, 1980

Breslow R, Kocsis J, Belkin B: Contribution of the depressive perspective to memory function in depression. Am J Psychiatry 138:227–230, 1981

Brittlebank AD, Scott J, Williams JM, et al: Autobiographical memory in depression: state or trait marker? Br J Psychiatry 162:118–121, 1993

Buckner RL: Beyond HERA: contributions of specific prefrontal brain areas to long-term memory retrieval. Psychon Bull Rev 3:149–158, 1996

Buckner RL, Petersen SE, Ojemann JG, et al: Functional anatomical studies of explicit and implicit memory retrieval tasks. J Neurosci 15:12–29, 1995

Buckner RL, Koutstaal W, Schacter DL, et al: Functional-anatomic study of episodic retrieval, II: selective averaging of event-related fMRI trials to test the retrieval success hypothesis. Neuroimage 7:163–175, 1998a

Buckner RL, Koutstaal W, Schacter DL, et al: Functional-anatomic study of episodic retrieval using fMRI, I: retrieval effort versus retrieval success. Neuroimage 7:151–162, 1998b

Buckner RL, Kelley WM, Petersen SE: Frontal cortex contributes to human memory formation. Nat Neurosci 2:311–314, 1999

Buckner RL, Koutstaal W, Schacter DL, et al: Functional MRI evidence for a role of frontal and inferior temporal cortex in amodal components of priming. Brain 123 Pt 3:620–640, 2000

Burke D, MacKay DG, Worthley JS, et al: On the tip of the tongue: what causes word findings failures in young and older adults. Journal of Memory and Language 30:542–579, 1991

Burt DB, Zembar MJ, Niederehe G: Depression and memory impairment: a meta-analysis of the association, its pattern, and specificity. Psychol Bull 117:285–305, 1995

Burt T, Prudic J, Peyser S, et al: Learning and memory in bipolar and unipolar major depression: effects of aging. Neuropsychiatry Neuropsychol Behav Neurol 13(4):246–253, 2000

Butters N, Heindel WC, Salmon DP: Dissociation of implicit memory in dementia: neurological implications. Bull Psychon Soc 28:230–246, 1990

Calev A: Recall and recognition in mildly disturbed schizophrenics: the use of matched tasks. Psychol Med 14:425–429, 1984

Calev A, Erwin P: Recall and recognition in depressives: use of matched tasks. Br J Clin Psychol 24:127–128, 1985

Callicott JH, Bertolino A, Mattay VS, et al: Physiological dysfunction of the dorsolateral prefrontal cortex in schizophrenia revisited. Cereb Cortex 10:1078–1092, 2000

Cavanaugh JC, Green EE: I believe, therefore I can: self-efficacy beliefs in memory aging, in Aging and Cognition: Mental Processes, Self-Awareness and Interventions. Edited by Lovelace EA. New York, Elsevier, 1990, pp 189–230

Channon S, Baker JE, Robertson MM: Effects of structure and clustering on recall and recognition memory in clinical depression. J Abnorm Psychol 102:323–326, 1993

Chapman LJ, Chapman JP: Disordered Thought in Schizophrenia. Englewood Cliffs, NJ, Prentice-Hall, 1973

Clare L, McKenna PJ, Mortimer AM, et al: Memory in schizophrenia: what is impaired and what is preserved? Neuropsychologia 31:1225–1241, 1993

Coffman JA, Bornstein RA, Olson SC, et al: Cognitive impairment and cerebral structure by MRI in bipolar disorder. Biol Psychiatry 27:1188–1196, 1990

Cohen NJ: Preserved learning capacity in amnesia: evidence for multiple memory systems, in The Neuropsychology of Memory. Edited by Squire LR, Butters N. New York, Guilford, 1984, pp 83–103

Cohen NJ, Corkin S: The amnesic patient H.M.: learning and retention of a cognitive skill (abstract). Abstr Soc Neurosci 7:235, 1981

Cohen NJ, Squire LR: Preserved learning and retention of pattern analyzing skill in amnesia: dissociation of knowing how and knowing that. Science 210:207–209, 1980

Coleman EA, Sackeim HA, Prudic J, et al: Subjective memory complaints before and after electroconvulsive therapy. Biol Psychiatry 39:346–356, 1996

Conway MA, Turk DJ, Miller SL, et al: A positron emission tomography (PET) study of autobiographical memory retrieval. Memory 7:679–702, 1999

Corkin S: Acquisition of motor skill after bilateral medial temporal lobe excision. Neuropsychologia 6:225–265, 1968

Corkin S: Lasting consequences of bilateral medial temporal lobectomy: clinical course and experimental findings in H.M. Semin Neurol 4:249–259, 1984

Corwin J, Peselow E, Feenan K, et al: Disorders of decision in affective disease: an effect of beta-adrenergic dysfunction? Biol Psychiatry 27:813–833, 1990

Craik FIM, Morris LW, Morris RG, et al: Relations between source amnesia and frontal lobe functioning in older adults. Psychol Aging 5:148–151, 1990

Cronholm B, Ottosson J-O: Memory functions in endogenous depression: before and after electroconvulsive therapy. Arch Gen Psychiatry 5:193–199, 1961

Davis H, Squire L: Protein synthesis and memory. Psychol Bull 96:518–559, 1984

DeMonbreun B, Craighead W: Selective recall of positive and neutral feedback. Cognit Ther Res 1:311–329, 1977

Dickey CC, McCarley RW, Voglmaier MM, et al: Schizotypal personality disorder and MRI abnormalities of temporal lobe gray matter. Biol Psychiatry 45:1393–1402, 1999

Donnelly EF, Murphy DL, Goodwin FK, et al: Intellectual function in primary affective disorder. Br J Psychiatry 140:633–636, 1982

Eich E, Macaulay D, Ryan L: Mood dependent memory for events of the personal past. J Exp Psychol Gen 123:201–215, 1994

Elvevag B, Egan MF, Goldberg TE: Paired-associate learning and memory interference in schizophrenia. Neuropsychologia 38:1565–1575, 2000

Fink GR, Markowitsch HJ, Reinkemeier M, et al: Cerebral representation of one's own past: neural networks involved in autobiographical memory. J Neurosci 16:4275–4282, 1996

Fisher C, Adams R: Transient global amnesia. Acta Neurol Scand 40 (suppl 9):1–83, 1964

Fleming K, Goldberg TE, Gold JM, et al: Verbal working memory dysfunction in schizophrenia: use of a Brown-Peterson paradigm. Psychiatry Res 56:155–161, 1995

Floyd M, Scoggin F: Effects of memory training on the subjective memory functioning and mental health of older adults: a meta-analysis. Psychol Aging 12:150–161, 1997

Gabrieli JDE: A systematic view of human memory processes. J Int Neuropsychol Soc 1:115–118, 1995

Gainotti G, Marra C: Some aspects of memory disorders clearly distinguish dementia of the Alzheimer's type from depressive pseudo-dementia. J Clin Exp Neuropsychol 16: 65–78, 1994

Gass C, Russell E: Differential impact of brain damage and depression on memory test performance. J Consult Clin Psychol 54:261–263, 1986

George MS, Lisanby SH, Sackeim HA: Transcranial magnetic stimulation: applications in psychiatry. Arch Gen Psychiatry 56:300–311, 1999

Gold JM, Blaxton TA, Hermann BP, et al: Memory and intelligence in lateralized temporal lobe epilepsy and schizophrenia. Schizophr Res 17:59–65, 1995

Goldberg TE, Gold JM: Neurocognitive deficits in schizophrenia, in Schizophrenia. Edited by Hirsch SR, Weinberger DR. Oxford, UK, Blackwell, 1995, pp 146–162

Goldberg TE, Greenberg R, Griffin S: The impact of clozapine on cognition and psychiatric symptoms in patients with schizophrenia. Br J Psychiatry 162:43–48, 1993

Goldman-Rakic PS: Working memory and the mind. Sci Am 267:110–117, 1992

Goldman-Rakic PS: Working memory dysfunction in schizophrenia. J Neuropsychiatry Clin Neurosci 6:348–357, 1994

Gorenstein C, Bernik MA, Pompeia S: Differential acute psychomotor and cognitive effects of diazepam on long-term benzodiazepine users. Int Clin Psychopharmacol 9:145–153, 1994

Graf P, Schacter DL: Implicit and explicit memory for new associations in normal and amnesic patients. J Exp Psychol Learn Mem Cogn 11:501–518, 1985

Gras-Vincendon A, Danion JM, Grange D, et al: Explicit memory, repetition priming and cognitive skill learning in schizophrenia. Schizophr Res 13:117–126, 1994

Gur RE, Turetsky BI, Cowell PE, et al: Temporolimbic volume reductions in schizophrenia. Arch Gen Psychiatry 57:769–775, 2000

Harvey PD, Powchik P, Mohs RC, et al: Memory functions in geriatric chronic schizophrenic patients: a neuropsychological study. J Neuropsychiatry Clin Neurosci 7:207–212, 1995

Hasher L, Zacks R: Automatic and effortful processes in memory. J Exp Psychol Gen 108:356–388, 1979

Heathfield K, Croft P, Swash M: The syndrome of transient global amnesia. Brain 96:729–736, 1973

Heaton R, Chelune G, Talley J, et al: Wisconsin Card Sorting Test (WCST) Manual, Revised and Expanded. Odessa, FL, Psychological Resources, 1993

Herman M: The use of intravenous sodium amytal in psychogenic amnesic states. Psychiatr Q 12:738–742, 1938

Hinkin CH, van Gorp WG, Satz P, et al: Actual versus self-reported cognitive dysfunction in HIV-1 infection: memory-metamemory dissociations. J Clin Exp Neuropsychol 18: 431–443, 1996

Hirayasu Y, McCarley RW, Salisbury DF, et al: Planum temporale and Heschl gyrus volume reduction in schizophrenia: a magnetic resonance imaging study of first-episode patients. Arch Gen Psychiatry 57:692–699, 2000

Hultsch DF, Hertzog C, Dixon RA, et al: Memory self-knowledge in the aged, in Cognitive Development in Adulthood: Progress in Cognitive Development Research. Edited by Howe ML, Brainerd CJ. New York, Springer, 1988, pp 65–92

Hyde TM, Nawroz S, Goldberg TE, et al: Is there cognitive decline in schizophrenia? a cross-sectional study. Br J Psychiatry 164:494–500, 1994

Jacobs DM, Sano M, Dooneief G, et al: Neuropsychological detection and characterization of preclinical Alzheimer's disease. Neurology 45:957–962, 1995

Jacoby LL, Lindsay DS, Toth JP: Unconscious influences revealed: attention, awareness, and control. Am Psychol 47:802–809, 1992

Johnson SD, Saykin AJ, Flashman LA, et al: Brain activation on fMRI and verbal memory ability: functional neuroanatomic correlates of CVLT performance. J Int Neuropsychol Soc 7:55–62, 2001

Jovin TG, Vitti RA, McCluskey LF: Evolution of temporal lobe hypoperfusion in transient global amnesia: a serial single photon emission computed tomography study. J Neuroimaging 10:238–241, 2000

Kapur N: Syndromes of retrograde amnesia: a conceptual and empirical synthesis. Psychol Bull 125:800–825, 1999

Kapur N, Millar J, Abbott P, et al: Recovery of function processes in human amnesia: evidence from transient global amnesia. Neuropsychologia 36:99–107, 1998

Kapur S, Craik FI, Jones C, et al: Functional role of the prefrontal cortex in retrieval of memories: a PET study. Neuroreport 6:1880–1884, 1995

Keane MM, Gabrieli JDE, Monti LA, et al: Amnesic patients show normal priming and a normal depth-of-processing effect in a conceptually driven implicit task (abstract). Abstr Soc Neurosci 19:1079, 1993

Keefe RS, Roitman SE, Harvey PD, et al: A pen-and-paper human analogue of a monkey prefrontal cortex activation task: spatial working memory in patients with schizophrenia. Schizophr Res 17:25–33, 1995

Kelly C, Sharkey V, Morrison G, et al: Nithsdale Schizophrenia Surveys. 20. Cognitive function in a catchment-area-based population of patients with schizophrenia. Br J Psychiatry 177:348–353, 2000

Kessing LV: Cognitive impairment in the euthymic phase of affective disorder. Psychol Med 28:1027–1038, 1998

Kindermann SS, Brown GG: Depression and memory in the elderly: a meta-analysis. J Clin Exp Neuropsychol 19:625–642, 1997

Kopelman MD: The "new" and the "old": components of the anterograde and retrograde memory loss in Korsakoff and Alzheimer patients, in Neuropsychology of Memory, 2nd Edition. Edited by Squire LR, Butters N. New York, Guilford, 1992, pp 130–146

Kopelman MD, Stanhope N, Kingsley D: Retrograde amnesia in patients with diencephalic, temporal lobe or frontal lesions. Neuropsychologia 37:939–958, 1999

Koriat A: How do we know that we know? The accessibility model of the feeling of knowing. Psychol Rev 100:609–639, 1993

Krueger RB, Sackeim HA, Gamzu ER: Pharmacological treatment of the cognitive side effects of ECT: a review. Psychopharmacol Bull 28:409–424, 1992

Lachner G, Engel RR: Differentiation of dementia and depression by memory tests: a meta-analysis. J Nerv Ment Dis 182:34–39, 1994

Larrabee GJ, Levin HS: Memory self-ratings and objective test performance in a normal elderly sample. J Clin Exp Neuropsychol 8:275–284, 1986

Lauria G, Gentile M, Fassetta G, et al: Transient global amnesia and transient ischemic attack: a community-based case-control study. Acta Neurol Scand 97:381–385, 1998

Lepage M, Habib R, Tulving E: Hippocampal PET activations of memory encoding and retrieval: the HIPER model. Hippocampus 8:313–322, 1998

Lepage M, Ghaffar O, Nyberg L, et al: Prefrontal cortex and episodic memory retrieval mode. Proc Natl Acad Sci U S A 97:506–511, 2000

Lewis SL: Aetiology of transient global amnesia. Lancet 352: 397–399, 1998

Light LL, La Voie D: Direct and indirect measures of memory in old age, in Implicit Memory. Edited by Graf P, Masson MEJ. Hillsdale, NJ, Erlbaum, 1993, pp 207–230

Lisanby SH, Maddox JH, Prudic J, et al: The effects of electroconvulsive therapy on memory of autobiographical and public events. Arch Gen Psychiatry 57:581–590, 2000

Lisanby SH, Schlaepfer TE, Fisch H-U, et al: Magnetic seizure therapy of major depression. Arch Gen Psychiatry 58(3): 303–305, 2001

Lloyd GG, Lishman WA: Effect of depression on the speed of recall of pleasant and unpleasant experiences. Psychol Med 5:173–180, 1975

Maguire EA, Mummery CJ: Differential modulation of a common memory retrieval network revealed by positron emission tomography. Hippocampus 9:54–61, 1999

Markowitsch HJ: Which brain regions are critically involved in the retrieval of old episodic memory? Brain Res Brain Res Rev 21:117–127, 1995

Markowitsch HJ: The neuroanatomy of memory, in The Oxford Handbook of Memory. Edited by Tulving E, Craik FIM. New York, Oxford University Press, 2000, pp 465–484

Marslen-Wilson WD, Teuber H: Memory for remote events in anterograde amnesia: recognition of public figures from news photographs. Neuropsychologia 13:353–364, 1975

Mason CF: Pre-illness intelligence of mental hospital patients. J Consult Psychol 20:297–300, 1956

McCarley RW, Wible CG, Frumin M, et al: MRI anatomy of schizophrenia. Biol Psychiatry 45:1099–1119, 1999

McElhiney MC, Moody BJ, Steif BL, et al: Autobiographical memory and mood: effects of electroconvulsive therapy. Neuropsychology 9:501–507, 1995

McKay AP, Tarbuck AF, Shapleske J, et al: Neuropsychological function in manic-depressive psychosis. Evidence for persistent deficits in patients with chronic, severe illness. Br J Psychiatry 167:51–57, 1995

McKenna PJ, Tamlyn D, Lund CE, et al: Amnesic syndrome in schizophrenia. Psychol Med 20:967–972, 1990

Meltzer HY, McGurk SR: The effects of clozapine, risperidone, and olanzapine on cognitive function in schizophrenia. Schizophr Bull 25:233–255, 1999

Milner B: The memory defect in bilateral hippocampal lesions. Psychiatr Res Rep Am Psychiatr Assoc11:43–52, 1959

Milner B, Petrides M, Smith ML: Frontal lobes and the temporal organization of memory. Hum Neurobiol 4:137–142, 1985

Moscovitch M: Memory and working with memory: evaluation of a component process model and comparisons with other models, in Memory Systems 1994. Edited by Schacter D, Tulving E. Cambridge, MA, MIT Press, 1994, pp 269–310

Mozley LH, Gur RC, Gur RE, et al: Relationships between verbal memory performance and the cerebral distribution of fluorodeoxyglucose in patients with schizophrenia. Biol Psychiatry 40:443–451, 1996

Nadel L, Moscovitch M: Memory consolidation, retrograde amnesia and the hippocampal complex. Curr Opin Neurol 7:217–227, 1997

Nemiah J: Dissociative amnesia: a clinical and theoretical reconsideration, in Functional Disorders of Memory. Edited by Kihlstrom J, Evans F. Hillsdale, NJ, Erlbaum, 1979, pp 303–323

Nopoulos P, Flashman L, Flaum M, et al: Stability of cognitive functioning early in the course of schizophrenia. Schizophr Res 14:29–37, 1994

Nyberg L, Cabeza R, Tulving E: PET studies of encoding and retrieval: the HERA model. Psychon Bull Rev 3:135–148, 1996a

Nyberg L, McIntosh AR, Cabeza R, et al: General and specific brain regions involved in encoding and retrieval of events: what, where, and when. Proc Natl Acad Sci U S A 93: 11280–11285, 1996b

Nyberg L, McIntosh AR, Houle S, et al: Activation of medial temporal structures during episodic memory retrieval. Nature 380:715–717, 1996c

Nyberg L, McIntosh AR, Tulving E: Functional brain imaging of episodic and semantic memory with positron emission tomography. J Mol Med 76:48–53, 1998

Nyberg L, Persson J, Habib R, et al: Large scale neurocognitive networks underlying episodic memory. J Cogn Neurosci 12:163–173, 2000

O'Donnell BF, McCarley RW, Potts GF, et al: Identification of neural circuits underlying P300 abnormalities in schizophrenia. Psychophysiology 36:388–398, 1999

Orne M: On the simulating subjects as a quasi-control group in hypnosis research: what, why, and how, in Hypnosis: Developments in Research and New Perspectives. Edited by Fromm E, Shor R. New York, Aldine, 1979, pp 519–565

Overall JE, Hoffmann NG, Levin H: Effects of aging, organicity, alcoholism, and functional psychopathology on WAIS subtest profiles. J Consult Clin Psychol 46:1315–1322, 1978

Pantoni L, Lamassa M, Inzitari D: Transient global amnesia: a review emphasizing pathogenic aspects. Acta Neurol Scand 102:275–283, 2000

Park S, Holzman PS: Association of working memory deficit and eye tracking dysfunction in schizophrenia. Schizophr Res 11:55–61, 1993

Parkin AJ, Walter BM, Hunkin NM: Relationships between normal aging, frontal lobe function, and memory for temporal and spatial information. Neuropsychology 9:304–312, 1995

Perley M, Guze S: Hysteria—the stability and usefulness of clinical criteria. N Engl J Med 266:421–426, 1962

Perry W, Light GA, Davis H, et al: Schizophrenia patients demonstrate a dissociation on declarative and non-declarative memory tests. Schizophr Res 46:167–174, 2000

Prudic J, Peyser S, Sackeim HA: Subjective memory complaints: a review of patient self-assessment of memory after electroconvulsive therapy. J ECT 16:121–132, 2000

Purdon SE: Cognitive improvement in schizophrenia with novel antipsychotic medications. Schizophr Res 35 (suppl):S51–60, 1999

Purdon SE, Jones BD, Stip E, et al: Neuropsychological change in early phase schizophrenia during 12 months of treatment with olanzapine, risperidone, or haloperidol. The Canadian Collaborative Group for Research in Schizophrenia. Arch Gen Psychiatry 57:249–258, 2000

Rees LM, Tombaugh TN, Gansler DA, et al: Five validation experiments of the Test of Memory Malingering (TOMM). Psychol Assess 10:10–20, 1998

Reitan R, Wolfson D: The Halstead-Reitan Neuropsychological Test Battery: Theory and Clinical Interpretation. Tuscon, AZ, Neuropsychology Press, 1985

Richardson JS, Keegan DL, Bowen RC, et al: Verbal learning by major depressive disorder patients during treatment with fluoxetine or amitriptyline. Int Clin Psychopharmacol 9:35–40, 1994

Riege WH: Self-report and tests of memory aging. Clin Gerontol 1:23–36, 1982

Roy-Byrne PP, Weingartner H, Bierer LM, et al: Effortful and automatic cognitive processes in depression. Arch Gen Psychiatry 43:265–267, 1986

Rush AJ, George MS, Sackeim HA, et al: Vagus nerve stimulation (VNS) for treatment-resistant depressions: a multicenter study. Biol Psychiatry 47:276–286, 2000

Russell WR, Nathan PW: Traumatic amnesia. Brain 69:280–300, 1946

Sackeim HA: The cognitive effects of electroconvulsive therapy, in Cognitive Disorders: Pathophysiology and Treatment. Edited by Moos WH, Gamzu ER, Thal LJ. New York, Marcel Dekker, 1992, pp 183–228

Sackeim HA: Memory and ECT: from polarization to reconciliation. J ECT 16:87–96, 2000a

Sackeim HA: Repetitive transcranial magnetic stimulation: what are the next steps? Biol Psychiatry 48:959–961, 2000b

Sackeim HA, Steif BL: The neuropsychology of depression and mania, in Depression and Mania. Edited by Georgotas A, Cancro R. New York, Elsevier, 1988, pp 265–289

Sackeim HA, Freeman J, McElhiney M, et al: Effects of major depression on estimates of intelligence. J Clin Exp Neuropsychol 14:268–288, 1992

Sackeim HA, Prudic J, Devanand DP, et al: Effects of stimulus intensity and electrode placement on the efficacy and cognitive effects of electroconvulsive therapy. N Engl J Med 328:839–846, 1993

Sackeim HA, Devanand DP, Nobler MS: Electroconvulsive therapy, in Psychopharmacology: The Fourth Generation of Progress. Edited by Bloom F, Kupfer D. New York, Raven, 1995, pp 1123–1142

Sackeim HA, Prudic J, Devanand DP, et al: A prospective, randomized, double-blind comparison of bilateral and right unilateral electroconvulsive therapy at different stimulus intensities. Arch Gen Psychiatry 57:425–434, 2000

Sackeim HA, Keilp JG, Rush AJ, et al: The effects of vagus nerve stimulation on cognitive performance in patients with treatment-resistant depression. Neuropsychiatry Neuropsychol Behav Neurol 14(1):53–62, 2001

Salisbury DF, Shenton ME, McCarley RW: P300 topography differs in schizophrenia and manic psychosis. Biol Psychiatry 45:98–106, 1999

Sander D, Winbeck K, Etgen T, et al: Disturbance of venous flow patterns in patients with transient global amnesia. Lancet 356:1982–1984, 2000

Saykin AJ, Shtasel DL, Gur RE, et al: Neuropsychological deficits in neuroleptic naive patients with first-episode schizophrenia. Arch Gen Psychiatry 51:124–131, 1994

Saykin AJ, Johnson SC, Flashman LA, et al: Functional differentiation of medial temporal and frontal regions involved in processing novel and familiar words: an fMRI study. Brain 122:1963–1971, 1999

Schacter DL: Perceptual representation systems and implicit memory: toward a resolution of the multiple memory systems debate. Ann N Y Acad Sci 608:543–571, 1990

Schacter DL, Church B: Auditory priming: implicit and explicit memory for words and voices. J Exp Psychol Learn Mem Cogn 18:915–930, 1992

Schacter DL, Wagner AD: Medial temporal lobe activations in fMRI and PET studies of episodic encoding and retrieval. Hippocampus 9:7–24, 1999

Schacter DL, Cooper LA, Delaney SM: Implicit memory for unfamiliar objects depends on access to structural descriptions. J Exp Psychol Gen 119:5–24, 1990

Schwartz BL, Benjamin AS, Bjork RA: The inferential and experiential bases of metamemory. Current Directions in Psychological Science 6:132–137, 1997

Shallice T, Fletcher P, Frith CD, et al: Brain regions associated with acquisition and retrieval of verbal episodic memory. Nature 368:633–635, 1994

Shelline YI, Sanghavi M, Mintun MA, et al: Depression duration but not age predicts hippocampal volume loss in medically healthy women with recurrent major depression. J Neurosci 19:5034–5043, 1999

Shimamura AP: Memory and frontal lobe function, in The Cognitive Neurosciences. Edited by Gazzaniga MS. Cambridge, MA, MIT Press, 1994, pp 803–813

Silver H, Geraisy N: Effects of biperiden and amantadine on memory in medicated chronic schizophrenic patients: a double-blind cross-over study. Br J Psychiatry 166:241–243, 1995

Singer JA, Salovey P: Mood and memory: evaluating the network theory of affect. Clin Psychol Rev 8:211–251, 1988

Slater E, Glithero E: A follow-up of patients diagnosed as suffering from "hysteria." J Psychosom Res 9:9–13, 1965

Small SA, Perera GM, DeLaPaz R, et al: Differential regional dysfunction of the hippocampal formation among elderly with memory decline and Alzheimer's disease. Ann Neurol 45:466–472, 1999

Sobin C, Sackeim HA, Prudic J, et al: Predictors of retrograde amnesia following ECT. Am J Psychiatry 152:995–1001, 1995

Squire LR: Memory functions as affected by electroconvulsive therapy. Ann N Y Acad Sci 462:307–314, 1986

Squire LR: Declarative and nondeclarative memory: multiple brain systems supporting learning and memory. J Cogn Neurosci 99:195–231, 1992

Squire LR, Wetzel CD, Slater PC: Memory complaint after electroconvulsive therapy: assessment with a new self-rating instrument. Biol Psychiatry 14:791–801, 1979

Squire L, Shimamura A, Graf P: Independence of recognition memory and priming effects: a neuropsychological analysis. J Exp Psychol Learn Mem Cogn 11:37–44, 1985

Staal WG, Hijman R, Hulshoff Pol HE, et al: Neuropsychological dysfunctions in siblings discordant for schizophrenia. Psychiatry Res 95:227–235, 2000

Steif BL, Sackeim HA, Portnoy S, et al: Effects of depression and ECT on anterograde memory. Biol Psychiatry 21:921–930, 1986

Stern Y, Moeller JR., Anderson, KE, et al: Different brain networks mediate task performance in normal aging and AD: defining compensation. Neurology 55:1291–1297, 2000

Sternberg DE, Jarvik ME: Memory function in depression: improvement with antidepressant medication. Arch Gen Psychiatry 33:219–224, 1976

Strous RD, Cowan N, Ritter W, et al: Auditory sensory (echoic) memory dysfunction in schizophrenia. Am J Psychiatry 152:1517–1519, 1995

Strupp M, Bruning R, Wu RH, et al: Diffusion-weighted MRI in transient global amnesia: elevated signal intensity in the left mesial temporal lobe in 7 of 10 patients. Ann Neurol 43:164–170, 1998

Stuss DT, Benson DF: The Frontal Lobes. New York, Raven, 1986

Sullivan EV, Shear PK, Zipursky RB, et al: A deficit profile of executive, memory, and motor functions in schizophrenia. Biol Psychiatry 36:641–653, 1994

Tanabe M, Watanabe T, Ishibashi M, et al: Hippocampal ischemia in a patient who experienced transient global amnesia after undergoing cerebral angiography: case illustration. J Neurosurg 91:347, 1999

Taylor JL, Tinklenberg JR: Cognitive impairment and benzodiazepines, in Psychopharmacology: The Third Generation of Progress. Edited by Meltzer H. New York, Raven, 1987, pp 1449–1454

Taylor MA, Abrams R: Cognitive dysfunction in schizophrenia. Am J Psychiatry 141:196–201, 1984

Tombaugh T: Test of Memory Malingering (TOMM). New York, Multi Health Systems, 1996

Tulving E: Episodic and semantic memory, in Organization of Memory. Edited by Tulving E, Donaldson W. New York, Academic Press, 1972, pp 381–403

Tulving E: Elements of Episodic Memory. Oxford, UK, Oxford University Press, 1983

Tulving E, Markowitsch HJ: Memory beyond the hippocampus. Curr Opin Neurobiol 7:209–216, 1997

Tulving E, Markowitsch HJ: Episodic and declarative memory: role of the hippocampus. Hippocampus 8:198–204, 1998

Tulving E, Schacter DL: Priming and human memory systems. Science 247:301–306, 1990

Tulving E, Kapur S, Craik FI, et al: Hemispheric encoding/retrieval asymmetry in episodic memory: positron emission tomography findings. Proc Natl Acad Sci U S A 91:2016–2020, 1994a

Tulving E, Kapur S, Markowitsch HJ, et al: Neuroanatomical correlates of retrieval in episodic memory: auditory sentence recognition. Proc Natl Acad Sci U S A 91:2012–2015, 1994b

Tulving E, Habib R, Nyberg L, et al: Positron emission tomography correlations in and beyond medial temporal lobes. Hippocampus 9:71–82, 1999

van Gorp WG, Altshuler L, Theberge DC, et al: Cognitive impairment in euthymic bipolar patients with and without prior alcohol dependence. A preliminary study. Arch Gen Psychiatry 55:41–46, 1998

Verdoux H, Liraud F: Neuropsychological function in subjects with psychotic and affective disorders. Relationship to diagnostic category and duration of illness. Eur Psychiatry 15:236–243, 2000

Victor M, Adams RD, Collins GH: The Wernicke-Korsakoff Syndrome, 2nd Edition. Philadelphia, PA, FA Davis, 1989

Voglmaier MM, Seidman LJ, Niznikiewicz MA, et al: Verbal and nonverbal neuropsychological test performance in subjects with schizotypal personality disorder. Am J Psychiatry 157:787–793, 2000

Watkins PC, Vache K, Verney SP, et al: Unconscious mood-congruent memory bias in depression. J Abnorm Psychol 105:34–41, 1996

Weickert TW, Goldberg TE, Gold JM, et al: Cognitive impairments in patients with schizophrenia displaying preserved and compromised intellect. Arch Gen Psychiatry 57:907–913, 2000

Weiner RD: Does ECT cause brain damage? Behavioral Brain Science 7:1–53, 1984

Weiner RD, Rogers HJ, Davidson JR, et al: Effects of stimulus parameters on cognitive side effects. Ann N Y Acad Sci 462:315–325, 1986

Weingartner H, Cohen R, Murphy D, et al: Cognitive processes in depression. Arch Gen Psychiatry 38:42–47, 1981

Weiskrantz L, Warrington EK: Conditioning in amnesic patients. Neuropsychologia 17:187–194, 1979

Welsh KA, Butters N, Hughes JP, et al: Detection and staging of dementia in Alzheimer's disease: use of the neuropsychological measures developed for the Consortium to Establish a Registry for Alzheimer's Disease. Arch Neurol 49:448–452, 1992

West RL: An application of prefrontal cortex function theory to cognitive aging. Psychol Bull 120:272–292, 1996

Wheeler MA, Stuss DT, Tulving E: Frontal lobe damage produces episodic memory impairment. J Int Neuropsychol Soc 1:525–536, 1995

Whitehead A: Verbal learning and memory in elderly depressives. Br J Psychiatry 123:203–208, 1973

Whitlock F: The etiology of hysteria. Acta Psychiatr Scand 43:144–162, 1967

Winokur G, Moscovitch M, Stuss DT: Explicit and implicit memory in the elderly: evidence for double dissociation involving medial temporal- and frontal-lobe functions. Neuropsychology 10:57–65, 1996

Zakzanis KK, Leach L, Kaplan E: On the nature and pattern of neurocognitive function in major depressive disorder. Neuropsychiatry Neuropsychol Behav Neurol 11:111–119, 1998

PART

III

Neuropsychiatric Disorders

Neuropsychiatric Aspects of Traumatic Brain Injury

Jonathan M. Silver, M.D.

Robert E. Hales, M.D., M.B.A.

Stuart C. Yudofsky, M.D.

Each year in the United States, more than 2 million people sustain a traumatic brain injury (TBI); 300,000 of these persons require hospitalization, and more than 80,000 of the survivors are afflicted with the chronic sequelae of such injuries (Kraus and Sorenson 1994). In this population, psychosocial and psychological deficits are commonly the major source of disability to the victims and of stress to their families. The psychiatrist, neurologist, and neuropsychologist are often called on by other medical specialists or the families to treat these patients. In this chapter, we review the role these professionals play in the prevention, diagnosis, and treatment of the cognitive, behavioral, and emotional aspects of TBI.

Epidemiology

It is commonly taught in introductory courses in psychiatry that suicide is the second most common cause of death among persons under age 35. What is often not stated is that the most common cause is injuries incurred during motor vehicle accidents. TBI accounts for 2% of all deaths and 26% of all injury deaths (Sosin et al. 1989). A conservative estimate of the annual incidence of TBI (including brain trauma and transient and persistent postconcussion syndromes) is 200 per 100,000 per year (Kraus and Sorenson 1994). In the United States, between 2.5 million and 6.5 million individuals live with the long-term consequences of TBI (NIH Consensus Development Panel 1999). Disorders arising from traumatic injuries to the brain are more common than any other neurologic disease, with the exception of headaches (Kurtzke 1984).

Those at the highest risk for brain injury are men 15–24 years old. Alcohol use is common in brain injury; a positive blood alcohol concentration was demonstrated in 56% of one sample of victims (Kraus et al. 1989). Motor vehicle accidents account for approximately one-half of traumatic injuries; other common causes are falls (21%), assaults and violence (20%), and accidents associated with sports and recreation (3%) (although as many as 90% of injuries in this category may be unreported) (NIH Consensus Development Panel 1999). Children are highly vulnerable to accidents as passengers, to falls as pedestrians, to impact from moving objects (e.g., rocks or baseballs), and to sports injuries. In the United States, as many as 5 million children sustain head injuries each year, and of this group 200,000 are hospitalized (Raphaely et al. 1980). As a result of bicycle accidents alone, 50,000 children sustain head injuries, and 400 children die each year (U.S. Department of Health and Human Services 1989). Tragically, among infants, most head injuries are the result of child abuse (64%) (U.S. Department of Health and Human Services 1989).

Statistics form only a piece of the picture of the cost of TBI. Mental health professionals must deal with individuals and families who have endured these tragic events. The psychological and social disability after brain injury can be dramatic. As with patients who have many psychiatric illnesses, and in distinction to patients with neurologic disorders such as stroke and Parkinson's disease, many survivors of TBI appear to be physically well (without sensorimotor impairment). In addition to the neurologic consequences of TBI, the cognitive, social, and behavioral problems result in significant impairment.

Neuroanatomy and Pathophysiology of Traumatic Brain Injury

Neuroanatomy

The patient who sustains brain injury from trauma may incur damage through several mechanisms, which are listed in Table 8–1. Contusions affect specific areas of the brain and usually occur as the result of low-velocity injuries, such as falls. Courville (1945) examined the neuroanatomic sites of contusions and found that most injuries were in the basal and polar portions of the temporal and frontal lobes. Most of these lesions were the result of the location of bony prominences that surround the orbital, frontal, and temporal areas along the base of the skull. Coup injuries occur at the site of impact due to local tissue strain. Contrecoup injuries occur away from the site of impact during sudden deceleration and translational and angular movements of the head. Impact is not required for contrecoup injuries to occur, and they usually occur in frontal and temporal areas (Gennarelli and Graham 1998).

TABLE 8–1. Mechanisms of neuronal damage in traumatic brain injury

Primary effects
  Contusions
  Diffuse axonal injury
Secondary effects
  Hematomas
    Epidural effects
    Subdural effects
    Intracerebral effects
  Cerebral edema
  Hydrocephalus
  Increased intracranial pressure
  Infection
  Hypoxia
  Neurotoxicity
  Inflammatory response
  Protease activation
  Calcium influx
  Excitotoxin and free radical release
  Lipid peroxidation
  Phospholipase activation

Diffuse axonal injury refers to mechanical or chemical damage to the axons in cerebral white matter that commonly occurs with lateral angular or rotational acceleration. The axon is vulnerable to injury during high-velocity accidents when there is twisting and turning of the brain around the brain stem (as can occur in "whiplash" car accidents). Axons are stretched, causing disruption of the cytoskeleton and impaired axoplasm transport. This results in axoplasmic swelling and detachment and in wallerian degeneration of the distal stump of the axon (Cassidy 1994). The disruption of axons can occur as long as 2 weeks after the injury (Gennarelli and Graham 1998). Chemically, metabolic changes occur, leading to axonal damage (discussion follows). The most vulnerable sites in the brain to axonal injury are the reticular formation, superior cerebellar peduncles, regions of the basal ganglia, hypothalamus, limbic fornices, and corpus callosum (Cassidy 1994).

Diffuse axonal injury often results in sudden loss of consciousness (LOC) and can occur in minor brain injury or *concussion* (Jane et al. 1985; Povlishock et al. 1983). Among cases of TBI without diffuse axonal injury, there is a lower incidence of skull fractures, contusions, and intracranial hematomas (Adams et al. 1982).

Subdural hematomas (acute, subacute, and chronic) and intracerebral hematomas have effects that are specific to their locations and degree of neuronal damage. In general, subdural hematomas affect arousal and cognition.

Pathophysiology

After TBI, the damaged neurons have an increased demand for energy. However, a decrease in cerebral blood flow occurs, which results in a mismatch between needed and available energy supply. These injured cells are more vulnerable to hypoxia, resulting in further neuronal damage (DeKosky et al. 1998). Secondary neurotoxicity is caused by calcium influx,

phospholipase activation, inflammatory response, protease activation, excitotoxin release, and lipid peroxidation that further damage axons and neuronal systems (DeKosky et al. 1998; Honig and Albers 1994). During hypoxia, free radicals and excitotoxic neurotransmitters, such as glutamate, are released and result in further neuronal damage (Becker et al. 1988; Faden et al. 1989), especially hippocampal damage to the CA1 neurons (Gennarelli and Graham 1998).

Studies in animals suggest that the hippocampal formation is differentially sensitive to injury relative to other regions of the brain, that the CA1 and CA3 subfields and the dentate hilar region are most commonly affected, that such injury can occur even in the absence of hypoxia or elevated intracranial pressure (Hicks et al. 1993; Lowenstein et al. 1992; D.H. Smith et al. 1991; Toulmond et al. 1993), and that functional alterations may occur without actual neuronal cell death (Reeves et al. 1995).

Animal models of TBI, including fluid percussion models in cats and rodents and controlled angular acceleration devices in nonhuman primates, suggest that even mild TBI can result in neuronal injury with the appearance of axonal edema, separation of proximal and distal portions of the injured axons, and subsequent wallerian degeneration of the distal axonal segment (Jane et al. 1985; Povlishock and Coburn 1989). This is accompanied by disruption of axoplasmic transport and by secondary deafferentation. These changes evolve over a broad period of time—for example, from hours to weeks in the cat model (Povlishock and Coburn 1989)—perhaps providing some rationale for evolving symptoms in the days and weeks following a mild TBI (Blumbergs et al. 1994; Gennarelli et al. 1982; Oppenheimer 1968).

There have been several studies of neurochemical changes after TBI. From these studies, it is evident that TBI can affect the neurotransmitter systems that mediate mood and affect, including norepinephrine, serotonin, dopamine, and acetylcholine (Bareggi et al. 1975; Clifton et al. 1981; DeAngelis et al. 1994; DeKosky et al. 1998; Dunn-Meynell et al. 1994; Hamill et al. 1987; Lyeth et al. 1994; Morrison et al. 1979; Porta et al. 1975; Van Woerkom et al. 1977; Vecht et al. 1975).

Neuropsychiatric Assessment of Traumatic Brain Injury

History Taking

Although brain injuries subsequent to serious automobile, occupational, or sports accidents may not result in diagnostic enigmas for the psychiatrist, less severe trauma may first present as relatively subtle behavioral or affective change. Patients may fail to associate the traumatic event with subsequent symptoms. Confusion, intellectual changes, affective lability, or psychosis may occur directly after the trauma or as long as many years afterward. Individuals who present for emergency treatment for blunt trauma may not be adequately screened for TBI (Chambers et al. 1996). Even individuals who identified themselves as "nondisabled" but who had experienced a blow to the head that left them at a minimum dazed and confused had symptoms and emotional distress similar to a group of individuals with known mild TBI (Gordon et al. 1998).

For all psychiatric patients, the clinician must specifically inquire whether the patient has been involved in situations that are associated with head trauma. The practitioner should ask about automobile, bicycle, or motorcycle accidents; falls; assaults; playground accidents; and participation in sports that are frequently asso-ciated with brain injury (e.g., football, soccer, rugby, and boxing). Patients must be asked whether there was any alteration in consciousness after they were injured, including feeling dazed or confused, losing consciousness, or experiencing a period of amnesia after the accident. The clinician should inquire as to whether the patients were hospitalized and whether they had posttraumatic symptoms, such as headache, dizziness, irritability, problems with concentration, and sensitivity to noise or light. Most patients will not volunteer this information without direct inquiry. Patients are usually unaware of the phenomenon of posttraumatic amnesia and may confuse posttraumatic amnesia with LOC. They assume that if they are unable to recall events, they must have been unconscious. Therefore, care must be taken to document the source of this observation (e.g., whether there were observers who witnessed the period of unconsciousness).

Because many patients either are unaware of, minimize, or deny the severity of behavioral changes that occur after TBI, family members also must be asked about the effects of injury on the behavior of their relative. Patients overestimate their level of functioning compared with the reporting of relatives, and they report more physical than nonphysical impairment (Sherer et al. 1998).

Documentation and Rating of Symptoms

Symptom rating scales, electrophysiological imaging, and neuropsychiatric assessments should be used to define symptoms and signs that result from TBI (Table 8–2). The severity of injury may be determined by several parameters, including duration of unconsciousness, initial score on the Glasgow Coma Scale (GCS) (Teasdale and Jennett 1974), and degree of posttraumatic amnesia. The GCS is a 15-point scale that documents eye opening, verbal responsiveness, and motor response to stimuli and may be used to measure the depth of coma, both initially and longitudinally. The Galveston Orientation and Amnesia Test (GOAT) (Levin et al. 1979) measures the extent of posttraumatic amnesia and can be used serially to document recovery of memory. Overall cognitive and behavioral recovery may be documented using the Rancho Los Amigos Cognitive Scale.

In severe TBI, posttraumatic amnesia or LOC may persist for at least 1 week or longer or, in extreme cases, may last weeks to months. GCS scores for severe TBI are less than 10. Mild head injury is usually defined as LOC for less than 15–20 minutes, a GCS score of 13–15, brief or no hospitalization, and no prominent residual neurobehavioral deficits. LOC is not required for the diagnosis of TBI; however, there must be some evidence of alteration in consciousness, including feeling dazed or experiencing a period of posttraumatic amnesia (Committee on Head Injury Nomenclature 1966; Quality Standards Subcommittee 1997). In fact, in analysis of 1,142 patients assessed after hospitalization for TBI, the simple presence or absence of LOC was not significantly related to performance on neuropsychological tests (Smith-Seemiller et al. 1996). Operationalized diagnostic criteria for mild TBI have been proposed (Mild Traumatic Brain Injury Committee 1993). A specific grading scale has been developed for concussions that occur during sports: Grade 1—confusion without amnesia and no LOC; Grade 2—confusion with amnesia and no LOC; and Grade 3—LOC (Kelly 1995).

Laboratory Evaluation

Imaging Techniques

Brain imaging techniques are frequently used to demonstrate the location and

TABLE 8–2. Assessment of traumatic brain injury

Behavioral assessment
  Structured interviews (e.g., Structured Clinical Interview for DSM-IV Diagnoses [SCID], Multinational Neuropsychiatric Inventory [MINI])
  Neurobehavioral Rating Scale (NBRS)
  Positive and Negative Symptom Scale (PANSS)
  Glasgow Coma Scale (GCS)
  Galveston Orientation and Amnesia Test (GOAT)
  Rancho Los Amigos Cognitive Scale
  Rating scales for depression (Hamilton)
  Rating scales for aggression (Overt Aggression Scale/Agitated Behavior Scale)
  Neuropsychiatric Inventory/Neuropsychiatric Inventory Questionnaire
  Brain Injury Symptom Questionnaire
  Rivermead Postconcussion Questionnaire
Brain imaging
  Computed tomography (CT)
  Magnetic resonance imaging (MRI) with fluid-attenuated inversion recovery (FLAIR)
  Functional magnetic resonance imaging (fMRI)
  Single photon emission computed tomography (SPECT)
  Regional cerebral blood flow (rCBF)
  Positron emission tomography (PET)
  Proton magnetic resonance spectroscopy (MRS)
Electrophysiological assessment
  Electroencephalogram (EEG), including special leads
  Computerized EEG
  Brain electrical activity mapping (BEAM)
Neuropsychological assessment
  Attention and concentration
  Premorbid intelligence
  Memory
  Executive functioning
  Verbal capacity
  Problem-solving skills

extent of brain lesions. Computed tomography (CT) is now widely available and may document contusions and hematomas and fractures. The timing of such imaging is important because lesions may be visualized months after the injury that cannot be seen during the acute phase. Thus, for a significant number of patients with severe brain injury, initial CT evaluations may not detect lesions that are observable on CT scans performed 1 and 3 months after the injury (Cope et al. 1988).

Magnetic resonance imaging (MRI) has been shown to detect clinically meaningful lesions in patients with severe brain injury when CT scans have not demonstrated anatomical bases for the degree of coma (Levin et al. 1987a; Wilberger et al. 1987). MRI is especially sensitive in detecting lesions in the frontal and temporal lobes that are not visualized by CT, and these loci are frequently related to the neuropsychiatric consequences of the injury (Levin et al. 1987a). MRI has been found to be more sensitive for the detection of contusions, shearing injury, and subdural and epidural hematomas (Orrison et al. 1994), and it has been able to document evidence of diffuse axonal injury in patients who have a normal CT scan after experiencing mild TBI (Mittl et al. 1994). When MRI is used, fluid-attenuated inversion recovery (FLAIR) is superior to T2-weighted spin-echo technique, especially in visualizing central diffuse axonal injury of the fornix and corpus callosum (Ashikaga et al. 1997). Morphometric analyses of individuals with TBI have revealed decreased thalamic volume (Anderson et al. 1996) and hippocampal atrophy (Bigler et al. 1997).

Functional techniques in brain imaging, such as regional cerebral blood flow (rCBF) and positron emission tomography (PET), can detect areas of abnormal function, when even CT and MRI scans fail to show any abnormalities of structure (Langfitt et al. 1987; Ruff et al. 1989). Single photon emission computed tomography (SPECT) also shows promise in documenting brain damage after TBI. Abnormalities are visualized in patients who have experienced mild TBI (Gross et al. 1996; Masdeu et al. 1994; Nedd et al. 1993) or who have chronic TBI (Nagamachi et al. 1995), even in the presence of normally appearing areas on CT scans. Abnormalities on SPECT appear to correlate with the severity of trauma (Jacobs et al. 1994). These techniques were utilized in examining a group of individuals with late whiplash syndrome (Bicik et al. 1998). Although there was significant frontopolar hypometabolism, it correlated significantly with scores on the Beck Depression Inventory. However, in individual cases, the reliability of the depiction of hypometabolism was low.

Caution must be observed in applying the findings in this literature to a clinical population. We are unable to determine the presence of abnormalities before the accident. Abnormalities on SPECT or PET have been demonstrated in individuals with psychiatric disorders who have no history of brain injury, including posttraumatic stress disorder (PTSD) (Rauch et al. 1996), somatization disorder (Lazarus and Cotterell 1989), major depression (Dolan et al. 1992), and chronic alcoholism (Kuruoglu et al. 1996). The American Academy of Neurology has concluded that there currently is insufficient evidence for the use of SPECT to diagnose TBI, and its use in this condition should be considered investigational (Therapeutics and Technology Assessment Subcommittee 1996). With the present state of the art, functional imaging results can only be used as part of an overall evaluation to confirm findings documented elsewhere (Silver and McAllister 1997).

Electrophysiological Techniques

Electrophysiological assessment of the patient after TBI may also assist in the evaluation. Electroencephalography can detect the presence of seizures or abnormal areas of functioning. To enhance the sensitivity of this technique, the electroencephalogram (EEG) should be performed after sleep deprivation, with photic stimulation and hyperventilation and with anterotemporal and/or nasopharyngeal leads (Goodin et al. 1990). Computed interpretation of the EEG and brain electrical activity mapping (BEAM) may be useful in detecting areas of dysfunction not shown in the routine EEG (Watson et al. 1995). There is controversy regarding the usefulness of these electrophysiological techniques. The American Academy of Neurology and the American Clinical Neurophysiology Society have concluded that "the evidence of clinical usefulness or consistency of results [is] not considered sufficient for us to support [the] use [of quantitative electroencephalography] in diagnosis of patients with postconcussion syndrome, or minor or moderate head injury" (Nuwer 1997). However, the EEG and Clinical Neuroscience Society addressed significant concerns regarding the interpretation of this report (Thatcher et al. 1999). In their opinion, there is significant scientific literature on the use and interpretation of quantitative electroencephalography, and several findings have been consistent (reduced amplitude of high-frequency electroencephalography, especially in the frontal lobes; a shift toward lower increased electroencephalographic frequencies; and changes in electroencephalographic coherence) (Thatcher et al. 1999). This area requires further examination.

Neuropsychological Testing

Neuropsychological assessment of the patient with TBI is essential to document cognitive and intellectual deficits and strengths. Tests are administered to assess the patient's attention, concentration, memory, verbal capacity, and executive functioning. This latter capacity is the most difficult to assess and includes problem-solving skills, abstract thinking, planning, and reasoning abilities. A valid interpretation of these tests includes assessment of the patient's preinjury intelligence and other higher levels of functioning. Because multiple factors affect the results of testing (Table 8–3), tests must be performed and interpreted by a clinician with skill and experience.

Patients' complaints may not be easily or accurately categorized as either functional (i.e., primarily due to a psychiatric disorder) or neurologic (i.e., primarily caused by the brain injury). Nonetheless, outside agencies (e.g., insurance companies and lawyers) may request a neuropsychiatric evaluation to assist with this "differential." In reality, most symptoms result from the interaction of many factors, including neurologic, social, emotional, educational, and vocational. Because important insurance and other reimbursement decisions may hinge on whether or not disabilities stem from brain injury, the clinician should take care that his or her impressions are based on data and are not misapplied to deprive the patient of deserved benefits. For example, mood disorders and cognitive sequelae of brain injury are often miscategorized as "mental illnesses" that are not covered by some insurance policies.

Clinical Features

The neuropsychiatric sequelae of TBI include problems with attention and arousal, concentration, and executive functioning; intellectual changes; memory impairment; personality changes; affec-

TABLE 8–3. Major factors affecting neuropsychological test findings

- Original endowment
- Environment
- Motivation (effort)
- Physical health
- Psychological distress
- Psychiatric disorders
- Medications
- Qualifications and experience of neuropsychologist
- Errors in scoring
- Errors in interpretation

Source. Reprinted from Simon RI: "Ethical and Legal Issues," in *Neuropsychiatry of Traumatic Brain Injury.* Edited by Silver JM, Yudofsky SC, Hales RE. Washington, DC, American Psychiatric Press, 1994, pp. 569–630. Used with permission.

TABLE 8–4. Factors influencing outcome after brain injury

- Severity of injury
- Type of injury
- Anosmia
- Intellectual functioning
- Psychiatric diagnosis
- Sociopathy
- Premorbid behavioral problems (children)
- Social support
- Substance use
- Neurologic disorder
- Age
- Apolipoprotein E status

tive disorders; anxiety disorders; psychosis; posttraumatic epilepsy; sleep disorders; aggression; and irritability. Physical problems such as headache, chronic pain, vision impairment, and dizziness complicate recovery. The severity of the neuropsychiatric sequelae of the brain injury is determined by multiple factors existing before, during, and after the injury (Dikmen and Machamer 1995) (Table 8–4). In general, prognosis is associated with the severity of injury. The duration of posttraumatic amnesia correlates with subsequent cognitive recovery (Levin et al. 1982). In addition, the symptoms of injury are correlated with the type of damage sustained. For example, those with diffuse axonal injury often experience problems with arousal, attention, and slow cognitive processing. The presence of total anosmia in a group of patients with closed head injury predicted major vocational problems at least 2 years after these patients had been given medical clearance to return to work (Varney 1988).

In a review by J.D. Corrigan (1995), patients with TBI who were intoxicated with alcohol at the time of the injury had longer periods of hospitalization, had more complications during hospitalization, and had a lower level of functioning at the time of discharge from the hospital compared with patients with TBI who had no detectable blood alcohol level at the time of hospitalization. One factor complicating the interpretation of these data is the fact that intoxication may produce decreased responsivity even without TBI, which can result in a GCS score that indicates greater severity of injury than is actually present. Furthermore, even a history of substance abuse is associated with increased morbidity and mortality rates.

Morbidity and mortality rates after brain injury increase with age. Elderly persons who experience TBI have longer periods of agitation and greater cognitive impairment and are more likely to develop mass lesions and permanent disability than are younger individuals (Fogel and Duffy 1994; Goldstein and Levin 1995; Katz and Alexander 1994; Rakier et al. 1995). Individuals who have a previous brain injury do not recover as well from subsequent injuries (Carlsson et al. 1987).

The interaction between the brain injury and the psychosocial factors cannot be underestimated. Demographic factors have been found to predict cognitive dysfunction after TBI (Smith-Seemiller et al. 1996). Preexisting emotional and behavioral problems are exacerbated after injury. Although many patients with TBI may not have a history of previous psychiatric problems, a significant percentage of patients do have histories of learning disabilities, attentional deficits, behavioral problems, and drug or alcohol abuse. Social conditions and support networks that existed before the injury affect the symptoms and course of recovery. In general, individuals with greater preinjury intelligence recover better after injury (G. Brown et al. 1981). Factors such as level of education, level of income, and socioeconomic status are positive factors in the ability to return to work after minor head injury (Rimel et al. 1981).

There have been several studies that have associated the presence of apolipoprotein E (ApoE) e4 with prognosis of recovery from TBI. Examining recovery in professional boxers, Jordan and colleagues (1997) found that the presence of ApoE e4 was associated with chronic neurologic deficits in "high-exposure" boxers. In individuals with TBI who were admitted to a neurosurgical unit, the presence of ApoE e4 predicted poor recovery after 6 months, even after controlling for severity of injury (Teasdale et al. 1997). Among individuals who were in a rehabilitation program subsequent to TBI, Friedman et al. (1999) found that ApoE e4 predicted poorer recovery. Although these results need additional confirmation, especially in those with mild TBI, they emphasize the fact that there are prognostic factors that influence recovery that we do not assess or that have not yet been determined. We must avoid "blaming the victim" or concluding that the individual does not "want" to improve (for psychological or monetary reasons), when there

may be biological factors that influence recovery. Our belief is that many more biological factors will be discovered that significantly affect recovery from TBI.

Personality Changes

Unlike many primary psychiatric illnesses that have gradual onset, TBI often occurs suddenly and devastatingly. Although some patients recognize that they no longer have the same abilities and potential that they had before the injury, many others with significant disabilities deny that there have been any changes. Prominent behavioral traits such as disorderliness, suspiciousness, argumentativeness, isolativeness, disruptiveness, and anxiousness often become more pronounced after brain injury.

Because of the vulnerability of the prefrontal and frontal regions of the cortex to contusions, injury to these regions is common and gives rise to changes in personality known as the frontal lobe syndrome. For the prototypic patient with frontal lobe syndrome, the cognitive functions are preserved while personality changes abound. Psychiatric disturbances associated with frontal lobe injury commonly include impaired social judgment, labile affect, uncharacteristic lewdness, inability to appreciate the effects of one's behavior or remarks on others, a loss of social graces (such as eating manners), a diminution of attention to personal appearance and hygiene, and boisterousness. Impaired judgment may take the form of diminished concern for the future, increased risk taking, unrestrained drinking of alcohol, and indiscriminate selection of food. Patients may appear shallow, indifferent, or apathetic, with a global lack of concern for the consequences of their behavior.

Certain behavioral syndromes have been related to damage to specific areas of the frontal lobe (Auerbach 1986). The orbitofrontal syndrome is associated with behavioral excesses, such as impulsivity, disinhibition, hyperactivity, distractibility, and mood lability. Injury to the dorsolateral frontal cortex may result in slowness, apathy, and perseveration. This may be considered similar to the negative (deficit) symptoms associated with schizophrenia, wherein the patient may exhibit blunted affect, emotional withdrawal, social withdrawal, passivity, and lack of spontaneity (Kay et al. 1987). As with TBI, deficit symptoms in patients with schizophrenia are thought to result from disordered functioning of the dorsolateral frontal cortex (Berman et al. 1988). Outbursts of rage and violent behavior occur after damage to the inferior orbital surface of the frontal lobe and anterior temporal lobes.

Although there have been studies examining personality changes after TBI, few have focused on Axis II psychopathology in individuals with TBI. In utilizing a structured clinical interview to diagnose personality disorders in 100 individuals with TBI, Hibbard and colleagues (2000) found that several personality disorders developed after TBI that were reflective of persistent challenges and compensatory coping strategies facing these individuals. Whereas before TBI, 24% of the sample population had personality disorders, 66% of the sample met criteria for personality disorders after TBI. The most common disorders were borderline, avoidant, paranoid, obsessive-compulsive, and narcissistic.

In DSM-IV-TR (American Psychiatric Association 2000), these personality changes would be diagnosed as personality change due to traumatic brain injury. Specific subtypes are provided as the most significant clinical problems (Table 8–5).

Intellectual Changes

Problems with intellectual functioning may be among the most subtle manifestations of brain injury. Changes can occur in the capacity to concentrate, use language, abstract, calculate, reason, remember, plan, and process information (Barth et al. 1983; Levin et al. 1985; Stuss et al. 1985). Problems with arousal can take the form of inattentiveness, distractibility, and difficulty switching and dividing attention (Ponsford and Kinsella 1992). Mental sluggishness, poor concentration, and memory problems are common complaints of both patients and relatives (Brooks et al. 1986; McKinlay et al. 1981; Thomsen 1984). High-level cognitive functions, termed *executive functions*, are frequently impaired, although such impairments are difficult to detect and diagnose with cursory cognitive testing (Table 8–6) (O'Shanick and O'Shanick 1994). Only specific tests that mimic real-life decision-making situations may objectively demonstrate the problems encountered in daily life (Bechara et al. 1994).

Studies suggest that among the long-term sequelae of brain trauma is Alzheimer's disease (Amaducci et al. 1986; Graves et al. 1990). Amyloid protein deposition has been found in the brains of patients who experienced severe TBI (Roberts et al. 1994; Sheriff et al. 1994). Several investigators have found this association in elderly persons who have brain injury (Mayeux et al. 1993; Van Duijn et al. 1992). Sustaining TBI reduced the time to onset of Alzheimer's disease among those who were at risk (Nemetz et al. 1999). There have been several studies that have examined the influence of ApoE status on the risk of developing Alzheimer's disease subsequent to TBI. Mayeux et al. (1995) found that the presence of the ApoE e4 allele combined with a history of head injury results in synergistic effect, increasing the risk from 2-fold with ApoE e4 alone to a 10-fold increase in risk with ApoE e4 and TBI. Katzman and colleagues (1996) determined that in

TABLE 8–5. DSM-IV-TR diagnostic criteria for personality change due to a general medical condition (e.g., traumatic brain injury)

A. A persistent personality disturbance that represents a change from the individual's previous characteristic personality pattern. (In children, the disturbance involves a marked deviation from normal development or a significant change in the child's usual behavior patterns lasting at least 1 year.)

B. There is evidence from the history, physical examination, or laboratory findings that the disturbance is the direct physiological consequence of a general medical condition.

C. The disturbance is not better accounted for by another mental disorder (including other mental disorders due to a general medical condition).

D. The disturbance does not occur exclusively during the course of a delirium.

E. The disturbance causes clinically significant distress or impairment in social, occupational, or other important areas of functioning.

Specify type:

    Labile type: if the predominant feature is affective lability

    Disinhibited type: if the predominant feature is poor impulse control as evidenced by sexual indiscretions, etc.

    Aggressive type: if the predominant feature is aggressive behavior

    Apathetic type: if the predominant feature is marked apathy and indifference

    Paranoid type: if the predominant feature is suspiciousness or paranoid ideation

    Other type: if the presentation is not characterized by any of the above subtypes

    Combined type: if more than one feature predominates in the clinical picture

    Unspecified type

Source. Reprinted from the *Diagnostic and Statistical Manual of Mental Disorders*, 4th Edition, Text Revision. Washington, DC, American Psychiatric Association, 2000. Copyright 2000, American Psychiatric Association. Used with permission.

TABLE 8–6. Executive functions

- Setting goals
- Assessing strengths and weaknesses
- Planning and/or directing activity
- Initiating and/or inhibiting behavior
- Monitoring current activity
- Evaluating results

Source. Reprinted from O'Shanick GJ, O'Shanick AM: "Personality and Intellectual Changes," in *Neuropsychiatry of Traumatic Brain Injury.* Edited by Silver JM, Yudofsky SC, Hales RE. Washington, DC, American Psychiatric Press, 1994, pp. 163–188. Used with permission.

their population, there was an additive effect. However, in another large family study, the influence of TBI on the development of Alzheimer's disease was greater among persons lacking ApoE e4 (Guo et al. 2000). This connection between these disorders is logical, given the pathological features of these disorders, and must be considered when reviewing the lifelong implications of recovery from TBI.

Children who survive head trauma often return to school with behavioral and learning problems (Mahoney et al. 1983). Children with behavioral disorders are much more likely to have a history of prior head injury (Michaud et al. 1993). In addition, children who sustained injury at or before age 2 years had significantly lower IQ scores (Michaud et al. 1993). The sequelae of mild TBI in children are controversial (Birmaher and Williams 1994). In a study of 43 children and adolescents who had sustained TBI, Max et al. (1998b) found that preinjury family functioning was a significant predictor of psychiatric disorders after 1 year. Whereas some investigators have demonstrated neuropsychological sequelae after mild TBI when carefully tested (Gulbrandsen 1984), others have shown that mild TBI produces virtually no clinically significant long-term deficits (Fay et al. 1993). In patients who survive moderate to severe brain injury, the degree of memory impairment often exceeds the level of intellectual dysfunction (Levin et al. 1988).

Psychiatric Disorders

Studies that utilize standard psychiatric diagnostic criteria have found that several psychiatric disorders are common in individuals with TBI (Deb et al. 1999; Fann et al. 1995; Hibbard et al. 1998; Jorge et al. 1993; van Reekum et al. 2000). In a group of patients referred to a brain injury rehabilitation center, Fann and colleagues (1995) found that 26% had current major depression, 14% had current dysthymia, 24% had current generalized anxiety disorder, and 8% had current substance abuse. There was a 12% occurrence of pre-TBI depression. Deb and colleagues (1999) performed a psychiatric evaluation of 196 individuals who were hospitalized after TBI. A psychiatric disorder was found in 21.7% versus 16.4% of a control population of individuals hospitalized for other reasons. Compared with the control group, the individuals with TBI had a higher rate of depression (13.9% vs. 2.1%) and panic disorder (9.0% vs. 0.8%). Factors associated with these psychiatric disorders included a history of psychiatric illness, preinjury alcohol use, unfavorable outcome, lower Mini-Mental State Exam scores, and fewer years of education. Hibbard and colleagues (1998) administered a structured psychiatric interview to 100 individuals with TBI. Major depression (61%), substance use disorder (28%), and PTSD (19%) were the most common psy-chiatric diagnoses elicited. Jorge and colleagues (1993) found that 26% of individuals had major depression 1 month after injury; 11% had comorbid generalized anxiety disorder.

In the New Haven portion of the National Institute of Mental Health Epidemiologic Catchment Area (ECA) program, individuals were administered standardized and validated structured interviews (Silver et al. 2001). Among 5,034 individuals interviewed, 361 admitted to a history of severe brain trauma with LOC or confusion (weighted rate of 8.5/100). When controlling for sociodemographic factors, quality-of-life indicators, and alcohol use, risk was increased for major depression, dysthymia, panic disorder, obsessive-compulsive disorder, phobic disorder, and drug abuse/dependence.

Several studies suggest that individuals who experience TBI have a higher than expected rate of preinjury psychiatric disorders. Histories of prior psychiatric disorders in individuals with TBI have varied between 17% and 44%, and pre-TBI substance use figures have ranged from 22% to 30% (Jorge et al. 1994; van Reekum et al. 1996). Fann and colleagues (1995) found that 50% of individuals who had sustained TBI reported a history of psychiatric problems prior to the injury. The Research and Training Center for the Community Integration of Individuals with TBI at Mt. Sinai Medical Center in New York found that in a group of 100 individuals with TBI, 51% had pre-TBI psychiatric disorders, most commonly major depression or substance use disorders, that occurred at rates more than twice those reported in community samples (Hibbard et al. 1998).

Affective Changes

Depression occurs frequently after TBI (Rosenthal et al. 1998). There are several diagnostic issues that must be considered in the evaluation of the patient who appears depressed after TBI. Sadness is a common reaction after TBI, as patients describe "mourning" the loss of their "former selves," often a reflection of deficits in intellectual functioning and motoric abilities. Careful psychiatric evaluation is required to distinguish grief reactions, sadness, and demoralization from major depression.

The clinician should endeavor to determine whether a patient may have been having an episode of major depression before an accident. Traumatic injury may occur as a result of the depression and suicidal ideation. Alcohol use, which frequently occurs with and complicates depressive illness, is also a known risk factor for motor vehicle accidents. One common scenario is depression leading to poor concentration, to substance abuse, and to risk taking (or even overt suicidal behavior), which together contribute to the motor vehicle accident and brain injury.

Prevalence of Depression After TBI

The prevalence of depression after brain injury has been assessed through self-report questionnaires, rating scales, and assessments by relatives. For mild TBI, estimates of depressive complaints range from 6% to 39%. For depression after severe TBI, in which patients often have concomitant cognitive impairments, reported rates of depression vary from 10% to 77%.

Robert Robinson and his colleagues have performed prospective studies of the occurrence of depression after brain injury (Federoff et al. 1992; Jorge et al. 1993). They evaluated 66 hospitalized patients who sustained acute TBI and followed the course of their mood over 1 year. Diagnoses were made using structured interviews and DSM-III-R (American Psychiatric Association 1987) criteria.

Patients were evaluated at 1 month, 3 months, 6 months, and 1 year after injury. At each period, approximately 25% of patients fulfilled criteria for major depressive disorder. The mean duration of depression was 4.7 months, with a range of 1.5–12 months. Of the entire group of patients, 42% developed major depression during the first year after injury. The researchers also found that patients with generalized anxiety disorder and comorbid major depression had longer lasting mood problems than did those patients with depression and no anxiety (Jorge et al. 1993). In an unselected population sample, major depression was found in 11.1% of those with a history of brain injury (Silver et al. 2001). Deb and colleagues (1999) found 13.9% of individuals developed depression after TBI. Major depression occurred in 61% of a sample of individuals with TBI who were administered a structured psychiatric interview (Hibbard et al. 1998). In a group of patients referred to a brain injury rehabilitation center, Fann and colleagues (1995) found that 26% had current major depression, and 14% had current dysthymia.

Studies consistently report increased risk of suicide subsequent to TBI (Tate et al. 1997). Silver et al. (2001) found that those with brain injury reported a higher frequency of suicide attempts than individuals without TBI (8.1% vs. 1.9%). This remained significant even after controlling for sociodemographic factors, quality-of-life variables, and the presence of any coexisting psychiatric disorder. Mann and colleagues (1999) found an increased occurrence of TBI in individuals who have made suicide attempts.

We believe that the high incidence of suicide attempts in this population is due to the combination of major depression with disinhibition secondary to frontal lobe injury. The medical team, family, and other caregivers must work closely together to gauge suicide risk on a regular and ongoing basis.

Mania After Traumatic Brain Injury

Manic episodes and bipolar disorder have also been reported to occur after TBI (Burstein 1993), although the occurrence is less frequent than that of depression after brain injury (Bakchine et al. 1989; Bamrah and Johnson 1991; Bracken 1987; Clark and Davison 1987; Nizamie et al. 1988). In the New Haven ECA sample, bipolar disorder occurred in 1.6% of those with brain injury, although the odds ratio was no longer significant when sociodemographic factors and quality of life were controlled (Silver et al. 2001). Predisposing factors for the development of mania after brain injury include damage to the basal region of the right temporal lobe (Starkstein et al. 1990) and right orbitofrontal cortex (Starkstein et al. 1988) in patients who have family histories of bipolar disorder.

Delirium

When a psychiatrist is consulted during the period when a patient with a brain injury is emerging from coma, the usual clinical picture is one of delirium with restlessness, agitation, confusion, disorientation, delusions, and/or hallucinations. As Trzepacz (1994) observed, this period of recovery is often termed posttraumatic amnesia in the brain injury literature and is classified as Rancho Los Amigos Cognitive Scale Level IV or V. Although delirium in patients with TBI is most often the result of the effects of the injury on brain tissue chemistry, the psychiatrist should be aware that there may be other causes for the delirium (such as side effects of medication, withdrawal, or intoxication from drugs ingested before the traumatic event) and environmental factors (such as sensory monotony). Table 8–7 lists common factors that can result in posttraumatic delirium.

TABLE 8–7. Causes of delirium in patients with traumatic brain injury

- Mechanical effects (acceleration or deceleration, contusion, and others)
- Cerebral edema
- Hemorrhage
- Infection
- Subdural hematoma
- Seizure
- Hypoxia (cardiopulmonary or local ischemia)
- Increased intracranial pressure
- Alcohol intoxication or withdrawal, Wernicke's encephalopathy
- Reduced hemoperfusion related to multiple trauma
- Fat embolism
- Change in pH
- Electrolyte imbalance
- Medications (barbiturates, steroids, opioids, and anticholinergics)

Source. Reprinted from Trzepacz P: "Delirium," in *Neuropsychiatry of Traumatic Brain Injury.* Edited by Silver JM, Yudofsky SC, Hales RE. Washington, DC, American Psychiatric Press, 1994, pp. 189–218. Used with permission.

Stuss et al. (1999) examined patients recovering from acute TBI using tests of attention and memory. Attention improved before performance on memory tasks, especially in individuals with mild TBI. The researchers concluded that the phenomenon currently termed posttraumatic amnesia is actually a confusional state and that the term *posttraumatic confusional state* should be used instead.

Psychotic Disorders

Psychosis can occur either immediately after brain injury or after a latency of many months of normal functioning. Smeltzer et al. (1994) reviewed the literature regarding the reports of the occurrence of psychosis in patients who had TBI and noted that a major difficulty in this literature was the absence of a standard definition of psychosis; therefore, comparison of studies is problematic. McAllister (1998) observed that psychotic symptoms may result from a number of different post-TBI disorders, including mania, depression, and epilepsy. Lishman (1987) reported schizophrenic-like symptoms of patients after TBI that were "indistinguishable" from symptoms of the "naturally occurring" disorder. The psychotic symptoms may persist despite improvement in the cognitive deficits caused by trauma (Nasrallah et al. 1981). Review of the literature published between 1917 and 1964 (Davison and Bagley 1969) revealed that 1%–15% of schizophrenic inpatients have histories of brain injury. Violon and De Mol (1987) found that of 530 head injury patients, 3.4% developed psychosis 1–10 years after the injury. Wilcox and Nasrallah (1987) found that a group of patients diagnosed with schizophrenia had a significantly greater history of brain injury with LOC before age 10 than did patients who were diagnosed with mania or depression or patients who were hospitalized for surgery. Achte et al. (1991) reported on a sample of 2,907 war veterans in Finland who sustained brain injury. They found that 26% of these veterans had psychotic disorders. In a detailed evaluation of 100 of these veterans, the authors found that 14% had paranoid schizophrenia. In a comparison of patients who developed symptoms of schizophrenia or schizoaffective disorder subsequent to TBI, left temporal lobe abnormalities were found only in the group who developed schizophrenia (Buckley et al. 1993). The rate of schizophrenia in the group of individuals with a history of TBI in the New Haven group in the ECA study was 3.4% (Silver et al. 2001). However, after controlling for alcohol abuse and dependence, the risk for the occurrence of schizophrenia was of borderline significance.

Patients with schizophrenia may have had brain injury that remains undetected unless the clinician actively elicits a history specific for the occurrence of brain trauma. One high-risk group is homeless mentally ill individuals. To examine the relationship of TBI to schizophrenia and homelessness, Silver et al. (1993) conducted a case-control study of 100 literally homeless and 100 never-homeless indigent schizophrenic men, and a similar population of women. In the group of men, 55 patients had a prior TBI (36 literally homeless, 19 domiciled, $P < 0.01$). In the group of women, 35 had previous TBI (16 literally homeless, 19 domiciled, $P = $ not significant). We believe that the cognitive deficits subsequent to TBI in conjunction with psychosis increase the risk for becoming homeless; in addition, being homeless, and living in a shelter, carries a definite risk for trauma (Kass and Silver 1990).

Posttraumatic Epilepsy

A varying percentage of patients, depending on the location and severity of injury, will have seizures during the acute period after the trauma. Posttraumatic epilepsy, with repeated seizures and the requirement for anticonvulsant medication, occurs in approximately 12%, 2%, and 1% of patients with severe, moderate, and mild head injuries, respectively, within 5 years of the injury (Annegers et al. 1980). Risk factors for posttraumatic epilepsy include skull fractures and wounds that penetrate the brain, a history of chronic alcohol use, intracranial hemorrhage, and increased severity of injury (Yablon 1993).

Salazar et al. (1985) studied 421 Vietnam veterans who had sustained brain-penetrating injuries and found that 53% had posttraumatic epilepsy. In 18% of these patients, the first seizure occurred after 5 years; in 7%, the first seizure occurred after 10 years. In addition, 26%

of the patients with epilepsy had an organic mental syndrome as defined in DSM-III (American Psychiatric Association 1980). In a study of World War II veterans (Corkin et al. 1984), patients with brain-penetrating injuries who developed posttraumatic epilepsy had a decreased life expectancy compared with patients with brain-penetrating injuries without epilepsy or compared with patients with peripheral nerve injuries. Patients who develop posttraumatic epilepsy have also been shown to have more difficulties with physical and social functioning and to require more intensive rehabilitation efforts (Armstrong et al. 1990).

Posttraumatic epilepsy is associated with psychosis, especially when seizures arise from the temporal lobes. Brief episodic psychoses may occur with epilepsy; about 7% of patients with epilepsy have persistent psychoses (McKenna et al. 1985). These psychoses exhibit a number of atypical features, including confusion and rapid fluctuations in mood. Psychiatric evaluation of 101 patients with epilepsy revealed that 8% had organic delusional disorder that, at times, was difficult to differentiate symptomatically from schizophrenia (Garyfallos et al. 1988).

Anticonvulsant drugs can produce cognitive and emotional symptoms (Reynolds and Trimble 1985; Rivinus 1992; M.C. Smith and Bleck 1991). Phenytoin has more profound effects on cognition than does carbamazepine (Gallassi et al. 1988), and negative effects on cognition have been found in patients who received phenytoin after traumatic injury (Dikmen et al. 1991). Minimal impairment in cognition was found with both valproate and carbamazepine in a group of patients with epilepsy (Prevey et al. 1996). Dikmen et al. (2000) found no adverse cognitive effects of valproate when it was administered for 12 months after TBI. The effects of phenytoin and carbamazepine in patients recovering from TBI were compared by K.R. Smith et al. (1994). They found that both phenytoin and carbamazepine had negative effects on cognitive performance, especially those that involved motor and speed performance. Although in the patient group as a whole the effects were of questionable clinical significance, some individual patients experienced significant effects. Intellectual deterioration in children undergoing long-term treatment with phenytoin or phenobarbital also has been documented (Corbett et al. 1985). Treatment with more than one anticonvulsant (polytherapy) has been associated with increased adverse neuropsychiatric reactions (Reynolds and Trimble 1985). Of the newer anticonvulsant medications, topiramate, but not gabapentin or lamotrigine, demonstrated adverse cognitive effects in healthy young adults (Martin et al. 1999). Hoare (1984) found that the use of multiple anticonvulsant drugs to control seizures resulted in an increase in disturbed behavior in children.

Patients who have a seizure immediately after brain injury are often given an anticonvulsant drug for seizure prophylaxis. Temkin et al. (1990) showed that the administration of phenytoin soon after traumatic injury had no prophylactic effect on seizures that occurred subsequent to the first week after injury. Similarly, valproate did not demonstrate any efficacy in preventing late posttraumatic seizures (Temkin et al. 1999). It should be noted that there was a nonsignificant trend toward a higher mortality rate. Anticonvulsant medications are not recommended after 1 week of injury for prevention of posttraumatic seizures (Brain Injury Special Interest Group 1998) Any patient with TBI who is treated with anticonvulsant medication requires regular reevaluations to substantiate continued clinical necessity.

Anxiety Disorders

Several anxiety disorders may develop after TBI. Epstein and Ursano (1994) compiled the results of 12 studies conducted from 1942 to 1990. Out of a group of 1,199 patients, 29% were diagnosed with clinical anxiety after TBI. Jorge et al. (1993) found that 11% of 66 patients with TBI developed generalized anxiety disorder in addition to major depression. Fann et al. (1995) evaluated 50 outpatients with TBI and found that 24% had generalized anxiety disorder. Deb et al. (1999) evaluated 196 individuals who were hospitalized after TBI. Panic disorder developed in 9%. Hibbard et al. (1998) found that 18% developed PTSD, 14% developed obsessive-compulsive disorder, 11% developed panic disorder, 8% developed generalized anxiety disorder, and 6% developed phobic disorder. All of these were more frequent after TBI compared with before TBI. In analysis of data from the New Haven portion of the ECA study, Silver et al. (2001) found that of individuals with a history of brain injury during their lifetime, the incidences of anxiety disorders were 4.7% for obsessive-compulsive disorder, 11.2% for phobic disorder, and 3.2% for panic disorder. Dissociative disorders, including depersonalization (Grigsby and Kaye 1993) and dissociative identity disorder (Sandel et al. 1990), may occur. It is our clinical observation that patients with histories of prior trauma are at higher risk for developing these disorders.

Because of the potential life-threatening nature of many of the causes of TBI, including motor vehicle accidents and assaults, one would expect that these patients are at increased risk of developing PTSD. There is a 9.2% risk of developing PTSD after exposure to trauma, highest for assaultive violence (Breslau et al. 1998). PTSD and acute stress response are not uncommon after serious motor vehicle accidents (Koren et al. 1999; Ursano et al. 1999a), including symptoms of peritraumatic dissociation (Ursano et al. 1999b).

PTSD has been found in individuals with TBI (Bryant 1996; McMillan 1996; Ohry et al. 1996; Parker and Rosenblum 1996; Rattok 1996; Silver et al. 1997). Using the Structured Clinical Interview for DSM-IV (SCID) (First et al. 1997) to evaluate 100 individuals with a history of TBI, Hibbard and colleagues found that 18% met criteria for PTSD (Hibbard et al. 1998). Harvey and Bryant conducted a 2-year study of 79 survivors of motor vehicle accidents who sustained mild TBI. They found that acute stress disorder developed in 14% of these patients at 1 month. After 2 years, 73% of the group with acute stress disorder developed PTSD (Harvey and Bryant 2000). Six months after severe TBI, 26 of 96 individuals (27.1%) developed PTSD (Bryant et al. 2000). Although few patients had intrusive memories (19.2%), 96.2% reported emotional reactivity. The authors suggested that traumatic experiences may be mediated at an implicit level. Similarly, in 47 subjects with moderate TBI who were amnestic for the traumatic event, Warden et al. (1995) found that no patients met the full criteria for the diagnosis of PTSD, which includes reexperiencing the event. However, 14% of patients had avoidance and arousal symptoms. Not all investigators have found that PTSD occurs with TBI. In evaluating a group of 70 patients diagnosed with PTSD or mild TBI, Sbordone and Liter (1995) found that no patients had both disorders (although the presence of subsyndromal PTSD was not assessed). Children are also susceptible to the development of PTSD after TBI. Max et al. (1998a) evaluated 50 children who were hospitalized after TBI. Although only 4%

of subjects developed PTSD, 68% had one PTSD symptom after 3 months, suggesting subsyndromal PTSD despite neurogenic amnesia.

Because of the overlap among symptoms of PTSD and mild TBI, it can be difficult to ascribe specific symptoms to the brain injury or to the circumstances of the accident. In studies of patients with PTSD, memory deficits consistent with temporal lobe injury have been demonstrated (Bremner et al. 1993). Imaging studies have shown smaller hippocampal volumes with PTSD (Bremner et al. 1995, 1997). It is therefore apparent that exposure to extreme stressors results in brain dysfunction that may be similar to that found after TBI.

Sleep Disorders

It is common for individuals with TBI to complain of disrupted sleep patterns, ranging from hypersomnia to difficulty maintaining sleep. Fichtenberg and colleagues (2000) assessed 91 individuals with TBI who were admitted to an outpatient neurorehabilitation clinic. The presence of depression (as indicated by score on the Beck Depression Inventory [Beck 1961]) and mild severity of the TBI were correlated with the occurrence of insomnia. Guilleminault and colleagues (2000) assessed 184 patients with head trauma and hypersomnia. Abnormalities were demonstrated on the Multiple Sleep Latency Test (MSLT). Sleep-disordered breathing was common (59/184 patients). Hypersomnia must be differentiated from lack of motivation and apathy. In addition, the contribution of pain to disruption of sleep must be considered. Although depression and sleep disorders can be related and have similarities in the sleep-endocrine changes (Frieboes et al. 1999), in our experience with depressed individuals after TBI, the sleep difficulties persist after successful treatment of the mood

disorder. In addition, we have seen patients who have developed sleep apnea or nocturnal myoclonus subsequent to TBI.

Mild Traumatic Brain Injury and the Postconcussion Syndrome

Patients with mild TBI may present with somatic, cognitive, perceptual, and emotional symptoms that have been characterized as the postconcussion syndrome (Table 8–8). By definition, mild TBI is associated with a brief duration of LOC (less than 20 minutes) or no LOC, and posttraumatic amnesia of less than 24 hours; the patient usually does not require hospitalization after the injury. For each patient hospitalized with mild TBI, probably four to five others sustain mild TBIs but receive treatment as outpatients or perhaps get no treatment at all. The psychiatrist is often called to assess the patient years after the injury, and the patient may not associate brain-related symptoms such as depression and cognitive dysfunction with the injury. The results of laboratory tests, such as structural brain imaging studies, often do not reveal significant abnormalities. However, as discussed previously, functional imaging studies such as SPECT (Masdeu et al. 1994; Nedd et al. 1993) and computerized electroencephalography and brain stem auditory evoked potential recordings have demonstrated abnormal findings (Watson et al. 1995). Diffuse axonal injury occurs with mild TBI, as demonstrated in the pathological examination of brains from patients who have died from systemic injuries (Oppenheimer 1968), as well as in nonhuman primates (Gennarelli et al. 1982).

Most studies of cognitive function subsequent to mild TBI suggest that patients report trouble with memory, attention, concentration, and speed of information processing, and patients can in fact be

TABLE 8–8. Postconcussion syndrome

Somatic symptoms
  Headache
  Dizziness
  Fatigue
  Insomnia
Cognitive symptoms
  Memory difficulties
  Impaired concentration
Perceptual symptoms
  Tinnitus
  Sensitivity to noise
  Sensitivity to light
Emotional symptoms
  Depression
  Anxiety
  Irritability

Source.   Adapted from Lishman 1988.

shown to have deficits in these areas shortly after their injury (1 week to 1 month) (S.J. Brown et al. 1994; McAllister 1994; McMillan and Glucksman 1987). In an evaluation of neuropsychological deficits in 53 patients who were experiencing postconcussive problems from 1 to 22 months after injury, Leininger et al. (1990) detected significantly poorer performance ($P < 0.05$) on tests of reasoning, information processing, and verbal learning than that found in a control population. Hugenholtz et al. (1988) reported that significant attentional and information processing impairment ($P < 0.01$) occurred in a group of adults after mild concussion. Although there was improvement over time, the patient group continued to have abnormalities 3 months after the injury.

Individuals with mild TBI have an increased incidence of somatic complaints, including headache, dizziness, fatigue, sleep disturbance, and sensitivity to noise and light (S.J. Brown et al. 1994; Dikmen et al. 1986; Levin et al. 1987b; Rimel et al. 1981). In the behavioral domain, the most common problems include irritability, anxiety, and depression (Dikmen et al. 1986; Fann et al. 1995; Hibbard et al. 1998).

The majority of individuals with mild TBI recover quickly, with significant and progressive reduction of complaints in all three domains (cognitive, somatic, and behavioral) at 1, 3, and certainly 6 months from the injury (Bernstein 1999). Unfortunately, good recovery is not universal. A significant number of patients continue to complain of persistent difficulties 6–12 months and even longer after their injury. For example, Keshavan et al. (1981) found that 40% of their patients had significant symptoms 3 months after injury. Levin et al. (1987c), in a multicenter study, found that 3 months postinjury, 47% complained of headache, 22% of decreased energy, and 22% of dizziness. In a review of this topic, Bohnen et al. (1992) found a range of 16%–49% of patients with persistent symptoms at 6 months, and 1%–50% with persistent symptoms at 1 year. Those with persistent symptoms have been found to have impaired cognitive function (Leininger et al. 1990). S.J. Brown et al. (1994) suggested that if symptoms are present at 3–6 months subsequent to injury, they tend to persist. Alves et al. (1993) prospectively assessed 587 patients with uncomplicated mild TBI for 1 year. The most frequent symptoms were headache and dizziness. The researchers found that fewer than 6% of these subjects complained of multiple symptoms consistent with postconcussion syndrome.

Therefore, there may be two groups of mild TBI patients: those who recover by 3 months and those who have persistent symptoms. It is not known whether the persistent symptoms are part of a cohesive syndrome or simply represent a collection of loosely related symptoms resulting from the vagaries of an individual injury (Alves et al. 1986). However, it is increasingly recognized that "mild" TBI and concussions that occur in sports injuries result in clinically significant neuropsychological impairment (Collins et al. 1999; Matser et al. 1999; Powell and Barber-Foss 1999).

Compensation and litigation do not appear to affect the course of recovery after "mild" brain injury (Bornstein et al. 1988), and many patients return to work despite the continuation of psychiatric symptoms (Hugenholtz et al. 1988). In fact, professional athletes who sustain mild TBI and have a negative financial incentive to stop playing have the same symptoms of postconcussion syndrome as do individuals who sustain mild TBI at work or in motor vehicle accidents. As McAllister (1994) has pointed out,

> there may be times when a patient's attorney gives clear encouragement to maintain symptoms when litigation extends over a period of several years.... [However,] there is virtually no evidence at this point to suggest that it is the primary factor in the overwhelming majority of patients with mild brain injury. (p. 375)

In an extensive review of the literature, Alexander (1995) highlighted several important aspects regarding patients who develop prolonged postconcussion syndrome: 1) they are more likely to have been under stress at the time of the accident, 2) they develop depression and/or anxiety soon after the accident, 3) they have extensive social disruption after the accident, and 4) they have problems with physical symptoms such as headache and dizziness.

The treatment of patients with mild TBI involves initiating several key interventions (Kay 1993). In the early phase of treatment, the major goal is prevention of the postconcussion syndrome. This involves providing information and education about understanding and predicting

symptoms and their resolution and actively managing a gradual process of return to functioning. Education about the postconcussion syndrome and its natural history improves prognosis (Wade et al. 1998). It is important to involve the patient's family or significant other, so that they understand the disorder and predicted recovery. After the postconcussion syndrome has developed, the clinician must develop an alliance with the patient and validate his or her experience of cognitive and emotional difficulties while not prematurely confronting emotional factors as primary. A combined treatment strategy is required that addresses the emotional problems along with cognitive problems.

Aggression

Individuals with TBI may experience irritability, agitation, and aggressive behavior (Silver and Yudofsky 1994a). These episodes range in severity from irritability to outbursts that result in damage to property or assaults on others. In severe cases, affected individuals cannot remain in the community or with their families and often are referred to long-term psychiatric or neurobehavioral facilities. Increased isolation and separation from others often occur.

In the acute recovery period, 35%–96% of patients are reported to have exhibited agitated behavior (Silver and Yudofsky 1994a). After the acute recovery phase, irritability or bad temper is common. There has been only one prospective study of the occurrence of agitation and restlessness that has been monitored by an objective rating instrument, the Overt Agression Scale (OAS) (Brooke et al. 1992b). These authors found that of 100 patients with severe TBI (GCS score less than 8, more than 1 hour of coma, and more than 1 week of hospitalization), only 11 patients exhibited agitated behavior.

Only 3 patients manifested these behaviors for more than 1 week. However, 35 patients were observed to be restless but not agitated. In a prospective sample of 100 patients admitted to a brain injury rehabilitation unit, 42% exhibited agitated behavior during at least one nursing shift (Bogner and Corrigan 1995). In follow-up periods ranging from 1 to 15 years after injury, these behaviors occurred in 31%–71% of patients who experienced severe TBI (Silver and Yudofsky 1994a). Studies of mild TBI have evaluated patients for much briefer periods of time; 1-year estimates from these studies range from 5% to 70% (Silver and Yudofsky 1994a). Carlsson et al. (1987) examined the relationship between the number of traumatic brain injuries associated with LOC and various symptoms, and they demonstrated that irritability increases with subsequent injuries. Of the men who did not have head injuries with LOC, 21% reported irritability, whereas 31% of men with one injury with LOC and 33% of men with two or more injuries with LOC admitted to this symptom ($P < 0.0001$).

Explosive and violent behaviors have long been associated with focal brain lesions as well as with diffuse damage to the central nervous system (Anderson and Silver 1999). The current diagnostic category in DSM-IV-TR is personality change due to a general medical condition (American Psychiatric Association 2000) (see Table 8–5). Patients with aggressive behavior would be specified as aggressive type, whereas those with mood lability are specified as labile type. Characteristic behavioral features occur in many individuals who exhibit aggressive behavior after brain injury (Yudofsky et al. 1990). Typically, violence seen in these patients is *reactive* (i.e., triggered by modest or trivial stimuli). It is *nonreflective*, in that it does not involve premeditation or planning, and *nonpurposeful*, in the sense that

the aggression serves no obvious long-term aims or goals. The violence is *periodic*, with brief outbursts of rage and aggression, interspersed between long periods of relatively calm behavior. The aggression is *ego-dystonic*, such that the individual is often upset or embarrassed after the episode. Finally, it is generally *explosive*, occurring suddenly with no apparent buildup.

Treatment

There are many useful therapeutic approaches available for people who have brain injuries. Brain-injured patients may develop neuropsychiatric symptoms based on the location of their injury, the emotional reaction to their injury, their preexisting strengths and difficulties, and social expectations and supports. Comprehensive rehabilitation centers address many of these issues with therapeutic strategies that are developed specifically for this population (Ben-Yishay and Lakin 1989; Binder and Rattok 1989; Pollack 1989; Prigatano 1989).

Although these programs meet many of the needs of patients with TBI, comprehensive neuropsychiatric evaluation (including the daily evaluation and treatment of the patient by a psychiatrist) is rarely available. Although we propose a multifactorial, multidisciplinary, collaborative approach to treatment, for purposes of exposition we have divided treatment into psychopharmacologic, behavioral, psychological, and social interventions.

Psychopharmacologic Treatment

It is critical to conduct a thorough assessment of the patient before any intervention is initiated. Two issues require particular attention in the evaluation of the potential use of medication. First, the presenting complaints must be carefully assessed and defined. Second, the current treatment must be reevaluated. Although consultation may be requested to decide whether medication would be helpful, it is often the case that 1) other treatment modalities have not been properly applied, 2) there has been misdiagnosis of the problem, or 3) there has been poor communication among treating professionals. On occasion, a potentially effective medication has not been beneficial because it has been prescribed in a dose that is too low or for a period of time that is too brief. In other instances, the most appropriate pharmacologic recommendation is that no medication is required and that other therapeutic modalities need to be reassessed. In reviewing the patient's current medication regimen, two key issues should be addressed: 1) the indications for all drugs prescribed and whether they are still necessary, and 2) the potential side effects of these medications. Patients who have had a severe brain trauma may be receiving many medications that result in psychiatric symptoms such as depression, mania, hallucinations, insomnia, nightmares, cognitive impairments, restlessness, paranoia, or aggression.

There are several general principles that should be followed in the pharmacologic treatment of the psychiatric syndromes that occur after TBI. Patients with brain injury of any type are far more sensitive to the side effects of medications than are patients who are not brain injured. Doses of psychotropic medications must be raised and lowered in small increments over protracted periods of time, although patients ultimately may require the same doses and serum levels that are used for patients without brain injury to achieve therapeutic response (Silver and Yudofsky 1994b).

When medications are prescribed, it is important that they are given in a manner to enhance the probability of benefit and to reduce the possibility of adverse reactions. Medications should be initiated at dosages that are lower than those usually administered to patients without brain injury. Dose increments should be made gradually, to minimize side effects and enable the clinician to observe adverse consequences. However, it is also critical that the medications be given sufficient time to work. Thus, when a decision to administer a medication is made, the patient must receive an adequate therapeutic trial of that medication in terms of dosage and duration of treatment.

Due to frequent changes in clinical status of patients after TBI, continuous reassessment is necessary to determine whether or not the medication is required. For conditions such as depression, the standard guidelines for the treatment of major depression should be used (i.e., continuation of medication for a minimum of 6 months after remission of symptoms). For other psychiatric conditions, the guidelines may not be so clear. For example, agitation that occurs during the early phases of recovery from TBI may last days, weeks, or months. The periods of underarousal and unresponsiveness may have similar variability of symptom duration. In general, if the patient has responded favorably to medication treatment, the clinician must use clinical judgment and apply risk/benefit determinations to each specific case in deciding just when to taper and attempt to discontinue the medication following TBI. There may be spontaneous remission or a carryover effect of the medication (i.e., its effects last longer than the duration of treatment).

Although individuals after TBI may be experiencing multiple neuropsychiatric symptoms (such as depressed mood, irritability, poor attention, fatigue, and sleep disturbances) that may all appear to result from a single "psychiatric diagnosis" such as major depression, we have found that many symptoms persist after the major "diagnosis" has been treated. Therefore, several medications may be required to alleviate distinct symptoms. However, medications must be initiated one at a time to determine the efficacy and side effects of each prescribed drug.

Studies of the effects of psychotropic medications in patients with TBI are few, and rigorous double-blind, placebo-controlled studies are rare (see Arciniegas et al. 2000a). Therefore, many of the recommendations are extensions of the known uses of these medications in the non-brain-injured psychiatric population or from studies on other types of brain injury (stroke, multiple sclerosis, etc.).

Affective Illness

Depression

Affective disorders subsequent to brain damage are common and are usually highly detrimental to a patient's rehabilitation and socialization. However, the published literature is sparse regarding the effects of antidepressant agents and/or electroconvulsive therapy (ECT) in the treatment of patients with brain damage in general and TBI in particular (Arciniegas et al. 1999; Bessette and Peterson 1992; Cassidy 1989; Saran 1985; Varney et al. 1987; see Silver and Yudofsky 1994b for review).

Guidelines for using antidepressants for patients with TBI. The choice of an antidepressant depends predominantly on the desired side-effect profile. Usually, antidepressants with the fewest sedative, hypotensive, and anticholinergic side effects are preferred. Thus, the selective serotonin reuptake inhibitors (SSRIs) are usually the first-line medications prescribed. These would be initiated at low dosages (e.g., fluoxetine starting at 10 mg/

day, sertraline starting at 25 mg/day, or citalopram starting at 10 mg/day). Fann and colleagues performed a single-blind placebo run-in trial of sertraline in 15 patients with major depression after TBI. Two-thirds of these patients achieved a Hamilton Rating Scale (Hamilton 1960) score consistent with remission by 2 months (Fann et al. 2000). In addition, those patients showed improvements in psychomotor speed, recent verbal memory, recent visual memory, and general cognitive efficiency (Fann et al. 2001). Other SSRIs, such as paroxetine and fluvoxamine, as well as venlafaxine and nefazodone, also appear effective. In a study comparing nortriptyline and fluoxetine in poststroke depression, nortriptyline was superior in efficacy to fluoxetine, and fluoxetine demonstrated no benefit above placebo (Robinson et al. 2000).

Side effects. The most common and disabling antidepressant side effects in patients with TBI, especially with the older heterocyclic antidepressants (HCAs), are the anticholinergic effects. These medications may impair attention, concentration, and memory, especially in patients with brain lesions. The antidepressants amitriptyline, trimipramine, doxepin, and protriptyline have high affinities for the muscarinic receptors and thus are highly anticholinergic and should be used only after careful consideration of alternative medications. Fluoxetine, sertraline, citalopram, mirtazapine, trazodone, venlafaxine, nefazodone, and bupropion all have minimal or no anticholinergic action. Several antidepressants (e.g., mirtazapine, doxepin, amitriptyline, trimipramine, imipramine, maprotiline, trazodone) are highly sedating and may result in significant problems of arousal in the TBI patient.

In some individuals, SSRIs may result in word-finding problems or apathy. This may be due to the effects of SSRIs on decreasing dopaminergic functioning, and it may be reversible with the addition of a dopaminergic or stimulant medication.

The available evidence suggests that, overall, antidepressants may be associated with a greater frequency of seizures in patients with brain injury. The antidepressants maprotiline and bupropion may be associated with a higher incidence of seizures (Davidson 1989; Pinder et al. 1977). Wroblewski et al. (1990) reviewed the records of 68 patients with TBI who received HCA treatment for at least 3 months. The frequencies of seizures were compared for the 3 months before treatment, during treatment, and after treatment. Seizures occurred in 6 patients (9%) during the baseline period, in 16 (24%) during HCA treatment, and in 4 (6%) after treatment was discontinued. Fourteen patients (19%) had seizures shortly after the initiation of HCA treatment. For 12 of these patients, no seizures occurred after HCA treatment was discontinued. Importantly, 7 of these patients were receiving anticonvulsant medication before and during HCA treatment. The occurrence of seizures was related to greater severity of brain injury. Other investigations have found that seizure control does not appear to worsen if psychotropic medication is introduced cautiously and if the patient is on an effective anticonvulsant regimen (Ojemann et al. 1987). Although there have been reports of seizures occurring with fluoxetine, Favale et al. (1995) demonstrated an anticonvulsant effect in patients with seizures. In our experience, few patients have experienced seizures during treatment with SSRIs and other newer antidepressants. Although antidepressants should be used with continuous monitoring in patients with severe TBI, we also believe that antidepressants can be used safely and effectively in patients with TBI.

Mania

Manic episodes that occur after TBI have been successfully treated with lithium carbonate, carbamazepine (Stewart and Nemsath 1988), valproic acid (Pope et al. 1988), clonidine (Bakchine et al. 1989), and ECT (Clark and Davison 1987). Because of the increased incidence of side effects when lithium is used in patients with brain lesions, we limit the use of lithium in patients with TBI to those with mania or with recurrent depressive illness that preceded their brain damage. Furthermore, to minimize lithium-related side effects, we begin with low doses (300 mg/day) and assess the response to low therapeutic blood levels (e.g., 0.2–0.5 mEq/L).

Lithium has been reported to aggravate confusion in patients with brain damage (Schiff et al. 1982), as well as to induce nausea, tremor, ataxia, and lethargy in this population. In addition, lithium may lower seizure threshold (Massey and Folger 1984). Hornstein and Seliger (1989) reported a patient with preexisting bipolar disorder who experienced a recurrence of mania after experiencing closed head injury. Before the injury, this patient's mania was controlled with lithium carbonate without side effects. However, after the brain injury, dysfunctions of attention and concentration emerged that reversed with lowering of the lithium dosage.

For patients with mania subsequent to TBI, valproic acid is begun at a dosage of 250 mg twice daily and is gradually increased to obtain plasma levels of 50–100 mg/mL. Tremor and weight gain are common side effects. Hepatotoxicity is rare and usually occurs in children who are treated with multiple anticonvulsants (Dreifuss et al. 1987). Carbamazepine should be initiated at a dosage of 200 mg twice daily and adjusted to obtain plasma levels of 8–12 g/mL. As for patients without histories of TBI, the clinician should be aware of the potential risks associated with carbamazepine treatment, particularly bone marrow suppression (including aplastic anemia) and hepatotoxicity. The most common signs of neurotoxicity include lethargy, confusion, drowsiness, weakness, ataxia, nystagmus, and increased seizures. Lamotrigine and gabapentin are other options, although evidence as to efficacy, especially in individuals with TBI, is sparse.

Lability of Mood and Affect

Antidepressants may be used to treat the labile mood that frequently occurs with neurologic disease. However, it appears that the control of lability of mood and affect may differ from that of depression, and the mechanism of action of antidepressants in treating mood lability in those with brain injuries may differ from that in the treatment of patients with "uncomplicated" depression (Lauterbach and Schweri 1991; Panzer and Mellow 1992; Ross and Rush 1981; Schiffer et al. 1985; Seliger et al. 1992; Sloan et al. 1992). Schiffer et al. (1985) conducted a double-blind crossover study with amitriptyline and placebo in 12 patients with pathologic laughing and weeping secondary to multiple sclerosis. Eight patients experienced a dramatic response to amitriptyline at a maximum dose of 75 mg/day.

There have been several reports of the beneficial effects of fluoxetine for "emotional incontinence" secondary to several neurologic disorders (K.W. Brown et al. 1998; Nahas et al. 1998; Panzer and Mellow 1992; Seliger et al. 1992; Sloan et al. 1992). K.W. Brown and colleagues (1998) treated 20 patients with post-stroke emotionalism with fluoxetine in a double-blind, placebo-controlled study. The individuals receiving fluoxetine exhibited statistically and clinically significant improvement. In our experience, all

SSRIs can be effective, and the dosage guidelines are similar to those used in the treatment of depression. Other antidepressants, such as nortriptyline, can also be effective for emotional lability. We emphasize that for many patients it may be necessary to administer these medications at standard antidepressant dosages to obtain full therapeutic effects, although response may occur for others within days of initiating treatment at relatively low doses.

Cognitive Function and Arousal

Stimulants, such as dextroamphetamine and methylphenidate, and dopamine agonists, such as amantadine and bromocriptine, may be beneficial in treating the patient with apathy and impaired concentration to increase arousal and to diminish fatigue. These medications all act on the catecholaminergic system but in different ways. Dextroamphetamine blocks the reuptake of norepinephrine and, in higher doses, also blocks the reuptake of dopamine. Methylphenidate has a similar mechanism of action. Amantadine acts both presynaptically and postsynaptically at the dopamine receptor and may also increase cholinergic and GABAergic activity (Cowell and Cohen 1995). In addition, amantadine is an N-methyl-D-aspartate (NMDA) glutamate receptor antagonist (Weller and Kornhuber 1992). Bromocriptine is a dopamine type 1 receptor antagonist and a dopamine type 2 receptor agonist. It appears to be a dopamine agonist at midrange doses (Berg et al. 1987). Assessment of improvement in attention and arousal may be difficult (Whyte 1992), and further work needs to be conducted in this area to determine whether these medications affect outcome. Therefore, careful objective assessment with appropriate neuropsychological tests may be helpful in determining response to treatment.

Dextroamphetamine and Methylphenidate

Several reports have indicated that impairments in verbal memory and learning, attention, and behavior are alleviated with either dextroamphetamine or methylphenidate (Bleiberg et al. 1993; Evans et al. 1987; Kaelin et al. 1996; Lipper and Tuchman 1976; Weinberg et al. 1987; Weinstein and Wells 1981). In a double-blind, placebo-controlled crossover study, Gualtieri and Evans (1988) studied 15 patients with TBI who were currently functioning at a Rancho Los Amigos Scale level of VII or VIII. Patients received a 2-week treatment with either placebo, methylphenidate 0.15 mg/kg body weight twice daily, or methylphenidate 0.30 mg/kg body weight twice daily. Of the 15 patients treated, 14 improved with active medication and had increased scores on ratings of mood and performance. The authors observed that this short-term response was not sustained over time. In a double-blind, placebo-controlled trial the administration of methylphenidate in the subacute setting to individuals with moderate to moderately severe TBI, Plenger and colleagues (1996) found that attention and performance were improved at 30 days but did not differ from a control group at 90 days. Therefore, the rate, but not the extent, of recovery was improved with stimulants. Speech et al. (1993) conducted a double-blind, placebo-controlled study of the effects of methylphenidate in 10 patients with chronic TBI. They found no significant increase in measures of attention, arousal, learning, cognitive processing speed, or behavior. Mooney and Haas (1993) found that methylphenidate improved anger and other personality problems after TBI. Whyte et al. (1997) performed a randomized, placebo-controlled trial of methylphenidate on 19 patients who exhibited attentional deficits after TBI. Although there was improvement in speed of mental processing, there were no improvements noted in orienting to distractions, sustained attention, and motor speed.

When used, methylphenidate should be initiated at 5 mg twice daily and dextroamphetamine at 2.5 mg twice daily. Maximum dosage of each medication is usually 60 mg/day, administered twice daily or three times daily. However, we have seen some patients who have required higher dosages of methylphenidate to obtain a reasonable serum level of 15 mg/mL.

Sinemet and Bromocriptine

Lal et al. (1988) reported on the use of L-dopa/carbidopa (Sinemet) in the treatment of 12 patients with brain injury (including anoxic damage). With treatment, patients exhibited improved alertness and concentration; decreased fatigue, hypomania, and sialorrhea; and improved memory, mobility, posture, and speech. Dosages administered ranged from 10/100 to 25/250 four times daily. Eames (1989) suggested that bromocriptine may be useful in treating cognitive initiation problems of brain-injured patients at least 1 year after injury. He recommended starting at 2.5 mg/day and administering treatment for at least 2 months at the highest dose tolerated (up to 100 mg/day). Other investigators have found that patients with nonfluent aphasia (Gupta and Mlcoch 1992), akinetic mutism (Echiverri et al. 1988), and apathy (Catsman-Berrevoets and Harskamp 1988) have improved after treatment with bromocriptine. Parks et al. (1992) suggested that bromocriptine exerts specific effects on the frontal lobe and increases goal-directed behaviors.

Amantadine

Amantadine may be beneficial in the treatment of anergia, abulia, mutism, and anhedonia subsequent to brain injury (Chandler et al. 1988; Cowell and Cohen 1995; Gualtieri et al. 1989; Nickels et al. 1994). Kraus and Maki (1997) administered amantadine 400 mg/day to six patients with TBI. Improvement was found in motivation, attention, and alertness, as well as executive function and dyscontrol. Dosages should initially be 50 mg twice daily and should be increased every week by 100 mg/day to a maximum dosage of 400 mg/day.

Tricyclic Antidepressants

Although the drugs involved are not in the category of stimulants or dopamine agonists, Reinhard and colleagues (1996) administered amitriptyline (one patient) and desipramine (two patients) and found improvement in arousal and initiation after TBI. The authors hypothesize that the improvement is from the noradrenergic effects of these drugs.

Side Effects of Medications for Impaired Concentration and Arousal

Adverse reactions to medications for impaired concentration and arousal are most often related to increases in dopamine activity. Dexedrine and methylphenidate may lead to paranoia, dysphoria, agitation, and irritability. Depression often occurs on discontinuation, so stimulants should be discontinued using a slow regimen. Interestingly, there may be a role for stimulants to increase neuronal recovery subsequent to brain injury (Crisostomo et al. 1988). Side effects of bromocriptine include sedation, nausea, psychosis, headaches, and delirium. Amantadine may cause confusion, hallucinations, edema, and hypotension; these reactions occur more often in elderly patients.

There is often concern that stimulant medications may lower seizure threshold in patients with TBI who are at increased risk for posttraumatic seizures. Wroblewski et al. (1992) reviewed their experience with methylphenidate in 30 patients with severe brain injury and seizures and examined changes in seizure frequency after initiation of methylphenidate. The number of seizures was monitored for 3 months before treatment with methylphenidate, for 3 months during treatment, and for 3 months after treatment was discontinued. The researchers found that whereas only 4 patients experienced more seizures during methylphenidate treatment, 26 had either fewer or the same number of seizures during treatment. The authors concluded that there is no significant risk in lowering seizure threshold with methylphenidate treatment in this high-risk group. Although many patients in this study were treated concomitantly with anticonvulsant medications that may have conferred some protection against the development of seizures, this does not explain why 13 patients had fewer seizures when treated with methylphenidate. In a double-blind, placebo-controlled study of the effects of methylphenidate (0.3 mg/kg twice daily) in 10 children with well-controlled seizures and attention-deficit/hyperactivity disorder, no seizures occurred during the 4 weeks of treatment either with active drug or with placebo. Dextroamphetamine has been used adjunctively in the treatment of refractory seizures (Livingston and Pauli 1975), and bromocriptine may also have some anticonvulsant properties (Rothman et al. 1990). Amantadine may lower seizure threshold (Gualtieri et al. 1989). We have also observed several patients who had not experienced seizures for months before the administration of amantadine to have had a seizure weeks after it was prescribed.

Problems with processing multiple stimuli. Although individuals with TBI may have difficulty with maintaining attention on single tasks, they can also have difficulty in processing multiple stimuli. This difficulty has been called an abnormality in auditory gating, and it is consistent with an abnormal response in processing auditory stimuli that are given 50 milliseconds apart (P50 response) (Arciniegas et al. 2000b). Preliminary evidence suggests that this response normalizes after treatment with donepezil 5 mg, which also results in symptomatic improvement (Arciniegas 2001).

Fatigue

Stimulants (methylphenidate and dextroamphetamine) and amantadine can diminish the profound daytime fatigue experienced by patients with TBI. Dosages utilized would be similar to those used for treatment of diminished arousal and concentration. Modafinil, a medication approved for the treatment of excessive daytime somnolence in patients with narcolepsy, also may have a role in treatment of post-TBI fatigue. There have been studies specifically in patients with multiple sclerosis that have shown benefit (Rammahan et al. 2000; Terzoudi et al. 2000). Dosages should start with 100 mg in the morning and can be increased to up to 600 mg/day administered in two doses (e.g., 400 mg in the morning and 200 mg in the afternoon).

Cognition

Cholinesterase Inhibitors

TBI may produce cognitive impairments via disruption of cholinergic function (Arciniegas et al. 1999), and the relative sensitivity of TBI patients to medications with anticholinergic agents has prompted speculation that cognitively impaired TBI patients may have a relatively reduced reserve of cholinergic function. This has prompted trials of procholinergic agents,

and in particular physostigmine, to treat behavioral dyscontrol and impaired cognition in TBI patients (Eames and Sutton 1995). However, the significant peripheral effects and narrow margin of safety of physostigmine have made treatment with this agent impractical. With the advent of relatively centrally selective acetylcholinesterase inhibitors such as donepezil, the issue of cholinergic augmentation strategies in the treatment of cognitive impairment following TBI is currently being revisited, and preliminary reports suggest that donepezil may improve memory and global functioning (Taverni et al. 1998). Doses of donepezil range from 5 to 10 mg/day. The most common side effects include sedation, insomnia, diarrhea, and dizziness, which are minimized by starting with the lower dosage and adjusting upward slowly. Although these adverse effects are generally transient, a few patients will be unable to tolerate the medication due to persistent, severe diarrhea.

Psychosis

The psychotic ideation resulting from TBI is generally responsive to treatment with antipsychotic medications. However, side effects such as hypotension, sedation, and confusion are common. Also, brain-injured patients are particularly subject to dystonia, akathisia, and other parkinsonian side effects—even at relatively low doses of antipsychotic medications (Wolf et al. 1989). Antipsychotic medications have also been reported to impede neuronal recovery after brain injury (Feeney et al. 1982). Therefore, we advise that antipsychotics should be used sparingly during the acute phases of recovery after the injury. Risperidone, olanzapine, and quetiapine have preferred therapeutic profiles over the conventional high-potency neuroleptics (such as haloperidol) because of decreased extrapyramidal effects. Therapeutic effect may not be evident for 3 weeks after treatment at each dosage. In general, we recommend a low-dose neuroleptic strategy for all patients with neuropsychiatric disorders. Clozapine is a novel and effective antipsychotic medication that does not produce extrapyramidal side effects. Although its use in patients with neuropsychiatric disorders has yet to be investigated fully, its side-effect profile poses many potential disadvantages. It is highly anticholinergic, produces significant sedation and hypotension, lowers seizure threshold profoundly, and is associated with a 1% risk of agranulocytosis that requires lifetime weekly monitoring of blood counts.

Among all the first-generation antipsychotic drugs, molindone and fluphenazine have consistently demonstrated the lowest potential for lowering the seizure threshold (Oliver et al. 1982). Clozapine treatment is associated with a significant dose-related incidence of seizures (ranging from 1% to 2% of patients who receive doses below 300 mg/day and 5% of patients who receive 600–900 mg/day); thus, in patients with TBI it must be used with extreme caution and for most carefully considered indications (Lieberman et al. 1989).

Sleep

Sleep patterns of patients with brain damage are often disordered, with impaired rapid eye movement (REM) recovery and multiple nocturnal awakenings (Prigatano et al. 1982). Hypersomnia that occurs after severe missile head injury most often resolves within the first year after injury, whereas insomnia that occurs in patients with long periods of coma and diffuse injury has a more chronic course (Askenasy et al. 1989). Barbiturates and long-acting benzodiazepines should be prescribed for sedation with great caution, if at all. These drugs interfere with REM and stage 4 sleep patterns and may contribute to persistent insomnia (Buysse and Reynolds 1990). Clinicians should warn patients of the dangers of using over-the-counter preparations for sleeping and for colds because of the prominent anticholinergic side effects of these agents.

Trazodone, a sedating antidepressant medication that is devoid of anticholinergic side effects, may be used for nighttime sedation. A dose of 50 mg should be administered initially; if this is ineffective, doses up to 150 mg may be prescribed. Nonpharmacologic approaches should be considered. These include minimizing daytime naps, adhering to regular sleep times, and engaging in regular physical activity during the day.

Aggression and Agitation

We suggest utilizing the Consensus Guidelines for the Treatment of Agitation in the Elderly with Dementia as a framework for the assessment and management of agitation and aggression after TBI (Alexopoulos et al. 1998). After appropriate assessment of possible etiologies of these behaviors, treatment is focused on the occurrence of comorbid neuropsychiatric conditions (depression, psychosis, insomnia, anxiety, and delirium) and whether the treatment is in the short-term (hours to days) or long-term (weeks to months) phase, and the severity of the behavior (mild to severe).

Acute Aggression and Agitation

In the treatment of agitation and of acute or severe episodes of aggressive behavior, medications that are sedating may be indicated. However, because these drugs are not specific in their ability to inhibit aggressive behavior, there may be detrimental effects on arousal and cognitive function. Therefore, the use of sedation-producing medications must be time limited to avoid the emergence of seriously disabling side effects ranging from oversedation to tardive dyskinesia.

Although there is no medication that is approved by the U.S. Food and Drug Administration specifically for the treatment of aggression, medications are widely used (and commonly misused) in the management of patients with acute or chronic aggression. After diagnosis and treatment of underlying causes of aggression and evaluation and documentation of aggressive behaviors (with the OAS), the use of pharmacologic interventions can be considered in two categories: 1) the use of the sedating effects of medications, as required in acute situations, so that the patient does not harm himself or herself or others; and 2) the use of nonsedating antiaggressive medications for the treatment of chronic aggression (Silver and Yudofsky 1994a; Yudofsky et al. 1995).

Antipsychotic drugs. In patients with brain injury and acute aggression, we recommend starting a neuroleptic such as risperidone at low doses of 0.5 mg orally, with repeated administration every hour until control of aggression is achieved. If after several administrations of risperidone the patient's aggressive behavior does not improve, the hourly dose may be increased until the patient is so sedated that he or she no longer exhibits agitation or violence. Once the patient is not aggressive for 48 hours, the daily dosage should be decreased gradually (i.e., by 25%/day) to ascertain whether aggressive behavior reemerges. In this case, consideration should then be made about whether it is best to increase the dose of risperidone and/or to initiate treatment with a more specific antiaggressive drug.

Sedatives and hypnotics. Benzodiazepines can produce amnesia, and preexisting memory dysfunction can be exacerbated by the use of benzodiazepines. Brain-injured patients may also experience increased problems with coor-

dination and balance with benzodiazepine use.

For treatment of acute aggression, lorazepam, 1–2 mg, may be administered every hour by either oral or intramuscular route until sedation is achieved (Silver and Yudofsky 1994a). Intramuscular lorazepam has been suggested as an effective medication in the emergency treatment of the violent patient (Bick and Hannah 1986). Intravenous lorazepam is also effective, although the onset of action is similar when administered intramuscularly. Caution must be taken with intravenous administration, and it should be injected in doses less than 1 mg/minute to avoid laryngospasm. As with neuroleptics, gradual tapering of lorazepam may be attempted when the patient has been in control for 48 hours. If aggressive behavior recurs, medications for the treatment of chronic aggression may be initiated. Lorazepam in 1- or 2-mg doses, administered either orally or by injection, may be administered, if necessary, in combination with a neuroleptic medication (haloperidol, 2–5 mg). Other sedating medications such as paraldehyde, chloral hydrate, or diphenhydramine may be preferable to sedative antipsychotic agents.

Chronic Aggression

If a patient continues to exhibit periods of agitation or aggression beyond several weeks, the use of specific antiaggressive medications should be initiated to prevent these episodes from occurring. Because no medication has been approved by the Food and Drug Administration for treatment of aggression, the clinician must use medications that may be antiaggressive but that have been approved for other uses (e.g., seizure disorders, depression, hypertension) (Silver and Yudofsky 1994a).

Antipsychotic medications. If, after thorough clinical evaluation, it is determined that the aggressive episodes result from psychosis, such as paranoid delusions or command hallucinations, then antipsychotic medications will be the treatment of choice. Risperidone has been used to treat agitation in elderly patients with dementia with good results (Goldberg and Goldberg 1995). Olanzapine appears to be more sedating, and quetiapine may have fewer extrapyramidal symptoms than does risperidone. Clozapine may have greater antiaggressive effects than other antipsychotic medications (Michals et al. 1993; Ratey et al. 1993). However, the increased risk of seizures must be carefully assessed.

Antianxiety medications. Serotonin appears to be a key neurotransmitter in the modulation of aggressive behavior. In preliminary reports, buspirone, a serotonin type 1A agonist, has been reported to be effective in the management of aggression and agitation for patients with head injury, dementia, and developmental disabilities and autism (Silver and Yudofsky 1994a). In rare instances, some patients become more aggressive when treated with buspirone. Therefore, buspirone should be initiated at low dosages (i.e., 5 mg twice daily) and increased by 5 mg every 3–5 days. Dosages of 45–60 mg/day may be required before there is improvement in aggressive behavior, although we have noted dramatic improvement within 1 week.

Clonazepam may be effective in the long-term management of aggression, although controlled, double-blind studies have not yet been conducted. Freinhar and Alvarez (1986) found that clonazepam decreased agitation in three elderly patients with organic brain syndromes. Keats and Mukherjee (1988) reported antiaggressive effects of clonazepam in a patient with schizophrenia and seizures. We use clonazepam when

pronounced aggression and anxiety occur together, or when aggression occurs in association with neurologically induced tics and similarly disinhibited motor behaviors. Doses should initially be 0.5 mg twice daily and may be increased to as high as 2–4 mg twice daily, as tolerated. Sedation and ataxia are frequent side effects.

Anticonvulsive medications. The anticonvulsant carbamazepine has been proved to be effective for the treatment of bipolar disorders and has also been advocated for the control of aggression in both epileptic and nonepileptic populations. Several open studies have indicated that carbamazepine may be effective in decreasing aggressive behavior associated with TBI dementia (Chatham-Showalter 1996), developmental disabilities, and schizophrenia and in patients with a variety of other organic brain disorders (Silver and Yudofsky 1994a). Carbamazepine can be a highly effective medication to treat aggression in the brain-injured patient, and we believe it is the drug of choice for patients who have aggressive episodes with concomitant seizures or epileptic foci. Reports also indicate that the antiaggressive response of carbamazepine can be found in patients with and without electroencephalographic abnormalities (Silver and Yudofsky 1994a; Yudofsky et al. 1998). Azouvi and colleagues (1999) found that 8 of 10 patients with aggressive behavior after TBI responded to carbamazepine.

In our experience and that of others, the anticonvulsant valproic acid may also be helpful to some patients with organically induced aggression (Geracioti 1994; Giakas et al. 1990; Horne and Lindley 1995; Mattes 1992; Wroblewski et al. 1997). For patients with aggression and epilepsy whose seizures are being treated with anticonvulsant drugs such as phenytoin and phenobarbital, switching to carbamazepine or to valproic acid may treat both conditions.

Gabapentin has been used effectively for the treatment of agitation in patients with dementia (Herrmann et al. 2000; Roane et al. 2000). Doses have ranged from 200 to 2,400 mg/day.

Antimanic medications. Although lithium is known to be effective in controlling aggression related to manic excitement, many studies suggest that it may also have a role in the treatment of aggression in selected nonbipolar patient populations (Yudofsky et al. 1998). Included are patients with TBI (Bellus et al. 1996; Glenn et al. 1989) as well as patients with mental retardation who exhibit self-injurious or aggressive behavior, children and adolescents with behavioral disorders, prison inmates, and patients with other organic brain syndromes.

Patients with brain injury have increased sensitivity to the neurotoxic effects of lithium (Hornstein and Seliger 1989; Moskowitz and Altshuler 1991). Because of lithium's potential for neurotoxicity and its relative lack of efficacy in many patients with aggression secondary to brain injury, we limit the use of lithium in patients whose aggression is related to manic effects or recurrent irritability related to cyclic mood disorders.

Antidepressants. The antidepressants that have been reported to control aggressive behavior are those that act preferentially (amitriptyline) or specifically (trazodone and fluoxetine) on serotonin. In open studies, Mysiw et al. (1988) and Jackson et al. (1985) reported that amitriptyline (maximum dose 150 mg/day) was effective in the treatment of patients with recent severe brain injury whose agitation had not responded to behavioral techniques. Trazodone has also been reported to be effective in the treatment

of aggression that occurs with organic mental disorders (Silver and Yudofsky 1994a; Yudofsky et al. 1998). Two individuals with Huntington's disease and aggressiveness were treated effectively with sertraline (Ranen et al. 1996). Thirteen patients who had irritability and aggression after TBI also exhibited improvement after treatment with sertraline (Kant et al. 1998). Fluoxetine, a potent serotonergic antidepressant, has been reported to be effective in the treatment of aggressive behavior in a patient who sustained brain injury as well as in patients with personality disorders and depression, and adolescents with mental retardation and self-injurious behavior (Silver and Yudofsky 1994a; Yudofsky et al. 1998). We have used SSRIs with considerable success in aggressive patients with brain lesions. The dosages used are similar to those for the treatment of mood lability and depression.

We have evaluated and treated many patients with emotional lability that is characterized by frequent episodes of tearfulness and irritability, and the full symptomatic picture of neuroaggressive syndrome (Silver and Yudofsky 1994a). These patients—who would be diagnosed under DSM-IV-TR as personality change, labile type, due to traumatic brain injury—have responded well to antidepressants. This is discussed above in the section on mood lability.

Antihypertensive medications: β-blockers. Since the first report of the use of β-adrenergic receptor blockers in the treatment of acute aggression in 1977, more than 25 articles have appeared in the neurologic and psychiatric literature reporting experience in using β-blockers with more than 200 patients with aggression (Yudofsky et al. 1987). Most of these patients had been unsuccessfully treated with antipsychotics, minor tranquilizers, lithium, and/or anticonvulsants before being treated with β-blockers. The β-blockers that have been investigated in controlled prospective studies include propranolol (a lipid-soluble, nonselective receptor antagonist), nadolol (a water-soluble, nonselective receptor antagonist), and pindolol (a lipid-soluble, nonselective β-receptor antagonist with partial sympathomimetic activity). A growing body of preliminary evidence suggests that β-adrenergic receptor blockers are effective agents for the treatment of aggressive and violent behaviors, particularly those related to organic brain syndrome. The effectiveness of propranolol in reducing agitation has been demonstrated during the initial hospitalization after TBI (Brooke et al. 1992a). Propranolol is initiated at a dosage of 60–80 mg/day with gradual dosage increments every several days; a total daily dosage of greater than 800 mg is not usually required. When a patient requires the use of a once-a-day medication because of compliance difficulties, long-acting propranolol (i.e., Inderal LA) or nadolol (Corgard) can be used. When patients develop bradycardia that prevents prescribing therapeutic dosages of propranolol, pindolol (Visken) can be substituted, using one-tenth the dosage of propranolol. The intrinsic sympathomimetic activity of pindolol stimulates the β receptor and restricts the development of bradycardia.

The major side effects of β-blockers when used to treat aggression are lowering of blood pressure and pulse rate. Because peripheral β receptors are fully blocked with doses of 300–400 mg/day, further decreases in these vital signs usually do not occur even when doses are increased to much higher levels. Despite reports of depression with the use of β-blockers, controlled trials and our experience indicate that it is a rare occurrence. Because the use of propranolol is associated with

TABLE 8–9. Pharmacotherapy of agitation

Acute agitation/severe aggression
  Antipsychotic drugs
  Benzodiazepines
Chronic agitation
  Atypical antipsychotics
  Anticonvulsants (VPA, CBZ, ?gabapentin)
  Serotoninergic antidepressants (SSRI, trazodone)
  Buspirone
  β-Blockers

Note. CBZ = carbamazepine; SSRI = selective serotonin reuptake inhibitor; VPA = valproic acid.

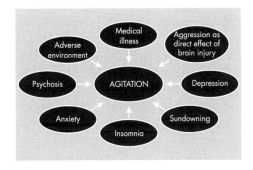

FIGURE 8–1. Factors associated with agitation in brain injury.

significant increases in plasma levels of thioridazine, which has an absolute dosage ceiling of 800 mg/day, the combination of these two medications should be avoided whenever possible.

Table 8–9 summarizes our recommendations for the use of various classes of medication in the treatment of chronic aggressive disorders associated with TBI. Acute aggression may be treated by using the sedative properties of neuroleptics or benzodiazepines. In treating aggression, the clinician, when possible, should diagnose and treat underlying disorders and should use, when possible, antiaggressive agents specific for those disorders (see Figure 8–1). When there is partial response after a therapeutic trial with a specific medication, adjunctive treatment with a medication with a different mechanism of action should be instituted. For example, a patient with partial response to β-blockers can have additional improvement with the addition of an anticonvulsant.

Behavioral and Cognitive Treatments

Behavioral treatments are important in the care of patients who have sustained TBI. These programs require careful design and execution by a staff well versed in behavioral techniques. Behavioral methods can be used in response to aggressive outbursts and other maladaptive social behaviors (Corrigan and Jakus 1994). One study (Eames and Wood 1985) found that behavior modification was 75% effective in dealing with disturbed behavior after severe brain injury.

After brain injury, patients may need specific cognitive strategies to assist with impairments in memory and concentration (Ben-Yishay and Diller 1993; Rattok and Ross 1994). As opposed to earlier beliefs that cognitive therapy should "exercise" the brain to develop skills that have been damaged, current therapies involve teaching the patient new strategies to compensate for lost or impaired functions. Salazar and colleagues (2000) for the Defense and Veterans Head Injury Program Study Group compared an intensive 8-week in-hospital cognitive rehabilitation program to a limited home program. Both groups improved, but there was no significant difference between the two treatments. (For more information on cognitive treatments, see Chapter 20 of this book.) We emphasize that, for most patients, treatment strategies are synergistic. For example, the use of β-adrenergic receptor antagonists to treat agitation and aggression may enhance a patient's ability

to benefit from behavioral and cognitive treatments.

Psychological and Social Interventions

In the broadest terms, psychological issues involving patients who incur brain injury revolve around four major themes: 1) psychopathology that preceded the injury, 2) psychological responses to the traumatic event, 3) psychological reactions to deficits brought about by brain injury, and 4) psychological issues related to potential recurrence of brain injury.

Preexisting psychiatric illnesses are most frequently intensified with brain injury. Therefore, the angry, obsessive patient or the patient with chronic depression will exhibit a worsening of these symptoms after brain injury. Specific coping mechanisms that were used before the injury may no longer be possible because of the cognitive deficits caused by the neurologic disease. Therefore, patients need to learn new methods of adaptation to stress. In addition, the social, economic, educational, and vocational status of the patient (and how these are affected by brain lesions) influence the patient's response to the injury.

The events surrounding brain injury often have far-reaching experiential and symbolic significance for the patient. Such issues as guilt, punishment, magical wishes, and fears crystallize about the nidus of a traumatic event. For example, a patient who sustains brain injury during a car accident may view his injury as punishment for long-standing violent impulses toward an aggressive father. In such cases, reassurance and homilies about his lack of responsibility for the accident are usually less productive than psychological exploration.

A patient's reactions to being disabled by brain damage have "realistic" as well as symbolic significance. When intense effort is required for a patient to form a word or to move a limb, frustration may be expressed as anger, depression, anxiety, or fear. Particularly in cases in which brain injury results in permanent impairment, a psychiatrist may experience countertransferential discomfort that results in failure to discuss directly with the patient and his or her family the implications of resultant disabilities and limitations. Gratuitous optimism, collaboration with denial of the patient, and facile solutions to complex problems are rarely effective and can erode the therapeutic alliance and ongoing treatment. Tyerman and Humphrey (1984) assessed 25 patients with severe brain injury for changes in self-concept. Patients viewed themselves as markedly changed after their injury but believed that they would regain preexisting capacities within a year. The authors concluded that these unrealistic expectations may hamper rehabilitation and adjustment of both the patient and his or her relatives. By gently and persistently directing the patient's attention to the reality of the disabilities, the psychiatrist may help the patient begin the process of acceptance and adjustment to the impairment. Clinical judgment will help the psychiatrist in deciding whether and when explorations of the symbolic significance of the patient's brain injury should be pursued. The persistence of anxiety, guilt, and fear beyond the normative stages of adjustment and rehabilitation may indicate that psychodynamic approaches are required (Drubach et al. 1994; Pollack 1994).

Families of patients with neurologic disorders are under severe stress. The relative with a brain injury may be unable to fulfill his or her previous role or function as parent or spouse, thus significantly affecting the other family members (Kay and Cavallo 1994). Oddy et al. (1978) evaluated 54 relatives of patients with brain injury within 1, 6, and 12 months of the traumatic event. Approximately 40% of the relatives showed depressive symptoms within 1 month of the event; 25% of the relatives showed significant physical or psychological illness within 6–12 months of the brain damage. Mood disturbances, especially anxiety, depression, and social role dysfunction, are also seen within this time (Kreutzer et al. 1994; Linn et al. 1994; Livingston et al. 1985a, 1985b). Family members may experience increased substance use, unemployment, and decreased financial status over time (Hall et al. 1994). By treating the psychological responses of relatives to the brain injury, the clinician can foster a supportive and therapeutic atmosphere for the patient as well as significantly help the relatives. In one study (Leach et al. 1994), teaching the family how to implement problem-solving techniques and behavioral coping strategies resulted in lower levels of depression in the person who sustained the injury.

For both patients and their families, severe TBI results in multifaceted losses, including the loss of dreams about and expectations for the future. The psychiatrist may be of enormous benefit in treating the family and patient by providing support, insight, and other points of view. A patient from a high-achieving family who lost his ability to do theoretical physics told one of us (S.C.Y.), "If I can't go to graduate school in physics at Princeton like my brother and my cousin, I am worthless."

Educational and supportive treatment of families can be therapeutic when used together with appropriate social skills training. Patient advocacy groups, such as the National Brain Injury Foundation, can provide important peer support for families. Many patients require clear, almost concrete statements describing their behaviors because insight and judgment may be impaired.

It is a distressing fact that brain injury can and often does recur. With repeated injury, there is an increase in the incidence of neuropsychiatric and emotional symptoms (Carlsson et al. 1987). In fact, trauma from accidents occurs more commonly in patients who have already experienced such events than in those who have not. Therefore, patients' fears and anxieties about recurrence of injury are more than simply efforts at magical control over terrifying conditions. Therapeutic emphasis should be placed on actions and activities that will aid in preventing recurrence, including compliance with appropriate medications and abstinence from alcohol and other substances of abuse.

Conclusions

Invariably, brain injury leads to emotional damage in the patient and in the family. In this chapter, we have reviewed the most frequently occurring psychiatric symptoms that are associated with TBI. We have emphasized how the informed psychiatrist is not only effective but essential in both the prevention of brain injury and, when it occurs, the treatment of its sequelae. In addition to increased efforts devoted to the prevention of brain injury, we advocate a multidisciplinary and multidimensional approach to the assessment and treatment of neuropsychiatric aspects of brain injury.

References

Achte K, Jarho L, Kyykka T, et al: Paranoid disorders following war brain damage: preliminary report. Psychopathology 24:309–315, 1991

Adams JH, Graham DI, Murray LS, et al: Diffuse axonal injury due to nonmissile head injury in humans: an analysis of 45 cases. Ann Neurol 12:557–563, 1982

Alexander MP: Mild traumatic brain injury: pathophysiology, natural history, and clinical management. Neurology 45:1253–1260, 1995

Alexopoulos GS, Silver JM, Kahn DA, et al: The Expert Consensus Guideline Series: Treatment of Agitation in Older Persons with Dementia. Postgrad Med (A Special Report). April 1998

Alves WM, Coloban ART, O'Leary TJ, et al: Understanding posttraumatic symptoms after minor head injury. J Head Trauma Rehabil 1:1–12, 1986

Alves W, Macciocchi SN, Barth JT: Postconcussive symptoms after uncomplicated mild head injury. J Head Trauma Rehabil 8:48–59, 1993

Amaducci LA, Fratiglioni L, Rocca WA, et al: Risk factors for clinically diagnosed Alzheimer's disease: a case control study of an Italian population. Neurology 36:922–931, 1986

American Psychiatric Association: Diagnostic and Statistical Manual of Mental Disorders, 3rd Edition. Washington, DC, American Psychiatric Association, 1980

American Psychiatric Association: Diagnostic and Statistical Manual of Mental Disorders, 3rd Edition, Revised. Washington, DC, American Psychiatric Association, 1987

American Psychiatric Association: Diagnostic and Statistical Manual of Mental Disorders, 4th Edition. Washington, DC, American Psychiatric Association, 1994

American Psychiatric Association: Diagnostic and Statistical Manual of Mental Disorders, 4th Edition, Text Revision. Washington, DC, American Psychiatric Association, 2000

Anderson KA, Silver JM: Neurological diseases and mental diseases, in Medical Management of the Violent Patient: Clinical Assessment and Therapy. Edited by Tardiff K. New York, Marcel Dekker, 1999, pp 87–124

Anderson CV, Wood DM, Bigler ED, et al: Lesion volume, injury severity, and thalamic integrity following head injury. J Neurotrauma 31(2):59–65, 1996

Annegers JF, Grabow JD, Groover RV, et al: Seizures after head trauma: a population study. Neurology 30:683–689, 1980

Arciniegas D, Adler L, Topkoff J, et al: Attention and memory dysfunction after traumatic brain injury: cholinergic mechanisms, sensory gating, and a hypothesis for further investigation. Brain Inj 13:1–13, 1999

Arciniegas D, Olincy A, Topkoff J, et al: Impaired auditory gating and P50 nonsuppression following traumatic brain injury. J Neuropsychiatry Clin Neurosci 12:77–85, 2000a

Arciniegas DB, Topkoff J, Silver JM: Neuropsychiatric aspects of traumatic brain injury. Curr Treat Options Neurol 2:169–186, 2000b

Arciniegas DB, Topkoff JL, Anderson CA, et al: Normalization of P50 physiology by donepezil hydrochloride in traumatic brain injury patients (abstract). J Neuropsychiatry Clin Neurosci 13:140, 2001

Armstrong KK, Sahgal V, Bloch R, et al: Rehabilitation outcomes in patients with posttraumatic epilepsy. Arch Phys Med Rehabil 71:156–160, 1990

Ashikaga R, Araki Y, Ishida O: MRI of head injury using FLAIR. Neuroradiology 39:239–242, 1997

Askenasy JJM, Winkler I, Grushkiewicz J, et al: The natural history of sleep disturbances in severe missile head injury. Journal of Neurologic Rehabilitation 3:93–96, 1989

Auerbach SH: Neuroanatomical correlates of attention and memory disorders in traumatic brain injury: an application of neurobehavioral subtypes. J Head Trauma Rehabil 1:1–12, 1986

Azouvi P, Jokic C, Attal N, et al: Carbamazepine in agitation and aggressive behaviour following severe closed head injury: results of an open trial. Brain Inj 13:797–804, 1999

Bakchine S, Lacomblez L, Benoit N, et al: Manic-like state after bilateral orbitofrontal and right temporoparietal injury: efficacy of clonidine. Neurology 39:777–781, 1989

Bamrah JS, Johnson J: Bipolar affective disorder following head injury. Br J Psychiatry 158:117–119, 1991

Bareggi SR, Porta M, Selenati A, et al: Homovanillic acid and 5-hydroxyindole-acetic acid in the CSF of patients after a severe head injury, I: lumbar CSF concentration in chronic brain post-traumatic syndromes. Eur Neurol 13:528–544, 1975

Barth JT, Macciocchi SN, Giordani B, et al: Neuropsychological sequelae of minor head injury. Neurosurgery 13:529–533, 1983

Bechara A, Damasio AR, Damasio H, et al: Insensitivity to future consequences following damage to human prefrontal cortex. Cognition 50:7–15, 1994

Beck AT, Ward CH, Mendelson M, et al: An inventory for measuring depression. Arch Gen Psychiatry 4:561–571, 1961

Becker DP, Verity MA, Povlishock J, et al: Brain cellular injury and recovery: horizons for improving medical therapies in stroke and trauma. West J Med 148:670–684, 1988

Bellus SB, Stewart D, Vergo JG, et al: The use of lithium in the treatment of aggressive behaviours with two brain-injured individuals in a state psychiatric hospital. Brain Inj 10:849–860, 1996

Ben-Yishay Y, Diller L: Cognitive remediation in traumatic brain injury: update and issues. Arch Phys Med Rehabil 74:204–213, 1993

Ben-Yishay Y, Lakin P: Structured group treatment for brain-injury survivors, in Neuropsychological Treatment After Brain Injury. Edited by Ellis DW, Christensen A-L. Boston, MA, Kluwer Academic, 1989, pp 271–295

Berg MJ, Ebert B, Willis DK, et al: Parkinsonism-drug treatment, I. Drug Intell Clin Pharm 21:10–21, 1987

Berman KF, Illowsky BP, Weinberger DR: Physiological dysfunction of dorsolateral prefrontal cortex in schizophrenia, IV: further evidence for regional and behavioral specificity. Arch Gen Psychiatry 45:616–622, 1988

Bernstein DM: Recovery from head injury. Brain Inj 13(3):151–172, 1999

Bessette RF, Peterson LG: Fluoxetine and organic mood syndrome. Psychosomatics 33:224–225, 1992

Bicik I, Radanov BP, Schafer N, et al: PET with 18-fluorodeoxyglucose and hexamethylpropylene amine oxime SPECT in late whiplash syndrome. Neurology 51:345–350, 1998

Bick PA, Hannah AL: Intramuscular lorazepam to restrain violent patients. Lancet 1:206–207, 1986

Bigler ED, Blatter DD, Anderson CV, et al: Hippocampal volume in normal aging and traumatic brain injury. AJNR Am J Neuroradiol 18(1):25–28, 1997

Binder LM, Rattok J: Assessment of the post-concussive syndrome after mild head trauma, in Assessment of the Behavioral Consequences of Head Trauma. Edited by Lezak MD. New York, Alan R Liss, 1989, pp 37–48

Birmaher B, Williams DT: Children and adolescents, in Neuropsychiatry of Traumatic Brain Injury. Edited by Silver JM, Yudofsky SC, Hales RE. Washington, DC, American Psychiatric Press, 1994, pp 393–412

Bleiberg J, Garmoe W, Cederquist J, et al: Effects of Dexedrine on performance consistency following brain injury: a double-blind placebo crossover case study. Neuropsychiatry Neuropsychol Behav Neurol 6:245–248, 1993

Blumbergs PC, Scott G, Manavis J, et al: Staining of amyloid precursor protein to study axonal damage in mild head injury. Lancet 344:1055–1056, 1994

Bogner J, Corrigan JD: Epidemiology of agitation following brain injury. Neurorehabilitation 5:293–297, 1995

Bohnen N, Twijnstra A, Jolles J: Post-traumatic and emotional symptoms in different subgroups of patients with mild head injury. Brain Inj 6:481–487, 1992

Bornstein RA, Miller HB, van Schoor T: Emotional adjustment in compensated head injury patients. Neurosurgery 23:622–627, 1988

Bracken P: Mania following head injury. Br J Psychiatry 150: 690–692, 1987

Brain Injury Special Interest Group of the American Academy of Physical Medicine and Rehabilitation: Practice parameter: antiepileptic drug treatment of posttraumatic seizures. Arch Phys Med Rehabil 79:594–597, 1998

Bremner JD, Scott TM, Delaney RC, et al: Deficits in short-term memory in posttraumatic stress disorder. Am J Psychiatry 150:1015–1019, 1993

Bremner JD, Randall P, Scott TM, et al: MRI-based measurement of hippocampal volume in patients with combat-related posttraumatic stress disorder. Am J Psychiatry 152:973–981, 1995

Bremner JD, Randall P, Vermetten E, et al: Magnetic resonance imaging–based measurement of hippocampal volume in posttraumatic stress disorder related to childhood physical and sexual abuse: a preliminary report. Biol Psychiatry 41:23–32, 1997

Breslau N, Kessler RC, Chilcoat HD, et al: Trauma and posttraumatic stress disorder in the community: the 1996 Detroit Area Survey of Trauma. Arch Gen Psychiatry 55: 626–632, 1998

Brooke MM, Patterson DR, Questad KA, et al: The treatment of agitation during initial hospitalization after traumatic brain injury. Arch Phys Med Rehabil 73:917–921, 1992a

Brooke MM, Questad KA, Patterson DR, et al: Agitation and restlessness after closed head injury: a prospective study of 100 consecutive admissions. Arch Phys Med Rehabil 73:320–323, 1992b

Brooks N, Campsie L, Symington C, et al: The five year outcome of severe blunt head injury: a relative's view. J Neurol Neurosurg Psychiatry 49:764–770, 1986

Brown G, Chadwick O, Shaffer D, et al: A prospective study of children with head injuries, III: psychiatric sequelae. Psychol Med 11:63–78, 1981

Brown KW, Sloan RL, Pentland B: Fluoxetine as a treatment for post-stroke emotionalism. Acta Psychiatr Scand 98:455–458, 1998

Brown SJ, Fann JR, Grant I: Postconcussional disorder: time to acknowledge a common source of neurobehavioral morbidity. J Neuropsychiatry Clin Neurosci 6:15–22, 1994

Bryant RA: Posttraumatic stress disorder, flashbacks, and pseudomemories in closed head injury. J Trauma Stress 9:621–629, 1996

Bryant RA, Marosszeky JE, Crooks J, et al: Posttraumatic stress disorder after severe traumatic brain injury. Am J Psychiatry 157:629–631, 2000

Buckley P, Stack JP, Madigan C, et al: Magnetic resonance imaging of schizophrenia-like psychoses associated with cerebral trauma: clinicopathological correlates. Am J Psychiatry 150:146–148, 1993

Burstein A: Bipolar and pure mania disorders precipitated by head trauma. Psychosomatics 34:194–195, 1993

Buysse DJ, Reynolds CF III: Insomnia, in Handbook of Sleep Disorders. Edited by Thorpy MJ. New York, Marcel Dekker, 1990, pp 373–434

Carlsson GS, Svardsudd K, Welin L: Long-term effects of head injuries sustained during life in three male populations. J Neurosurg 67:197–205, 1987

Cassidy JW: Fluoxetine: a new serotonergically active antidepressant. J Head Trauma Rehabil 4:67–69, 1989

Cassidy JW: Neuropathology, in Neuropsychiatry of Traumatic Brain Injury. Edited by Silver JM, Yudofsky SC, Hales RE. Washington, DC, American Psychiatric Press, 1994, pp 43–80

Catsman-Berrevoets CE, Harskamp FV: Compulsive pre-sleep behavior and apathy due to bilateral thalamic stroke: response to bromocriptine. Neurology 38:647–649, 1988

Chambers J, Cohen SS, Hemminger L, et al: Mild traumatic brain injuries in low-risk trauma patients. J Trauma 41:976–979, 1996

Chandler MC, Barnhill JL, Gualtieri CT: Amantadine for the agitated head-injury patient. Brain Inj 2:309–311, 1988

Chatham-Showalter PE: Carbamazepine for combativeness in acute traumatic brain injury. J Neuropsychiatry Clin Neurosci 8:96–99, 1996

Clark AF, Davison K: Mania following head injury: a report of two cases and a review of the literature. Br J Psychiatry 150:841–844, 1987

Clifton GL, Ziegler MG, Grossman RG: Circulating catecholamines and sympathetic activity after head injury. Neurosurgery 8:10–14, 1981

Collins MW, Grindel SH, Lovell MR, et al: Relationship between concussion and neuropsychological performance in college football players. JAMA 282:964–970, 1999

Committee on Head Injury Nomenclature: Report of the Ad Hoc Committee to study head injury nomenclature: proceedings of the Congress of Neurological Surgeons in 1964. Clin Neurosurg 12:386–394, 1966

Cope DN, Date ES, Mar EY: Serial computerized tomographic evaluations in traumatic head injury. Arch Phys Med Rehabil 69:483–486, 1988

Corbett JA, Trimble MR, Nichol TC: Behavioral and cognitive impairments in children with epilepsy: the long-term effects of anticonvulsant therapy. J Am Acad Child Psychiatry 24:17–23, 1985

Corkin S, Sullivan EV, Carr A: Prognostic factors for life expectancy after penetrating head injury. Arch Neurol 41:975–977, 1984

Corrigan JD: Substance abuse as a mediating factor in outcome from traumatic brain injury. Arch Phys Med Rehabil 76:302–309, 1995

Corrigan PW, Jakus MR: Behavioral treatment, in Neuropsychiatry of Traumatic Brain Injury. Edited by Silver JM, Yudofsky SC, Hales RE. Washington, DC, American Psychiatric Press, 1994, pp 733–769

Courville CB: Pathology of the Nervous System, 2nd Edition. Pacific Press Publications, 1945

Cowell LC, Cohen RF: Amantadine: a potential adjuvant therapy following traumatic brain injury. J Head Trauma Rehabil 10:91–94, 1995

Crisostomo EA, Duncan PW, Propst M, et al: Evidence that amphetamine with physical therapy promotes recovery of motor function in stroke patients. Ann Neurol 23:94–97, 1988

Davidson J: Seizures and bupropion: a review. J Clin Psychiatry 50:256–261, 1989

Davison K, Bagley CR: Schizophrenic-like psychoses associated with organic disorders of the central nervous system: a review of the literature, in Current Problems in Neuropsychiatry: Schizophrenia, Epilepsy, the Temporal Lobe. Edited by Herrington RN. Br J Psychiatry (special publication no 4), 1969, pp 113–184

DeAngelis MM, Hayes RL, Lyeth BG: Traumatic brain injury causes a decrease in M2 muscarinic cholinergic receptor binding in the rat brain. Brain Res 653:39–44, 1994

Deb S, Lyons I, Koutzoukis C, et al: Rate of psychiatric illness 1 year after traumatic brain injury. Am J Psychiatry 156: 374–378, 1999

DeKosky ST, Kochanek PM, Clark RS, et al: Secondary injury after head trauma: subacute and long-term mechanisms. Semin Clin Neuropsychiatry 3:176–185, 1998

Dikmen S, Machamer JE: Neurobehavioral outcomes and their determinants. J Head Trauma Rehabil 10:74–86, 1995

Dikmen S, McLean A, Temkin N: Neuropsychological and psychosocial consequences of minor head injury. J Neurol Neurosurg Psychiatry 49:1227–1232, 1986

Dikmen SS, Temkin NR, Miller B, et al: Neurobehavioral effects of phenytoin prophylaxis of posttraumatic seizures. JAMA 265:1271–1277, 1991

Dikmen SS, Machamer JE, Win HR, et al: Neuropsychological effects of valproate in traumatic brain injury: a randomized trial. Neurology 54:895–902, 2000

Dolan RJ, Bench CJ, Brown RG, et al: Regional cerebral blood flow abnormalities in depressed patients with cognitive impairment. J Neurol Neurosurg Psychiatry 55:768–773, 1992

Dreifuss FE, Santilli N, Langer DH, et al: Valproic acid hepatic fatalities: a retrospective review. Neurology 37:379–385, 1987

Drubach D, McAlaster R, Hartman P: The use of a psychoanalytic framework in the rehabilitation of patients with traumatic brain injury. Am J Psychoanal 54:255–263, 1994

Dunn-Meynell A, Pan S, Levin BE: Focal traumatic brain injury causes widespread reductions in rat brain norepinephrine turnover from 6 to 24 h. Brain Res 660:88–95, 1994

Eames P: The use of Sinemet and bromocriptine. Brain Inj 3:319–320, 1989

Eames P, Sutton A: Protracted post-traumatic confusional state treated with physostigmine. Brain Inj 9:729–734, 1995

Eames P, Wood R: Rehabilitation after severe brain injury: a follow-up study of a behavior modification approach. J Neurol Neurosurg Psychiatry 48:613–619, 1985

Echiverri HC, Tatum WO, Merens TA, et al: Akinetic mutism: pharmacologic probe of the dopaminergic mesencephalo-frontal activating system. Pediatr Neurol 4:228–230, 1988

Epstein RS, Ursano RJ: Anxiety disorders, in Neuropsychiatry of Traumatic Brain Injury. Edited by Silver JM, Yudofsky SC, Hales RE. Washington, DC, American Psychiatric Press, 1994, pp 285–312

Evans RW, Gualtieri CT, Patterson D: Treatment of chronic closed head injury with psychostimulant drugs: a controlled case study and an appropriate evaluation procedure. J Nerv Ment Dis 175:106–110, 1987

Faden AI, Demediuk P, Panter S, et al: The role of excitatory amino acids and NMDA receptors in traumatic brain injury. Science 244:798–800, 1989

Fann JR, Katon WJ, Uomoto JM, et al: Psychiatric disorders and functional disability in outpatients with traumatic brain injuries. Am J Psychiatry 152:1493–1499, 1995

Fann JR, Uomoto JM, Katon WJ: Sertraline in the treatment of major depression following mild traumatic brain injury. J Neuropsychiatry Clin Neurosci 12:226–232, 2000

Fann JR, Uomoto JM, Katon WJ: Cognitive improvement with treatment of depression following mild traumatic brain injury. Psychosomatics 42:48–54, 2001

Favale E, Rubino V, Mainaardi P, et al: Anticonvulsant effect of fluoxetine in humans. Neurology 45:1926–1927, 1995

Fay GC, Jaffe KM, Polissar NL, et al: Mild pediatric brain injury: a cohort study. Arch Phys Med Rehabil 74:895–901, 1993

Federoff PJ, Starkstein SE, Forrester AW, et al: Depression in patients with acute traumatic brain injury. Am J Psychiatry 149:918–923, 1992

Feeney DM, Gonzalez A, Law WA: Amphetamine, haloperidol, and experience interact to affect rate of recovery after motor cortex injury. Science 217:855–857, 1982

Fichtenberg NL, Millis SR, Mann NR, et al: Factors associated with insomnia among post-acute traumatic brain injury survivors. Brain Inj 14:659–667, 2000

First MB, Spitzer RL, Gibbon M, et al: Structured Clinical Interview for DSM-IV (SCID) User's Guide. Washington, DC, American Psychiatric Press, 1997

Fogel BS, Duffy J: Elderly patients, in Neuropsychiatry of Traumatic Brain Injury. Edited by Silver JM, Yudofsky SC, Hales RE. Washington, DC, American Psychiatric Press, 1994, pp 413–442

Freinhar JP, Alvarez WA: Clonazepam treatment of organic brain syndromes in three elderly patients. J Clin Psychiatry 47:525–526, 1986

Frieboes R-M, Muller U, Murck H, et al: Nocturnal hormone secretion and the sleep EEG in patients several months after traumatic brain injury. J Neuropsychiatry Clin Neurosci 11:354–360, 1999

Friedman G, Froom P, Sazbon ML, et al: Apolipoprotein E-epsilon4 genotype predicts a poor outcome in survivors of traumatic brain injury. Neurology 52:244–248, 1999

Gallassi R, Morreale A, Lorusso S, et al: Carbamazepine and phenytoin: comparison of cognitive effects in epileptic patients during monotherapy and withdrawal. Arch Neurol 45:892–894, 1988

Garyfallos G, Manos N, Adamopoulou A: Psychopathology and personality characteristics of epileptic patients: epilepsy, psychopathology and personality. Acta Psychiatr Scand 78:87–95, 1988

Gennarelli TA, Graham DI: Neuropathology of the head injuries. Semin Clin Neuropsychiatry 3:160–175, 1998

Gennarelli TA, Thibault LE, Adams JH, et al: Diffuse axonal injury and traumatic coma in the primate. Ann Neurol 12:564–574, 1982

Geracioti TD: Valproic acid treatment of episodic explosiveness related to brain injury. J Clin Psychiatry 55:416–417, 1994

Giakas WJ, Seibyl JP, Mazure CM: Valproate in the treatment of temper outbursts (letter). J Clin Psychiatry 51:525, 1990

Glenn MB, Wroblewski B, Parziale J, et al: Lithium carbonate for aggressive behavior or affective instability in ten brain-injured patients. Am J Phys Med Rehabil 68:221–226, 1989

Goldberg RJ, Goldberg JS: Low-dose risperidone for dementia related disturbed behavior in nursing home. Paper presented at the annual meeting of the American Psychiatric Association, Miami, FL, May 20–25, 1995

Goldstein FC, Levin HS: Neurobehavioral outcome of traumatic brain injury in older adults: initial findings. J Head Trauma Rehabil 10:57–73, 1995

Goodin DS, Aminoff MJ, Laxer KD: Detection of epileptiform activity by different noninvasive EEG methods in complex partial epilepsy. Ann Neurol 27:330–334, 1990

Gordon WA, Brown M, Sliwinski M, et al: The enigma of "hidden" traumatic brain injury. J Head Trauma Rehabil 13(6):1–18, 1998

Graves AB, White E, Koepsell TD, et al: The association between head trauma and Alzheimer's disease. Am J Epidemiol 131:491–501, 1990

Grigsby J, Kaye K: Incidence and correlates of depersonalization following head trauma. Brain Inj 7:507–513, 1993

Gross H, Kling A, Henry G, et al: Local cerebral glucose metabolism in patients with long-term behavioral and cognitive deficits following mild traumatic brain injury. J Neuropsychiatry Clin Neurosci 8:324–334, 1996

Gualtieri CT, Evans RW: Stimulant treatment for the neurobehavioural sequelae of traumatic brain injury. Brain Inj 2:273–290, 1988

Gualtieri T, Chandler M, Coons TB, et al: Amantadine: a new clinical profile for traumatic brain injury. Clin Neuropharmacol 12:258–270, 1989

Guilleminault C, Yuen KM, Gulevich MG, et al: Hypersomnia after head-neck trauma: a medicolegal dilemma. Neurology 54:653–659, 2000

Gulbrandsen GB: Neuropsychological sequelae of light head injuries in older children 6 months after trauma. J Clin Neuropsychol 6:257–268, 1984

Guo Z, Cupples LA, Kurz A, et al: Head injury and the risk of AD in the MIRAGE study. Neurology 54:1316–1323, 2000

Gupta SR, Mlcoch AG: Bromocriptine treatment of nonfluent aphasia. Arch Phys Med Rehabil 73:373–376, 1992

Hall KM, Karzmark P, Stevens M, et al: Family stressors in traumatic brain injury: a two-year follow-up. Arch Phys Med Rehabil 75:876–884, 1994

Hamill RW, Woolf PD, McDonald JV, et al: Catecholamines predict outcome in traumatic brain injury. Ann Neurol 21:438–443, 1987

Hamilton M: A rating scale for depression. J Neurol Neurosurg Psychiatry 23:56–62, 1960

Harvey AG, Bryant RA: Two-year prospective evaluation of the relationship between acute stress disorder and posttraumatic stress disorder following mild traumatic brain injury. Am J Psychiatry 15:626–628, 2000

Herrmann N, Lanctot K, Myszak M: Effectiveness of gabapentin for the treatment of behavioral disorders in dementia. J Clin Psychopharmacol 20:90–93, 2000

Hibbard MR, Uysal S, Kepler K, et al: Axis I psychopathology in individuals with traumatic brain injury. J Head Trauma Rehabil 13(4):24–39, 1998

Hibbard MR, Bogdany J, Uysal S, et al: Axis II psychopathology in individuals with traumatic brain injury. Brain Inj 14(1):45–61, 2000

Hicks RR, Smith DH, Lowenstein DH, et al: Mild experimental brain injury in the rat induces cognitive deficits associated with regional neuronal loss in the hippocampus. J Neurotrauma 10:405–414, 1993

Hoare P: The development of psychiatric disorder among schoolchildren with epilepsy. Dev Med Child Neurol 26:3–13, 1984

Honig LS, Albers GW: Neuropharmacological treatment for acute brain injury, in Neuropsychiatry of Traumatic Brain Injury. Edited by Silver JM, Yudofsky SC, Hales RE. Washington, DC, American Psychiatric Press, 1994, pp 771–804

Horne M, Lindley SE: Divalproex sodium in the treatment of aggressive behavior and dysphoria in patients with organic brain syndromes. J Clin Psychiatry 56:430–431, 1995

Hornstein A, Seliger G: Cognitive side effects of lithium in closed head injury (letter). J Neuropsychiatry Clin Neurosci 1:446–447, 1989

Hugenholtz H, Stuss DT, Stethem LL, et al: How long does it take to recover from a mild concussion? Neurosurgery 22:853–858, 1988

Jackson RD, Corrigan JD, Arnett JA: Amitriptyline for agitation in head injury. Arch Phys Med Rehabil 66:180–181, 1985

Jacobs A, Put E, Ingels M, et al: Prospective evaluation of technetium-99m-HMPAO SPECT in mild and moderate traumatic brain injury. J Nucl Med 35:942–947, 1994

Jane JA, Steward O, Gennarelli T: Axonal degeneration induced by experimental noninvasive minor injury. J Neurosurg 62:96–100, 1985

Jordan BD, Relkin NR, Ravdin LD, et al: Apolipoprotein E epsilon4 associated with chronic traumatic brain injury in boxing. JAMA 278:136–140, 1997

Jorge RE, Robinson RG, Starkstein SE, et al: Depression and anxiety following traumatic brain injury. J Neuropsychiatry Clin Neurosci 5:369–374, 1993

Jorge RE, Robinson RG, Starkstein SE, et al: Influence of major depression on 1-year outcome in patients with traumatic brain injury. J Neurosurg 81:726–733, 1994

Kaelin DL, Cifu DX, Matthies B: Methylphenidate effect on attention deficit in the acutely brain-injured adult. Arch Phys Med Rehabil 77:6–9, 1996

Kant R, Smith-Seemiller L, Zeiler D: Treatment of aggression and irritability after head injury. Brain Inj 12:661–666, 1998

Kass F, Silver JM: Neuropsychiatry and the homeless. J Neuropsychiatry Clin Neurosci 2:15–19, 1990

Katz DI, Alexander MP: Traumatic brain injury: predicting course of recovery and outcome for patients admitted to rehabilitation. Arch Neurol 51:661–670, 1994

Katzman R, Galasko DR, Saitoh T, et al: Apolipoprotein-epsilon4 and head trauma: synergistic or additive risks? Neurology 46:889–891, 1996

Kay SR, Fiszbein A, Opler LA: The Positive and Negative Syndrome Scale (PANSS) for schizophrenia. Schizophr Bull 13:261–276, 1987

Kay T: Neuropsychological treatment of mild traumatic brain injury. J Head Trauma Rehabil 8:74–85, 1993

Kay T, Cavallo MM: The family system: impact, assessment, and intervention, in Neuropsychiatry of Traumatic Brain Injury. Edited by Silver JM, Yudofsky SC, Hales RE. Washington, DC, American Psychiatric Press, 1994, pp 533–568

Keats MM, Mukherjee S: Antiaggressive effect of adjunctive clonazepam in schizophrenia associated with seizure disorder. J Clin Psychiatry 49:117–118, 1988

Kelly JP: Concussion, in Current Therapy in Sports Medicine, 3rd Edition. Edited by Torg JS, Shephard RJ. Philadelphia, PA, CV Mosby, 1995, pp 21–24

Keshavan MS, Channabasavanna SM, Narahana Reddy GN: Post-traumatic psychiatric disturbances: patterns and predictors of outcome. Br J Psychiatry 138:157–160, 1981

Koren D, Arnon I, Klein E: Acute stress response and posttraumatic stress disorder in traffic victims: a one-year prospective, follow-up study. Am J Psychiatry 156:367–373, 1999

Kraus JF, Sorenson SB: Epidemiology, in Neuropsychiatry of Traumatic Brain Injury. Edited by Silver JM, Yudofsky SC, Hales RE. Washington, DC, American Psychiatric Press, 1994, pp 3–41

Kraus JF, Morgenstern H, Fife D, et al: Blood alcohol tests, prevalence of involvement, and outcomes following brain injury. Am J Public Health 79:294–299, 1989

Kraus MF, Maki PM: Effect of amantadine hydrochloride on symptoms of frontal lobe dysfunction in brain injury: case studies and review. J Neuropsychiatry Clin Neurosci 9:222–230, 1997

Kreutzer JS, Gervasio AH, Camplair PS: Primary caregivers' psychological status and family functioning after traumatic brain injury. Brain Inj 8:197–210, 1994

Kurtzke JF: Neuroepidemiology. Ann Neurol 16:265–277, 1984

Kuruoglu AC, Arikan Z, Vural G, et al: Single photon emission computerized tomography in chronic alcoholism: antisocial personality disorder may be associated with decreased frontal perfusion. Br J Psychiatry 169:348–354, 1996

Lal S, Merbitz CP, Grip JC: Modification of function in head-injured patients with Sinemet. Brain Inj 2:225–233, 1988

Langfitt TW, Obrist WD, Alavi A, et al: Regional structure and function in head-injured patients: correlation of CT, MRI, PET, CBF, and neuropsychological assessment, in Neurobehavioral Recovery From Head Injury. Edited by Levin HS, Grafman J, Eisenberg HM. New York, Oxford University Press, 1987, pp 30–42

Lauterbach EC, Schweri MM: Amelioration of pseudobulbar affect by fluoxetine: possible alteration of dopamine-related pathophysiology by a selective serotonin reuptake inhibitor. J Clin Psychopharmacol 11:392–393, 1991

Lazarus A, Cotterell KP: SPECT scan reveals abnormality in somatization disorder patient. J Clin Psychiatry 50:475–476, 1989

Leach LR, Frank RG, Bouman DE, et al: Family functioning, social support and depression after traumatic brain injury. Brain Inj 8:599–606, 1994

Leininger BE, Gramling SE, Farrell AD, et al: Neuropsychological deficits in symptomatic minor head injury patients after concussion and mild concussion. J Neurol Neurosurg Psychiatry 53:293–296, 1990

Levin HS, O'Donnell VM, Grossman RG: The Galveston Orientation and Amnesia Test: a practical scale to assess cognition after head injury. J Nerv Ment Dis 167:675–684, 1979

Levin HS, Benton AL, Grossman RG: Neurobehavioral Consequences of Closed Head Injury. New York, Oxford University Press, 1982

Levin HS, High WM, Meyers CA, et al: Impairment of remote memory after closed head injury. J Neurol Neurosurg Psychiatry 48:556–563, 1985

Levin HS, Amparo E, Eisenberg HM, et al: Magnetic resonance imaging and computerized tomography in relation to the neurobehavioral sequelae of mild and moderate head injuries. J Neurosurg 66:706–713, 1987a

Levin HS, Mattis S, Ruff RM, et al: Neurobehavioral outcome following minor head injury: a three-center study. J Neurosurg 66:234–243, 1987b

Levin HS, Goldstein FC, High WM Jr, et al: Disproportionately severe memory deficit in relation to normal intellectual functioning after closed head injury. J Neurol Neurosurg Psychiatry 51:1294–1301, 1988

Lieberman JA, Kane JM, Johns CA: Clozapine: guidelines for clinical management. J Clin Psychiatry 50:329–338, 1989

Linn RT, Allen K, Willer BS: Affective symptoms in the chronic stage of traumatic brain injury: a study of married couples. Brain Inj 8:135–147, 1994

Lipper S, Tuchman MM: Treatment of chronic post-traumatic organic brain syndrome with dextroamphetamine: first reported case. J Nerv Ment Dis 162:266–371, 1976

Lishman WA: Organic Psychiatry: The Psychological Consequences of Cerebral Disorder, 2nd Edition. Boston, MA, Blackwell Scientific, 1987

Lishman WA: Physiogenesis and psychogenesis in the "post-concussional syndrome." Br J Psychiatry 153:460–469, 1988

Livingston MG, Brooks DN, Bond MR: Patient outcome in the year following severe head injury and relatives' psychiatric and social functioning. J Neurol Neurosurg Psychiatry 48:876–881, 1985a

Livingston MG, Brooks DN, Bond MR: Three months after severe head injury: psychiatric and social impact on relatives. J Neurol Neurosurg Psychiatry 48:870–875, 1985b

Livingston S, Pauli LL: Dextroamphetamine for epilepsy. JAMA 233:278–279, 1975

Lowenstein DH, Thomas MJ, Smith DH, et al: Selective vulnerability of dentate hilar neurons following traumatic brain injury: a potential mechanistic link between head trauma and disorders of the hippocampus. J Neurosci 12:4846–4853, 1992

Lyeth BG, Jiang JY, Delahunty TM, et al: Muscarinic cholinergic receptor binding in rat brain following traumatic brain injury. Brain Res 640:240–245, 1994

Mahoney WJ, D'Souza BJ, Haller JA, et al: Long-term outcome of children with severe head trauma and prolonged coma. Pediatrics 71:754–762, 1983

Mann JJ, Waternaux C, Haas GL, et al: Toward a clinical model of suicidal behavior in psychiatric patients. Am J Psychiatry 156:181–189, 1999

Martin R, Kuzniecky R, Ho S, et al: Cognitive effects of topiramate, gabapentin, and lamotrigine in healthy young adults. Neurology 52:321–327, 1999

Masdeu JC, Van Heertum RL, Kleiman A, et al: Early single-photon emission computed tomography in mild head trauma: a controlled study. J Neuroimaging 4:177–181, 1994

Massey EW, Folger WN: Seizures activated by therapeutic levels of lithium carbonate. South Med J 77:1173–1175, 1984

Matser EJT, Kessels AG, Lezak MD, et al: Neuropsychological impairment in amateur soccer players. JAMA 282:971–973, 1999

Mattes JA: Valproic acid for nonaffective aggression in the mentally retarded. J Nerv Ment Dis 180:601–602, 1992

Max JE, Castillo CS, Robin DA, et al: Posttraumatic stress symptomatology after childhood traumatic brain injury. J Nerv Ment Dis 186:589–596, 1998a

Max JE, Robin DA, Lindgren SD, et al: Traumatic brain injury in children and adolescents: psychiatric disorders at one year. J Neuropsychiatry Clin Neurosci 10:290–297, 1998b

Mayeux R, Ottman R, Tang MX, et al: Genetic susceptibility and head injury as risk factors for Alzheimer's disease among community-dwelling elderly persons and their first-degree relatives. Ann Neurol 33:494–501, 1993

Mayeux R, Ottman R, Maestre G, et al: Synergistic effects of traumatic head injury and apolipoprotein-epsilon 4 in patients with Alzheimer's disease. Neurology 45:555–557, 1995

McAllister TW: Mild traumatic brain injury and the postconcussive syndrome, in Neuropsychiatry of Traumatic Brain Injury. Edited by Silver JM, Yudofsky SC, Hales RE. Washington, DC, American Psychiatric Press, 1994, pp 357–392

McAllister TW: Traumatic brain injury and psychosis: what is the connection? Semin Clin Neuropsychiatry 3:211–223, 1998

McKenna PJ, Kane JM, Parrish K: Psychotic syndromes in epilepsy. Am J Psychiatry 142:895–904, 1985

McKinlay WW, Brooks DN, Bond MR, et al: The short-term outcome of severe blunt head injury as reported by the relatives of the injured person. J Neurol Neurosurg Psychiatry 44:527–533, 1981

McMillan TM: Post-traumatic stress disorder following minor and severe closed head injury: 10 single cases. Brain Inj 10:749–758, 1996

McMillan TM, Glucksman EE: The neuropsychology of moderate head injury. J Neurol Neurosurg Psychiatry 50:393–397, 1987

Michals ML, Crismon ML, Roberts S, et al: Clozapine response and adverse effects in nine brain-injured patients. J Clin Psychopharmacol 13:198–203, 1993

Michaud LJ, Rivara FP, Jaffe KM, et al: Traumatic brain injury as a risk factor for behavioral disorders in children. Arch Phys Med Rehabil 74:368–375, 1993

Mild Traumatic Brain Injury Committee of the Head Injury Interdisciplinary Special Interest Group of the American Congress of Rehabilitation Medicine: Definition of mild traumatic brain injury. J Head Trauma Rehabil 8:86–87, 1993

Mittl RL, Grossman RI, Hiehle JF, et al: Prevalence of MR evidence of diffuse axonal injury in patients with mild head injury and normal head CT findings. AJNR Am J Neuroradiol 15:1583–1589, 1994

Mooney GF, Haas LJ: Effect of methylphenidate on brain injury–related anger. Arch Phys Med Rehabil 74:153–160, 1993

Morrison JH, Molliver ME, Grzanna R: Noradrenergic innervation of cerebral cortex: widespread effects of local cortical lesions. Science 205:313–316, 1979

Moskowitz AS, Altshuler L: Increased sensitivity to lithium-induced neurotoxicity after stroke: a case report. J Clin Psychopharmacol 11:272–273, 1991

Mysiw WJ, Jackson RD, Corrigan JD: Amitriptyline for post-traumatic agitation. Am J Phys Med Rehabil 67(1):29–33, 1988

Nagamachi S, Nichikawa T, Ono S, et al: A comparative study of 123I-IMP SPET and CT in the investigation of chronic-stage head trauma patients. Nucl Med Commun 16:17–25, 1995

Nahas Z, Arlinghaus KA, Kotrla KJ, et al: Rapid response of emotional incontinence to selective serotonin reuptake inhibitors. J Neuropsychiatry Clin Neurosci 10:453–455, 1998

Nasrallah HA, Fowler RC, Judd LL: Schizophrenia-like illness following head injury. Psychosomatics 22:359–361, 1981

Nedd K, Sfakianakis G, Ganz W, et al: 99mTc-HMPAO SPECT of the brain in mild to moderate traumatic brain injury patients: compared with CT—a prospective study. Brain Inj 7:469–479, 1993

Nemetz PN, Leibson C, Naessens JM, et al: Traumatic brain injury and time to onset of Alzheimer's disease: a population-based study. Am J Epidemiol 149:32–40, 1999

Nickels JL, Schneider WN, Dombovy ML, et al: Clinical use of amantadine in brain injury rehabilitation. Brain Inj 8: 709–718, 1994

NIH Consensus Development Panel on Rehabilitation of Persons With Traumatic Brain Injury: Rehabilitation of persons with traumatic brain injury. JAMA 282:974–983, 1999

Nizamie SH, Nizamie A, Borde M, et al: Mania following head injury: case reports and neuropsychological findings. Acta Psychiatr Scand 77:637–639, 1988

Nuwer MR: Assessment of digital EEG, quantitative EEG and EEG brain mapping: report of the American Academy of Neurology and the American Clinical Neurophysiology Society. Neurology 49: 277–292, 1997

Oddy M, Humphrey M, Uttley D: Stresses upon the relatives of head-injured patients. Br J Psychiatry 133:507–513, 1978

Ohry A, Rattok J, Solomon Z: Post-traumatic stress disorder in brain injury patients. Brain Inj 10:687–695, 1996

Ojemann LM, Baugh-Bookman C, Dudley DL: Effect of psychotropic medications on seizure control in patients with epilepsy. Neurology 37:1525–1527, 1987

Oliver AP, Luchins DJ, Wyatt RJ: Neuroleptic-induced seizures: an in vitro technique for assessing relative risk. Arch Gen Psychiatry 39:206–209, 1982

Oppenheimer DR: Microscopic lesions in the brain following head injury. J Neurol Neurosurg Psychiatry 31:299–306, 1968

Orrison WW, Gentry LR, Stimac GK, et al: Blinded comparison of cranial CT and MR in closed head injury evaluation. AJNR Am J Neuroradiol 15:351–356, 1994

O'Shanick GJ, O'Shanick AM: Personality and intellectual changes, in Neuropsychiatry of Traumatic Brain Injury. Edited by Silver JM, Yudofsky SC, Hales RE. Washington, DC, American Psychiatric Press, 1994, pp 163–188

Panzer MJ, Mellow AM: Antidepressant treatment of pathologic laughing or crying in elderly stroke patients. J Geriatr Psychiatry Neurol 4:195–199, 1992

Parker RS, Rosenblum A: IQ loss and emotional dysfunctions after mild head injury in a motor vehicle accident. J Clin Psychol 52:32–43, 1996

Parks RW, Crockett DJ, Manji HK, et al: Assessment of bromocriptine intervention for the treatment of frontal lobe syndrome: a case study. J Neuropsychiatry Clin Neurosci 4:109–110, 1992

Pinder RM, Brogden RN, Speight TM, et al: Maprotiline: a review of its pharmacological properties and therapeutic efficacy in mental states. Drugs 13:321–352, 1977

Plenger PM, Dixon CE, Castillo RM, et al: Subacute methylphenidate treatment for moderate to moderately severe traumatic brain injury: a preliminary double-blind placebo-controlled study. Arch Phys Med Rehabil 77:536–540, 1996

Pollack IW: Traumatic brain injury and the rehabilitation process: a psychiatric perspective, in Neuropsychological Treatment After Brain Injury. Edited by Ellis D, Christensen A-L. Boston, MA, Kluwer Academic, 1989, pp 105–127

Pollack IW: Individual psychotherapy, in Neuropsychiatry of Traumatic Brain Injury. Edited by Silver JM, Yudofsky SC, Hales RE. Washington, DC, American Psychiatric Press, 1994, pp 671–702

Ponsford J, Kinsella G: Attention deficits following closed head injury. J Clin Exp Neuropsychol 14:822–838, 1992

Pope HG Jr, McElroy SL, Satlin A, et al: Head injury, bipolar disorder, and response to valproate. Compr Psychiatry 29:34–38, 1988

Porta M, Bareggi SR, Collice M, et al: Homovanillic acid and 5-hydroxyindole-acetic acid in the CSF of patients after a severe head injury, II: ventricular CSF concentrations in acute brain post-traumatic syndromes. Eur Neurol 13: 545–554, 1975

Povlishock JT, Coburn TH: Morphopathological change associated with mild head injury, in Mild Head Injury. Edited by Levin HS, Eisenberg HM, Benton AL. New York, Oxford University Press, 1989, pp 37–53

Povlishock JT, Becker DP, Cheng CLY, et al: Axonal change in minor head injury. J Neuropathol Exp Neurol 42:225–242, 1983

Powell JW, Barber-Foss KD: Traumatic brain injury in high school athletes. JAMA 282: 958–963, 1999

Prevey ML, Delany RC, Cramer JA, et al: Effect of valproate on cognitive functioning: comparison with carbamazepine. Arch Neurol 53:1008–1016, 1996

Prigatano GP: Work, love, and play after brain injury. Bull Menninger Clin 53:414–431, 1989

Prigatano GP, Stahl ML, Orr WC, et al: Sleep and dreaming disturbances in closed head injury patients. J Neurol Neurosurg Psychiatry 45:78–80, 1982

Quality Standards Subcommittee, American Academy of Neurology: Practice parameter. Neurobiology (Bp) 48:1–5, 1997

Rakier A, Guilburd JN, Sousteil JF, et al: Head injuries in the elderly. Brain Inj 9:187–193, 1995

Rammahan KW, Rosenberg JH, Pollak CP, et al: Modafinil: efficacy for the treatment of fatigue in patients with multiple sclerosis (abstract). Neurology 54 (suppl 3):A24, 2000

Ranen NG, Lipsey JR, Treisman G, et al: Sertraline in the treatment of severe aggressiveness in Huntington's disease. J Neuropsychiatry Clin Neurosci 8:338–340, 1996

Raphaely RC, Swedlow DB, Downes JJ, et al: Management of severe pediatric head trauma. Pediatr Clin North Am 27:715–727, 1980

Ratey JJ, Leveroni C, Kilmer D, et al: The effects of clozapine on severely aggressive psychiatric inpatients in a state hospital. J Clin Psychiatry 54:219–223, 1993

Rattok J: Do patients with mild brain injuries have posttraumatic stress disorder, too? J Head Trauma Rehabil 11:95–97, 1996

Rattok J, Ross BP: Cognitive rehabilitation, in Neuropsychiatry of Traumatic Brain Injury. Edited by Silver JM, Yudofsky SC, Hales RE. Washington, DC, American Psychiatric Press, 1994, pp 703–732

Rauch SL, van Der Kolk BA, Fisler RE, et al: A symptom provocation study of posttraumatic stress disorder using positron emission tomography and script-driven imagery. Arch Gen Psychiatry 53:380–387, 1996

Reeves TM, Lyeth BG, Povlishock JT: Long-term potentiation deficits and excitability changes following traumatic brain injury. Exp Brain Res 106:248–256, 1995

Reinhard DL, Whyte J, Sandel ME: Improved arousal and initiation following tricyclic antidepressant use in severe brain injury. Arch Phys Med Rehabil 77:80–83, 1996

Reynolds EH, Trimble MR: Adverse neuropsychiatric effects of anticonvulsant drugs. Drugs 29:570–581, 1985

Rimel RW, Giordani B, Barht JT, et al: Disability caused by minor head injury. Neurosurgery 9:221–228, 1981

Rivinus TM: Psychiatric effects of the anticonvulsant regimens. J Clin Psychopharmacol 2:165–192, 1992

Roane DM, Feinberg TE, Meckler L, et al: Treatment of dementia-associated agitation with gabapentin. J Neuropsychiatry Clin Neurosci 12:40–43, 2000

Roberts GW, Gentleman SM, Lynch A, et al: Beta amyloid protein depositions in the brain after severe head injury: implications for the pathogenesis of Alzheimer's disease. J Neurol Neurosurg Psychiatry 57:419–423, 1994

Robinson RG, Schultz SK, Castillo C, et al: Nortriptyline versus fluoxetine in the treatment of depression and in short-term recovery after stroke: a placebo-controlled, double-blind study. Am J Psychiatry 157:351–359, 2000

Rosenthal M, Christensen BK, Ross TP: Depression following traumatic brain injury. Arch Phys Med Rehabil 79:90–103, 1998

Ross ED, Rush AJ: Diagnosis and neuroanatomical correlates of depression in brain-damaged patients: implications for a neurology of depression. Arch Gen Psychiatry 38:1344–1354, 1981

Rothman KJ, Funch DP, Dreyr NA: Bromocriptine and puerperal seizures. Epidemiology 1:232–238, 1990

Ruff RM, Buchsbaum MS, Troster AI, et al: Computerized tomography, neuropsychology, and positron emission tomography in the evaluation of head injury. Neuropsychiatry Neuropsychol Behav Neurol 2:103–123, 1989

Salazar AM, Jabbari B, Vance SC, et al: Epilepsy after penetrating head injury, I: clinical correlates: a report of the Vietnam head injury study. Neurology 35:1406–1414, 1985

Salazar AM, Warden DL, Schwab K, et al: Cognitive rehabilitation for traumatic brain injury: a randomized trial. Defense and Veterans Head Injury Program (DVHIP) Study Group. JAMA 283:3075–3081, 2000

Sandel ME, Weiss B, Ivker B: Multiple personality disorder: diagnosis after a traumatic brain injury. Arch Phys Med Rehabil 71:523–535, 1990

Saran AS: Depression after minor closed head injury: role of dexamethasone suppression test and antidepressants. J Clin Psychiatry 46:335–338, 1985

Sbordone RJ, Liter JC: Mild traumatic brain injury does not produce post-traumatic stress disorder. Brain Inj 9:405–412, 1995

Schiff HB, Sabin TD, Geller A, et al: Lithium in aggressive behavior. Am J Psychiatry 139:1346–1348, 1982

Schiffer RB, Herndon RM, Rudick RA: Treatment of pathologic laughing and weeping with amitriptyline. N Engl J Med 312:1480–1482, 1985

Seliger GM, Hornstein A, Flax J, et al: Fluoxetine improves emotional incontinence. Brain Inj 6:267–270, 1992

Sherer M, Boake C, Levin E, et al: Characteristics of impaired awareness after traumatic brain injury. J Int Neuropsychol Soc 4:380–387, 1998

Sheriff FE, Bridges LR, Sivaloganaathan S: Early detection of axonal injury after human head trauma using immunocytochemistry for beta-amyloid precursor protein. Acta Neuropathol (Berl) 87:55–62, 1994

Silver JM, McAllister TW: Forensic issues in the neuropsychiatric evaluation of the patient with mild traumatic brain injury. J Neuropsychiatry Clin Neurosci 9:102–113, 1997

Silver JM, Yudofsky SC: Aggressive disorders, in Neuropsychiatry of Traumatic Brain Injury. Edited by Silver JM, Yudofsky SC, Hales RE. Washington, DC, American Psychiatric Press, 1994a, pp 313–356

Silver JM, Yudofsky SC: Psychopharmacology, in Neuropsychiatry of Traumatic Brain Injury. Edited by Silver JM, Yudofsky SC, Hales RE. Washington, DC, American Psychiatric Press, 1994b, pp 631–670

Silver JM, Caton CM, Shrout PE, et al: Traumatic brain injury and schizophrenia. Paper presented at the annual meeting of the American Psychiatric Association, San Francisco, CA, May 22–27, 1993

Silver JM, Rattok J, Anderson K: Posttraumatic stress disorder and traumatic brain injury. Neurocase 3:151–157, 1997

Silver JM, Kramer R, Greenwald S, et al: The association between head injuries and psychiatric disorders: findings from the New Haven NIMH Epidemiologic Catchment Areas Study. Brain Inj 15:935–945, 2001

Sloan RL, Brown KW, Pentland B: Fluoxetine as a treatment for emotional lability after brain injury. Brain Inj 6:315–319, 1992

Smeltzer DJ, Nasrallah HA, Miller SC: Psychotic disorders, in Neuropsychiatry of Traumatic Brain Injury. Edited by Silver JM, Yudofsky SC, Hales RE. Washington, DC, American Psychiatric Press, 1994, pp 251–284

Smith DH, Okiyama K, Thomas MJ, et al: Evaluation of memory dysfunction following experimental brain injury using the Morris water maze. J Neurotrauma 8:259–269, 1991

Smith KR, Goulding PM, Wilderman D, et al: Neurobehavioral effects of phenytoin and carbamazepine in patients recovering from brain trauma: a comparative study. Arch Neurol 51:653–660, 1994

Smith MC, Bleck TP: Convulsive disorders: toxicity of anticonvulsants. Clin Neuropharmacol 14:97–115, 1991

Smith-Seemiller L, Lovell MR, Smith SS: Cognitive dysfunction after closed head injury: contributions of demographics, injury severity and other factors. Appl Neuropsychol 3:41–47, 1996

Sosin DM, Sacks JJ, Smith SM: Head injury-associated deaths in the United States from 1979–1986. JAMA 262:2251–2255, 1989

Speech TJ, Rao SM, Osmon DC, et al: A double-blind controlled study of methylphenidate treatment in closed head injury. Brain Inj 7:333–338, 1993

Starkstein SE, Boston JD, Robinson RG: Mechanisms of mania after brain injury: 12 case reports and review of the literature. J Nerv Ment Dis 176:87–100, 1988

Starkstein SE, Mayberg HS, Berthier ML, et al: Mania after brain injury: neuroradiological and metabolic findings. Ann Neurol 27:652–659, 1990

Stewart JT, Nemsath RH: Bipolar illness following traumatic brain injury: treatment with lithium and carbamazepine. J Clin Psychiatry 49:74–75, 1988

Stuss DT, Ely P, Hugenholtz H, et al: Subtle neuropsychological deficits in patients with good recovery after closed head injury. Neurosurgery 17:41–47, 1985

Stuss DT, Binns MA, Carruth FG, et al: The acute period of recovery from traumatic brain injury: posttraumatic amnesia or posttraumatic confusional state? J Neurosurg 90:635–643, 1999

Tate R, Simpson G, Flanagan S, et al: Completed suicide after traumatic brain injury. J Head Trauma Rehabil 12(6):16–20, 1997

Taverni JP, Seliger G, Lichtman SW: Donepezil mediated memory improvement in traumatic brain injury during post acute rehabilitation. Brain Inj 12:77–80, 1998

Teasdale G, Jennett B: Assessment of coma and impaired consciousness: a practical scale. Lancet 2:81–84, 1974

Teasdale GM, Nicoll JAR, Murray G, et al: Association of apolipoprotein E polymorphism with outcome after head injury. Lancet 350:1069–1071, 1997

Temkin NR, Dikmen SS, Wilensky AJ, et al: A randomized, double-blind study of phenytoin for the prevention of post-traumatic seizures. N Engl J Med 323:497–502, 1990

Temkin NR, Dikmen SS, Anderson GD, et al: Valproate therapy for prevention of post-traumatic seizures: a randomized trial. J Neurosurg 91:593–600, 1999

Terzoudi M, Gavrielidou P, Heilakos G, et al: Fatigue in multiple sclerosis: evaluation of a new pharmacological approach (abstract). Neurology 54 (suppl 3):A61–A62, 2000

Thatcher RW, Moore N, John ER, et al: QEEG and traumatic brain injury: rebuttal of the American Academy of Neurology 1997 Report by the EEG and Clinical Neuroscience Society. Clin Electroencephalogr 30:94–98, 1999

Therapeutics and Technology Assessment Subcommittee of the American Academy of Neurology: Assessment of brain SPECT. Neurology 46:278–285, 1996

Thomsen IV: Late outcome of very severe blunt head trauma: a 10–15 year second follow-up. J Neurol Neurosurg Psychiatry 47:260–268, 1984

Toulmond S, Duval D, Serrano A, et al: Biochemical and histological alterations induced by fluid percussion brain injury in the rat. Brain Res 620:24–31, 1993

Trzepacz P: Delirium, in Neuropsychiatry of Traumatic Brain Injury. Edited by Silver JM, Yudofsky SC, Hales RE. Washington, DC, American Psychiatric Press, 1994, pp 189–218

Tyerman A, Humphrey M: Changes in self-concept following severe head injury. Int J Rehabil Res 7:11–23, 1984

Ursano RJ, Fullerton CS, Epstein RS, et al: Acute and chronic posttraumatic stress disorder in motor vehicle accident victims. Am J Psychiatry 156:589–595, 1999a

Ursano RJ, Fullerton CS, Epstein RS, et al: Peritraumatic dissociation and posttraumatic stress disorder following motor vehicle accidents. Am J Psychiatry 156:1808–1810, 1999b

U.S. Department of Health and Human Services: Interagency Head Injury Task Force Report. Washington, DC, U.S. Department of Health and Human Services, 1989

Van Duijn CM, Tanja TA, Haaxma R, et al: Head trauma and the risk of Alzheimer's disease. Am J Epidemiol 135:775–782, 1992

van Reekum R, Bolago I, Finlayson MA, et al: Psychiatric disorders after traumatic brain injury. Brain Inj 10:319–327, 1996

van Reekum R, Cohen T, Wong J: Can traumatic brain injury cause psychiatric disorders? J Neuropsychiatry Clin Neurosci 12:316–327, 2000

Van Woerkom TCAM, Teelken AW, Minderhoud JM: Difference in neurotransmitter metabolism in frontotemporal-lobe contusion and diffuse cerebral contusion. Lancet 1:812–813, 1977

Varney NR: Prognostic significance of anosmia in patients with closed-head trauma. J Clin Exp Neuropsychol 10:250–254, 1988

Varney NR, Martzke JS, Roberts RJ: Major depression in patients with closed head injury. Neuropsychology 1:7–9, 1987

Vecht CJ, Van Woerkom TCAM, Teelken AW, et al: Homovanillic acid and 5-hydroxyindoleacetic acid cerebrospinal fluid levels. Arch Neurol 32:792–797, 1975

Violon A, De Mol J: Psychological sequelae after head trauma in adults. Acta Neurochir (Wien) 85:96–102, 1987

Wade DT, King NS, Crawford S, et al: Routine follow up after head injury: a second randomised clinical trial. J Neurol Neurosurg Psychiatry 65(2):177–183, 1998

Warden DL, Labbate LA, Salazar AM, et al: PTSD symptoms in moderate traumatic brain injury. Paper presented at the annual meeting of the American Psychiatric Association, Miami Beach, FL, May 20–25, 1995

Watson MR, Fenton GW, McClelland RJ, et al: The post-concussional state: neurophysiological aspects. Br J Psychiatry 167:514–521, 1995

Weinberg RM, Auerbach SH, Moore S: Pharmacologic treatment of cognitive deficits: a case study. Brain Inj 1:57–59, 1987

Weinstein GS, Wells CE: Case studies in neuropsychiatry: post-traumatic psychiatric dysfunction—diagnosis and treatment. J Clin Psychiatry 42:120–122, 1981

Weller M, Kornhuber J: A rationale for NMDA receptor antagonist therapy of the neuroleptic malignant syndrome. Med Hypotheses 38:329–333, 1992

Whyte J: Neurologic disorders of attention and arousal: assessment and treatment. Arch Phys Med Rehabil 73:1094–1103, 1992

Whyte J, Hart T, Schuster K, et al: Effects of methylphenidate on attentional function after traumatic brain injury: a randomized placebo-controlled trial. Am J Phys Med Rehabil 76:440–450, 1997

Wilberger JE, Deeb A, Rothfus W: Magnetic resonance imaging in cases of severe head injury. Neurosurgery 20:571–576, 1987

Wilcox JA, Nasrallah HA: Childhood head trauma and psychosis. Psychiatry Res 21:303–306, 1987

Wolf B, Grohmann R, Schmidt LG, et al: Psychiatric admissions due to adverse drug reactions. Compr Psychiatry 30:534–545, 1989

Wroblewski BA, McColgan K, Smith K, et al: The incidence of seizures during tricyclic antidepressant drug treatment in a brain-injured population. J Clin Psychopharmacol 10:124–128, 1990

Wroblewski BA, Leary JM, Phelan AM, et al: Methylphenidate and seizure frequency in brain-injured patients with seizure disorders. J Clin Psychiatry 53:86–89, 1992

Wroblewski BA, Joseph AB, Kupfer J, et al: Effectiveness of valproic acid on destructive and aggressive behaviours in patients with acquired brain injury. Brain Inj 11:37–47, 1997

Yablon SA: Posttraumatic seizures. Arch Phys Med Rehabil 74:983–1001, 1993

Yudofsky SC, Silver JM, Schneider SE: Pharmacologic treatment of aggression. Psychiatr Ann 17:397–407, 1987

Yudofsky SC, Silver JM, Hales RE: Pharmacologic management of aggression in the elderly. J Clin Psychiatry 51 (suppl 10):22–28, 1990

Yudofsky SC, Silver JM, Hales RE: Psychopharmacology of aggression, in American Psychiatric Press Textbook of Psychopharmacology. Edited by Schatzberg AF, Nemeroff CB. Washington, DC, American Psychiatric Press, 1995, pp 735–751

Yudofsky SC, Silver JM, Hales RE: Treatment of agitation and aggression, in Textbook of Psychopharmacology, 2nd Edition. Edited by Schatzberg AF, Nemeroff CB. Washington, DC, American Psychiatric Press, 1998, pp 881–900

Neuropsychiatric Aspects of Seizure Disorders

Gary J. Tucker, M.D.

Seizure Disorders

Seizures and Epilepsy

Epilepsy is a term applied to a broad group of disorders. The defining feature of any of the epilepsies is the seizure. A seizure can have almost protean manifestations, and it is usually defined as having all or parts of the following: an impairment of consciousness, involuntary movements, behavioral changes, and/or altered perceptual experiences.

Classification of Seizures

The latest classification of epileptic seizures, as recognized by the International League Against Epilepsy (ILAE) in 1981, ignores anatomical aspects; for example, the term *temporal lobe epilepsy* technically no longer exists. Furthermore, the classification ignores attempts at explaining pathology and does not take into account age and sex. It makes a descriptive attempt at classifying epilepsy as generalized or partial and describes the progression of firing; for example, seizures may begin as simple partial, progress to complex partial, and then secondarily generalize.

Temporal Lobe Epilepsy

Although the term *temporal lobe epilepsy* has formally become an anachronism, in practice it is still commonly used in the absence of an adequate alternative. The phenomena of temporal lobe epilepsy are *not* synonymous with those of its proposed, nonanatomical replacement, complex partial seizures (CPSs), because CPSs are restricted to patients who have focal firing with defects of consciousness.

In practice, many patients with temporal lobe epilepsy have no defect of consciousness and have simple partial seizures (e.g., olfactory hallucinations), which may derive from the temporal lobes. In addition, they may have simple partial seizures with psychic symptomatology (e.g., cognitive alterations, such as flashbacks or déjà vu experiences occurring in clear consciousness). Temporal lobe epilepsy may also manifest with the *temporal lobe absence* or behavioral arrest that is associated with a brief loss of consciousness of 10–30 seconds. These episodes may be associated with minor automatisms (e.g., chewing movements) and at times with "drop attacks" (the falling associated with loss of muscle tone). Patients with temporal lobe epilepsy often appear to be staring and after the episode may be aware that there was a loss of consciousness. They may experience postictal features such as headache and sleepiness. Thus, the temporal lobe absence differs from petit mal, as the latter is a shorter episode, without muscle movements and postictal features (Fenton 1986).

Temporal lobe epilepsy may also manifest with psychomotor automatisms alone, which are no longer regarded as a form of CPS. Psychomotor automatisms may involve a psychic (cognitive-affective, somatosensory, or perceptual) phase followed by a motor phase. The psychic phase may be very brief and not recognized by the patient, who may be amnestic for it. It may be associated with many perceptual alterations, such as an auditory buzz or hum, complex verbalizations, or aphasias. Visual abnormalities include diplopia, misperceptions of movement, and changes in perceived object size or shape. Other alterations may include illusions, tactile distortions, olfactory phenomena (e.g., generally unpleasant, burning, or rotting smells), gustatory phenomena (e.g., metallic tastes), and somatosensory autonomic symptoms (e.g., piloerection, gastric sensations, or nausea). Flashbacks and alterations of consciousness (jamais vu, depersonalization, derealization, and déjà vu) may occur. These are followed by automatisms of various degrees of complexity. There may be simple buttoning or unbuttoning or masticatory movements, more complex "wandering" fugue states, furor-type anger (which is very rare), or speech automa-

tisms (which are far more common than is recognized).

The features of temporal lobe epilepsy are varied and protean (Bear 1986; Blumer 1975). Table 9–1 describes some of the symptoms that have often been associated with temporal lobe disturbances.

TABLE 9–1. Behavioral symptoms often associated with seizures, particularly temporal lobe epilepsy

Hallucinations: all sensory modalities
Illusions
Déjà vu
Jamais vu
Depersonalization
Repetitive thoughts and nightmares
Flashbacks and visual distortions
Epigastric sensations
Automatisms
Affective and mood changes
Catatonia
Cataplexy
Amnestic episodes

Epidemiology of Seizure Disorders

Most researchers seem to agree that the prevalence of active epilepsy is in the range of 4–10 in 1,000 people. A large study (Hauser et al. 1993) from Rochester, Minnesota, showed that the highest prevalence of epilepsy was before age 10 and after age 65, with a cumulative incidence of epilepsy at age 70 as high as 2%–3% of the population. The disparity between the cumulative incidence and the prevalence raises interesting questions concerning the natural history and prognosis of epilepsy. Shovron and Reynolds (1986) presented convincing data that the majority of patients developing seizures enter long-term remission. Goodridge and Shovron (1983) reported that 122 patients from a sample of 6,000 suffered at least one epileptic seizure (excluding febrile seizures), and 70% of these patients, after 15 years following the initial diagnosis, were in long-term remission. The earlier the remission of seizures after onset, the more likely it was that the patient would have a permanent remission. Those whose seizures continued beyond 2 years were more likely to have seizures at the end of the longitudinal study. A more recent study by Sillanpaa et al. (1995) confirms these findings.

Psychosocial Facets of Epilepsy

The epileptic patient encounters major psychosocial stressors. First is the stress of having a chronic illness. Studies comparing the epileptic patient with groups of patients with other chronic illnesses, such as rheumatic heart disease, diabetes mellitus, and cancer, have concluded that each of these conditions has its own special stressors (Dodrill and Batzel 1986). However, when comparing any of these populations to patients with organic brain disease, there are specific problems in that damage to the central nervous system (CNS), in and of itself, leads to unique consequences (Szatmari 1985).

A special difficulty of the epileptic patient is the often paroxysmal (or episodic) element to the illness. Between episodes, the person with epilepsy may be functioning normally. There is a substantial covert stress that leads the person with epilepsy to be afraid of performing normal social activities, such as dating during adolescence. The fear of a seizure is greater than the occurrence. In addition, the witnessing of an actual tonic-clonic seizure is a frightening experience for many members of the general population, and there is much folklore associated with seizures (Temkin 1979). Consequently, conceptions of epilepsy may be distorted thereafter, and even an isolated seizure may have grave consequences on interpersonal relations.

Diagnosis

The diagnosis of epilepsy is basically a clinical one, much as is the diagnosis of schizophrenia. Although an electroencephalogram (EEG) can often be confirmatory, 20% of patients with epilepsy will have normal EEGs and 2% of patients without epilepsy will have spike and wave formations (Engel 1992). The best diagnostic test for seizures is the observation of the patient or the report of someone who has observed the patient having a seizure. Thus, the history taken from the patient and the family is crucial. Key factors important in the history of these patients are the age at onset of seizures, any history of illness or trauma to the nervous system that could cause seizures, a family history of epilepsy, and some idea of whether the condition is progressive or static. Attempts should be made to determine whether the seizures are idiopathic or secondary.

Laboratory

Finding an elevated prolactin level is the only major chemical diagnostic test for the diagnosis of seizures. After a seizure, usually within 15–20 minutes after a generalized tonic-clonic seizure, there will be an abrupt rise in prolactin levels. As a rule, the prolactin level decreases to normal within 60 minutes; therefore, blood should be drawn 15–20 minutes after the seizure. These levels are typically three to four times the patient's baseline prolactin level. This response of prolactin is seen more often in major motor seizures and less frequently in partial complex seizures. Widespread activation of the temporal lobe structures, however, is often associated with increasing prolactin levels. There are some data indicating that repeated seizures and the frequency of seizure decreases the prolactin response (Malkowicz et al. 1995). It is also important to remember that neuroleptics can also raise prolactin levels.

Imaging

Magnetic resonance imaging (MRI) and computed tomography (CT) scans are crucial for the evaluation of symptomatic epilepsies. Another important use of these imaging modalities is to evaluate presurgical patients to determine the locations of lesions. Functional imaging such as single photon emission computed tomography (SPECT) and positron emission tomography (PET) has been valuable in evaluating ictal events and blood flow to focal lesions during a seizure. However, postictal and interictal evaluations are much less informative. SPECT studies are very reliable for localizing ictal events. PET is somewhat better in the detection of interictal temporal lobe hypermetabolism (Ho et al. 1995). Undoubtedly, as these instruments become more sensitive, they will be used more frequently in the evaluation of seizure disorders.

Electroencephalogram

The EEG is one of the most important tests in the evaluation of seizures, suspected seizures, or episodic behavioral disturbances. In this day of major advances in imaging, the EEG is also frequently overlooked and often, when it is used, it is misinterpreted. The paroxysmal interictal EEG with spikes and wave complexes can confirm the clinical diagnosis of a seizure disorder. It can, when positive, differentiate between seizure types (e.g., absence seizures from generalized seizures) and indicate the possibility of a structural lesion when there are focal findings in the EEG. However, a normal EEG cannot eliminate the possibility of a seizure disorder being present in a particular patient. The EEG is a reflection of surface activity in the cortex and may not reflect seizure activity deep in the brain. Most clinicians, when confronted with a behavior disorder that does not fit the usual clinical picture of a schizophrenic psychosis (particularly if the disorder is episodic), will obtain an EEG. If the EEG is negative, the clinicians may then be deterred from further pursuing the idea that this episodic behavior may represent a seizure disorder. It is important to remember that the diagnosis of epilepsy (as with schizophrenia) is a clinical one and that although the EEG can confirm the diagnosis, it cannot exclude it. Even with elaborate recordings (i.e., 24-hour EEGs) and concomitant videotaping, a diagnosis of a seizure disorder cannot always be made.

A sleep EEG can evoke electroencephalographic abnormalities. In this method, the yield of actual ictal-related events is not substantially increased. However, the potential for detecting a particular focus or focal abnormality may increase because of the extra synchronization that may occur. Phases of sleep may differ in threshold for inducing seizures (i.e., less potentiality for seizures), and it is during such phases that focal abnormalities may be more evident (Brodsky et al. 1983).

The preferred means of evaluating brain wave activity during sleep is the natural induction of sleep. However, in a laboratory situation this is often not practical, and at times (e.g., overnight) the patient is sleep deprived so that no medication need be given. Such a practice is a good one but is not applicable to the psychiatric patient who is generally disturbed enough to require a sedative. The alternative is the administration of chloral hydrate, 1–3 g, as premedication before the sleep record. The chloral hydrate has little effect on the EEG and does not prevent the demonstration of focal abnormalities.

Certain medications should be particularly avoided when obtaining electroencephalographic studies. The first are those in the benzodiazepine group, which may have, by virtue of their strong antiepileptic effects, profound effects in normalizing the EEG. The second medication to avoid for sleep is L-tryptophan. Adamec and Stark (1983) demonstrated that L-tryptophan has some effect in raising the seizure threshold during electroconvulsive therapy (ECT). Some psychotropic medications, such as neuroleptics, the tricyclic and heterocyclic antidepressants, and the benzodiazepines (Pincus and Tucker 1985), may also increase synchronization of the EEG (leading to a seizurelike pattern). One report (Ryback and Gardner 1991) describes a small series in which procaine activation of the EEG was useful in identifying patients with episodic behavioral disorders responsive to anticonvulsants.

Differential Diagnosis of Behavioral Symptoms Associated With Epilepsy

There is a range of medical conditions that must be distinguished from seizures: panic disorder, hyperventilation, hypoglycemia, various transient cerebral ischemias, migraine, narcolepsy, malingering, and conversion reactions. The defining characteristics of temporal lobe epilepsy are typically subjective experiences or feelings, automatisms, and, more rarely, catatonia or cataplexy. Because the symptoms are usually related to a focal electrical discharge in the brain, they are usually consistent and few in number. Although the list of possible symptoms may be quite large (see Table 9–1), each patient will have a limited number of specific symptoms, for example, auditory hallucinations (usually voices), repetitive sounds, or visual hallucinations and misperceptions that are of a consistent type that include a visual disturbance. The automatisms, as related previously, are simple (e.g., chewing, swallowing, pursing of the lips, looking around, smiling, grimacing, crying). Other types of automatisms are attempting to sit up, examining or fumbling with objects, and buttoning or unbuttoning clothes. Complex, goal-directed behavior is unusual during these episodes. Aggressive behavior is also rare. The only time the patient will sometimes become aggressive is when there is an attempt to restrain or prevent ambulation (Rodin 1973). Typical attacks usually consist of a cessation of activity, followed by automatism and impairment of consciousness. The entire episode usually lasts from 10 seconds to as long as 30 minutes. The motor phenomena and postural changes, such as catatonia, are more rare (Fenton 1986; Kirubakaran et al. 1987).

The profile of patients who present primarily with behavioral symptoms is usually of episodic "brief" disturbances lasting for variable periods of time (hours to days). Historically, the patient often states that such episodes have occurred mainly once a month or once every 3 months. The patient seeks psychiatric attention when the frequency of the episodes increases to daily or several times per day and, as a result, functioning becomes impaired. Critical factors helpful in the diagnosis of temporal lobe epilepsy are shown in Table 9–2.

A final term that requires clarification does not refer to epileptic seizures at all. The term *pseudoseizures* is used synonymously with *hysteroepilepsy* and *nonepileptic seizure* or *conversion reaction*. The differentiation of these conditions from true seizures is, at times, extremely difficult (Table 9–3).

However, patients will at times have episodes that are extremely difficult to interpret. These episodes may be very short-lived, lasting seconds or minutes, but on occasion can last for days. Such patients behave out of character and usually exhibit a profound lability of affect, with disturbances ranging from depres-

TABLE 9–2. Factors helpful in the diagnosis of temporal lobe epilepsy

Does the patient describe typical subjective alterations?

Has the patient been observed performing characteristic automatisms?

Was the patient confused during the episode?

Is the patient's memory for events that occurred impaired?

Did the patient experience postictal depression?

Has the patient had other lapses during which he or she engaged in nearly identical behavior?

TABLE 9–3. General features of nonepileptic seizures ("pseudoseizures")

Setting
Environmental gain (audience usually present)
Seldom sleep related
Often triggered (e.g., by stress)
Suggestive profile on Minnesota Multiphasic Personality Inventory (Hathaway and McKinley 1989)

Attack
Atypical movements, often bizarre or purposeful
Seldom results in injury
Often starts and ends gradually
Out-of-phase movements of extremities
Pelvic thrusting or side-to-side movements

Examination
Restraint accentuates the seizure
Inattention decreases over time
Plantar flexor reflexes
Reflexes intact (corneal, pupillary, and blink)
Consciousness preserved
Autonomic system uninvolved
Autonomically intact

After attack
No postictal features (lethargy, tiredness, abnormal electroencephalogram)
Prolactin normal (after 30 minutes)
No or little amnesia
Memory exists (hypnosis or amobarbital sodium)

sion through mania. The patients may appear markedly thought disordered, delusional, or to be hallucinating. Very often, these episodes are repetitive and of the same quality each time. These patients may exhibit behavioral alterations perceived as characterological disorders. Clinically these nonepileptic seizures often occur in young women and consist of significant amounts of staring, shaking, blacking out without falling, and stiffening without loss of consciousness (Devinsky et al. 1996). Pelvic thrusting can occur in many types of seizures and is not alone diagnostic of nonepileptic seizures (Geyer et al. 2000).

In such episodes, EEGs or 24-hour monitoring may not reveal any additional information. However, if the patients have temporal spikes, even if they do not correlate with video monitoring, they may respond to anticonvulsant medication. But in most cases the patient will be left with the label of having nonepileptic seizures. Twenty percent of intractable seizures remain as nonepileptic seizures (Krumholz 1999). Kanner et al. (1999) studied 45 patients with the diagnosis of nonepileptic seizures. Interestingly, 29% of the patients stopped having seizures after being told that the seizures were psychogenic. Twenty-seven percent had only brief recurrences, and in 44% the seizures persisted. The patients in whom the seizures persisted often had psychiatric diagnoses of recurrent affective disorder, dissociative disorders, or personality disorders. However, an abnormal MRI predicted the recurrence of seizures with 75% accuracy, which may indicate some covert biological basis for the nonepileptic seizure.

Frontal lobe epilepsy can also present with bizarre behavioral symptoms and can be confused with nonepileptic seizures.

Laskowitz et al. (1995) noted that the symptoms often appear as spells with an aura of panic symptoms, with weird vocalizations and with bilateral limb movements but no periods of postictal tiredness and no confusion; there are also no oral or alimentary movements. These spells last about 60–70 seconds. Fortunately, most of these seizures are symptomatic of a CNS lesion, and usually the correct diagnosis is made with the EEG or imaging studies. Thomas et al. (1999) described a form of nonconvulsive status epilepticus of frontal origin. These patients often presented with a mood disturbance similar to hypomania, subtle cognitive impairments, some disinhibition, and some indifference.

Comorbid Psychiatric Syndromes

Psychosis

It is clear that *all* of the symptoms described in schizophrenic patients can occur in patients with seizure disorders (Toone et al. 1982). The classic study by Slater et al. (1963) conducted at Maudsley Hospital in London evaluated patients hospitalized for psychosis who had seizure disorders. These patients had all the symptoms associated with schizophrenia. A community sample studied by Perez and Trimble (1980) showed that 50% of the patients with epilepsy and psychosis met diagnostic criteria for schizophrenia by standardized rating scales. However, the question of definition remains. There are similarities in the cognitive deficits noted in both epileptic patients and schizophrenic patients. Mellers et al. (2000) compared a group of patients with epilepsy and psychosis, epilepsy alone, and schizophrenia with a group of neuropsychologically healthy control subjects using neuropsychological testing. Patients

with psychosis and epilepsy had almost identical neuropsychological test patterns. Often, what patients with seizure disorders and behavioral problems describe is a single complaint such as auditory hallucinations or a solitary perceptual change. The patients with these single symptoms are frequently classified by clinicians as psychotic. Conversely, psychiatric patients with several symptoms are sometimes dubiously labeled as epileptic based on a history of a seizure disorder, a solitary seizure, seizures associated with alcohol or other substance withdrawal, or vaguely described and poorly characterized "blackouts." Such cases are difficult to interpret, but there seems to be no denying the relationship of seizures to psychopathology. Kanner et al. (1996) studied patients admitted to a video electroencephalographic monitoring unit for evaluation of their seizures. As part of the evaluation, all anticonvulsants were stopped. The researchers found that of the 140 patients admitted to the unit, there was a 7.8% incidence of postictal psychiatric events; 6.4% were psychotic and 1.4% were nonpsychotic. The psychotic events were mostly depressive, hypomanic, or delusional, and all seemed to take place in a confused state. These episodes responded to psychotropic medication and lasted about 69 hours on average. A similar finding was noted by Ketter et al. (1994), who described increased anxiety and depressive symptoms in 38% of 32 patients withdrawn from their anticonvulsant medications in order to enter a controlled trial.

Despite more than 100 publications in the scientific literature dealing with core issues of epilepsy in relation to psychosis, the cause of the increased psychopathology in epileptic conditions remains unclear, and a precise clinical picture has not been established (Diehl 1989; McKenna et al. 1985; Neppe 1986). Betts

(1974), Ey (1954), Gibbs and Gibbs (1952), Gudmundsson (1966), Krohn (1961), Lindsay et al. (1979), Sengoku et al. (1983), Slater et al. (1963), and Wilensky and Neppe (1986) have all described a clear association between these two conditions.

Clinically, there seem to be three psychotic presentations that one sees with seizure disorders. One is an episodic course usually manifested by perceptual changes, alterations in consciousness, and poor memory for the events. A chronic psychotic condition also occurs in which the patient may have simple auditory hallucinations, paranoia, or other perceptual changes. The third type is simply a variation in which the patient usually has some type of persistent experience of depersonalization or visual distortion that, for lack of a better name, is usually labeled as psychotic. The latter is probably a variant of the chronic psychotic state.

Treatment of Psychotic Conditions

The major treatment of the episodic psychotic conditions is usually the appropriate use of anticonvulsant medications. The treatment of chronic conditions involves not only anticonvulsant medications but neuroleptics and other antipsychotic medications as well. In general, the use of medication in these patients is difficult in that very small doses of any medication often cause an increase in symptoms that diminishes over time. Consequently, very small doses and infrequent changes seem to be the major guidelines in treating these patients. For example, when adding a neuroleptic to the anticonvulsant medications, a clinician often begins with a small dose, such as 1 mg of haloperidol, and waits 6–8 weeks before changing the dose. Although all of the neuroleptics can lower the seizure threshold, haloperidol, fluphenazine, molindone, pimozide, and trifluoperazine

seem to lower the seizure threshold the least. The propensity for clozapine to lower the seizure threshold is quite well known. Although seizures have been reported with the use of risperidone, quetiapine, and olanzapine, the rate is quite low, and it would seem safe to use these new atypical neuroleptics in patients with seizures and psychosis (Alldredge 1999).

With anticonvulsant drugs, it is best to adjust their doses as far as possible to the top range of the therapeutic window. Because all of the anticonvulsants can cause cognitive side effects, it is important to distinguish between toxicity from the drugs and a worsening in behavior (Armon et al. 1996; Hamer et al. 2000; Martin et al. 1999; Meador et al. 1995). Vigabatrin has been reported to have a side-effect profile that shows a 2.5% incidence of psychotic symptoms and a 17.1% incidence of affective symptoms (Levinson and Devinsky 1999).

Anxiety Disorders

The correspondence between seizure disorders and anxiety disorders is a fascinating topic, and the substantial overlapping of symptoms often makes differentiation between these classes of disorders complex. Either type of syndrome can be confused with the other, and the same class of medications (benzodiazepines) helps to reduce the symptoms and subsequent impairment of both types. Panic disorder and CPSs are each included in the differential diagnosis of the other. Although many symptoms overlap, evidence of neurophysiological linkage between anxiety and seizure disorder remains tenuous, except that both involve underlying limbic dysfunction (Fontaine et al. 1990). This connection appears to be more relevant between partial seizure and CPS than other seizure disorders, and it has been speculated that there is a subgroup of patients who have panic disorder that has a pathophysiological relation to epilepsy (Dantendorfer et al. 1995). This relationship is not surprising given that modulation of fear is associated with the temporal lobes; others have hypothesized relationships between the parietal and frontal lobe neural circuits and panic attacks (Alemayehu et al. 1995; McNamara and Fogel 1990).

Little is known about the prevalence of comorbidity. A post hoc analysis of the Epidemiologic Catchment Area data suggested a mild association between panic disorder and seizures (Neugebauer et al. 1993). On the other hand, Spitz (1991) reported that in a clinical sample there was no association between panic disorder and CPS. The relationship between posttraumatic stress disorder, obsessive-compulsive disorder, generalized anxiety, social phobia, and simple phobias has not been articulated. As is the case with panic disorder, there are overlapping symptoms. Table 9–4 lists many of the symptoms that overlap between CPS and anxiety disorders.

Roth and Harper (1962) pointed out some of the similarities between epilepsy and anxiety disorders. Both are episodic disorders with sudden onset without a precipitating event; both sometimes present with dissociative symptoms (depersonalization, derealization, and déjà vu); both often present with abnormal perceptual and emotional disturbance, such as intense fear and terror; and both have associated physical symptoms.

There are significant clinical differences between panic disorder and CPS that help to differentiate the two. In panic disorders consciousness is usually preserved, olfactory hallucinations are unusual, there is a positive family history, electroencephalographic results are usually normal, and many patients do not respond well to anticonvulsants (Handal et al. 1995). Individuals with CPS do not

TABLE 9–4. Anxiety disorder symptoms that overlap with those of seizure disorder

Panic disorder
    Fear
    Depersonalization
    Derealization
    Déjà vu
    Jamais vu
    Misperceptions
    Illusions
    Dizziness
    Paresthesias
    Chills or hot flashes
Obsessive-compulsive disorder
    Obsessions, forced or intrusive
Posttraumatic stress disorder
    Recurrent memories or distressing
      recollections
    Flashback-like episodes
    Irritability
    Difficulty concentrating
Agoraphobia
    Fear of recurrent episodes that leads to
      restriction of activities

generally have agoraphobia, they may have automatisms, their attacks are generally shorter, they often have abnormal brain scans, and antidepressants may worsen the course of their illness (Roth and Harper 1962). Patients with refractory anxiety, in particular panic disorder, and patients who have atypical responses to psychotropic medications should be reevaluated for a seizure disorder. A pilot study by Weilburg et al. (1995) found that in patients with atypical panic attacks, ambulatory electroencephalographic monitoring helped to identify an underlying seizure disorder. Electroencephalographic changes occurred in 33% of the subjects ($N = 15$), and among subjects with "captured" panic attacks, 45% showed focal paroxysmal electroencephalographic changes. Two of these five subjects previously had a normal routine EEG.

Treatment of Comorbid Anxiety

Patients with seizure disorders and comorbid anxiety disorder should receive treatment for their anxiety. Most anxiety disorders can be treated using psychotherapeutic approaches, for example, behavioral, cognitive-behavioral, and short-term symptom-focused therapies. Patients with more severe or refractory anxiety disorders may require pharmacological intervention. Most antianxiety agents and selective serotonin reuptake inhibitors (SSRIs) and other newer antidepressants are tolerated by patients with seizure disorders. The principal reason for not treating epileptic patients with benzodiazepines (although they can be used if needed) is the concern of developing tolerance and dependence and promoting withdrawal-related seizures.

Mood Disorders

CNS disorders and chronic medical illnesses are frequently associated with increased incidence of mood disorders (Silver et al. 1990); however, there seems to be a distinct relationship between mood disorders and epilepsy. Suicide is of special concern because its prevalence is more common than in the general population (Gehlert 1994; Robertson 1986). Barraclough (1981) reported a 25-fold increase in suicide risk for patients with temporal lobe epilepsy. Most studies of major depression from clinical samples suggest an increase in depressive symptoms using self-report measures (Guze and Gitlin 1994; Robertson et al. 1994), but there are some exceptions (Fiordelli et al. 1993). Little is known about the prevalence of bipolar disorder and dysthymia and comorbid seizure disorders. It is also unknown whether there is an increased vulnerability to depression due to type, frequency, or age at onset of seizures. Several studies have identified a link between left-sided epileptogenic lesions and depression (Mendez et al. 1994; Victoroff et al. 1994). Partial seizures, male gender, and depressive symptoms have also been associated with a left epileptogenic focus (Altshuler et al. 1990; Septien et al. 1993; Strauss et al. 1992). Blumer et al. (1995) evaluated 97 patients admitted to a neurodiagnostic electroencephalographic/video monitoring unit and noted that 34% had atypical depression and 22% had nonepileptic seizures. He defined eight key symptoms that he thought were characteristic of the affective disorders of these patients: depressed mood, anergy, irritability, euphoria, pain, insomnia, fear, and anxiety. These patients also had a history of suicide attempts and hallucinations. Blumer believes this is an epilepsy-specific syndrome, but again many of these symptoms are associated with many types of insult to the CNS. Altshuler et al. (1999) did a 10-year follow-up of 49 patients who had undergone surgery for refractory temporal lobe seizures. The incidence of affective disorder in these patients was quite high: 45% had a lifetime history of depression, 77% had a prior history of depression, 10% developed depression for the first time after surgery, and 50% showed complete remission of their depression after surgery. Forty-seven percent had no recurrence of their depression after surgery. This study certainly implicates the temporal lobes as an anatomical area of some interest in affective disorder.

There are several features of depression in epilepsy that require special consideration before one diagnoses a patient as having a comorbid affective disorder. Sometimes it can be difficult to distinguish affective symptoms from symptoms related to the seizure disorder or the underlying pathology. For example, depressive symptoms for some patients may represent an aura preceding an ictal event or a characteristic postictal phase (Robertson 1986). Similarly, emotional lability or affective instability are symptoms that span both the "neurologic" and "psychiatric" spectrum of epilepsy.

In evaluating depression in a patient with epilepsy, it is very important to examine the medications the patient is taking. Anticonvulsants have been identified as causal agents of depression and cognitive impairments; phenobarbital, the anticonvulsant vigabatrin, and multiple combinations of anticonvulsants appear to contribute to mood disturbance (Bauer and Elger 1995; Brent et al. 1990; Levinson and Devinsky 1999; Mendez et al. 1993). Other anticonvulsants have minimal effect, and some, such as carbamazepine and lamotrigine, may have beneficial effects on mood.

Treatment of Comorbid Mood Disorders

The role of psychotherapeutic approaches seems intuitively beneficial, but there are few empirical studies that have evaluated this topic. Several studies have suggested that psychological interventions help children and adults with seizure disorders to comply with medications, accept and manage the illness, cope with stressful events, and develop improved self-esteem (Fenwick 1994; Mathers 1992; Regan et al. 1993). A study by Gillham (1990) demonstrated that psychological intervention with education to improve coping skills could be helpful in reducing seizure frequency and psychological symptoms (as well as depressive symptoms) in patients with refractory seizures.

Some patients with seizure disorders and comorbid depression are frequently taking many medications and may respond to careful anticonvulsant monotherapy, especially with carbamazepine (Carrieri et al. 1993). An open study of partial seizure patients with depression refractory to tricyclic antidepressants demonstrated that a subgroup responded very well to carbamazepine (Varney et al. 1993). For patients with a bipolar diathesis or suspected mood lability, monotherapy using carbamazepine or valproic acid (or now lamotrigine) may suffice to prevent episodes, decrease severity of symptoms, and minimize overall decompensation.

It has been well documented that most of the tricyclic antidepressants lower the seizure threshold. This is particularly true of amitriptyline, maprotiline, and clomipramine. Bupropion is also very likely to cause seizures. However, doxepin, trazodone, and the monoamine oxidase inhibitors have less of a tendency to lower the seizure threshold (Rosenstein et al. 1993). All of the SSRIs and other new antidepressants (nefazodone and mirtazapine; venlafaxine and fluvoxamine have slightly higher incidences of seizures) have had seizures reported with their use, but the incidence is low (Alldredge 1999). Most of the seizures reported with any of these medications are dose related; therefore, blood level monitoring in these patients can be quite useful. Consequently, it is important to start any medication with smaller doses than are conventionally given, with gradual increases over time. In most cases, treating the depression often improves seizure control. In an open study evaluating the use of fluoxetine as an adjunctive medication in patients with CPSs, six patients showed a dramatic improvement, and the others had a 30% reduction in their seizure frequency over 14 months (Favale et al. 1995). To date there is no evidence that any one particular antidepressant is more effective than another, and the choice should be made on clinical grounds. Patients with refractory or severe depression should be considered for ECT, but this is another area lacking data from well-designed studies

(Zwil and Pelchat 1994). Blumer (1997) reported a series of depressed epileptic patients who responded to a combination of a tricyclic antidepressant and an SSRI; he advocates this regimen for psychotic epileptic patients as well, because he sees the psychosis as an interictal dysphoric disorder (Blumer et al. 2000).

Behavioral and Personality Disturbances

The literature and clinical experience clearly point to an association between seizure disorders and behavioral disturbances, particularly in patients who have had a chronic course (Neppe and Tucker 1988). Evidence for personality pathology with seizure disorders is sparse because of methodological constraints, but many case reports cite personality disturbance (Blumer 1999; Blumer et al. 1995). Hermann and Riel (1981) underscored the issues that have perpetuated misunderstanding of the relationship between personality and seizures. Methods of measuring personality pathology and comparisons among epilepsy and control groups have not been uniform. There are no longitudinal studies that have assessed behavior and personality before the onset of a seizure disorder. Most of our knowledge in this area comes from cross-sectional case control studies, case reports, and tertiary centers that treat the most severe cases. As a result, it is difficult to extricate the relationship between personality formation and the course of a seizure disorder. Several factors such as stigma of the illness, adverse social factors, level of social support, cultural acceptability, consequences of the illness on psychosocial adaptation, and interpersonal relationships play an important role in shaping patterns of behavior and have a significant impact on the integrity of personality development. Factors that may assume a role in the pathogenesis of personality and behavioral disturbance are the age at onset of the seizure disorder, the type of seizure disorder, the location and the laterality, the frequency of the seizures, the etiology, the presence of a structural lesion, the presence of another medical illness or behavior dysfunction, and the ongoing administration of anticonvulsants.

It is unlikely that there is an epileptic personality (Dam and Dam 1986; Devinsky and Najjar 1999), and there is only a tenuous link between any formal DSM-IV-TR (American Psychiatric Association 2000) personality disorders and seizure disorders. Some have suggested that neurologic dysfunction, including epilepsy, may play a role in the development of symptoms in subtypes of borderline personality disorder (Andrulonis et al. 1982; Gunderson and Zanarini 1989). Maladaptive personality characteristics and specific personality profiles have been described—preoccupation with philosophical and moral concerns; a belief in a personal destiny; dependency; and traits such as humorlessness (circumstantially), hypergraphia, hyposexuality, religiosity, viscosity, and paranoia (Bear and Fedio 1977; Hermann and Riel 1981; Waxman and Geschwind 1975)— but large-scale studies do not confirm these case reports or even that there is a specific personality type associated with seizure disorders (Mungus 1982; Rodin and Schmaltz 1984; Stark-Adamec et al. 1985; Stevens 1975).

An increase in episodic and impulsive aggression has also been associated with seizure disorders, particularly CPS (Blake et al. 1995; Mann 1995). Following the postictal period, uncooperative and aggressive behavior may occur when a confused patient is restrained or may occur in a patient who develops a postictal paranoid psychosis (Rodin 1973). Aggressive behavior during a seizure is very unusual, and aggressive activity is usually carried out in a disordered, uncoordinated, and nondirected way (Fenwick 1986). The relationship between aggression and seizure disorders has traditionally been controversial because of methodological concerns. The prevalence of interictal aggression is increased in some seizure disorders, CPS, and generalized seizure disorders but may be an epiphenomenon of epilepsy. This probably can be accounted for by other factors associated with violence and aggression: exposure to violence as a child, male sex, low IQ, low socioeconomic status, adverse social factors, focal or diffuse neurologic lesions, refractory seizures, cognitive impairment, history of institutionalization, and drug use (Devinsky and Vazquez 1993).

The manner in which a particular seizure disorder promotes psychopathic behavioral syndromes is not well understood. Auras have been hypothesized as manifestations of an underlying mechanism that contributes to the development of personality disturbance (Mendez et al. 1993). There is evidence that patients with chronic seizure disorders develop brain neuropathology, and histologic studies of the temporal lobes in CPS demonstrate neuronal loss (Sloviter and Tamminga 1995).

Devinsky and Vazquez (1993) emphasized the diversity of symptoms, behaviors, and profiles, and that the most important characteristic of patients with a seizure disorder is the tendency for extremes of behavior to be accentuated in numerous manners. Not all of the symptoms and consequences of a seizure disorder are debilitating, and some may play an even positive role. It is the maladaptive consequences and dysfunctional traits that should be of paramount importance in treatment.

Overall Guidelines for the Treatment of Comorbid Psychiatric Syndromes

With any chronic illness, there are basic principles that should be applied in developing a treatment plan. Seizure disorders are no exception, and guidelines for treatment are summarized in Table 9–5.

Most patients will require treatment of psychiatric syndromes. Individual, group, family, or couple therapies can provide specific syndrome-focused treatments. Psychotherapeutic approaches have many advantages. They avoid drug interactions, circumvent the tendency of psychotropic medications to alter seizure thresholds, and can teach patients behavior and coping skills that can have a positive impact on symptoms and dysfunction.

TABLE 9–5.   Basic principles of treating patients with a seizure disorder and concomitant psychiatric symptoms

Perform a thorough assessment of biopsychosocial factors that aggravate neuropsychiatric symptoms.

Evaluate the need for adjustment of the anticonvulsant.

Consider psychotherapeutic approaches (individual, group, family) that are specific for the syndrome or that target behaviors or stressors.

Preferably—but not always—use anticonvulsant monotherapy.

Optimize the addition of psychotropic medication by targeting specific psychiatric symptoms.

Start with smaller than usual dose and wait until symptoms stabilize (often weeks) before changing doses.

Anticipate interactions between anticonvulsant and psychotropic medications.

Collaborate with other caregivers.

Many patients will require pharmacotherapy, either combined with psychotherapeutic approaches or alone. Patients with temporal lobe epilepsy display a wide variety of mood, anxiety, dissociative, psychotic, and behavioral disturbances that frequently resemble psychiatric disorders. Discriminating the symptoms of previous seizures from target psychiatric symptoms will ensure a greater likelihood of response to medication.

Although we recommend an aggressive approach for the treatment of comorbid psychiatric syndromes, we are judicious with the dosing of psychotropics and prefer gradual increases. Clinical experience shows that many patients with seizure disorders seem to respond to smaller doses. Given the concern about anticonvulsant and psychotropic drug interactions, such an approach is warranted. Any time a new drug is added it is mandatory for the clinician to be aware of potential drug interactions. Many anticonvulsants will lower the serum drug level of psychotropics through enzyme induction (Perucca et al. 1985), and psychotropics may increase the levels of anticonvulsants secondary to increased P450 hepatic enzyme competition (Cloyd et al. 1986). For patients receiving tricyclic antidepressants, monitoring of serum levels is recommended, and avoiding elevated blood levels may prevent seizure promotion (Preskorn and Fast 1992). Initially, anticonvulsant blood levels should be monitored weekly and then monthly, after the addition of a psychotropic. After a few months, serum levels can be checked less frequently. Thereafter, any changes in the dosage of medications require reexamination of serum blood levels.

Finally, the importance of coordinating care with other professionals and health care providers cannot be overemphasized. It behooves the psychiatrist to work with a neurologist (if available) to develop a long-term strategy. Often, psychiatrists will assume the role of supervising all treatment planning (Schoenenberger et al. 1995).

Specific Aspects of Anticonvulsant Use

It is important to recognize that in many of the patients who have suspected seizure disorders, the psychiatrist will be left to manage the anticonvulsants. Often, even when the patient has a documented seizure disorder and the major persistent symptoms are behavioral, the psychiatrist will also be managing these medications alone. Until the psychiatrist is comfortable with these medications, collaboration with a neurologist is not only helpful but is a good learning technique. However, as valproic acid and carbamazepine have become more common in the treatment of bipolar illness, the basic principles are known to most psychiatrists (McElroy et al. 1988; Neppe et al. 1988).

Pharmacokinetic Interactions

Anticonvulsant administration is particularly important and particularly difficult by virtue of enzyme induction and inhibition occurring in the liver. This enzyme induction tends to affect predominantly the P450 cytochrome enzyme system in the liver. This implies that both the metabolism of anticonvulsants (particularly carbamazepine) and the metabolism of other lipid-soluble compounds are accelerated (Alldredge 1999; Post et al. 1985). However, some of the new anticonvulsants—oxcarbazepine, gabapentin, and vigabatrin—have few drug interactions (Dichter and Brodie 1996).

Of the major anticonvulsants, phenobarbital, phenytoin, carbamazepine, lamotrigine, topiramate, and tiagabine have potent drug interactions. Table 9–6 indicates what is known about some interactions and demonstrates the complexity of these drug interactions (Bertilsson 1978; Birkhimer et al. 1985; Bramhall and Levine 1988; Dichter and Brodie 1996; Dorn 1986; Jann et al. 1985; Kidron et al. 1985; Shukla et al. 1984; Zimmerman 1986).

New Antiepileptic Drugs

There are many new antiepileptic drugs (AEDs): gabapentin, felbamate, oxcarbazepine, tiagabine, topiramate, vigabatrin, and lamotrigine. Most of these drugs for which the actions are known affect either the inhibitory γ-aminobutyric acid system (gabapentin, tiagabine, vigabatrin) or the excitatory glutaminergic system (felbamate, lamotrigine). Many of these have been well studied throughout the world and in the United States, and all have various mild to serious side effects (Table 9–7) (Dichter and Brodie 1996; Ketter et al. 1999).

Conclusions

Psychopathology occurs only in a minority of persons with epilepsy. Attempted etiologic explanations such as kindling, lateralization, localization, and biochemical changes are all, therefore, explanations for a small proportion of the epileptic population. Medications used to treat seizure disorders often do not alleviate behavior changes, and at times agents such as neuroleptics and antidepressants help behavior change but not seizure disturbances. The exact etiology of these conditions remains to be determined. Clinical judgment in the individual case remains the essential standard of care in the absence of

TABLE 9–6. Known interactions between carbamazepine and other drugs

Drugs that increase carbamazepine level
>   Isoniazid
>   Valproic acid (increased free carbamazepine in vitro)
>   Carbamazepine epoxide only
>   Troleandomycin
>   Propoxyphene
>   Erythromycin
>   Nicotinamide
>   Cimetidine
>   Viloxazine

Drugs that decrease carbamazepine level
>   Phenobarbital
>   Phenytoin
>   Primidone and phenobarbital
>   Carbamazepine itself (autoinduction)
>   Alcohol (chronic use)
>   Cigarettes

Conditions caused by carbamazepine
>   Pregnancy test failure
>   Escape from dexamethasone suppression
>   Oral contraceptive failure

Substances whose effects are decreased by carbamazepine
>   Vitamin D, calcium, and folate; causes possible hyponatremia
>   Clonazepam
>   Dicumarol
>   Doxycycline
>   Phenytoin
>   Sodium valproate
>   Theophylline
>   Ethosuximide
>   Haloperidol
>   Isoniazid

Note. Because enzyme induction is the mechanism in most of these interactions, it can be hypothesized that there are similar effects with phenytoin, phenobarbital, and primidone.

solid evidence for specific indications and protocols for the use of anticonvulsant/psychotropic combinations in specific populations.

TABLE 9–7. Selected clinical aspects of the new anticonvulsants

Felbamate[a,b]
    Irritability, insomnia, stimulant effects
    Aplastic anemia, hepatitis
Gabapentin
    Weight gain
    Few drug interactions
    Anxiolytic
Lamotrigine[a,b]
    No weight gain
    Occasional tourettism
    Rash
    Does not induce P450 system
    Can increase neurotoxicity of
        carbamazepine
Oxcarbazepine
    Few drug interactions (not affected by
        enzyme inducers)
    Induces 3A family of P450 system weakly
    Hyponatremia
Tiagabine
    Confusion, fatigue
    Does not induce P450 system
Topiramate[a]
    Hyperammonemic encephalopathy when
        combined with valproate
    Cognitive impairments
    Weak effect on P450 system
Vigabatrin[a]
    Increased incidence of depression and
        psychosis
    Weight gain
    Possible retinal damage
    No drug interactions

[a]Can affect phenytoin, carbamazepine, and phenobarbital levels.
[b]Valproate decreases levels of this compound.

References

Adamec RE, Stark AC: Limbic kindling and animal behavior: implications for human psychopathology associated with complex partial seizures. Biol Psychiatry 18:269–293, 1983

Alemayehu S, Bergey GK, Barry E, et al: Panic attacks as ictal manifestations of parietal lobe seizures. Epilepsia 36:824–830, 1995

Alldredge BK: Seizure risk associated with psychotropic drugs: clinical and pharmacokinetic considerations. Neurology 53 (suppl 2):S68–S75, 1999

Altshuler LL, Devinsky O, Post RM, et al: Depression, anxiety, and temporal lobe epilepsy: laterality of focus and symptoms. Arch Neurol 47:284–288, 1990

Altshuler LL, Rausch R, Delrahim S, et al: Temporal lobe epilepsy, temporal lobectomy, major depression. J Neuropsychiatry Clin Neurosci 11:436–443, 1999

American Psychiatric Association: Diagnostic and Statistical Manual of Mental Disorders, 4th Edition, Text Revision. Washington, DC, American Psychiatric Association, 2000

Andrulonis PA, Glueck BC, Stroebel CF, et al: Borderline personality subcategories. J Nerv Ment Dis 170:670–679, 1982

Armon C, Shin M, Miller P, et al: Reversible parkinsonism and cognitive impairment with chronic valproate use. Neurology 47:626–635, 1996

Barraclough B: Suicide and epilepsy, in Epilepsy and Psychiatry. Edited by Reynolds EH, Trimble MR. Edinburgh, UK, Churchill Livingstone, 1981, pp 72–76

Bauer J, Elger CE: Anticonvulsive drug therapy: historical and current aspects. Nervenarzt 66:403–411, 1995

Bear DM: Behavioural changes in temporal lobe epilepsy: conflict, confusion challenge, in Aspects of Epilepsy and Psychiatry. Edited by Trimble MR, Bolwig TG. Chichester, UK, Wiley, 1986, pp 19–29

Bear DM, Fedio P: Quantitative analysis of interictal behavior in temporal lobe epilepsy. Arch Neurol 34:454–467, 1977

Bertilsson L: Clinical pharmacokinetics of carbamazepine. Clin Pharmacokinet 3:128–143, 1978

Betts TA: A follow-up study of a cohort of patients with epilepsy admitted to psychiatric care in an English city, in Epilepsy: Proceedings of the Hans Berger Centenary Symposium, Edinburgh, 1973. Edited by Harris P, Mawdsley C. New York, Churchill Livingstone, 1974

Birkhimer LJ, Curtis JL, Jann MW: Use of carbamazepine in psychiatric disorders. Clinical Pharmacology 4:425–434, 1985

Blake P, Pincus J, Buckner C: Neurologic abnormalities in murderers. Neurology 45: 1641–1647, 1995

Blumer D: Temporal lobe epilepsy and its psychiatric significance, in Psychiatric Aspects of Neurological Disease. Edited by Benson FD, Blumer D. New York, Grune & Stratton, 1975, pp 171–198

Blumer D: Antidepressant and double antidepressant treatment for the affective disorder of epilepsy. J Clin Psychiatry 58:3–11, 1997

Blumer D: Evidence supporting the temporal lobe epilepsy personality syndrome: Neurology 53 (suppl 2):S9–S12, 1999

Blumer D, Montouris G, Hermann B: Psychiatric morbidity in seizure patients on a neurodiagnostic monitoring unit. J Neuropsychiatry Clin Neurosci 7:445–456, 1995

Blumer D, Wakhulu S, Montouris G, et al: Treatment of the interictal psychoses. J Clin Psychiatry 61:110–122, 2000

Bramhall D, Levine M: Possible interaction of ranitidine with phenytoin. Drug Intell Clin Pharm 22:979–980, 1988

Brent DA, Crumrine PK, Varma R, et al: Phenobarbital treatment and major depressive disorder in children with epilepsy: a naturalistic follow-up. Pediatrics 85: 1086–1091, 1990

Brodsky L, Zuniga JG, Casenas ER, et al: Refractory anxiety: a masked epileptiform disorder. Psychiatr J Univ Ott 8:42–45, 1983

Carrieri PB, Provitera V, Iacovitti B, et al: Mood disorders in epilepsy. Acta Neurol (Napoli) 15:62–67, 1993

Cloyd JC, Levy RH, Wedlund RH: Relationship between carbamazepine concentration and extent of enzyme autoinduction (abstract). Epilepsia 27:592, 1986

Dam M, Dam AM: Is there an epileptic personality? in Aspects of Epilepsy and Psychiatry. Edited by Trimble MR, Bolwig TG. New York, Wiley, 1986, pp 9–18

Dantendorfer K, Amering M, Baischer W, et al: Is there a pathophysiological and therapeutic link between panic disorder and epilepsy? Acta Psychiatr Scand 91:430–432, 1995

Devinsky O, Najjar S: Evidence against the existence of a temporal lobe epilepsy personality syndrome. Neurology 53 (suppl 2):S12–S25, 1999

Devinsky O, Vazquez B: Behavioral changes associated with epilepsy. Neurol Clin 11:127–149, 1993

Devinsky O, Sanchez-Villasenor F, Vazquez B, et al: Clinical profile of patients with epileptic and nonepileptic seizures. Neurology 46:1530–1533, 1996

Dichter M, Brodie M: New antiepileptic drugs. N Engl J Med 334:1583–1590, 1996

Diehl LW: Schizophrenic syndromes in epilepsies. Psychopathology 22:65–140, 1989

Dodrill CB, Batzel LW: Interictal behavioral features of patients with epilepsy. Epilepsia 27 (suppl 2):S64–S76, 1986

Dorn JM: A case of phenytoin toxicity possibly precipitated by trazodone. J Clin Psychiatry 47:89–90, 1986

Engel J: The epilepsies, in Cecil's Textbook of Medicine, 19th Edition. Edited by Wyngoorden J, Smith L, Bennet C. Philadelphia, PA, WB Saunders, 1992, pp 2202–2213

Ey H: Etudes psychiatriques. Paris, Desclee de Brouwer, 1954

Favale E, Rubino P, Mainardi P, et al: Anticonvulsant effect of fluoxetine in humans. Neurology 45:1926–1927, 1995

Fenton GW: The EEG, epilepsy and psychiatry, in What Is Epilepsy? Edited by Trimble MR, Reynolds EH. Edinburgh, UK, Churchill Livingstone, 1986, pp 139–160

Fenwick P: In dyscontrol epilepsy, in What Is Epilepsy? Edited by Trimble MR, Reynolds EH. Edinburgh, UK, Churchill Livingstone, 1986, pp 161–182

Fenwick P: The behavioral treatment of epilepsy generation and inhibition of seizures. Neurol Clin 12:175–202, 1994

Fiordelli E, Beghi E, Bogliun G, et al: Epilepsy and psychiatric disturbance: a cross-sectional study. Br J Psychiatry 163: 446–450, 1993

Fontaine R, Breton G, D'ery R, et al: Temporal lobe abnormalities in panic disorder: an MRI study. Biol Psychiatry 27:304–310, 1990

Gehlert S: Perceptions of control in adults with epilepsy. Epilepsia 35:81–88, 1994

Geyer J, Payne T, Drury I: The value of pelvic thrusting in the diagnosis of seizures and pseudoseizures. Neurology 54:227–229, 2000

Gibbs FA, Gibbs EL: Atlas of Electroencephalography. Cambridge, MA, Addison-Wesley, 1952

Gillham RA: Refractory epilepsy: an evaluation of psychological methods in outpatient management. Epilepsia 31:427–432, 1990

Goodridge DMG, Shovron SD: Epileptic seizures in a population of 6000. Br Med J 287:641–644, 1983

Gudmundsson G: Epilepsy in Iceland. Acta Neurol Scand 43 (suppl 25):1–124, 1966

Gunderson JG, Zanarini MC: Pathogenesis of borderline personality, in American Psychiatric Press Review of Psychiatry, Vol 8. Edited by Tasman A, Hales RE, Frances AJ. Washington, DC, American Psychiatric Press, 1989, pp 25–48

Guze BH, Gitlin M: The neuropathologic basis of major affective disorders: neuroanatomic insights. J Neuropsychiatry Clin Neurosci 6:114–121, 1994

Hamer H, Knake S, Schomburg M, et al: Valproate induced hyperammonemic encephalopathy in the presence of topiramate. Neurology 54:230–232, 2000

Handal N, Masand P, Weilburg J: Panic disorder and complex partial seizures: a truly complex relationship. Psychosomatics 36:498–502, 1995

Hathaway SR, McKinley JC: Minnesota Multiphasic Personality Inventory—2. Minneapolis, MN, University of Minnesota, 1989

Hauser WA, Annegers J, Kurland L: Incidence of epilepsy and unprovoked seizures in Rochester, MN. Epilepsia 34:453–468, 1993

Hermann BP, Riel P: Interictal personality and behavioral traits in temporal lobe and generalized epilepsy. Cortex 17:125–128, 1981

Ho S, Berkovic S, Berlangieri S, et al: Comparison of ictal SPECT and interictal PET in the presurgical evaluation of TLE. Ann Neurol 37:738–745, 1995

International League Against Epilepsy Commission: Proposal for revised clinical and electroencephalographic classification of epileptic seizures. Epilepsia 22:489–501, 1981

Jann MW, Ereshefsky L, Saklad SR, et al: Effects of carbamazepine on plasma haloperidol levels. J Clin Psychopharmacol 5:106–109, 1985

Kanner A, Stagno S, Kotagal P, et al: Postictal psychiatric events during prolonged video-EEG monitoring studies. Arch Neurol 53:258–263, 1996

Kanner A, Parra J, Frey M, et al: Psychiatric and neurologic predictors of psychogenic seizure outcome. Neurology 53: 933–938, 1999

Ketter T, Malow B, Flamini R, et al: Anticonvulsant withdrawal emergent psychopathology. Neurology 44:55–61, 1994

Ketter T, Post R, Theodore W: Positive and negative psychiatric effects of antiepileptic drugs in patients with seizure disorders. Neurology 53 (suppl 2):S53–S67, 1999

Kidron R, Averbuch I, Klein E, et al: Carbamazepine-induced reduction of blood levels of haloperidol in chronic schizophrenia. Biol Psychiatry 20:219–222, 1985

Kirubakaran V, Sen S, Wilkinson C: Catatonic stupor: unusual manifestation of TLE. Psychiatr J Univ Ott 12:244–246, 1987

Krohn W: A study of epilepsy in Northern Norway: its frequency and character. Acta Psychiatr Scand (suppl 150):215–225, 1961

Krumholz A: Nonepileptic seizures: diagnosis and management. Neurology 53 (suppl 2):S76–S83, 1999

Laskowitz D, Sperling M, French J, et al: The syndrome of frontal lobe epilepsy. Neurology 45:780–787, 1995

Levinson D, Devinsky O: Psychiatric events during vigabatrin therapy. Neurology 53:1503–1511, 1999

Lindsay J, Ounstead C, Richards P: Long-term outcome in children with temporal lobe seizures, III: psychiatric aspects in childhood and adult life. Dev Med Child Neurol 21:630–636, 1979

Malkowicz D, Legido A, Jackel R, et al: Prolactin secretion following repetitive seizures. Neurology 45:448–452, 1995

Mann JJ: Violence and aggression, in Psychopharmacology: The Fourth Generation of Progress. Edited by Bloom FE, Kupfer DJ. New York, Raven, 1995, pp 1919–1928

Martin R, Kuzniecky R, Ho S, et al: Cognitive effects of topiramate, gabapentin, and lamotrigine in healthy young adults. Neurology 52:321–327, 1999

Mathers CB: Group therapy in the management of epilepsy. Br J Med Psychol 65:279–287, 1992

McElroy S, Keck P, Pope H, et al: Valproate in primary psychiatric disorders, in Use of Anticonvulsants in Psychiatry. Edited by McElroy S, Pope H. Clifton, NJ, Oxford Health Care, 1988, pp 25–42

McKenna PJ, Kane JM, Parrish K: Psychotic syndromes in epilepsy. Am J Psychiatry 142:895–904, 1985

McNamara ME, Fogel BS: Anticonvulsant-responsive panic attacks with temporal lobe EEG abnormalities. J Neuropsychiatry Clin Neurosci 2:193–196, 1990

Meador KJ, Loring D, Moore E, et al: Comparative effects of phenobarbital, phenytoin, and valproate in healthy adults. Neurology 45:1494–1499, 1995

Mellers J, Toone B, Lishman A: A neuropsychological comparison of schizophrenia and schizophrenia-like psychosis of epilepsy. Psychol Med 30:325–335, 2000

Mendez MF, Doss RC, Taylor JL, et al: Depression in epilepsy: relationship to seizures and anticonvulsant therapy. J Nerv Ment Dis 181:444–447, 1993

Mendez MF, Taylor JL, Doss RC, et al: Depression in secondary epilepsy: relation to lesion laterality. J Neurol Neurosurg Psychiatry 57:232–233, 1994

Mungus D: Interictal behavior abnormality in temporal lobe epilepsy. Arch Gen Psychiatry 39:108–111, 1982

Neppe VM: Epileptic psychosis: a heterogeneous condition (letter). Epilepsia 27:634, 1986

Neppe VM, Tucker GJ: Modern perspectives on epilepsy in relation to psychiatry: behavioral disturbances of epilepsy. Hosp Community Psychiatry 39:389–396, 1988

Neppe VM, Tucker GJ, Wilensky AJ: Fundamentals of carbamazepine use in neuropsychiatry. J Clin Psychiatry 49 (suppl 4):4–6, 1988

Neugebauer R, Weissman MM, Ouellette R, et al: Comorbidity of panic disorder and seizures: affinity or artifact? J Anxiety Disord 7:21–35, 1993

Perez MM, Trimble MR: Epileptic psychosis: psychopathological comparison with process schizophrenia. Br J Psychiatry 137:245–249, 1980

Perucca E, Manzo L, Crema A: Pharmacokinetic interactions between antiepileptic and psychotropic drugs, in The Psychopharmacology of Epilepsy. Edited by Trimble M. Chichester, UK, Wiley, 1985, pp 95–105

Pincus JH, Tucker GJ: Behavioral Neurology, 3rd Edition. New York, Oxford University Press, 1985

Post RM, Uhde TW, Joffe RT, et al: Anticonvulsant drugs in psychiatric illness: new treatment alternatives and theoretical implications, in The Psychopharmacology of Epilepsy. Edited by Trimble MR. Chichester, UK, Wiley, 1985, pp 141–171

Preskorn SH, Fast GA: Tricyclic antidepressant-induced seizures and plasma drug concentration. J Clin Psychiatry 53: 160–162, 1992

Regan KJ, Banks GK, Beran RG: Therapeutic recreation programmes for children with epilepsy. Seizure 2:195–200, 1993

Robertson MM: Ictal and interictal depression in patients with epilepsy, in Aspects of Epilepsy and Psychiatry. Edited by Trimble MR, Bolwig TG. Chichester, UK, Wiley, 1986, pp 213–234

Robertson MM, Channon S, Baker J: Depressive symptomatology in a general hospital sample of outpatients with temporal lobe epilepsy: a controlled study. Epilepsia 35:771–777, 1994

Rodin EA: Psychomotor epilepsy and aggressive behavior. Arch Gen Psychiatry 28:210–213, 1973

Rodin EA, Schmaltz S: The Bear-Fedio personality inventory and temporal lobe epilepsy. Neurology 34:591–596, 1984

Rosenstein DL, Nelson JC, Jacobs SC, et al: Seizures associated with antidepressants: a review. J Clin Psychiatry 54:289–299, 1993

Roth M, Harper M: Temporal lobe epilepsy and the phobic anxiety-depersonalization syndrome, II: practical and theoretical considerations. Compr Psychiatry 3:215–226, 1962

Ryback R, Gardner E: Limbic system dysrhythmia: a diagnostic EEG procedure utilizing procaine activation. J Neuropsychiatry Clin Neurosci 3:321–329, 1991

Schoenenberger R, Tonasijevic M, Jha A, et al: Appropriateness of antiepileptic drug level monitoring. JAMA 274:1622–1626, 1995

Sengoku A, Yagi K, Seino M, et al: Risks of occurrence of psychoses in relation to the types of epilepsies and epileptic seizures. Folia Psychiatr Neurol Jpn 37:221–225, 1983

Septien L, Giroud M, Didi-Roy R, et al: Depression and partial epilepsy: relevance of laterality of the epileptic focus. Neurol Res 15:136–138, 1993

Shovron SD, Reynolds EH: The nature of epilepsy: evidence from studies of epidemiology, temporal patterns of seizures, prognosis and treatment, in What Is Epilepsy? Edited by Trimble MR, Reynolds EH. Edinburgh, UK, Churchill Livingstone, 1986, pp 36–45

Shukla S, Godwin CD, Long LE, et al: Lithium-carbamazepine neurotoxicity and risk factors. Am J Psychiatry 141:1604–1606, 1984

Sillanpaa M, Camfield P, Camfield C: Predicting long-term outcome of childhood epilepsy in Nova Scotia, Canada and Turku, Finland. Arch Neurol 52:589–592, 1995

Silver JM, Hales RE, Yudofsky SC: Psychopharmacology of depression in neurologic disorders. J Clin Psychiatry 51:33–39, 1990

Slater E, Beard AW, Glithero E: The schizophrenia-like psychoses of epilepsy. Br J Psychiatry 109:95–150, 1963

Sloviter RS, Tamminga CA: Cortex, VII: the hippocampus in epilepsy (letter). Am J Psychiatry 152:659, 1995

Spitz MC: Panic disorder in seizure patients: a diagnostic pitfall. Epilepsia 32:33–38, 1991

Stark-Adamec C, Adamec RE, Graham JM, et al: Complexities in the complex partial seizures personality controversy. Psychiatr J Univ Ott 10:231–236, 1985

Stevens JR: Interictal clinical manifestations of complex partial seizures, in Advances in Neurology. Edited by Penry JK, Daly DD. New York, Raven, 1975, pp 85–107

Strauss E, Wada J, Moll A: Depression in male and female subjects with complex partial seizures. Arch Neurol 49:391–392, 1992

Szatmari P: Some methodologic criteria for studies in developmental neuropsychiatry. Psychiatr Dev 3:153–170, 1985

Temkin O: The Falling Sickness, 2nd Edition. Baltimore, MD, Johns Hopkins University Press, 1979

Thomas P, Zifkin B, Migneco O, et al: Nonconvulsive status epilepticus of frontal origin. Neurology 52:1174–1183, 1999

Toone BK, Garralda ME, Ron MA: The psychoses of epilepsy and the functional psychoses: a clinical and phenomenological comparison. Br J Psychiatry 141:256–261, 1982

Varney NR, Garvey MJ, Cook BL, et al: Identification of treatment-resistant depressives who respond favorably to carbamazepine. Ann Clin Psychiatry 5:117–122, 1993

Victoroff JI, Benson F, Grafton ST, et al: Depression in complex partial seizures. Arch Neurol 51:155–163, 1994

Waxman SG, Geschwind N: The interictal behavior syndrome of temporal lobe epilepsy. Arch Gen Psychiatry 32:1580–1586, 1975

Weilburg JB, Schacter S, Worth J, et al: EEG abnormalities in patients with atypical panic attacks. J Clin Psychiatry 56:358–362, 1995

Wilensky AJ, Neppe VM: Acute interictal psychoses in epileptic patients (letter). Epilepsia 27:634, 1986

Zimmerman AW: Hormones and epilepsy. Neurol Clin 4:853–861, 1986

Zwil AS, Pelchat RJ: ECT in the treatment of patients with neurological and somatic disease. Int J Psychiatry Med 24:1–29, 1994

Neuropsychiatric Aspects of Sleep and Sleep Disorders

Max Hirshkowitz, Ph.D., A.B.S.M.

The most fundamental concept for understanding sleep is realizing that sleep is a brain process. Furthermore, it is not one process. There are several sleep states, each having distinctly different neuronal generators, regulatory mechanisms, and electroencephalographic correlates. Moreover, some of the sleep processes involve cortical activation. Thus, at times sleep is active rather than passive (Chase 1972; Kleitman 1972).

The first continuous overnight electroencephalographic recordings in humans were published by Loomis et al. (1937). Using the tracings from their giant 8-foot-long drum polygraph, they developed a sleep stage classification system (stages A, B, C, D, and E) and graphically illustrated sleep stages in a manner remarkably similar to that currently used. They defined sleep stages according to sleep electroencephalogram (EEG) frequency bands, including beta activity (>13 Hz), sleep spindles (bursts of 12–14 Hz), alpha rhythm (8–13 Hz, sometimes slower), theta rhythm (4–7 Hz, more common in adolescents than adults), sawtooth theta waves (4–7 Hz, with notched appearance), delta rhythm (<4 Hz), and slow waves (≤2 Hz).

The next major milestone was Eugene Aserinsky's discovery of periodic electrooculogram (EOG) activity episodes during sleep. These activity episodes occurred approximately every 90–120 minutes. At first called jerky eye movements (JEMs), the phenomenon was renamed rapid eye movement (REM) sleep, reportedly by William C. Dement (a medical student at that time). Subsequent studies revealed that individuals awakened from REM sleep reported dreaming on 20 of the 27 instances (Aserinsky and Kleitman 1953).

The discovery of a connection between REM sleep and dreaming generated tremendous excitement in the psychiatric community. Freud had characterized dreams as "the royal road to the unconscious" (Freud 1950). The sleep EEG-EOG recording technique held promise as an objective way to explore the mysteries of the unconscious mind. Hundreds of studies attempted to exploit this paradigm; however, no unified "dream theory" emerged. Many of the concepts forwarded by Freud were verified (for example, daytime residue), whereas others were not. Modern theoretical framework varies widely. The neurophysiologically grounded "activation-synthesis hypothesis" casts dreams as epiphenomena arising from the cortex making its best attempt to interpret random subcortical activation. By contrast, the cognitive theories consider dreaming an extension of daytime thought, albeit governed by a different grammar and looser rules (Foulkes 1982; Hobson and McCarley 1977).

In the late 1950s, Michel Jouvet introduced the concept that REM sleep was a third state of consciousness and not just another component of the basic rest activity cycle (BRAC) (Jouvet et al. 1959). He observed postural changes in the cat associated with different states of sleep, and using electromyographic recordings he found muscle atonia accompanying REM sleep in normal animals. This discovery of "functional paralysis" using electromyographic recording was the final step toward development of what is now standard recording practice. The final transition step that helped launch modern sleep research was the development and publication of *A Manual of Standardized Terminology, Techniques and Scoring System for Sleep Stages of Human Subjects* (Rechtschaffen and Kales 1968).

Physiology of Normal Human Sleep

Stages of Sleep

In humans, sleep stages are differentiated on the basis of activity occurring in central (C3 or C4) and occipital (O3 or O4) EEGs, right and left eye EOGs (recorded from the outer canthi), and submental electromyograms (EMGs). Traditional sleep recordings were paper polygraphic tracings usually made at a chart speed of 10 mm/second. The resulting polysomnogram (PSG) represented each 30 seconds of recording (1 epoch) as one polygraph page. It is for this reason that standard practice was designed to classify each 30-second epoch as either awake or one or another of the stages of sleep. The practice of epoch classification according to sleep stage continues even though computerized polygraph systems allow page resizing and temporal resolution alteration (Rechtschaffen and Kales 1968).

Stage W (also called wakefulness or stage 0), is characterized by an EEG containing predominantly alpha activity and/or low-voltage, mixed-frequency activity. Muscle activity is fairly high, and both rapid and slow eye movements may occur. The sleep-onset epoch is defined when the duration of alpha activity decreases below 50% of an epoch and/or a vertex wave, a K complex, a sleep spindle, or delta activity occurs. The K complex is a high-voltage biphasic slow or sharply contoured wave that begins with a negative component and is followed by a positive component. The sleep spindle is a burst of 11.5–16 Hz waves with a duration greater than 0.5 seconds. If a sleep spindle or K complex occurs and high-amplitude (75 µV or greater) delta electroencephalographic activity occupies less than 20% of an epoch, Stage II is scored. If there is 20%–50% delta activity, Stage III is designated, and if there is more than 50% delta activity the epoch is classified as sleep Stage IV. Stage I is an intermediate, non-alpha state that has low-voltage, mixed-frequency electroencephalographic activity that is a deltaless, spindleless stage that does not have K complexes. Rapid eye movements and muscle atonia accompanying stage 1 EEG define REM sleep. Sawtooth theta is another common electroencephalographic feature of REM

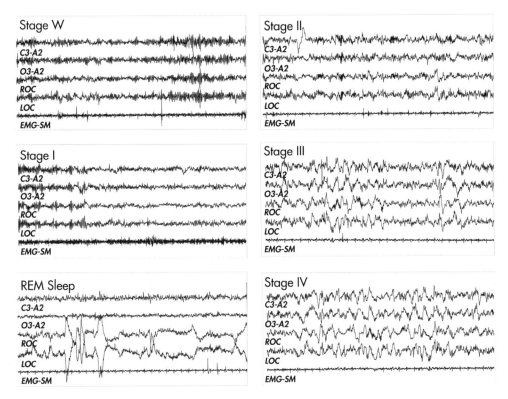

FIGURE 10–1. Polysomnographic recordings of the stages of sleep.

TABLE 10–1. Comparison of NREM and REM sleep activity

Physiologic measure	NREM sleep	REM sleep
Heart and breathing rate	Regular, slow	Variable
Oxygen consumption	Low	High
Cerebral blood flow	Low	High
Penile blood flow (erections)	Absent	Present
Vaginal blood flow and uterine activity	Low	Increased
Breathing response to O_2	Similar to awake	Similar to awake
Breathing response to CO_2	Similar to awake	Depressed
Electrodermal activity	Present, active	Absent
Temperature regulation	Homeothermic	Poikilothermic
Mental activity	Thoughtlike	Dreamlike

Note. REM=rapid eye movement; NREM=non–rapid eye movement.

sleep. Figure 10–1 shows an example of each stage.

Stages I, II, III, and IV are sometimes collectively referred to as non-REM (NREM) sleep. Stages III and IV are often combined and called slow-wave sleep. NREM and REM sleep differ for a wide variety of physiological measures (Table 10–1).

Normal Sleep Pattern: Generalizations

Figure 10–2 shows the nightly percentages for each stage. Sleeping for the first

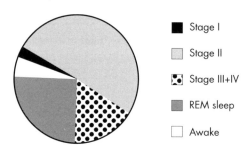

FIGURE 10–2. Sleep stage percentages in a healthy young adult.

time in a new environment (for example, a sleep laboratory) is usually associated with delayed sleep onset, general disruption, and decreased percentages of REM and/or slow-wave sleep. This adaptation-related phenomenon is termed the *first-night effect*. Nonetheless, age-specific normative values have been derived empirically for both first and succeeding nights. Such data are useful for clinical sleep assessments (Hirshkowitz et al. 1992; Roffwarg et al. 1966; Williams et al. 1974).

Sleep architecture refers to the progression and continuity of sleep through a given night. Figure 10–3 is a graphical representation of a typical night with normal sleep architecture in a healthy young adult. The following five generalizations can be made about sleep architecture: 1) sleep is entered through NREM sleep; 2) NREM and REM sleep alternate approximately every 90 minutes; 3) slow-wave sleep predominates in the first third of the night; 4) REM sleep predominates in the last third of the night; and 5) REM sleep occurs in 4–6 discrete episodes each night, with episodes generally being longer later in the sleep period.

Sleep pattern changes occur across the lifespan; the most global change is the gradual decline in overall total sleep time. REM sleep percentage (of total sleep time) decreases from birth to adolescence and then stabilizes at 20%–25%; however,

some additional decline may occur after age 65. By contrast, slow-wave sleep begins to decline after adolescence and continues that trend with age, disappearing completely in some elderly individuals. Aging, especially after middle age, is associated with greater wakefulness intermixed with sleep (fragmentation) and increased incidence of sleep-related breathing and movement disorders. Figure 10–4 shows changes in sleep stage composition from adulthood to old age.

Mechanisms Regulating Sleep

There are three basic factors involved in the general coordination of sleep and wakefulness: 1) autonomic nervous system balance, 2) homeostatic sleep drive, and 3) circadian rhythms (Hirshkowitz et al. 1997).

Autonomic Nervous System Balance

In general, sleep depends on decreasing sympathetic activation and increasing parasympathetic balance. Consequently, activities and influences that increase sympathetic outflow have the potential to disturb sleep. It does not matter whether the cause of sympathetic activation is exogenous or endogenous. That is, ingesting stimulants before bedtime (exogenous) and anxious rumination when trying to sleep (endogenous) work via similar autonomic mechanisms.

Another property of autonomic activation is that it commences rapidly but dissipates slowly. Rituals are often helpful during the presleep period to promote progressive relaxation and gradual reorientation away from daytime stressors and toward nocturnal tranquility. In children who sleep well, elaborate presleep rituals are common. Such rituals may include bedtime stories, a light

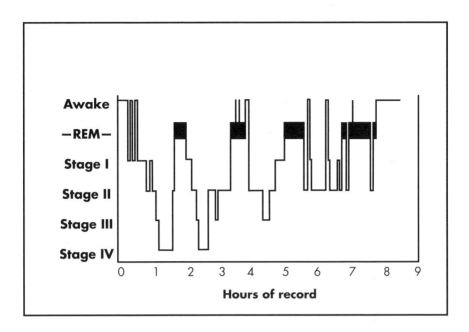

FIGURE 10–3. Sleep stage histogram for a healthy young adult.

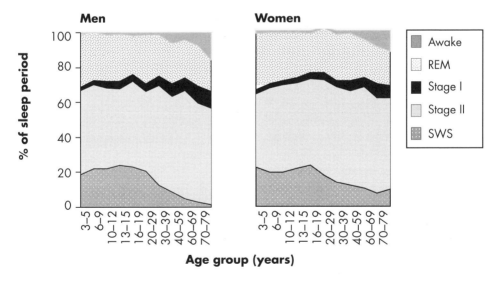

FIGURE 10–4. Sleep macroarchitecture (stages) as a function of age.
SWS = slow-wave sleep.

snack, teeth brushing, prayers, and having a favorite stuffed animal, toy, pillow, and blanket. The latter act as sleep-onset association stimuli and likely also play a role in respondent conditioning.

Autonomic activities are susceptible to classical conditioning. Pavlov was able to condition a dog to salivate by ringing a bell that had been paired with the presentation of food (which automatically produces canine salivation). Conditioning sleep onset to the stimulus properties surrounding it is therefore possible. The bed can become a conditioned stimulus for falling asleep, or in some cases it can become a cue for becoming aroused and alert (as in psychophysiological insomnia). Similarly, if a parent becomes the infant's conditioned stimulus for sleep onset, the parent may find himself or herself having to rock the baby back to sleep at any and all times of the night.

Homeostatic Sleep Drive

In general, the longer an individual remains awake, the sleepier he or she becomes. Such are the dynamics of sleep debt. If one attempts continuous, uninterrupted prolonged wakefulness, sleep eventually becomes irresistible.

Sleep deprivation studies explore changes resulting from stretching the homeostatic mechanism beyond its normal limits. Such studies ultimately hope to gain insight into the role or function of sleep by examining deficits produced by its loss. Sleep loss not only increases sleepiness, it adversely affects a variety of coping mechanisms. Sleep-deprived individuals become irritable and easily frustrated. As sleep deprivation continues, attention becomes impaired and performance lapses occur on tasks that challenge the ability to remain vigilant. Psychomotor impairment may occur, and mood suffers. Longer-term sleep deprivation can, in some individuals, produce hallucinations and on rare occasions seizures. After 72 hours of total sleep deprivation, executive function may deteriorate. Some individuals and most children lose their impulse control and suffer attention deficits when sleepy (Binks et al. 1999; Dinges 1992; Horne 1988).

However, in your own experience you may have noticed that during an extended wakeful vigil, sleepiness waxes and wanes.

Sometimes after staying up all night, the chronobiological self-abuser will note a surge of energy at daybreak. This indicates the presence of another sleep-wake mechanism: the circadian rhythm.

Circadian Rhythms

An approximate daylong or 24-hour rhythm is called a circadian rhythm (from the Latin *circa*, around + *dias*, day). There are many circadian rhythms; however, the one that regulates the sleep-wake cycle is superimposed on the homeostatic mechanisms. The biological clock believed to regulate the sleep-wake circadian rhythm is located in the suprachiasmatic nucleus (SCN). SCN firing patterns oscillate in concert and persist even in isole preparations (in vitro). Because the daily core body temperature cycle is entrained to this sleep-wake oscillator, the temperature cycle is commonly used as a marker of circadian rhythm. Lack of synchrony between scheduled bedtime and the sleepiness biological rhythm could mean less than optimal sleep and/or less than optimal daytime alertness (some degree of daytime drowsiness) (Aschoff 1965; Borbely and Achermann 1992; Moore-Ede et al. 1982).

Sleep in Patients With Psychiatric Conditions

Thirty-five percent of patients seen in sleep disorders centers with a chief complaint of insomnia had a psychiatric disorder (Coleman et al. 1982). Half of these patients had a major depressive disorder (MDD). Moreover, 90% of patients with MDD have insomnia (Reynolds and Kupfer 1987). Sleep problems are a risk factor (or marker) for worsening or recurrence of depression episodes. Sleep disturbances identified using electroencephalographic criteria in MDD include

1) generalized sleep disturbance (increase sleep latency, increased nocturnal awakenings, and early-morning awakenings), 2) slow-wave sleep decrease in the first NREM-REM cycle with delta activity shifts to the second NREM period, 3) latency to REM sleep shortened, 4) REM sleep occurring earlier in the night, and 5) REM density increase (especially early in the night). Selective REM sleep deprivation alleviates depression. Furthermore, this antidepressant action can persist for several days or more. Interestingly, most antidepressant medications suppress REM sleep (including selective serotonin reuptake inhibitors, tricyclic antidepressants, and monoamine oxidase inhibitors). Arecoline (a cholinergic agonist) infusion will induce REM sleep in depressed patients, and scopolamine withdrawal mimics depression in normal subjects (including electroencephalographic sleep changes). These data support the cholinergic-aminergic imbalance theory of major depression. Although it still holds that any drug capable of suppressing REM sleep has potential antidepressant properties, a couple of newer antidepressants do not suppress REM sleep (i.e., bupropion and nefazodone). Thus, a piece is missing from the theory. Restated, REM suppression is sufficient but not necessary for antidepressant action (Benca et al. 1992; Ford and Kamerow 1989; Hirshkowitz, in press; Vogel et al. 1980).

Patients with *mania* and *hypomania* seldom complain of sleep problems even though they sleep only a short time (2–4 hours per night), have very prolonged latency to sleep, and sometimes have reduced slow-wave sleep. Patients with *schizophrenia* have no consistent electroencephalographic sleep changes except that they do not have REM sleep rebound in response to REM sleep deprivation. The only other consistent finding is that patients with schizophrenia frequently deny having slept even though sleep appears normal on the EEG-EOG-EMG. Patients with *anxiety* and *personality* disorders often have sleep-onset and sleep-maintenance insomnia (Culebras 1996; Joseph et al. 1989; Zarcone 1989).

Sleep Disorders Overview and Classification Systems

Several classification systems have been developed to categorize sleep disorders, including the International Classification of Diseases (ICD), the Diagnostic and Statistical Manual of Mental Disorders (DSM), and the International Classification of Sleep Disorders (ICSD). The most complete nosology is ICSD (American Sleep Disorders Association 1997; see also Yudofsky and Hales 2002, p. 704), which details 84 individual sleep disorders and is organized into four sections: dyssomnias, parasomnias, sleep disorders associated with medical and psychiatric disorders, and proposed sleep disorders.

For instructional purposes, however, it is useful to consider sleep disorders categorized according to presenting complaint; that is, insomnia (disorders of initiating or maintaining sleep), hypersomnia (disorders of excessive sleepiness), and parasomnias (disorders of arousal). The national cooperative study (Coleman et al. 1982) of patients ($N = 5,000$) seen in accredited sleep disorders centers found that 31% of patients had insomnias, 51% had hypersomnias, and 15% had parasomnias. In addition, 3% of patients had disorders of the sleep-wake schedule (circadian dysrhythmia).

Insomnia

According to DSM-IV (American Psychiatric Association 1994), insomnia is diffi-

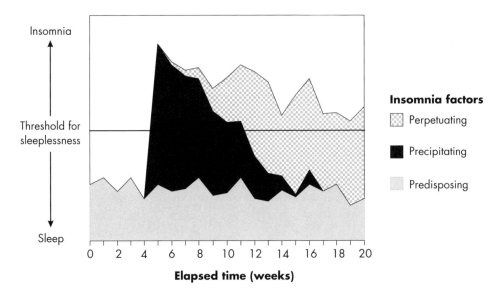

FIGURE 10–5. Spielman's dynamic model of insomnia.
Source. Adapted from Spielman et al. 1987a.

culty initiating sleep or maintaining sleep, or experiencing nonrestorative sleep for 1 month or more. The insomnia or resulting sleepiness must cause clinically significant impairment or distress. To be considered primary insomnia, the etiology of the insomnia must not be rooted in psychiatric conditions, parasomnias, substance use or abuse, sleep-disordered breathing, or circadian rhythm disorders. However, insomnia usually has multiple and overlapping causes, and ruling in the assorted contributors is more helpful clinically for devising a treatment plan than is ruling out factors for the sake of diagnostic purity.

Essentially, insomnia is a symptom. It is neither a disease nor a specific condition. Insomnia can accompany a wide variety of sleep, medical, and psychiatric disorders. When possible, the goal is to treat the cause(s); however, in some cases, symptomatic relief is desirable while therapeutic modalities progress. Approximately a third of the American population has several serious bouts of insomnia yearly, and

in 9% insomnia is a chronic condition. More than 40% of individuals with chronic insomnia will self-medicate with over-the-counter drugs, alcohol, or both (Gallup Organization 1991; Mellinger et al. 1985).

Spielman et al. (1987a) conceptualized insomnia in terms of the dynamic model depicted in Figure 10–5. In this model, an individual's generalized threshold for sleeplessness acts in conjunction with three factors: 1) predisposition, 2) precipitating event, and 3) perpetuating factors. In the preclinical state, every person falls within some range from being a very *sound sleeper* to a *light sleeper*. A light sleeper may have a lower sleeplessness threshold such that even minor changes in routine or mildly disquieting daytime events will trigger insomnia. The sound sleeper may be conceptualized as having a high threshold for sleeplessness and thus has no difficulty sleeping even in novel or environmentally adverse conditions. Nonetheless, a precipitating factor may usher in an episode of insomnia regardless of the individual trait disposition for sound or light sleep. Precipitating factors can vary widely. Examples include job stress, relocation, anxiety about taking an examination, undergoing a tax audit, being sued, development of a medical condition, change in medication, separation or divorce, or grief reaction. Over time, the impact of most of these factors will wane and one would expect the sleeplessness to follow suit; however, the insomnia often persists. The persistence of sleeplessness, notwithstanding diminution of the influence of the original causes (for example, having taken the examination and passed), is considered to result from perpetuating factors. Examples of perpetuating factors are ongoing use of alcohol as a sleep aid, developing habits that are inconsistent with good quality sleep (e.g., watching television in bed), or having a grief reaction evolve into depression. In some cases, the bed and bedroom become conditioned stimuli for wakefulness, and psychophysiological insomnia is the perpetuating factor.

Psychophysiological Insomnia

The patient with psychophysiological insomnia has developed a conditioned arousal associated with the thought of sleeping. Objects related to sleep (e.g., the bed, the bedroom) likewise have become conditioned stimuli that evoke insomnia. Daytime adaptation is usually good. Work and relationships are satisfying; however, there can be extreme tiredness and the individual can become desperate. By contrast, daytime adaptation in patients with psychiatrically related insomnia is often impaired. Other features of psychophysiological insomnia include 1) excessive worry about not being able to sleep, 2) trying too hard to sleep, 3) rumination, inability to clear one's mind while trying to sleep, 4) increased muscle tension when getting into bed, 5) other somatic manifestations

of anxiety, 6) ability to fall asleep when not trying to (e.g., while watching television), and 7) sleeping better away from one's own bedroom (including in the sleep laboratory). In one sense, the individual has developed a performance anxiety concerning the ability to sleep and autonomic nervous system conditioning reinforces the situation. Stimulus control therapy is well suited for treating psychophysiological insomnia (American Sleep Disorders Association 1997; Hauri and Fisher 1986). (See the section "Insomnia Treatment Options," Behavioral Treatments, later in this chapter.)

Drug and Alcohol Dependence

Use of alcohol and hypnotic drugs initially promotes sleep onset because of the sedating properties of these substances. Sleep later in the night, however, is fragmented by arousals. As tolerance develops to the alcohol, greater amounts are needed to sustain the effects. Furthermore, during withdrawal or after tolerance has developed, the sleep disturbance can rebound to a level more severe than the initial problem.

Barbiturates and, later, benzodiazepines represent the most commonly used prescription medications for insomnia during the twentieth century. Both have potential for abuse and dependency, especially those producing euphoria. Except in rare cases, sedative-hypnotic medicines are not recommended for long-term use. Benzodiazepines that alter sleep architecture and produce rebound insomnia on withdrawal tend to be habit-forming and can act as a perpetuating factor for insomnia.

Restless Legs Syndrome and Periodic Limb Movement Disorder

Restless legs syndrome is characterized by the irresistible urge to move the legs when at rest or while trying to fall asleep.

Patients often report crawling feelings in their legs. Moving the legs or walking helps alleviate the discomfort.

Another type of leg movement disorder associated with insomnia is periodic limb movement disorder (PLMD). PLMD involves brief, stereotypic, repetitive, nonepileptiform movements of the limbs, usually the legs. It occurs primarily in NREM sleep and involves an extension of the big toe. Partial flexion of the ankle, knee, and hip may also occur. The leg movements are frequently associated with brief arousals from sleep. The prevalence of PLMD increases with age and can occur in association with folate deficiency, renal disease, anemia, and the use of antidepressants (American Sleep Disorders Association 1997; Ekbom 1960; Lugaresi et al. 1986; Walters 1995; Walters et al. 1991).

Sleep-State Misperception

Most individuals are under the mistaken impression that mental activity necessarily ceases during sleep. However, most people readily acknowledge dreaming and understand that dreams constitute mental activity. Under normal circumstances sleep and unconsciousness are coupled, but they can dissociate. Anxiety can provoke sleep-state misperception, and ruminative worry about not sleeping adds fuel to the fire (American Sleep Disorders Association 1997; Carskadon et al. 1976).

Often a psychoeducational approach that attempts to explain the dissociability between physiological brain correlates of sleep and the perception of sleep is helpful.

Sleep-Disordered Breathing

Sleep-related breathing disorders are more commonly associated with excessive daytime sleepiness than with insomnia. In some individuals, particularly if the breathing disorder is mild or at an early stage of development, the predominant complaint will be insomnia.

Idiopathic Insomnia

Persons with idiopathic insomnia have a lifelong inability to obtain adequate sleep. The insomnia must predate any psychiatric condition, and other etiologies must be ruled out or treated, including psychophysiological insomnia, environmental sleep disturbances, and practices that would constitute poor sleep hygiene. If the insomnia persists, then it is assumed that there is a defect in the neurologic mechanisms that govern the sleep-wake system. That is, the sleep homeostatic process is dysfunctional. Sleep restriction therapy may provide some benefit and will also give the clinician a clue to the limits of the patient's homeostatic process (see "Insomnia Treatment Options," sleep restriction therapy, later in this chapter). Unfortunately, patients with idiopathic insomnia never slept well and will likely never have normal sleep. Although it is controversial, this group may require long-term pharmacotherapeutic intervention.

Circadian Rhythm Dyssomnias

In an optimal schedule, hours in bed must coincide with the sleepy phase of the circadian cycle. *Advanced sleep phase* is when the circadian rhythm cycle is shifted earlier. Therefore, the sleepiness cycle is advanced with respect to clock time. Individuals with advanced sleep phase are drowsy in the evening, want to retire to bed earlier, awaken earlier, and are more alert in the early morning. Individuals with this pattern of advanced sleep phase are sometimes called "larks." By contrast, the biological clock may run slow or be shifted later than the desired schedule. This produces a *phase delay* in the sleepiness-alertness cycle. Individuals with delayed sleep phase are more alert in the

TABLE 10–2.   Sleep hygiene and affected systems

Presumed mechanism of action	Sleep hygiene recommendation
Strengthens circadian rhythm	Maintain a regular sleep-wake schedule
	Get a steady daily amount of exercise
Avoids endogenous ANS activation	Do not try to fall asleep, let sleep come
	A light snack before bedtime may be helpful
Avoids exogenous ANS activation	Insulate the bedroom against loud noises
	Make sure bedroom is not excessively warm
	Do not eat a heavy meal close to bedtime
	Avoid caffeine in the evening
	Quit smoking or avoid smoking near bedtime
Avoids developing dependence	Avoid ongoing use of sleeping pills as a sleep aid
	Avoid ongoing use of alcohol as a sleep aid

Note.   ANS = autonomic nervous system.

evening and early nighttime, stay up later, and are more tired in the morning. These individuals are referred to as "owls" (Moore-Ede et al. 1982; Zammit 1997).

In the past, chronotherapy was used to reentrain the circadian rhythm; however, it has largely been replaced by bright light therapy (see Behavioral Treatments, below) (Czeisler et al. 1989).

Insomnia Treatment Options

Behavioral Treatments

Behavioral treatments for insomnia include universal sleep hygiene, relaxation training, stimulus control therapy, sleep restriction therapy, and bright light therapy.

Universal sleep hygiene.   Many individuals with insomnia, regardless of the underlying cause, make things worse with poor sleep hygiene. Essentially, they have developed bad habits with respect to sleep. These habits may operate through autonomic, homeostatic, or circadian mechanisms. When these habits are a primary etiology, inadequate sleep hygiene can be diagnosed. Universal sleep hygiene essentially involves recommending that the individual promote sleep-enhancing

habits and avoid sleep-destroying behaviors. Table 10–2 lists some recommendations to improve sleep hygiene.

Relaxation training.   This type of behavioral therapy takes many forms, including progressive relaxation, breathing exercises (or yoga), biofeedback, and guided visualization. The goal of relaxation training is twofold. Primarily, it provides a systematic technique for reducing tension and stress. Thus, it acts through the autonomic mechanisms that can enhance or impede sleep. Additionally, however, it provides a distraction such that the individual thinks about something other than his or her inability to sleep. The therapy must be properly performed and overlearned before it is applied. The clinician should monitor the progress during training to ensure that the technique is performed correctly and to judge when it is time for it to be applied in the sleepless bed (Espie et al. 1989; Lichstein and Riedel 1994).

Stimulus control therapy.   For individuals with psychophysiological insomnia, stimulus control directly addresses the underlying autonomic conditioning. Secondarily it arranges homeostatic and circadian factors so that they will work in concert with attempts to recondition sleep onset. Stimulus control therapy directives attempt to enhance stimulus cues for sleeping and diminish bedroom stimulus associations with sleeplessness. The instructions are simple; however, following them consistently and keeping sleep diaries are the keys to success. The first rule is to go to bed only when sleepy. Second, use the bed only for sleeping. That is, in bed one should not eat, read, talk on the telephone, watch television, do paperwork, write letters, exercise, argue with one's spouse, or worry about things that happened in the past or are expected to happen in the future. If the individual is unable to sleep, rule three instructs him or her to get up, go to another room, and do something nonarousing until he or she becomes sleepy. One should not watch the clock; in fact, the clock should be hidden from view so that when nocturnal arousals occur the time is not known. Nonetheless, if one feels that he or she has been unable to sleep for more than a few minutes, getting out of bed avoids increasing frustration with the inability to sleep. Ultimately, the goal is to associate the bed and bedroom with rapid sleep onset (Bootzin 1972, 1977).

Sleep restriction therapy.   Sleep restriction therapy is designed to enhance sleep through the homeostatic mechanism. The initial step is to have a patient keep a diary of bedtimes, arising times, and the amount of time spent actually sleeping. From this, the total sleep time can be estimated. Sometimes, patients will spend an inordinate amount of time in bed in an attempt to increase their sleep time, only to find their sleep becoming more and more fragmented. I have seen patients who spend 11 hours in bed to attain a reported 6 hours of sleep. The second step in sleep restriction therapy is to compress the sleep schedule to the reported

sleep time. Thus, in a patient reporting 6 hours of sleep in an 11-hour total bedtime, I set arising time at 6 hours after retiring time. It should be noted that restricting bedtime schedule to less than four hours per night is not advised. In addition, patients must be advised that they will likely be very sleepy the next day and must exercise extreme care, especially when performing potentially dangerous actions (e.g., driving). Sleep at other times during the day must be avoided, except in elderly persons, who may take a 30-minute nap. Each night, the amount of time spent asleep is reported and the clinician calculates sleep efficiency (the ratio of total sleep time to total bed time). If the patient attains a five-night moving average sleep efficiency of 0.85 or greater, time in bed is increased by 15 minutes (some clinicians use a three-night average). In this manner, time awake in bed is controlled while time asleep gradually and steadily increases. Moreover, when the sleep efficiency plateaus, the clinician has an empirical estimate of the patient's homeostatic drive limit and can better judge if idiopathic insomnia is present. Nonetheless, greater sleep consolidation is achieved and the patient spends less time lying in bed becoming frustrated by his or her inability to sleep (Morin et al. 1994; Spielman et al. 1987b).

Bright light therapy.   Bright light appears to be the critical factor in controlling the biological clock. With precise timing of bright light exposure, the biological clock may be phase advanced, phase delayed, or even stopped and reset. In general, bright light in the evening will delay the sleep phase, and bright light in the morning will advance the sleep phase. Thus, the phase-delayed "owl" who stays up surfing the Internet until 2:00 A.M. with his or her face less than a meter from a 19-inch video monitor is probably further phase delaying the sleep-wake cycle. What the phase-delaying "owl" needs to do is avoid bright light in the evening and replace it with bright light in the early morning (Czeisler et al. 1989; Zammit 1997).

Drug Treatments

Specific drug therapies have been applied for PLMD and restless legs syndrome. Currently, the most popular pharmacotherapy is with the dopaminergic agents carbidopa-levodopa, pramipexole, and ropinirole. However, clonazepam and narcotics are in common use and can be effective (Chockroverty 2000).

It should go without saying that antidepressants are indicated if depression is comorbid. Most antidepressants, however, alter sleep architecture and exacerbate the leg movement disorders. Tricyclic antidepressants and selective serotonin reuptake inhibitors suppress REM sleep (especially clomipramine and amitriptyline). Amitriptyline, doxepin, and trazodone have strong sedative properties. Most tricyclics increase slow-wave sleep, whereas serotonin reuptake inhibitors generally decrease or do not change slow-wave activity. Monoamine oxidase inhibitors are powerful REM-sleep suppressors and also diminish slow-wave sleep. By contrast, nefazodone and bupropion are not associated with decreased REM sleep (Hirshkowitz, in press).

The more general, nonspecific, drug-therapy approach to insomnia involves using sedative-hypnotic medications. The profile for an ideal hypnotic is shown in Table 10–3. Sleep-promoting substances have been used since antiquity (e.g., opium and alcohol), but in the 1860s chloral hydrate was formulated as a sleeping pill. In essence it represented alcohol in pill form, and it gained widespread acceptance. At the turn of the last century, barbiturates became available. As

TABLE 10–3. Profile for an ideal hypnotic

Desired effect	Parameter
Increase	Sleep efficiency
	Total sleep time
Decrease	Latency to sleep onset
	Wake after sleep onset time
	Number of awakenings
Remain unchanged	Sleep macroarchitecture (stages)
	Sleep microarchitecture
Avoid producing	Carryover—hangover
	Early morning rebound insomnia
	Withdrawal rebound insomnia
	Psychomotor impairment
	Cognitive impairment
	Dependency

strong partial γ-aminobutyric acid (GABA) agonists, barbiturates were very effective at producing sedation and immediately became popular, notwithstanding their toxic liability. Most of the barbiturates have a large REM sleep suppression effect and a smaller slow-wave sleep suppression effect. Sleep latency decreases, sleep efficiency increases, and there are fewer awakenings after sleep onset. The toxic liability, however, spurred further development, and in the 1960s a new class of GABA partial agonists, the benzodiazepines, largely replaced barbiturates for treating insomnia. Their wide dose safety range, minimum side effects, and milder abstinence syndrome on withdrawal made benzodiazepines far more attractive than previously available medications. Perhaps the most clinically salient advantage of benzodiazepines compared with barbiturates was the increased dose-range margin of safety (that is, a much wider effective dose to lethal dose [ED:LD] ratio). The safety range for toxicity is critically important, because many patients with MDD present with a complaint of insomnia. Barbiturates have a long legacy of lethality. Nonetheless, even with benzodiazepines, long-term use is considered problematic.

Pharmaceutical companies developed a wide variety of benzodiazepines, differing in speed of onset, half-life, and presence or absence of active metabolites. Benzodiazepines are very effective at decreasing sleep latency, increasing sleep efficiency, and decreasing awakenings after sleep onset; however, they also alter sleep macroarchitecture with suppression of slow-wave sleep and, to a lesser extent, REM sleep. Benzodiazepines can powerfully increase sleep spindle activity. Longer-acting benzodiazepines (especially those with active metabolites) often have carry-over effects (hangover) in terms of both residual sedation and diminished psychomotor performance. The efficacy of shorter-acting benzodiazepines is marred by early morning rebound and withdrawal rebound insomnia.

Pharmaceutical development continued, and a class of more specific benzodiazepine receptor agonists was developed, cyclopyrrolones (zopiclone) and imadazopyridine (zolpidem) in the 1980s and pyrazolopyrimidine (zaleplon) in the 1990s. These further pharmacological strides have been made because the newer medications target specific GABA receptor subtypes. These hypnotics now dominate the market. These drugs are effective hypnotics and appear to produce fewer rebound problems. The newer drugs tend to have very rapid onset, be short acting, and have little or no effect on sleep macroarchitecture. Zolpidem and zaleplon are also associated with fewer side effects, most notably the lack of residual sedation (due to their short half-lives and nonactive metabolites). Amnesia, however, persists as a side effect (less in zaleplon than zolpidem, but present in both). There is evidence that memory effects may be related

to sleep induction (inasmuch as sleep itself produces amnesia). Consequently, it may not be possible to entirely eliminate amnesia as an undesirable effect of sleep-promoting substances (Morgan and Closs 1999; Shneerson 2000).

Current Recommendations

Short-term insomnia treatment recommendations include several areas of intervention. First, it is important to review and address any behaviors or habits that are counterproductive to a good night's sleep by initiating a sleep hygiene program. Next, if other factors are identified as contributory to perpetuating sleeplessness (for example, psychophysiological insomnia), they should be treated aggressively. If pharmacotherapy is intended, the lowest effective dose of a short-acting sedative-hypnotic should be used. Finally, treatment course should usually be less than 3 weeks in duration, and intermittent dosing is preferred.

Treatment is more difficult for chronic insomnia. First, the underlying condition(s), if present, that predispose the individual to sleeplessness must be identified and treated. For example, if underlying depression exists, treating only the insomnia is ill-advised. Similarly, any perpetuating factors (e.g., inadequate sleep hygiene, ongoing use of alcohol, conditioned insomnia) should be a main therapeutic target. In chronic insomnia it is important to improve sleep behaviorally as much as possible even if other treatments are planned. Thus, combined behavioral, psychological, and pharmacological treatment can be used concurrently.

Clinicians should be cautious when prescribing hypnotic medications for patient who are elderly; who have a history of heavy snoring; who have renal, hepatic, or pulmonary disease; or who are using concomitant psychoactive medications (especially depressants). Caution is also warranted when prescribing sedating drugs for patients who use alcohol regularly, have suicidal tendencies, or work in hazardous occupations. If a person needs to be able to become alert rapidly during their usual sleep period (for example, a physician on call), sedative-hypnotics are generally contraindicated unless they are ultra-short-acting. Sedative-hypnotic medications are clearly contraindicated during pregnancy and in patients who have sleep-disordered breathing or who use alcohol to excess.

Hypersomnia

Excessive sleepiness is a serious, debilitating, potentially life-threatening, noncommunicable condition. It affects not only the afflicted individuals but also their families and co-workers and the public at large. Sleepiness can be a consequence of insufficient sleep, disrupted sleep, or nonrestorative sleep. The sleep debt produced by insufficient sleep is cumulative. If one reduces sleep duration by 1–2 hours per night and continues this regimen for a week, sleepiness will reach pathological levels. When sleep debt is added to sleep disruption or nonrestorative sleep, there is increasing risk that an individual will lapse unexpectedly into sleep. Sleep onset in such circumstances characteristically occurs without warning. Sleepiness can be episodic and can occur as irresistible sleep attacks, can occur in the morning as sleep drunkenness, or be chronic. Fatigue, tiredness, and sleepiness are terms that are used by most people synonymously; however, one can be tired but not sleepy, sleepy but not tired, or sleepy and tired.

Sleep-Disordered Breathing

Sleep-disordered breathing includes disorders ranging from upper-airway resistance syndrome to severe obstructive sleep apnea. An episode of sleep apnea is defined as a cessation of breathing for 10 seconds or more during sleep. A reduction in breathing is termed *hypopnea*. These sleep-related breathing impairments are most often caused by airway obstruction; however, sometimes respiratory reduction results from central (brain stem) changes in ventilatory control, metabolic factors, or heart failure. Each sleep-disordered breathing event is classified as either *central, obstructive,* or *mixed.* Central apnea or hypopnea is the absence of breathing due to lack of respiratory effort. In obstructive events, respiratory effort continues but airflow stops due to reduction in or loss of airway patency. Mixed apnea or hypopnea episodes contain components of both, often beginning as central apnea and progressing to obstructive apnea.

Sleep-disordered breathing events may be accompanied by oxygen desaturation and cardiac arrhythmias. Clinical features associated with obstructive sleep apnea (the most common form of sleep-disordered breathing) include 1) excessive daytime sleepiness, 2) loud snoring with frequent awakenings, 3) awakening with choking and/or gasping for breath, 4) morning dry mouth, and 5) witnessed apnea. Predisposing factors include 1) being male, 2) reaching middle age, 3) obesity, 4) micrognathia or retrognathia and nasal pharyngeal abnormalities, and 5) hypothyroidism and acromegaly. Other features and comorbidities include sleep choking, morning headaches, nocturnal sweating, sleepwalking, sleep talking, nocturia, enuresis, impotence, memory impairment, impaired quality of life, depression, hearing loss, automatic behaviors, hypertension, polycythemia, and right-sided heart failure (Flemons and Tsai 1997; Guilleminault et al. 1988; Robinson and Guilleminault 1999).

Treatment

Many treatments are available for sleep-disordered breathing, including weight loss, positive airway pressure therapy, use of oral appliances, and surgery. Weight loss is difficult to achieve and maintain; therefore, it is recommended but not relied on (Fairbanks et al. 1987; Loube et al. 1999; Sanders 2000; Thorpy and Ledereich 1990).

Positive airway pressure. Currently, the most popular therapy is positive airway pressure. Positive airway pressure comes in three varieties: continuous, bilevel, and sleep-adjusting. Continuous positive airway pressure (CPAP) is the most common and represents the preferred treatment. It delivers fan-generated flow at a set pressure to the nares, usually via a nasal mask. In so doing it creates a "pneumatic splint" and thereby maintains airway patency. It is highly effective in most patients; however, it requires nightly utilization. Patients who have more severe sleep-disordered breathing or who are sleepier at baseline are the most compliant with this therapy.

Oral appliances. For patients who cannot tolerate positive airway pressure, other options include oral appliances or surgery. Oral appliances were developed to treat snoring and have also been found to be sometimes effective for upper-airway resistance syndrome and mild to moderate obstructive sleep apnea. Most appliances in current use either manipulate the position of the mandible, retain the tongue, or both. Breathing, although improved, may not reach satisfactory levels; therefore, follow-up sleep studies are needed.

Surgery. The earliest surgical intervention for severe obstructive sleep apnea was trachcostomy. There was little doubt that tracheostomy succeeded in creating an airway. Although it is no longer a preferred treatment, it remains a standard against which newer therapies are judged. The next generation of surgical intervention was uvulopalatopharyngoplasty (UPPP). Initial results indicated that this modification of the soft palate was effective. More recent studies have tempered the initial enthusiasm. Clinically significant improvement is attained with UPPP in approximately 50% of patients with sleep apnea. The soft palate surgeries are also sometimes performed using a laser. Nonetheless, predicting success is difficult, and complications may occur. Another surgical intervention includes maxillomandibular advancement. This procedure seems particularly effective in retrognathic patients or in patients with cephalometrics revealing compromised posterior airway space. Finally, the most recent anatomic alteration performed for sleep-disordered breathing, called somnoplasty, uses radiofrequency ablation.

Other treatments. Position-dependent sleep-disordered breathing, although rare, is sometimes encountered. Typically, breathing will be impaired when the patient sleeps supine. In such cases, tennis balls sewn onto or placed into pockets on the back of the nightshirt may prevent the patient from sleeping on his or her back. Finally, it would be a great advantage if a medication to treat sleep apnea were discovered. Methoxyprogesterone acetate was once thought to be helpful but is seldom used now. Similarly, tricyclic antidepressants (e.g., protriptyline) may decrease apnea severity by increasing upper-airway tone and/or reducing REM sleep (the sleep stage in which the worst sleep-disordered breathing usually occurs). Theophylline also reportedly reduces sleep-disordered breathing; however, further study is needed.

Narcolepsy

Narcolepsy is characterized by a tetrad of symptoms: 1) excessive daytime sleepiness, 2) cataplexy, 3) sleep paralysis, and 4) hypnagogic hallucinations. Patients with narcolepsy often have an abnormal sleep architecture in which REM sleep occurs soon after sleep onset both at night and during daytime naps. This, in connection with the symptom tetrad, makes narcolepsy appear to be a REM sleep intrusion syndrome, presumably resulting from dysfunction of REM sleep generator gating mechanisms. The features of the tetrad match REM sleep characteristics. The sleep paralysis is similar to the muscle atonia that occurs during REM sleep. The hypnagogic hallucinations are vivid "dreams" that occur while the patient is still conscious or partially conscious. However, not all patients have the full constellation of symptoms. Narcolepsy is estimated to afflict 10–60 individuals per 10,000. Symptoms commonly appear in the second decade of life. Strong emotions usually act as the "trigger" for cataplexy. Common emotional triggers include laughter and anger (Aldrich 1996; Fry 1998; Standards of Practice Committee 1994).

Treatment

In general, the ancillary symptoms of narcolepsy (cataplexy, sleep paralysis, and hypnagogia) are treated with REM-suppressing medications.

The excessive daytime sleepiness associated with narcolepsy presents a greater challenge. Stimulant medications are used palliatively to provide symptom relief. Until recently, methylphenidate was the usual first-line treatment, followed by amphetamines if it was ineffective. The introduction of modafinil, a nonstimulant somnolytic, provides clinicians with an alternative option for treating sleepiness in narcolepsy. Modafinil's benign side-effect profile makes it more attractive for long-term use than traditional stimulants.

Idiopathic Hypersomnia

Idiopathic hypersomnia is another disorder of excessive sleepiness; however, patients do not have the ancillary symptoms associated with narcolepsy. Unlike in narcolepsy, sleep is usually well preserved, and sleep efficiency remains high even with very extended sleep schedules (12 hours or more). Furthermore, the patient readily falls asleep if given an opportunity to nap the following day. The proportion of slow-wave sleep is often increased; however, the electroencephalographic sleep pattern is essentially the same as that seen in healthy individuals who are sleep deprived. Unlike a sleep-deprived individual, however, the sleep pattern continues in this profile even after several nights of extended sleep. As the name indicates, the etiology of idiopathic hypersomnia is not known; however, a central nervous system cause is presumed. Age at onset is characteristically between 15 and 30 years, and the dyssomnia becomes a lifelong problem. In addition to the prolonged, undisturbed, and unrefreshing sleep, idiopathic hypersomnia is associated with long nonrefreshing naps, difficulty awakening, sleep drunkenness, and automatic behaviors with amnesia. Other symptoms suggesting autonomic nervous system dysfunction, including migraine-like headaches, fainting spells, syncope, orthostatic hypotension, and Raynaud's-type phenomena with cold hands and feet, are typical (Aldrich 1996; Guilleminault and Pelayo 2000).

Treatment

The sleepiness is treated palliatively in a similar fashion to the approach used in narcolepsy. However, the stimulants are usually less effective than in narcolepsy, and prophylactic napping does not seem to be as beneficial. Modafinil has not been tested in patients with idiopathic hypersomnia. However, in pivotal clinical trials in the United States, modafinil was equally effective for patients with and without cataplexy who nonetheless were diagnosed with narcolepsy.

Parasomnia

Parasomnias are sometimes referred to as disorders of partial arousal. In general, the parasomnias are a large and diverse collection of sleep disorders characterized by physiological or behavioral phenomena that occur during or that are potentiated by sleep. One conceptual framework posits many parasomnias as overlapping or intrusion of one basic sleep-wake state into another (Figure 10–6). Wakefulness, NREM sleep, and REM sleep can be characterized as the three basic states that differ in their neurologic organization. In the awake state, both the body and brain are active, whereas in NREM sleep, both the body and brain are inactive. REM sleep involves an inactive body (atonic, in fact) and an active brain (capable of creating elaborate dream fantasies). Regional cerebral blood flow studies have confirmed increased brain activation during REM sleep. It certainly appears that in some parasomnias there are state boundary violations. For example, all of the arousal disorders (confusional arousals, sleepwalking, and sleep terrors) involve momentary or partial wakeful behaviors suddenly occurring in NREM (slow-wave) sleep. Similarly, isolated sleep paralysis is the persistence of REM sleep atonia into the wakefulness transition, whereas REM sleep behavior disorder is the failure of the mechanism creating paralytic atonia such that individuals literally act out their dreams (American Sleep Disorders Association 1997).

The nosologic classification for parasomnias has evolved over the years, and the system used in the multicenter cooperative study differed from today's nosology. Figure 10–7 shows recalculated percentages of occurrence of different parasomnias among patients seen at sleep disorders centers using the cooperative study data (Coleman et al. 1982). According to this study, the most commonly encountered parasomnias are secondary to nocturnal seizure activity (33.7%). After that, the most common conditions currently classified as parasomnias include sleepwalking, sleep terrors, sleep-related enuresis, nightmares, familial sleep paralysis, head banging (rhythmic movement disorder), bruxism, and other parasomnias.

Sleepwalking

Sleepwalking in its classic form is, as the name implies, a condition in which an individual arises from bed and ambulates without awakening. Sleepwalking individuals can engage in a variety of complex behaviors while unconscious. Sleepwalking usually occurs during slow-wave sleep and lies in the middle of a parasomnia continuum that ranges from confused arousal to sleep terror. Sleep deprivation and interruption of slow-wave sleep appear to exacerbate, or even provoke, sleepwalking in susceptible individuals. Sleepwalking episodes may range from sitting up and attempting to walk to conducting an involved sequence of semipurposeful actions. The sleepwalker can often successfully interact with the environment (for example, avoiding tripping over objects in his or her path). However, the sleepwalker will often interact with the environment inappropriately, which sometimes results in injury (for example, stepping out of an upstairs window or walking into the roadway). There are cases in which sleepwalkers have committed acts of violence. An individual who is

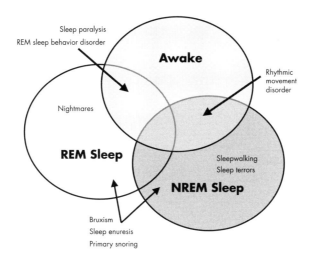

FIGURE 10–6. The relationship of common parasomnias to REM sleep, NREM sleep, and the awake state.

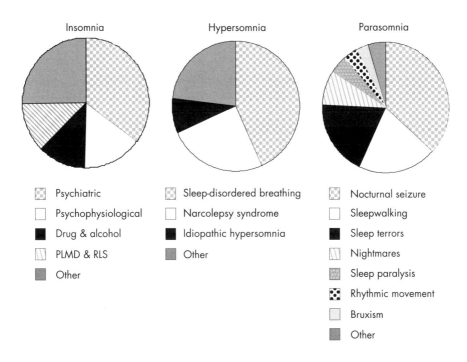

FIGURE 10–7. Proportions for the most common insomnias, hypersomnias, and parasomnias seen in sleep disorders centers.

PLMD = periodic limb movement disorder; RLS = restless legs syndrome.

Source. Adapted from Coleman et al. 1982.

sleepwalking is difficult to awaken. Once awake, the sleepwalker will usually appear confused. Sleepwalking in adults is rare,

has a familial pattern, and may occur as a primary parasomnia or secondary to another sleep disorder (for example, sleep apnea). By contrast, sleepwalking is very common in children, with peak prevalence between ages 4 and 8 years. After adolescence it usually disappears spontaneously. Nightly to weekly sleepwalking episodes associated with physical injury to the patient and others are considered severe (American Sleep Disorders Association 1997; Kales et al. 1966, 1980b).

Sleep Terrors

Sleep terror (sometimes called pavor nocturnus, incubus, or night terror) is characterized by a sudden arousal with intense fearfulness. It may begin with a piercing scream or cry. Autonomic and behavioral correlates of fright typically mark the experience. An individual experiencing a sleep terror usually sits up in bed, is unresponsive to stimuli, and if awakened is confused or disoriented. Vocalizations may occur, but they are usually incoherent. Notwithstanding the intensity of these events, amnesia for the episodes usually occurs. Like sleepwalking, these episodes usually arise from slow-wave sleep. Fever and withdrawal from central nervous system depressants can potentiate sleep terror episodes. Unlike nightmares in which an elaborate dream sequence unfolds, sleep terrors may be devoid of images or contain only fragments of very brief and frighteningly vivid but sometimes static images. A familial pattern has been reported. Like other slow-wave sleep parasomnias, sleep terrors can be provoked or exacerbated by sleep deprivation. Psychopathology is seldom associated with sleep terrors in children; however, a history of traumatic experience or frank psychiatric problems is often comorbid in adults with this disorder. Severity ranges from less than once per month to almost nightly occurrence (with injury to patient or others) (American Sleep Disorders Association

1997; Fisher et al. 1973; Hartmann 1988).

Sleep Enuresis

Sleep enuresis is a disorder in which the individual urinates during sleep while in bed. Bedwetting, as it is commonly called, has primary and secondary forms. In children, primary sleep enuresis is the continuance of bedwetting since infancy. Secondary enuresis refers to relapse after toilet training was complete and there was a period when the child remained dry. Usually, after toilet training bedwetting spontaneously resolves before age 6 years. Prevalence progressively declines from 30% at age 4 to 10% at age 6 to 5% at age 10 and 3% at age 12 years. If a parent had primary enuresis, it increases the likelihood that the children will be enuretic. A single recessive gene is suspected. Secondary enuresis in children may occur with the birth of a sibling and represent a "cry for attention." Secondary enuresis can also be associated with nocturnal seizures, sleep deprivation, and urologic anomalies. In adults, sleep enuresis is occasionally seen in patients with sleep-disordered breathing. In most cases, embarrassment is the most serious consequence. Nonetheless, if sleep enuresis is not addressed, it may leave psychosocial scars. A variety of medications have also been used to treat sleep enuresis and include imipramine, oxybutynin chloride, and synthetic vasopressin. Behavioral treatments—including bladder training, use of conditioning devices (bell and pad), and fluid restriction—reportedly have good success when properly administered. Other treatments include psychotherapy, motivational strategies, and hypnotherapy. Frequency ranges from nightly to monthly, and severity ranges from mild embarrassment to severe shame and guilt (Nino-Murcia and Keenan 1987; Scharf et al. 1987).

Nightmares

Nightmares are frightening or terrifying dreams. Sometimes called dream anxiety attacks, they produce sympathetic activation that ultimately awaken the dreamer. Nightmares occur in REM sleep and usually evolve from a long, complicated dream that becomes increasingly frightening. Having aroused to wakefulness, the individual typically remembers the dream content (in contrast to sleep terrors). Some nightmares are recurrent, and—reportedly when occurring in association with posttraumatic stress disorder—they may be recollections of actual events. Common in children ages 3–6 (prevalence estimates range from 10%–50%), nightmares are rare in adults (1% or less). Frequent and distressing nightmares are sometimes responsible for insomnia because the individual is afraid to sleep. In Freudian terms, the nightmare is an example of the failure of the dream process that defuses the emotional content of the dream by disguising it symbolically, thus preserving sleep. Most patients who experience nightmares are free from psychiatric conditions. Nonetheless, individuals at risk for nightmares include those with schizotypal personality, borderline personality disorder, schizoid personality disorder, and schizophrenia. Hartmann (1984) posits that nightmares are more common in individuals with "thin boundaries," who are open and trusting, and who often have creative or artistic inclinations. Having thin boundaries makes these individuals more vulnerable; furthermore, they may be at risk for schizophrenia. Traumatic events are known to induce nightmares, sometimes immediately but at other times delayed. The nightmares can persist for many years. Several medications, including levodopa, β-adrenergic blockers, and withdrawal from REM suppressant medications, are known to sometimes provoke nightmares. Finally, drug or alcohol abuse is associated with nightmares (Ermin 1987; Hartmann 1984, 1998; Kales et al. 1980a)

Frequently occurring nightmares often produce a "fear of sleeping" type of insomnia. In turn, the insomnia may provoke sleep deprivation, which is known to exacerbate nightmares. In this manner, a vicious cycle is created. Treatment using behavioral techniques can be helpful. Universal sleep hygiene, stimulus control therapy, lucid dream therapy, and cognitive therapy reportedly improve sleep and reduce nightmares. In patients with nightmares related to posttraumatic stress disorder, nefazodone (an atypical antidepressant) reportedly provides therapeutic benefit. Benzodiazepines may also be helpful; however, systematic controlled trials are lacking (Hirshkowitz and Moore 2000).

Sleep Paralysis

Sleep paralysis is, as the name implies, an inability to make voluntary movements during sleep. It becomes a parasomnia when it occurs at sleep onset or on awakening, a time when the individual is partially conscious and aware of his or her surroundings. This inability to move can be extremely distressing, especially when it is coupled with the feeling that there is an intruder in the house or when hypnagogic hallucinations are occurring. Sleep paralysis is one of the tetrad of symptoms associated with narcolepsy; however, it is known to occur (with or without hypnagogia) in individuals who have neither cataplexy nor excessive daytime sleepiness. Although it is sometimes frightening, sleep paralysis is a feature of normal REM sleep briefly intruding into wakefulness. The paralysis may last from one to several minutes.

It is interesting that the occurrence of sleep paralysis with hypnagogia may account for a variety of experiences in which the sleeper is confronted or attacked by some sort of creature. The common description is that a "presence" is felt to be near; the individual is paralyzed; and the creature talks, attacks, or sits on the sleeper's chest and then vanishes. Whether it is called incubus, "Old Hag," vampire, ghost oppression (*kanashibari*), witch riding, or alien encounter, elements common to sleep paralysis are seen.

Irregular sleep, sleep deprivation, psychological stress, and shift work are thought to increase the likelihood of sleep paralysis occurring. Occasional sleep paralysis occurs in 7%–8% of young adults. Estimates of at least one experience of sleep paralysis during the lifetime range from 25% to 50%. Improving sleep hygiene and ensuring sufficient sleep are first-line therapies. Sometimes, if the individual voluntarily makes very rapid eye movements or is touched by another person, the episode will terminate (Broughton 1982; Ness 1978; Wing et al. 1994).

REM Sleep Behavior Disorder

REM sleep behavior disorder involves a failure of the atonia mechanism (sleep paralysis) during REM sleep. The result is that the patient literally enacts his or her dreams. Under normal circumstances, the dreamer is immobilized by REM-related hypopolarization of alpha and gamma motor neurons. Without this paralysis or with intermittent atonia, punching, kicking, leaping, and running from bed occur during attempted dream enactment. The activity has been correlated with dream imagery, and unlike during sleepwalking, the individual seems unaware of the actual environment. Although complex behaviors can be performed, the individual is acting on the dream sensorium. Thus, a

sleepwalker may calmly go to a bedroom window, open it, and step out. By contrast, a person with REM sleep behavior disorder would more likely dive through the window thinking it to be a dream-visualized lake. Patients and bed partners frequently sustain injuries, sometimes serious ones (e.g., lacerations, fractures).

Animal research ascribes REM sleep atonia to the peri–locus coeruleus exerting an excitatory influence on the medulla (reticularis magnocellularis nucleus), which in turn paralyzes spinal motor neurons. Cats with pontine tegmental lesions perform a variety of behaviors during REM sleep. Neurologic examinations of patients with REM sleep behavior disorder suggest diffuse lesions of the hemispheres, bilateral thalamic abnormalities, or primary brain stem lesions.

Biperiden, tricyclic antidepressants, monoamine oxidase inhibitors, caffeine, venlafaxine, selegiline, and serotonin agonists can precipitate or exacerbate REM behavior disorder. In addition, REM behavior disorder may occur during withdrawal from alcohol, meprobamate, pentazocine, and nitrazepam. A variety of neurologic conditions, including Parkinson's disease, dementia, progressive supranuclear palsy, Shy-Drager syndrome, and narcolepsy, have been associated with this parasomnia. Other conditions that may provoke a secondary REM sleep behavior disorder include sleepwalking, sleep terrors, sleep-disordered breathing, posttraumatic stress disorder, and nocturnal seizures.

REM sleep behavior disorder is rare. Severity ranges from a mild form in which nonviolent episodes occur less than once a month to a severe form in which injury-associated episodes occur more than once a week (Schenck et al. 1986, 1989).

References

Aldrich M: The clinical spectrum of narcolepsy and idiopathic hypersomnia. Neurology 46:393–401, 1996

American Psychiatric Association: Diagnostic and Statistical Manual of Mental Disorders, 4th Edition. Washington, DC, American Psychiatric Association, 1994

American Sleep Disorders Association: The International Classification of Sleep Disorders, Revised: Diagnostic and Coding Manual. Rochester, MN, American Sleep Disorders Association, 1997

Aschoff J: Circadian rhythms in man. Science 148:1427–1432, 1965

Aserinsky E, Kleitman N: Regularly occurring periods of eye motility, and concomitant phenomena. Science 118:273–274, 1953

Benca RM, Obermeyer WH, Thisted RA, et al: Sleep and psychiatric disorders: a meta-analysis. Arch Gen Psychiatry 49:651–668, 1992

Binks GP, Waters FW, Hurry M: Short-term total sleep deprivations does not selectively impair higher cortical functioning. Sleep 22:328–334, 1999

Bootzin RR: A stimulus control treatment for insomnia. Proc Am Psychol Assoc 7:395–396, 1972

Bootzin RR: Effects of self-control procedures for insomnia, in Behavioral Self-Management: Strategies, Techniques, and Outcomes. Edited by Stuart RB. New York, Brunner/Mazel, 1977, pp 176–195

Borbely AA, Achermann P: Concepts and models of sleep regulation: an overview. J Sleep Res 1:63–79, 1992

Broughton RJ: Neurology and dreaming. Psychiatr J Univ Ott 7:101–110, 1982

Carskadon M, Dement WC, Mitler M, et al: Sleep report versus sleep laboratory findings in 122 drug free subjects with the complaint of chronic insomnia. Am J Psychiatry 133: 1382–1388, 1976

Chase MH (ed): The Sleeping Brain. Los Angeles, CA, Brain Information Service/Brain Research Institute, University of California–Los Angeles, 1972

Chockroverty S: Clinical Companion to Sleep Disorders Medicine, 2nd Edition. Boston, MA, Butterworth-Heinemann, 2000

Coleman RM, Roffwarg HP, Kennedy SJ, et al: Sleep-wake disorders based on a polysomnographic diagnosis. A national cooperative study. JAMA 247:997–1003, 1982

Culebras A: Sleep disorders associated with psychiatric, medical and neurologic disorders, in Clinical Handbook of Sleep Disorders. Edited by Culebras A. Boston, MA, Butterworth-Heinemann, 1996, pp 233–282

Czeisler CA, Kronauer RE, Allan JS, et al: Bright light induction of strong (type 0) resetting of the human circadian pacemaker. Science 244:1328–1333, 1989

Dinges D: Proving the limits of functional capability: the effects of sleep loss on short-duration tasks, in Sleep, Arousal, and Performance. Edited by Broughton RJ, Ogilvie RD. Boston, MA, Birkhauser, 1992, pp 177–188

Ekbom KA: Restless legs syndrome. Neurology 10:868–873, 1960

Ermin MK: Dream anxiety attacks (nightmares). Psychiatr Clin North Am 10:667–674, 1987

Espie CA, Lindsay WR, Brooks DN, et al: A controlled comparative investigation of psychological treatments for chronic sleep-onset insomnia. Behav Res Ther 27: 79–88, 1989

Fairbanks DNF, Fujita S, Ikematsu T, et al: Snoring and Obstructive Sleep Apnea. New York, Raven, 1987

Fisher C, Kahn E, Edwards A: A psychophysiological study of nightmares and night terrors, I: psychophysiological aspects of the stage 4 terror. J Nerv Ment Dis 157:75–98, 1973

Flemons WW, Tsai W: Quality of life consequences of sleep-disordered breathing. J Allergy Clin Immunol 99: S750–S756, 1997

Ford DE, Kamerow DB: Epidemiologic study of sleep disturbances and psychiatric disorders: an opportunity for prevention? JAMA 262:1479–1484, 1989

Foulkes D: A cognitive-psychological model of REM dream production. Sleep 5:169–187, 1982

Freud S: The Interpretation of Dreams. New York, Random House, 1950

Fry JM: Treatment modalities for narcolepsy. Neurology 50: S43–48, 1998

Gallup Organization: Sleep in America. Princeton, NJ, Gallup, 1991

Guilleminault C, Pelayo R: Idiopathic central nervous system hypersomnia, in Principles and Practice of Sleep Medicine, 3rd Edition. Edited by Kryger MH, Roth T, Dement WC. Philadelphia, PA, WB Saunders, 2000, pp 687–692

Guilleminault C, Partinen MD, Quera-Salva MA, et al: Determinants of daytime sleepiness in obstructive sleep apnea. Chest 9 (1):32–37, 1988

Hartmann E: The Nightmare: The Psychology and Biology of Terrifying Dreams. New York, Basic Books, 1984

Hartmann E: Two case reports: night terrors with sleep-walking a potentially lethal disorder. J Nerv Ment Dis 171:503–550, 1988

Hartmann E: Dreams and Nightmares. New York, Plenum, 1998

Hauri PJ, Fisher J: Persistent psychophysiological (learned) insomnia. Sleep 2:38–53, 1986

Hirshkowitz M: Somnopharmacology. J Am Osteopath Assoc (in press)

Hirshkowitz M, Moore CA: Nightmares, in Encyclopedia of Stress, Vol 3. Edited by Fink G. San Diego, CA, Academic Press, 2000, pp 49–53

Hirshkowitz M, Moore CA, Hamilton CR, et al: Polysomnography of adults and elderly: sleep architecture, respiration, and leg movements. J Clin Neurophysiol 9:56–63, 1992

Hirshkowitz M, Moore CA, Minhoto G: The basics of sleep, in Understanding Sleep: The Evaluation and Treatment of Sleep Disorders. Edited by Pressman MR, Orr WC. Washington, DC, American Psychological Association, 1997, pp 11–34

Hobson JA, McCarley R: The brain as a dream stage generator: an activation-synthesis hypothesis of the dream process. Am J Psychiatry 134:1335–1348, 1977

Horne J: Why We Sleep. Oxford, UK, Oxford University Press, 1988

Joseph KC, Dube D, Sitaram N: Sleep electroencephalographic characteristics of anxiety disorders, in Principles and Practice of Sleep Medicine. Edited by Kryger MH, Roth T, Dement WC. Philadelphia, PA, WB Saunders, 1989, pp 424–425

Jouvet M, Michel F, Courjon J: Sur un stade d'activite electrique cerebrale rapide au cours du sommeil physiologique. C R Seances Soc Biol Fil 153:1024–1028, 1959

Kales A, Jacobson A, Paulson MJ, et al: Somnambulism: psychophysiological correlates, I: all-night EEG studies. Arch Gen Psychiatry 14:586–594, 1966

Kales A, Soldatos C, Caldwell A, et al: Nightmares: clinical characteristics and personality patterns. Am J Psychiatry 137:1197–1201, 1980a

Kales A, Soldatos CR, Caldwell AB, et al: Sleepwalking. Arch Gen Psychiatry 37:1406–1410, 1980b

Kleitman N: Sleep and Wakefulness, 2nd Edition. Chicago, IL, University of Chicago, 1972

Lichstein KL, Riedel BW: Behavioral assessment and treatment of insomnia: a review with an emphasis on clinical application. Behav Ther 25:659–688, 1994

Loomis AL, Harvey N, Hobart GA: Cerebral states during sleep, as studied by human brain potentials. J Exper Psychol 21:127–144, 1937

Loube DI, Gay PC, Strohl KP, et al: Indications for positive airway pressure treatment of adult obstructive sleep apnea patients: a consensus statement. Chest 115:863–866, 1999

Lugaresi E, Cirgnotta F, Coccagna G, et al: Nocturnal myoclonus and restless legs syndrome. Adv Neurol 43:295–306, 1986

Mellinger GD, Balter MB, Uhlenhuth EH: Insomnia and its treatment: prevalence and correlates. Arch Gen Psychiatry 42:225–232, 1985

Moore-Ede MC, Sulzman FM, Fuller CA: The Clocks That Time Us. Cambridge, MA, Harvard University Press, 1982

Morgan K, Closs SJ: Hypnotic drugs in the treatment of insomnia, in Sleep Management in Nursing Practice. Edinburgh, UK, Churchill Livingstone, 1999, pp 143–159

Morin CM, Culbert JP, Schwartz SM: Nonpharmacological interventions for insomnia: a meta-analysis of treatment efficacy. Am J Psychiatry 151:1172–1180, 1994

Ness RC: The old hag phenomenon as sleep paralysis: a biocultural interpretation. Cult Med Psychiatry 2:15–39, 1978

Nino-Murcia G, Keenan SA: Enuresis and sleep, in Sleep and Its Disorders in Children. Edited by Guilleminault C. New York, Raven, 1987, pp 253–267

Rechtschaffen A, Kales A (eds): A manual of standardized terminology, techniques and scoring system for sleep stages of human subjects (NIH Publ No 204). Washington, DC, U.S. Government Printing Office, 1968

Reynolds CF, Kupfer DJ: Sleep research in affective illness: state of the art circa 1987. Sleep 10:199–215, 1987

Robinson A, Guilleminault C: Obstructive sleep apnea syndrome, in Sleep Disorders Medicine. Edited by Chokroverty S. Boston, MA, Butterworth-Heinemann, 1999, pp 331–354

Roffwarg HP, Muzio JN, Dement WC: Ontogenetic development of the human sleep-dream cycle. Science 152:604–619, 1966

Sanders MH: Medical therapy for obstructive sleep apnea-hypopnea syndrome, in Principles and Practice of Sleep Medicine, 3rd Edition. Edited by Kryger MH, Roth T, Dement WC. Philadelphia, PA, WB Saunders, 2000, pp 879–893

Scharf MB, Pravda MF, Jennings SW, et al: Childhood enuresis: a comprehensive treatment program. Psychiatr Clin North Am 10:655–674, 1987

Schenck CH, Bundlie SR, Ettinger MG, et al: Chronic behavioral disorders of human REM sleep: a new category of parasomnia. Sleep 9:293–308, 1986

Schenck CH, Hurwitz TD, Bundlie SR, et al: Sleep-related injury in 100 adult patients: a polysomnographic and clinical report. Am J Psychiatry 146:1166–1173, 1989

Shneerson JM: Handbook of Sleep Medicine. Oxford, UK, Blackwell Science, 2000

Spielman AJ, Caruso LS, Glovinsky PB: A behavioral perspective on insomnia treatment. Psychiatr Clin North Am 10:541–553, 1987a

Spielman AJ, Saskin P, Thorpy MJ: Treatment of chronic insomnia by restriction of time in bed. Sleep 10:45–65, 1987b

Standards of Practice Committee of the American Sleep Disorders Association: Practice parameters for the use of stimulants in the treatment of narcolepsy. Sleep 17:348–351, 1994

Thorpy MJ, Ledereich PS: Medical treatment of obstructive sleep apnea, in Handbook of Sleep Disorders. Edited by Thorpy MJ. New York, Marcel Dekker, 1990, pp 285–309

Vogel GW, Vogel F, McAbee RS, et al: Improvement of depression by REM sleep deprivation. Arch Gen Psychiatry 37:247–253, 1980

Walters AS: Toward a better definition of the restless legs syndrome. International Restless Legs Syndrome Study Group. Mov Disord 10:634–642, 1995

Walters AS, Hening W, Rubinstein, et al: A clinical and polysomnographic comparison of neuroleptic-induced akathisia and the idiopathic restless legs syndrome. Sleep 14:339–345, 1991

Williams RL, Karacan I, Hursch CJ: EEG of Human Sleep: Clinical Applications. New York, Wiley, 1974

Wing YK, Lee ST, Chen CN: Sleep paralysis in Chinese: ghost oppression phenomenon in Hong Kong. Sleep 17:609–613, 1994

Yudofsky SC, Hales RE (eds): The American Psychiatric Publishing Textbook of Neuropsychiatry and Clinical Neurosciences, Fourth Edition. Washington, DC, American Psychiatric Publishing, 2002

Zammit GK: Delayed sleep phase syndrome and related conditions, in Understanding Sleep: The Evaluation and Treatment of Sleep Disorders. Edited by Pressman MR, Orr WC. Washington, DC, American Psychological Association, 1997, pp 229–248

Zarcone V: Sleep abnormalities in schizophrenia, in Principles and Practice of Sleep Medicine. Edited by Kryger MH, Roth T, Dement WC. Philadelphia, PA, WB Saunders, 1989, pp 422–423

Neuropsychiatric Aspects of Cerebrovascular Disorders

Robert G. Robinson, M.D.

Sergio E. Starkstein, M.D., Ph.D.

Stroke is the most common serious neurologic disorder in the world and accounts for half of all the exigent hospitalizations for neurologic disease. The age-specific incidence of stroke varies dramatically over the life course (Figure 11–1). In Rochester, Minnesota, the annual incidence in those under age 35 was 1 per 10,000 population, whereas among those over age 85 the incidence was almost 200 per 10,000 population (Bonita 1992).

The neuropsychiatric complications of cerebrovascular disease include a wide range of emotional and cognitive disturbances.

Historical Perspective

The first reports of emotional reactions after brain damage (usually caused by cerebrovascular disease) were made by neurologists and psychiatrists in case descriptions. Meyer (1904) warned that new discoveries of cerebral localization in the early 1900s of such capacities as language function led to an overhasty identification of centers and functions. He identified several disorders such as delirium, dementia, and aphasia that were the direct result of brain injury. In keeping with his view of biopsychosocial causes of most mental "reactions," however, he saw manic-depressive illness and paranoiac conditions as arising from a combination of head injury (specifically citing left frontal lobe and cortical convexities) along with a family history of psychiatric disorder and premorbid personal psychiatric disorders, thus producing the specific mental reaction.

In contrast to psychiatric disorders seen in patients with or without brain injury, Goldstein (1939) described an

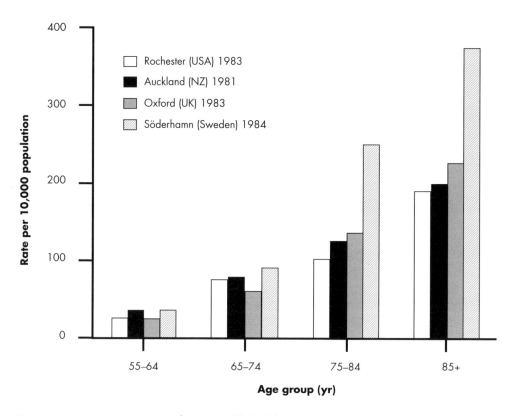

FIGURE 11–1.   Average annual age-specific incidence of stroke in selected studies around the world.

In all studies, the incidence of stroke increased with increasing age.

Source.   Reprinted with permission from Elsevier. Bonita R: "Epidemiology of Stroke." *The Lancet* 339:342–344, 1992. The Rochester 1983 study refers to Broderick et al. 1989; the Auckland 1981 study to Bonita et al. 1984; the Oxford 1983 study to Bamford et al. 1988; and the Söderhamn 1984 study to Terent 1988.

emotional disorder thought to be uniquely associated with brain disease. He termed this disorder *catastrophic reaction*, which is an emotional outburst characterized by various degrees of anger, frustration, depression, tearfulness, refusal, shouting, swearing, and sometimes aggressive behavior. Goldstein ascribed this reaction to the inability of the subject to cope when faced with a serious defect in physical or cognitive functions. In his extensive studies of brain injuries in war, Goldstein (1942) described two symptom clusters: those related directly to physical damage of a circumscribed area of the brain and those related secondarily to the subject's psychological response to injury. Emo-

tional symptoms, therefore, represented the latter category (i.e., the psychological response of a subject struggling with physical or cognitive impairments). (Catastrophic reaction is also discussed later in this chapter under "Neuropsychiatric Syndromes Associated With Cerebrovascular Disease.")

A second emotional abnormality, also thought to be characteristic of brain injury, was the indifference reaction Babinski (1914) noted that patients with right hemisphere disease often displayed the symptoms of anosognosia, euphoria, and indifference. The indifference reaction, associated with right hemisphere lesions, consisted of symptoms of indifference toward failures, lack of interest in family and friends, enjoyment of foolish jokes, and minimization of physical difficulties (Denny-Brown et al. 1952; Haecen et al. 1951).

Two primary lines of thought have emerged in the study of emotional disorders associated with cerebrovascular disease. One attributes emotional disorders to an understandable psychological reaction to the associated impairment; the other, based on a lack of association between severity of impairment and severity of emotional disorder, suggests a direct causal connection between cerebrovascular disease and neuropsychiatric disorders.

Classification of Cerebrovascular Disease

There are many ways to classify the wide range of disorders that constitute the spectrum of cerebrovascular disease.

From the perspective of schematizing its neuropsychiatric complications, however, probably the most pragmatic way of classifying cerebrovascular disease is not to focus on the anatomic-pathologic processes or the interactive mechanisms but to examine the means by which parenchymal changes in the brain occur. The first of these, ischemia, may occur either with or without infarction of parenchyma and includes transient ischemic attacks (TIAs), atherosclerotic thrombosis, cerebral embolism, and hemorrhage. The last of these may cause either direct parenchymal damage by extravasation of blood into the surrounding brain tissue, as in intracerebral hemorrhage (ICH), or indirect damage by hemorrhage into the ventricles, subarachnoid space, extradural area, or subdural area. These changes result in a common mode of expression, defined by Adams and Victor (1985) as a sudden,

convulsive, focal neurologic deficit, or stroke.

To expand slightly on this categorization (i.e., the means by which parenchymal changes occur), there are two categories of ischemic disorders and three categories of hemorrhagic disorders (Table 11–1). These include atherosclerotic thrombosis, cerebral embolism, lacunae, and ICH. In various studies of the incidence of cerebrovascular disease (e.g., Wolf et al. 1977), the ratio of infarcts to hemorrhages has been shown to be about 5:1. Atherosclerotic thrombosis and cerebral embolism each accounts for approximately one-third of all incidents of stroke. Finally, there are several less common types of intracranial disease. These may lead to intraparenchymal damage, but frequently bleeds on the surface of the brain (e.g., subdural hematoma) do not produce permanent parenchymal damage.

Atherosclerotic Thrombosis

Atherosclerotic thrombosis is often the result of a dynamic interaction between hypertension and the atherosclerotic deposition of hyaline-lipid material in the walls of peripheral, coronary, and cerebral arteries. Risk factors in the development of atherosclerosis include hyperlipidemia, diabetes mellitus, hypertension, and cigarette smoking. Atheromatous plaques tend to propagate at the branchings and curves of the internal carotid artery or the carotid sinus, in the cervical part of the vertebral arteries and their junction to form the basilar artery, in the posterior cerebral arteries as they wind around the midbrain, and in the anterior cerebral arteries as they curve over the corpus callosum. These plaques may lead to stenosis of one or more of these cerebral arteries or to complete occlusion. TIAs, defined as periods of transient focal ischemia associated with reversible neurologic deficits, almost always indicate that a thrombotic

TABLE 11–1. Classification of cerebrovascular disease

Ischemic phenomena (85%)
  Infarction
    Atherosclerotic thrombosis
    Cerebral embolism
    Lacunae
    Other causes (arteritis [e.g., infectious or connective tissue disease], cerebral thrombophlebitis, fibromuscular dysplasia, venous occlusions)
  Transient ischemic attacks
Hemorrhagic phenomena (15%)
  Intraparenchymal hemorrhage
    Primary (hypertensive) intracerebral hemorrhage
    Other causes (hemorrhagic disorders [e.g., thrombocytopenia, clotting disorders], trauma)
  Subarachnoid or intraventricular hemorrhage
    Ruptured saccular aneurysm or arteriovenous malformation
    Other causes
  Subdural or epidural hematoma

process is occurring. Only rarely is embolism or ICH preceded by transient neurologic deficits. Thrombosis of virtually any cerebral or cerebellar artery can be associated with TIAs.

Cerebral Embolism

Of all the types of stroke, those due to cerebral embolism develop most rapidly. In general, there are no warning episodes; embolism can occur at any time. A large embolus may occlude the internal carotid artery or the stem of the middle cerebral artery, producing a severe hemiplegia. More often, however, the embolus is smaller and passes into one of the branches of the middle cerebral artery. This may produce infarction distal to the site of the arterial occlusion, which is characterized by a pattern of neurologic deficits consistent with that vascular distribution, or may result in a

transient neurologic deficit that resolves as the embolus fragments and travels into smaller, more distal arteries.

Lacunae

Lacunae, which account for nearly one-fifth of strokes, are the result of occlusion of small penetrating cerebral arteries. They are infarcts that may be so small as to produce no recognizable deficits or, depending on their location, may be associated with pure motor or sensory deficits. Lacunae are strongly associated with both atherosclerosis and hypertension, suggesting that lacunar infarction is the result of the extension of the atherosclerotic process into small-diameter vessels.

Intracerebral Hemorrhage

ICH is the fourth most frequent cause of stroke. The main causes of ICH that present as acute stroke include hypertension, rupture of saccular aneurysms or arteriovenous malformations (AVMs), a variety of hemorrhagic disorders of assorted etiologies, and trauma. Primary (hypertensive) ICH occurs within the brain tissue when the extravasation of blood forms a roughly circular or oval-shaped mass that disrupts and displaces the parenchyma. Adjacent tissue is compressed, and seepage into the ventricular system usually occurs, producing bloody cerebrospinal fluid in more than 90% of cases.

Severe headache is generally considered to be a constant accompaniment of ICH, but this occurs in only about 50% of cases. The prognosis for ICH is grave: 70%–75% of patients die within 30 days (Adams and Victor 1985).

Aneurysms and Arteriovenous Malformations

Aneurysms are usually located at arterial bifurcations and are presumed to result from developmental defects in the formation of the arterial wall. Rupture occurs when the intima bulges outward and eventually breaks through the adventitia. AVMs consist of a tangle of dilated vessels that form an abnormal communication between the arterial and venous systems. They are developmental abnormalities consisting of embryonic patterns of blood vessels. Most AVMs are clinically silent but ultimately bleed.

Subdural and Epidural Hematomas

Chronic subdural hematomas (SDHs) are frequently (60%), but not exclusively, caused by head trauma, followed by a gradual progression of signs and symptoms during the subsequent days to weeks. These manifestations include confusion, inattention, apathy, memory loss, drowsiness, and coma.

Epidural hematomas usually follow a temporal or parietal skull fracture that causes a laceration or avulsion of the middle meningeal artery or vein or a tear of the aural venous sinus. Acute SDH is usually caused by the avulsion of bridging veins or laceration of pial arteries. Both conditions produce loss of consciousness or a brief period of lucidity followed by a loss of consciousness, hemiparesis, cranial nerve palsies, and death, usually secondary to respiratory compromise, if the hematoma is not emergently evacuated.

Other Types of Cerebrovascular Disease

Another cause of cerebrovascular disease is fibromuscular dysplasia, which leads to narrowed arterial segments caused by degeneration of elastic tissue, disruption and loss of the arterial muscular coat, and an increase in fibrous tissue. Inflammatory diseases of the arterial system can also lead to stroke. These diseases include meningovascular syphilis, pyogenic or tuberculous meningitis, temporal arteritis, and systemic lupus erythematosus.

Neuropsychiatric Syndromes Associated With Cerebrovascular Disease

A number of emotional disorders have been associated with cerebrovascular disease, including poststroke depression, poststroke mania, poststroke bipolar disorder, poststroke anxiety disorder, poststroke psychosis, apathy, catastrophic reaction, pathologic emotions, and aprosody. Table 11–2 summarizes the prevalence, clinical symptoms, and associated lesion location of these syndromes.

Poststroke Depression

Diagnosis

Although strict diagnostic criteria have not been used in some studies of emotional disorders associated with cerebrovascular disease (Andersen et al. 1993), most studies have used structured interviews and diagnostic criteria defined by DSM-III-R or DSM-IV (American Psychiatric Association 1987, 1994) or Research Diagnostic Criteria (Eastwood et al. 1989; Morris et al. 1990; Robinson et al. 1983a; Spitzer et al. 1978). Poststroke major depression (Table 11–2) is now categorized in DSM-IV-TR (American Psychiatric Association 2000) as mood disorder due to stroke with major depressive-like episode. For patients with less severe forms of depression, there are "research criteria" in DSM-IV for minor depression (i.e., subsyndromal major depression; depression or anhedonia with at least one but fewer than four additional symptoms of major depression) (see Table 11–2) or, alternatively, a diagnosis of mood disorder due to stroke with depressive features.

TABLE 11–2. Clinical syndromes associated with cerebrovascular disease

Syndrome	Prevalence	Clinical symptoms	Associated lesion location
Major depression	20%	Depressed mood, diurnal mood variation, loss of energy, anxiety, restlessness, worry, weight loss, decreased appetite, early-morning awakening, delayed sleep onset, social withdrawal, and irritability	Left frontal lobe and left basal ganglia during the acute period after stroke
Minor depression	10%–40%	Depressed mood, anxiety, restlessness, worry, diurnal mood variation, hopelessness, loss of energy, delayed sleep onset, early-morning awakening, social withdrawal, weight loss, and decreased appetite	Left posterior parietal and occipital regions during the acute poststroke period
Mania	Unknown, rare	Elevated mood, increased energy, increased appetite, decreased sleep, feeling of well-being, pressured speech, flight of ideas, grandiose thoughts	Right basotemporal or right orbitofrontal lesions
Bipolar mood disorder	Unknown, rare	Symptoms of major depression alternating with mania	Right basal ganglia or right thalamic lesions
Anxiety disorder	27%	Symptoms of major depression plus intense worry and anxious foreboding in addition to depression, associated light-headedness or palpitations and muscle tension or restlessness, and difficulty concentrating or falling asleep	Left cortical lesions, usually dorsolateral frontal lobe
Psychotic disorder	Unknown, rare	Hallucinations or delusions	Right temporoparietal-occipital junction
Apathy			
Without depression	22%	Loss of drive, motivation, interest, low energy, unconcern	Posterior internal capsule
With depression	11%		
Pathologic laughing and crying	20%	Frequent, usually brief laughing and/or crying; crying not caused by sadness or out of proportion to it; and social withdrawal secondary to emotional outbursts	Frequently, bilateral hemispheric lesions; can occur with almost any lesion location
Anosognosia	24%–43%	Denial of impairment related to motor function, sensory perception, visual perception, or other modality with an apparent lack of concern	Right hemisphere and enlarged ventricles

TABLE 11–2. Clinical syndromes associated with cerebrovascular disease *(continued)*

Syndrome	Prevalence	Clinical symptoms	Associated lesion location
Catastrophic reaction	19%	Anxiety reaction, tears, aggressive behavior, swearing, displacement, refusal, renouncement, and compensatory boasting	Left anterior-subcortical region
Aprosodias			
Motor	Unknown	Poor expression of emotional prosody and gesturing, good prosodic comprehension and gesturing, and denial of feelings of depression	Right hemisphere posterior inferior frontal lobe and basal ganglia
Sensory	32%–49%	Good expression of emotional prosody and gesturing, poor prosodic comprehension and gesturing, and difficulty empathizing with others	Right hemisphere posterior inferior parietal lobe and posterior superior temporal lobe

The frequencies of vegetative symptoms in hospital and at each of the follow-up visits are shown in Figure 11–2. Throughout the 2-year follow-up, depressed patients showed a higher frequency of both vegetative and psychological symptoms compared with the nondepressed patients. The only vegetative symptoms that were not more frequent in the depressed than in the nondepressed patients were weight loss and early awakening at the initial evaluation; weight loss and early-morning awakening at 6 months; weight loss, early-morning awakening, anxious foreboding, and loss of libido at 1 year; and weight loss and loss of libido at 2 years. Among the psychological symptoms, the depressed patients had a higher frequency of most psychological symptoms throughout the 2-year follow-up. The only psychological symptoms that were not significantly more frequent in the depressed than in the nondepressed group were suicide plans, simple ideas of reference, and pathologic guilt at 3 months; pathologic guilt at 6 months; pathologic guilt, suicide plans, guilty ideas of reference, and irritability at 1 year; and pathologic guilt and self-depreciation at 2 years.

The sensitivity of unmodified DSM-IV criteria consistently showed a sensitivity of 100% and a specificity that ranged from 95% to 98% compared with criteria using only specific symptoms. Thus, one could reasonably conclude that modifying DSM-IV criteria because of the existence of an acute medical illness is probably unnecessary.

These findings also suggest that the nature of poststroke depression (PSD) may change over time. Since the symptoms that were specific to depression changed over time, this may reflect an alteration in the underling etiology of PSD associated with early-onset depression compared with the late or chronic poststroke period (see Figure 11–2).

Phenomenology

Lipsey et al. (1986) examined the frequency of depressive symptoms in a group of 43 patients with major PSD compared with that in a group of 43 age-matched patients with "functional" (i.e., no known brain pathology) depression. The main finding was that both groups showed almost identical profiles of symptoms, including those that were not part of the diagnostic criteria (Figure 11–3). More than 50% of the patients who met the diagnostic criteria for major PSD reported sadness, anxiety, tension, loss of interest and concentration, sleep disturbances with early-morning awakening, loss of appetite with weight loss, difficulty concentrating and thinking, and thoughts of death.

Prevalence

During the past 10 years, there have been a large number of studies around the world examining the prevalence of PSD. These publications indicate an increasing interest among clinicians caring for poststroke patients in the frequency and significance of depression following stroke. The findings of many of these studies are shown in Table 11–3. In general, these studies have found similar rates of major and minor depression among patients hospitalized for acute stroke, in rehabilitation hospitals, and in outpatient clinics. The mean frequency of major depression among patients in acute and rehabilitation hospitals was 22% for major depression and 17% for minor depression. Among patients studied in community settings, however, the mean prevalence of major depression was 13% and the mean prevalence of minor depression was 10%. Thus, PSD is common both among patients who are receiving treatment for stroke and among community samples. The higher rates of depression among patients who were receiving treatment for stroke is probably related to the greater severity of

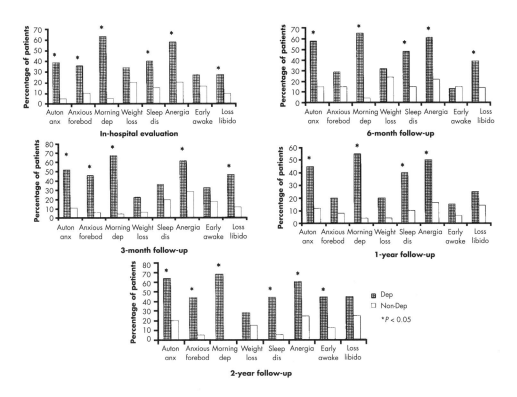

FIGURE 11–2. The frequency of vegetative symptoms of depression in patients with depressed mood (Dep) and without depressed mood (Non-Dep) following stroke.

Symptom frequency is shown over the 2-year follow-up. Morning depression (i.e., diurnal mood variation) and anergia were associated with depression throughout the entire 2-year period. Loss of libido was only seen early in the follow-up, whereas early-morning awakening was only seen late in the follow-up. These findings suggest changes over time in both the effects of chronic medical illness and the phenomenology of depression following stroke.

Auton anx = autonomic anxiety; Anxious forebod = anxious foreboding; Morning dep = morning depression; Sleep dis = sleep disturbance; Early awake = early-morning awakening; Loss libido = loss of libido.

Source. Reprinted with the permission of Cambridge University Press from Robinson RG: *The Clinical Neuropsychiatry of Stroke.* New York, Cambridge University Press, 1998 (data taken from Paradiso et al. 1997).

stroke seen in treatment settings compared with community settings, in which many patients have no physical or intellectual impairment.

Duration

The percentage of patients with major depression who had improved to a diagnosis of minor depression by 1-year follow-up is shown in Figure 11–4. Although all studies found that the majority of depressions were less than 1 year in duration, the mean frequency of major depression that was persistent beyond 1 year was 26%.

Two factors have been identified that can influence the natural course of PSD. One is treatment of depression with antidepressant medications (discussed below). The second factor is lesion location. Starkstein et al. (1988c) compared two groups of depressed patients: one group ($n = 6$) had spontaneously recovered from depression by 6 months after stroke, whereas the other group ($n = 10$) remained depressed at this point. There were no significant between-group differ-

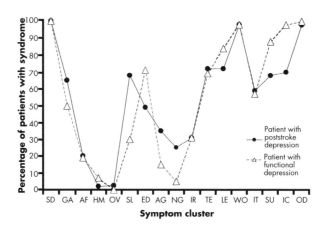

FIGURE 11–3. Patients with major depression after acute stroke (*n*=43) were compared with age-comparable patients hospitalized for functional primary depression (*n*=43).

The symptom clusters are "syndromes" derived from the semistructured interview of the present state examination (PSE). SD=simple depression; GA=general anxiety; AF=affective flattening; HM=hypomania; OV=overactivity; SL=slowness; ED=special features of depression; AG=agitation; NG=self-neglect; IR=ideas of reference; TE=tension; LE=lack of energy; WO=worrying; IT=irritability; SU=social unease; IC=loss of interest and concentration; OD=other symptoms of depression. Patients with primary and poststroke depression showed the same frequency of all syndromes except slowness (stroke patients showed a higher frequency) and loss of interest and concentration (primary depression patients showed a higher frequency).

Source. Reprinted with the permission of Cambridge University Press from Robinson RG: *The Clinical Neuropsychiatry of Stroke.* New York, Cambridge University Press, 1998 (modified from Lipsey et al. 1986).

ences in important demographic variables, such as age, sex, and education, and both groups had similar levels of social functioning and degrees of cognitive dysfunction. There were, however, two significant between-group differences. One was lesion location: the recovered group had a higher frequency of subcortical and cerebellar–brain stem lesions; the nonrecovered group had a higher frequency of cortical lesions (*P*<0.01).

The available data suggest that PSD is not transient but is usually a long-standing disorder with a natural course of approximately 9–10 months for most cases of major depression. Depression lasting more than 2 years, however, does occur in some patients with major or minor depression.

Relationship to Lesion Variables

The first study to report a significant clinical-pathologic correlation in PSD was an investigation by Robinson and Szetela (1981) of 29 patients with left hemisphere brain injury secondary to stroke (*n* = 18) or to traumatic brain injury (*n* = 11). Based on localization of the lesion by computed tomography, there was a significant inverse correlation between the severity of depression and the distance of the anterior border of the lesion from the frontal pole (*r*=0.76). This surprising finding led to a number of subsequent examinations of this phenomenon in other populations. Robinson et al. (1984) found a significant correlation in 10 patients with left-frontal acute stroke who were right-handed and had no known risk factors for depression (*r*=0.92; *P*<0.05). Thus, the location of the lesion along the anterior-posterior dimension appears to be an important variable in the severity of depression after stroke.

In addition, however, lesion location

TABLE 11–3. Prevalence studies of poststroke depression

Investigators	Patient population	N	Criteria	% Major	% Minor	Total %
Folstein et al. 1977	Rehab hospital	20	PSE & items			45
Finklestein et al. 1982	Rehab hospital	25	Cutoff score			48
Sinyor et al. 1986	Rehab hospital	35	Cutoff score			36
Finset et al. 1989	Rehab hospital	42	Cutoff score			36
Eastwood et al. 1989	Rehab hospital	87	SADS, RDC	10	40	50
Morris et al. 1990	Rehab hospital	99	CIDI, DSM-III	14	21	35
Schubert et al. 1992	Rehab hospital	18	DSM-III-R	28	44	72
Gainotti et al. 1999	Rehab hospital	153	DSM-III-R	31	NR	31+
Schwartz et al. 1993	Rehab hospital	91	DSM-III	40		40[a]
Feibel and Springer 1982	Outpatient (6 months)	91	Nursing evaluation			26
Robinson and Price 1982	Outpatient (6 months–10 years)	103	Cutoff score			29
Collin et al. 1987	Outpatient	111	Cutoff score			42
Astrom et al. 1993a, 1993b	Outpatient (3 months)	73	DSM-III	31	NR	31[a]
	(1 year)	73	DSM-III	16	NR	16[a]
	(2 years)	57	DSM-III	19	NR	19[a]
	(3 years)	49	DSM-III	29	NR	29[a]
Robinson 1998	Outpatient (3 months)	77	PSE, DSM-III	20	13	33
	(6 months)	80	PSE, DSM-III	21	21	42
	(1 year)	70	PSE, DSM-III	11	16	27
	(2 years)	67	PSE, DSM-III	18	17	35
Pohjasvaara et al. 1998	Outpatient	277	DSM-III-R	26	14	40
Dennis et al. 2000	Outpatient (6 months)	309	Cutoff score			38

TABLE 11–3. Prevalence studies of poststroke depression (*continued*)

Investigators	Patient population	N	Criteria	% Major	% Minor	Total %
N. Herrmann et al. 1998	Outpatient					
	(3 months)	150	Cutoff score			27
	(1 year)	136				22
Kotila et al. 1998	Outpatient					
	(3 months)	321	Cutoff score			47
	(1 year)	311				48
Wade et al. 1987	Community	379	Cutoff score			30
House et al. 1991	Community	89	PSE, DSM-III	11	12	23
Burvill et al. 1995	Community	294	PSE, DSM-III	15	8	23
Robinson et al. 1983b	Acute hospital	103	PSE, DSM-III	27	20	47
Ebrahim et al. 1987	Acute hospital	149	Cutoff score			23
Fedoroff et al. 1991	Acute hospital	205	PSE, DSM-III	22	19	41
Castillo et al. 1995	Acute hospital	291	PSE, DSM-III	20	18	38
Starkstein et al. 1992	Acute hospital	80	PSE, DSM-III	16	13	29
Astrom et al. 1993a, 1993b	Acute hospital	80	DSM-III	25	NR	25[a]
M. Herrmann et al. 1993	Acute hospital	21	RDC	24	14	38
Andersen et al. 1994	Acute hospital or outpatient	285	Ham-D cutoff	10	11	21
			Mean	20	21	34[a]

[a]Because minor depression was not included, these values may be low.

Note. PSE = Present State Examination; SADS = Schedule for Affective Disorders and Schizophrenia; RDC = Research Diagnostic Criteria; CIDI = Composite International Diagnostic Interview; DSM-III = Diagnostic and Statistical Manual of Mental Disorders, 3rd Edition; DSM-III-R = Diagnostic and Statistical Manual of Mental Disorders, 3rd Edition, Revised; NR = not reported; Ham-D = Hamilton Rating Scale for Depression.

Source. Reprinted with the permission of Cambridge University Press from Robinson RG: *The Clinical Neuropsychiatry of Stroke.* New York, Cambridge University Press, 1998.

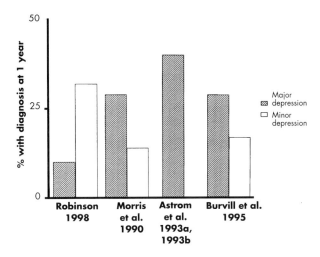

FIGURE 11–4. The percentage of patients with an initial assessment diagnosis of major poststroke depression who continued to have a diagnosis of major depression or who had improved to a diagnosis of minor depression at 1-year follow-up.

Note that the number of chronic cases varies between studies, probably reflecting a mixture of etiologies among the group with an in-hospital diagnosis of major poststroke depression. The mean frequency of persistent major depression at 1-year follow-up across all studies was 26%.

Source. Reprinted with the permission of Cambridge University Press from Robinson RG: *The Clinical Neuropsychiatry of Stroke.* New York, Cambridge University Press, 1998.

influences the frequency of depression. In a study of 45 patients with single lesions restricted to either cortical or subcortical structures in the left or right hemisphere, Starkstein et al. (1987b) found that 44% of patients with left cortical lesions were depressed, whereas 39% of patients with left subcortical lesions, 11% of patients with right cortical lesions, and 14% of patients with right subcortical lesions were depressed. Thus, patients with lesions in the left hemisphere had significantly higher rates of depression than did those with lesions in the right hemisphere, regardless of the cortical or subcortical location of the lesion. These findings supported the hypothesis that depressive disorders after stroke are more frequent among patients with acute left hemisphere lesions than in those with right hemisphere lesions ($P<0.05$).

Astrom et al. (1993a, 1993b) similarly found that among patients with acute

stroke, 12 of 14 with left anterior lesions had major depression, compared with only 2 of 7 patients with left posterior lesions ($P=0.017$) and 2 of 23 with right hemisphere lesions ($P<0.001$). House et al. (1990a, 1990b) found only 4 cases of major depression among 40 patients with acute stroke in a community survey and did not find an association with left anterior lesions. M. Herrmann et al. (1993), however, found major depression in 7 of 10 patients with nonfluent aphasia and left anterior lesions, compared with 0 of 7 patients with fluent aphasia and left posterior lesions ($P=0.0014$), but only during the acute poststroke period.

Numerous studies, however, have failed to replicate these findings. Some of these findings are shown in Figure 11–5. For example, Gainotti et al. (1999) examined lesion location in 53 patients using magnetic resonance or computed tomographic scans. Among patients with left

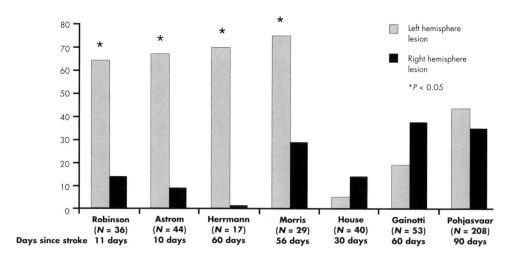

FIGURE 11–5. The frequency of major depression among patients with single lesions of left or right hemisphere.

The association of left (anterior) lesions with major depression was found among patients who were studied within 2 months of their acute stroke. Numerous studies have not found this association with left hemisphere lesions. Most, but not all, of these studies examined patients more than 2 months following stroke. Longitudinal follow-up in the Robinson et al. and Astrom et al. studies found no lateralized differences in frequency of depression at 3-month follow-up.

anterior lesions who were less than 2 months poststroke, only 1 of 9 patients had major depression, although 3 of 7 patients with right anterior lesions had major depression.

Shimoda and Robinson (1999) examined the relationship between lesion location and time since stroke using a longitudinally studied patient population. This study examined 60 patients with single lesions involving either the right or left middle cerebral artery distribution that were visible on computed tomographic scan and who had follow-up at 3 or 6 months (short-term follow-up) and at 12 or 24 months (long-term follow-up). There were no statistically significant differences between the patients with right and left hemisphere lesions in their age, gender, race, marital status, or other background characteristics. The frequency of depression in patients during the initial evaluation was significantly higher for both major and minor depression among

patients with left hemisphere stroke compared with patients with right hemisphere stroke $(P=0.0006)$ (Figure 11–6). At short- and long-term follow-up, however, there were no significant differences between groups with right hemisphere and left hemisphere lesions in terms of the frequency of major or minor depression.

This study suggests that the failure of other investigators to replicate the association of left anterior lesion location with increased frequency of depression may in most cases be related to time since stroke.

Although it is uncertain why this temporal dynamic occurs in the relationship between severity of depression and lesion location, it suggests that if physiologic changes such as depletion of biogenic amines occur in patients with left anterior lesions that lead to depression, these changes are hemisphere-specific for only a few weeks. By 2–3 months after stroke (i.e., short-term follow-up) similar alter-

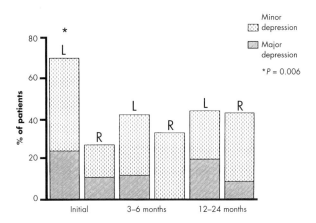

FIGURE 11–6.   The frequency of major and minor depression defined by DSM-IV criteria associated with single lesions of the right (R) or left (L) hemisphere during the acute stroke period and at follow-up.

The lateralized effect of left hemisphere lesions on both major and minor depression was found only during the acute stroke period. At short-term and long-term follow-up, there were no hemispheric lesion effects on the frequency of depression.

Source.   Reprinted with the permission of Cambridge University Press from Robinson RG: *The Clinical Neuropsychiatry of Stroke.* New York, Cambridge University Press, 1998.

native mechanisms occur in patients with right frontal lesions that lead to correlation of depression severity with proximity of the lesion to the frontal pole.

Premorbid Risk Factors

The studies reviewed above indicate that although a significant proportion of patients with left anterior or right posterior lesions develop PSD, not every patient with a lesion in these locations develops a depressive mood. This observation raises the question of why clinical variability occurs and why some but not all patients with lesions in these locations develop depression.

Starkstein et al. (1988b) examined these questions by comparing 13 patients with major PSD with 13 stroke patients without depression, all of whom had lesions of the same size and location. Eleven pairs of patients had left hemisphere lesions, and two pairs had right hemisphere lesions. Damage was cortical in 10 pairs and subcortical in 3 pairs. The groups did not differ on important demographic variables, such as age, sex, socioeconomic status, or education. They also did not differ on family or personal history of psychiatric disorders or neurologic deficits. Patients with major PSD, however, had significantly more subcortical atrophy ($P < 0.05$), as measured both by the ratio of third ventricle to brain (i.e., the area of the third ventricle divided by the area of the brain at the same level) and by the ratio of lateral ventricle to brain (i.e., the area of the body of the lateral ventricle contralateral to the brain lesion divided by the brain area at the same level). It is likely that the subcortical atrophy preceded the stroke. Thus, a mild degree of subcortical atrophy may be a premorbid risk factor that increases the risk of developing major depression following a stroke.

In summary, lesion location is not the only factor that influences the development of PSD. Subcortical atrophy that probably precedes the stroke and a family or personal history of affective disorders also seem to play an important role.

Relationship to Physical Impairment

Numerous investigators, including Robinson et al. (1983b), Eastwood et al. (1989), and N. Herrmann et al. (1998), have reported a low but significant correlation between depression and functional physical impairment (i.e., activities of daily living [ADL]). This association, however, might be construed as the severe functional impairment producing depression or, alternatively, the severity of depression influencing the severity of functional impairment. Several studies lend support to the latter suggestion.

Parikh et al. (1990) compared a consecutive series of 63 stroke patients who had major or minor depression with nondepressed stroke patients during a 2-year follow-up. Although both groups had similar impairments in ADL during the time they were in hospital, the depressed patients had significantly less improvement by 2-year follow-up than did the nondepressed patients. This finding held true after the authors controlled for important variables such as the type and extent of in-hospital and rehabilitation treatment, the size and location of the lesion, the patients' demographic characteristics, the nature of the stroke, the occurrence of another stroke during the follow-up period, and medical history.

A recent study by Chemerinski and Robinson (2000) included a consecutive series of patients with PSD ($N = 55$) divided into those whose mood improved at 3- to 6-month follow-up and those who had not improved ($n = 34$). This study found significantly greater improvement in ADL scores among patients whose major or minor depression improved compared with those whose depression did not. In addition, patients with minor depression showed the same degree of improvement with remission of their depression as did patients with major depression.

Relationship to Cognitive Impairment

This issue was first examined in patients with PSD by Robinson et al. (1986). Patients with major depression after a left hemisphere infarct were found to have significantly lower (i.e., more impaired) scores on the Mini-Mental State Exam (MMSE) (Folstein et al. 1975) than did a comparable group of nondepressed patients. Both the size of the patients' lesions and their depression scores correlated independently with severity of cognitive impairment.

In a second study (Starkstein et al. 1988b), stroke patients with and without major depression were matched for lesion location and volume. Of 13 patients with major PSD, 10 had an MMSE score lower than that of their matched control subjects, 2 had the same score, and only 1 patient had a higher score ($P < 0.001$). Thus, even when patients were matched for lesion size and location, depressed patients were more cognitively impaired.

In a follow-up study, Bolla-Wilson et al. (1989) administered a comprehensive neuropsychological battery and found that patients with major depression and left hemisphere lesions had significantly greater cognitive impairments than did nondepressed patients with comparable left hemisphere lesions ($P < 0.05$). These cognitive deficits primarily involved tasks of temporal orientation, language, and executive motor and frontal lobe functions. On the other hand, among patients with right hemisphere lesions, patients with major depression did not differ from nondepressed patients on any of the measures of cognitive impairment.

Treatment studies of PSD have consistently failed to show an improvement in cognitive function even when poststroke mood disorders responded to antidepressant therapy (Andersen et al. 1996). Kimura et al. (2000) examined this issue in a study comparing nortriptyline and placebo using a double-blind treatment methodology among patients with major ($n = 33$) or minor ($n = 14$) PSD. When patients were divided into those who responded to treatment (i.e., greater than 50% decline in Ham-D score (Hamilton 1960) and no longer meeting depression diagnosis criteria) and those who did not respond, there was a significantly greater improvement in MMSE score among patients who responded to treatment ($n = 24$) compared with patients who did not respond to treatment ($n = 23$). The responding group included 16 patients treated with nortriptyline and 8 treated with placebo, whereas the nonresponding group included 5 patients treated with nortriptyline and 18 treated with placebo.

There were no significant differences between the two groups in baseline Ham-D scores, demographic characteristics, stroke characteristics, or neurologic findings. A repeated measures analysis of variance (ANOVA) demonstrated a significant group by time interaction ($P = 0.005$), and planned post hoc comparisons demonstrated that the responders had significantly less impaired MMSE scores than did the nonresponders, at nortriptyline doses of 75 mg ($P = 0.036$) and 100 mg ($P = 0.024$). When the effect of major versus minor depression was examined, patients with major depression who responded to treatment ($n = 15$) showed significantly greater improvement in MMSE scores than did patients with major depression who did not respond ($n = 18$) ($P = 0.0087$) (Figure 11–7). Among patients with minor depression (9 responders and 5 nonresponders), repeated measures ANOVA of MMSE scores showed no significant group by time interaction.

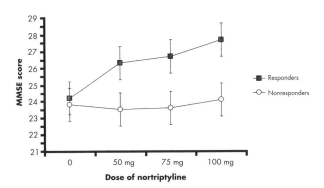

FIGURE 11–7. Change in Mini-Mental State Exam (MMSE) scores in patients with post-stroke major depression during a double-blind treatment study of nortriptyline versus placebo.

Treatment responders ($n = 15$) showed significantly great improvement in cognitive function than nonresponders ($n = 18$) ($P = 0.0087$). Error bars represent standard errors of mean (SE).

Source. Reprinted from Kimura M, Robinson RG, Kosier JT: "Treatment of Cognitive Impairment After Poststroke Depression." *Stroke* 31:1482–1486, 2000. Used with permission.

Mechanism of PSD

Although the cause of PSD remains unknown, one of the mechanisms that has been hypothesized to play an etiologic role is dysfunction of the biogenic amine system. The noradrenergic and serotonergic cell bodies are located in the brain stem and send ascending projections through the median forebrain bundle to the frontal cortex. The ascending axons then arc posteriorly and run longitudinally through the deep layers of the cortex, arborizing and sending terminal projections into the superficial cortical layers (Morrison et al. 1979). Lesions that disrupt these pathways in the frontal cortex or the basal ganglia may affect many downstream fibers. Based on these neuroanatomic facts and the clinical findings that the severity of depression correlates with the proximity of the lesion to the frontal pole, Robinson et al. (1984) suggested that PSD may be the consequence of depletions of norepinephrine and/or serotonin produced by lesions in the frontal lobe or basal ganglia.

In support of this hypothesis, laboratory investigations in rats have demonstrated that the biochemical response to ischemic lesions is lateralized. Right hemisphere lesions produce depletions of norepinephrine and spontaneous hyperactivity, whereas comparable lesions of the left hemisphere do not (Robinson 1979). More recently, a similar lateralized biochemical response to ischemia in human subjects was reported by Mayberg et al. (1988). Patients with stroke lesions in the right hemisphere had significantly higher ratios of ipsilateral to contralateral spiperone binding (presumably serotonin type 2 receptor binding) in noninjured temporal and parietal cortex than did patients with comparable left hemisphere strokes. Patients with left hemisphere lesions, on the other hand, showed a significant inverse correlation between the amount of spiperone binding in the left temporal cortex and depression scores (i.e., higher depression scores were associated with lower serotonin receptor binding).

Treatment of PSD

There have been four placebo-controlled, randomized, double-blind treatment studies on the efficacy of single-antidepressant treatment of PSD. In the first study, Lipsey et al. (1984) examined 14 patients treated with nortriptyline and 20 patients given placebo. The 11 patients treated with nortriptyline who completed the 6-week study showed significantly greater improvement in their Ham-D scores than did 15 placebo-treated patients ($P < 0.01$). Successfully treated patients had serum nortriptyline levels of 50–150 ng/mL. Three patients experienced side effects (including delirium, confusion, drowsiness, and agitation) that were severe enough to require the discontinuation of nortriptyline. Similarly, Reding et al. (1986) reported that patients with PSD (defined as having an abnormal dexamethasone suppression test) taking trazodone had greater improvement in Barthel ADL scores (Granger et al. 1979) than did placebo-treated control subjects ($P < 0.05$). In another double-blind controlled trial in which the selective serotonin reuptake inhibitor (SSRI) citalopram was used, it was found that Ham-D scores were significantly more improved over 6 weeks in patients receiving active treatment ($n = 27$) than in those receiving placebo ($n = 32$) (Andersen et al. 1994). At both 3 and 6 weeks, the group receiving active treatment had significantly lower Ham-D scores than did the group receiving placebo. This study established for the first time the efficacy of an SSRI in the treatment of PSD.

The most recent treatment study, however, was conducted by Robinson et al. (2000). This study compared depressed patients treated with fluoxetine ($n = 23$), nortriptyline ($n = 16$), or placebo ($n = 17$) in a double-blind, randomized treatment design. Patients were enrolled if they had a diagnosis of either major or minor PSD and had no contraindication to the use of fluoxetine or nortriptyline such as intracerebral hemorrhage (fluoxetine) or cardiac induction abnormalities (nortriptyline). Patients in the fluoxetine group were treated with 10-mg doses for the first 3 weeks, 20 mg for weeks 4–6, 30 mg for weeks 6–9, and 40 mg for weeks 9–12. The patients in the nortriptyline group were given 25 mg for the first week, 50 mg for weeks 2 and 3, 75 mg for weeks 3–6, and 100 mg for weeks 6–12. Patients treated with placebo were given identical capsules in the same number used for the actively treated patients. Intention-to-treat analysis demonstrated significant time by treatment interaction, with patients treated with nortriptyline showing a significantly greater decline in Ham-D scores than either the placebo-treated or the fluoxetine-treated patients at 12 weeks of treatment. There were no significant differences between the fluoxetine and the placebo groups (Figure 11–8).

Electroconvulsive therapy has also been reported to be effective for treating PSD (Murray et al. 1987). It causes few side effects and no neurologic deterioration. Psychostimulants have also been reported in open-label trials to be effective for the treatment of PSD. Finally, psychological treatment—including cognitive-behavioral therapy (Hibbard et al. 1990), group therapy, and family therapy—has also been reported to be useful (Oradei and Waite 1974; Watzlawick and Coyne 1980). However, controlled studies for these treatment modalities have not been conducted.

Psychosocial Adjustment

Kotila et al. (1998) examined depression after stroke in the Finnstroke study. This study examined the effect of active rehabilitation programs after discharge together with support and social activities on the frequency of depression among patients and caregivers at 3 months and 1 year after stroke. At both 3 months and 1 year, the frequency of depression was significantly lower among patients receiving active outpatient treatment than among patients without active rehabilitation programs (41% vs. 54% at 3 months and 42% vs. 55% at 1 year).

Poststroke Mania

Although poststroke mania occurs much less frequently than depression (we have observed only three cases among a consecutive series of more than 300 stroke patients), manic syndromes are sometimes associated with stroke.

Phenomenology of Secondary Mania

Starkstein et al. (1988a) examined a series of 12 consecutive patients who met DSM-III criteria (American Psychiatric Association 1980) for an organic affective syndrome, manic type. These patients, who developed mania after a stroke, traumatic brain injury, or tumors, were compared with patients with functional (i.e., no known neuropathology) mania (Starkstein et al. 1987a). Both groups of patients showed similar frequencies of elation, pressured speech, flight of ideas, grandiose thoughts, insomnia, hallucinations, and paranoid delusions. Thus, the symptoms of mania that occurred after brain damage (secondary mania) appeared to be the same as those found in patients with mania without brain damage (primary mania).

Lesion Location

Robinson et al. (1988) reported on 17 patients with secondary mania. Most of the patients had right hemisphere lesions involving either cortical limbic areas, such

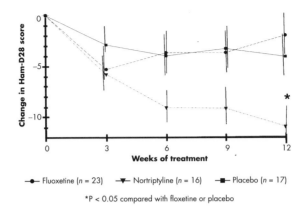

FIGURE 11–8. Intention-to-treat analysis.

Change in (28-item) Hamilton Rating Scale for Depression score over 12 weeks of treatment for all patients who were entered in the study.

Source. Reprinted from Robinson RG, Schultz SK, Castillo C, et al.: "Nortriptyline Versus Fluoxetine in the Treatment of Depression and in Short Term Recovery After Stroke: A Placebo Controlled, Double-Blind Study." *American Journal of Psychiatry* 157:351–359, 2000. Used with permission.

as the orbitofrontal cortex and the basotemporal cortex, or subcortical nuclei, such as the head of the caudate nucleus or the thalamus. The frequency of right hemisphere lesions was significantly greater than it was among patients with major depression, who tended to have left-frontal or basal ganglia lesions.

These findings have been replicated in another study of eight patients with secondary mania (Starkstein et al. 1990b). All eight patients had right hemisphere lesions (seven unilateral and one bilateral injury). Lesions were either cortical (basotemporal cortex in four patients and orbitofrontal cortex in one patient) or subcortical (frontal white matter, head of the caudate nucleus, and anterior limb of the internal capsule in one patient each). Positron emission tomography scans with (^{18}F)fluorodeoxyglucose were carried out in the three patients with purely subcortical lesions. They all showed a focal hypometabolic deficit in the right basotemporal cortex.

Risk Factors

Not every patient with a lesion in limbic areas of the right hemisphere will develop secondary mania. Therefore, there must be risk factors for this disorder.

In one study (Robinson et al. 1988), patients with secondary mania were compared with patients with secondary major depression. Results indicated that patients with secondary mania had a significantly higher frequency of positive family history of affective disorders than did depressed patients or patients with no mood disturbance ($P < 0.05$). Therefore, it appears that genetic predisposition to affective disorders may constitute a risk factor for mania.

In another study (Starkstein et al. 1987a), patients with secondary mania were compared with patients with no mood disturbance who were matched for size, location, and etiology of brain lesion. The groups were also compared with patients with primary mania and control subjects. No significant between-group differences were found either in demographic variables or neurologic evaluation. Patients with secondary mania, however, had a significantly greater degree of subcortical atrophy, as measured by bifrontal-to-brain ratio and third ventricle–to-brain ratio ($P < 0.001$).

Mechanism of Secondary Mania

A case report by Starkstein et al. (1989) suggested that the mechanism of secondary mania is not related to the release of trans-callosal inhibitory fibers (i.e., the release of left limbic areas from tonic inhibition due to a right hemisphere lesion). A patient who developed secondary mania after bleeding from a right basotemporal AVM underwent a Wada test before the therapeutic embolization of the malformation. Injection of amobarbital in the left carotid artery did not abolish the manic symptoms (which would be expected if the "release" theory were correct).

Although the mechanism of secondary mania remains unknown, both lesion studies and metabolic studies suggest that the right basotemporal cortex may play an important role. A combination of biogenic amine system dysfunction and release of tonic inhibitory input into the basotemporal cortex and lateral limbic system may lead to the production of mania.

Treatment of Secondary Mania

Although no systematic treatment studies of secondary mania have been conducted, one report suggested several potentially useful treatment modalities. Bakchine et al. (1989) carried out a double-blind, placebo-controlled treatment study in a single patient with secondary mania. Clonidine (0.6 mg/day) rapidly reversed the manic symptoms, whereas carbamazepine (1,200 mg/day) was associated with no mood changes and levodopa (375 mg/day) was associated with an increase in manic symptoms. In other treatment studies, however, the anticonvulsants valproic acid and carbamazepine as well as neuroleptics and lithium therapy have been reported to be useful in treating secondary mania (Starkstein et al. 1991). None of these treatments, however, have been evaluated in double-blind, placebo-controlled studies.

Poststroke Bipolar Disorder

Although some patients have one or more manic episodes after brain injury, other manic patients also have depression after brain injury. In an effort to examine the crucial factors in determining which patients have bipolar as opposed to unipolar disorder, Starkstein et al. (1991) examined 19 patients with the diagnosis of secondary mania. The bipolar (manic-depressive) group consisted of patients who, after the occurrence of the brain lesion, met DSM-III-R criteria for organic mood syndrome, mania, followed or preceded by organic mood syndrome, depressed. The unipolar-mania group consisted of patients who met the criteria for mania described previously (i.e., DSM-III-R organic mood syndrome, mania), not followed or preceded by depression. All the patients had computed tomographic scan evidence of vascular, neoplastic, or traumatic brain lesion and no history of other neurologic, toxic, or metabolic conditions.

Patients in the bipolar group were found to have significantly greater intellectual impairment as measured by MMSE scores ($P < 0.05$). Almost half of the patients in the bipolar group had recurrent episodes of depression, whereas approximately one-fourth of patients in both the unipolar and bipolar groups had recurrent episodes of mania.

Of the 7 patients with bipolar disorder, 6 had lesions restricted to the right hemisphere, which involved the head of the caudate nucleus (2 patients); the thalamus (3 patients); and the head of the caudate nucleus, the dorsolateral frontal cortex, and the basotemporal cortex (1 patient). The remaining patient developed bipolar illness after surgical removal of a pituitary adenoma. In contrast to the primarily subcortical lesions in the bipolar group, 8 of 12 patients in the unipolar mania group had lesions restricted to the right hemisphere, which involved the basotemporal cortex (6 patients), the orbitofrontal cortex (1 patient), and the head of the caudate nucleus (1 patient). The remaining 4 patients had bilateral lesions involving the orbitofrontal cortex (3 patients) and the orbitofrontal white matter (1 patient).

Poststroke Anxiety Disorder

Starkstein et al. (1990a) examined a consecutive series of patients with acute stroke lesions for the presence of both anxiety and depressive symptoms. Slightly modified DSM-III criteria for generalized anxiety disorder (GAD) (i.e., excluding 6-month duration criteria) were used for the diagnosis of anxiety disorder. The presence of anxious foreboding and excessive worry were required, as were one or more symptoms of motor tension (i.e., muscle tension, restlessness, and easy fatigability), one or more symptoms of autonomic hyperactivity, and one or more symptoms of vigilance and scanning (i.e., feeling keyed up or on edge, difficulty concentrating because of anxiety, trouble falling or staying asleep, and irritability). Of a consecutive series of 98 patients with first-episode acute stroke lesions, only 6 met the criteria for GAD in the absence of any other mood disorder. On the other hand, 23 of 47 patients with major depression also met the criteria for GAD. Patients were then divided into those with anxiety only ($n = 6$), anxiety and depression ($n = 23$), depression only ($n = 24$), and no mood disorder ($n = 45$).

Examination of patients with positive computed tomographic scans revealed that anxious-depressed patients had a significantly higher frequency of cortical lesions (16 of 19 patients) than did either the depression-only group (7 of 15 patients) or the control group (13 of 27 patients). On the other hand, the depres-

sion-only group showed a significantly higher frequency of subcortical lesions than did the anxious-depressed group.

Astrom (1996) examined 71 acute stroke patients for anxiety disorder and observed these patients over 3 years. The strongest correlates of GAD were the absence of social contacts outside the family and dependence of patients on others to perform their primary ADL. These factors were significantly more common in the GAD population than in the non-GAD population at 3 months, 1 year, 2 years, and 3 years after stroke. No other impairment or demographic factors distinguished the GAD patients from the non-GAD patients throughout the follow-up period. At 3-year follow-up, however, GAD was associated with both cortical atrophy (7 of 7 GAD patients had cortical atrophy vs. 19 of 39 non-GAD patients) and greater subcortical atrophy (as measured by frontal horn ratios on computed tomographic scan, $P = 0.03$).

A study by Shimoda and Robinson (1998a, 1998b) examined the effect of GAD on outcome in patients with stroke. A group of 142 patients examined during hospitalization for acute stroke and followed up for 2 years were diagnosed with either GAD ($n = 9$), major depressive disorder alone ($n = 10$), both GAD and major depression ($n = 10$), or neither GAD nor depression ($n = 36$). An examination of the effect of GAD and major depression at the time of the initial hospital evaluation on recovery in ADL at short-term follow-up (i.e., 3–6 months) demonstrated a significant effect of major depression but no significant effect of GAD and no interaction. At long-term follow-up (1–2 years), however, there was a significant interaction between major depression and GAD to inhibit recovery in ADL.

A recent treatment study examined the effect of nortriptyline on GAD that is

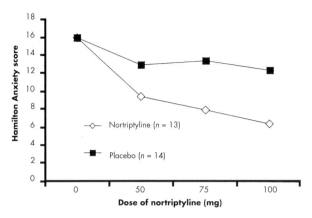

FIGURE 11–9. Mean Hamilton Anxiety Scale scores in patients with generalized anxiety disorder with comorbid depression after stroke following treatment with nortriptyline or placebo.

comorbid with PSD (Kimura and Robinson, unpublished observations, 2001). The study included 29 patients who met criteria for GAD (17 with comorbid major depression, 10 with minor depression, and 2 with no depression). Analysis of the 27 GAD patients with comorbid depression used an intention-to-treat analysis that included 4 patients who dropped out of the study. There were no significant differences between the patients treated with nortriptyline and the patients treated with placebo in background characteristics including age, education, and time since stroke. There were also no significant differences between actively treated and placebo-treated patients in their neurologic findings or the nature of the stroke lesion. In the group treated with nortriptyline, 54% of the patients had right hemisphere lesions; 64% of the placebo group had similar lesions. Motor impairments were present in 77% of the nortriptyline-treated patients and in 86% of the placebo-treated patients. Aphasia was found in 23% of the nortriptyline-treated patients and in 14% of the placebo patients. Because some patients in the study had been treated for 6 weeks whereas others

had been treated for 12 weeks, they were combined based on the dose of nortriptyline that they were receiving.

A repeated measures ANOVA of Hamilton Anxiety Scale (Ham-A) scores using an intention-to-treat analysis demonstrated a significant group by time interaction ($P=0.002$) (i.e., the nortriptyline group improved more quickly than the placebo group) (see Figure 11–9). Planned comparisons revealed that the nortriptyline group was significantly more improved than the placebo group at nortriptyline doses of 50 mg, 75 mg, and 100 mg. Nine of 13 (69%) of the nortriptyline-treated group had more than a 50% reduction in Ham-A scores, whereas only 3 of 14 placebo-treated patients (21%) had a similar reduction ($P=0.017$). At 50 mg of nortriptyline (i.e., 2–3 weeks), there was a 39% improvement in Ham-A scores and only a 14% improvement in Ham-D scores ($P=0.03$). This suggests that anxiety symptoms were responding more rapidly than depressive symptoms with nortriptyline therapy.

Poststroke Psychosis

In a study of acute organic psychosis occurring after stroke lesions, Rabins et al.

(1991) found a very low prevalence of psychosis among stroke patients (only 5 in more than 300 consecutive admissions). All 5 of these patients, however, had right hemisphere lesions, primarily involving frontoparietal regions. When compared with 5 age-matched patients with cerebrovascular lesions in similar locations but no psychosis, patients with secondary psychosis had significantly greater subcortical atrophy, as manifested by significantly larger areas of both the frontal horn of the lateral ventricle and the body of the lateral ventricle (measured on the side contralateral to the brain lesion). Several investigators have also reported a high frequency of seizures among patients with secondary psychosis (Levine and Finklestein 1982). These seizures usually started after the occurrence of the brain lesion but before the onset of psychosis. The study by Rabins et al. (1991) found seizures in 3 of 5 patients with poststroke psychosis, compared with none of 5 poststroke, nonpsychiatric control subjects.

It has been hypothesized that three factors may be important in the mechanism of organic hallucinations: 1) a right hemisphere lesion involving the temporoparietal cortex, 2) seizures, and/or 3) subcortical brain atrophy (Starkstein et al. 1992).

Apathy

Apathy is the absence or lack of feeling, emotion, interest, or concern and has been reported frequently among patients with brain injury. Using the Apathy Scale, Starkstein et al. (1993a) examined a consecutive series of 80 patients with single-stroke lesions and no significant impairment in comprehension. Of 80 patients, 9 (11%) showed apathy as their only psychiatric disorder, whereas another 11% had both apathy and depression. The only demographic correlate of apathy was age, as apathetic patients (with or without

depression) were significantly older than nonapathetic patients. In addition, apathetic patients showed significantly more severe deficits in ADL, and a significant interaction was noted between depression and apathy on ADL scores, with the greatest impairment found in patients who were both apathetic and depressed.

Patients with apathy (without depression) showed a significantly higher frequency of lesions involving the posterior limb of the internal capsule than did patients without apathy (Starkstein et al. 1993a).

Catastrophic Reaction

As described under Historical Perspective earlier in this chapter, *catastrophic reaction* is a term coined by Goldstein (1939) to describe the "inability of the organism to cope when faced with physical or cognitive deficits." Catastrophic reaction is expressed by anxiety, tears, aggressive behavior, swearing, displacement, refusal, renouncement, and sometimes compensatory boasting. Starkstein et al. (1993b) assessed a consecutive series of 62 patients, using the Catastrophic Reaction Scale, which was developed to assess the existence and severity of catastrophic reaction. The Catastrophic Reaction Scale has been demonstrated to be a reliable instrument in the measurement of symptoms of catastrophic reaction.

Catastrophic reactions occurred in 12 of 62 (19%) consecutive patients with acute stroke lesions (Starkstein et al. 1993b). Three major findings emerged from this study. First, patients with catastrophic reaction were found to have a significantly higher frequency of familial and personal history of psychiatric disorders (mostly depression) than were patients without catastrophic reaction. Second, catastrophic reaction was not significantly more frequent among aphasic (33%) than among nonaphasic (66%) patients. This finding does not support the contention that catastrophic reaction is an understandable psychological response of "frustrated" aphasic patients (Gainotti 1972). Third, 9 of the 12 patients with catastrophic reaction also had major depression, 2 had minor depression, and only 1 was not depressed. On the other hand, among the 50 patients without catastrophic reaction, 7 had major depression, 6 had minor depression, and 37 were not depressed. Thus, catastrophic reaction was significantly associated with major depression, but it does not support the proposal by Gainotti et al. (1999) that the catastrophic reaction is an integral part of PSD. It is rather a comorbid condition that occurs in some but not all patients with PSD or may characterize a subgroup of patients with PSD.

Pathologic Emotions

Emotional lability is a common complication of stroke lesions. It is characterized by sudden, easily provoked episodes of crying that, although frequent, generally occur in appropriate situations and are accompanied by a congruent mood change. Pathologic laughing and crying is a more severe form of emotional lability and is characterized by episodes of laughing and/or crying that are not appropriate to the context. They may appear spontaneously or may be elicited by nonemotional events and do not correspond to underlying emotional feelings. These disorders have also been termed *emotional incontinence* and *pathologic emotions*.

Robinson et al. (1993) examined the clinical correlates and treatment of emotional lability (including pathologic laughter and crying) in 28 patients with either acute or chronic stroke. A Pathological Laughter and Crying Scale (PLACS) (Robinson et al. 1993) was developed.

A double-blind treatment trial of nortriptyline versus placebo was con-ducted. The doses of nortriptyline were 25 mg for 1 week, 50 mg for 2 weeks, 70 mg for 1 week, and 100 mg for the last 2 weeks of the study. One patient dropped out during the study, 2 patients withdrew before initiation of the study, and 28 completed the 6-week protocol. Patients receiving nortriptyline showed significant improvements in PLACS scores compared with the placebo-treated patients. These differences became statistically significant at 4 and 6 weeks. Although a significant improvement in depression scores was also observed, improvements in PLACS scores were significant for both depressed and nondepressed patients with pathologic laughing and crying, indicating that treatment response was not simply related to an improvement in depression (Robinson et al. 1993).

Andersen et al. (1993) also conducted a double-blind study using the SSRI citalopram to treat pathologic crying. This study evaluated 16 patients using a crossover design. Three of the patients were dropped from the study—1 who was given placebo because of a generalized seizure on day 28, and 2 others who were also taking placebo because of a lack of response to treatment after the first week. The protocol consisted of 1 week as a baseline, 3 weeks of treatment, and 1 week of washout, followed by 1 week as a second baseline, then 3 weeks of the crossover treatment. The number of crying episodes was recorded daily by the patients in their journals as the measure of treatment efficacy. Their response to treatment is shown in Figure 11–10. The response to citalopram was nearly immediate, with patients reporting a 50% or greater reduction in the frequency of crying episodes during the first week of treatment; 8 patients reported response within 24 hours, 3 patients reported response within 3 days, and only 4 patients took more than a week to respond.

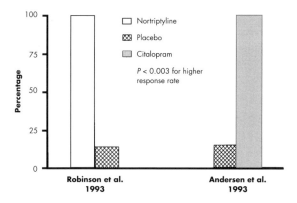

FIGURE 11–10.   Comparison of double-blind treatment studies using nortriptyline or citalopram in patients with pathologic crying.

Both nortriptyline and citalopram produced improvement in 100% of the cases, whereas placebo treatment produced improvement in about 15% of the cases. These findings suggest that nortriptyline and citalopram produce similar reductions in severity measures as well as similar response rates for pathologic crying.

Source.   Reprinted with the permission of Cambridge University Press from Robinson RG: *The Clinical Neuropsychiatry of Stroke.* New York, Cambridge University Press, 1998.

Aprosody

Ross and Mesulam (1979) described aprosody as abnormalities in the affective components of language, encompassing prosody and emotional gesturing. Prosody can be defined as the "variation of pitch, rhythm, and stress of pronunciation that bestows certain semantic and emotional meaning to speech" (Ross and Mesulam 1979, p. 144).

Motor aprosody consists of marked difficulty in spontaneous use of emotional inflection in language (e.g., an absence of normal prosodic variations in speech) or emotional gesturing, whereas comprehension of emotional inflection or gesturing remains intact. Sensory aprosody, on the other hand, is manifested by intact spontaneous emotional inflection in language and gesturing, whereas comprehension of emotional inflection or gesturing is markedly impaired. In a manner analogous to the organization of propositional language in the left hemisphere, expression and comprehension of emotional inflection have been associated respectively with frontal and temporoparietal regions of the right hemisphere (Ross and Mesulam 1979).

Starkstein et al. (1994) examined prosody comprehension in 59 patients with acute stroke lesions. With the use of tapes expressing verbal emotion and photographs of emotional facial expressions, impaired comprehension of emotion was found in a mild form in 10 patients (17%) and in a severe form in 19 patients (32%). Severe aprosody was associated with the following three clinical variables: 1) neglect for tactile stimulation, 2) lesions of the right hemisphere, including the basal ganglia and temporoparietal cortex, and 3) significantly larger third ventricle to brain ratio. Although Ross and Rush (1981) suggested that patients with sensory aprosody might not be able to recognize their own depressed mood, major depression was found in 2 of 19 patients (11%) with severe aprosody and 7 of 30 patients (23%) without aprosody (*P* not significant).

Conclusions

There are numerous emotional and behavioral disorders that occur after cerebrovascular lesions (see Table 11–2). Depression occurs in about 40% of stroke patients, with approximately equal distributions of major depression and minor depression. Major depression is significantly associated with left frontal and left basal ganglia lesions during the acute stroke period and may be successfully treated with nortriptyline or citalopram. Treatment of depression has also been shown to improve poststroke cognitive function.

Mania is a rare complication of stroke and is strongly associated with right hemisphere damage involving the orbitofrontal cortex, basal temporal cortex, thalamus, or basal ganglia. Risk factors for mania include a family history of psychiatric disorders and subcortical atrophy. Bipolar disorders are associated with subcortical lesions of the right hemisphere, whereas right cortical lesions lead to mania without depression.

GAD, which is present in about 27% of stroke patients, is associated with depression in the vast majority of cases. Among the few patients with poststroke anxiety and no depression, there is a high frequency of alcoholism and lesions of the right hemisphere. A recent treatment study demonstrated that GAD can be treated effectively with nortriptyline.

Apathy is present in about 20% of stroke patients. It is associated with older age, more severe deficits in ADL, and a significantly higher frequency of lesions involving the posterior limb of the internal capsule.

Psychotic disorders are rare complications of stroke lesions. Poststroke hallucinations are associated with right hemisphere temporoparietal lesions, sub-cortical brain atrophy, and seizures.

Catastrophic reactions occur in about 20% of stroke patients. These reactions are not related to the severity of impairments or the presence of aphasia but may represent a symptom for one clinical type of poststroke major depression. Catastrophic reactions are associated with anterior subcortical lesions and may result from a "release" of emotional display in a subgroup of depressed patients. Pathologic laughing and crying is another common complication of stroke lesions that may sometimes coexist with depression and may be successfully treated with nortriptyline or citalopram.

References

Adams RD, Victor M: Principles of Neurology. New York, McGraw-Hill, 1985

American Psychiatric Association: Diagnostic and Statistical Manual of Mental Disorders, 3rd Edition. Washington, DC, American Psychiatric Association, 1980

American Psychiatric Association: Diagnostic and Statistical Manual of Mental Disorders, 3rd Edition, Revised. Washington, DC, American Psychiatric Association, 1987

American Psychiatric Association: Diagnostic and Statistical Manual of Mental Disorders, 4th Edition. Washington, DC, American Psychiatric Association, 1994

American Psychiatric Association: Diagnostic and Statistical Manual of Mental Disorders, 4th Edition, Text Revision. Washington, DC, American Psychiatric Association, 2000

Andersen G, Vestergaard K, Riis J: Citalopram for poststroke pathological crying. Lancet 342(8875):837–839, 1993

Andersen G, Vestergaard K, Lauritzen L: Effective treatment of poststroke depression with the selective serotonin reuptake inhibitor citalopram. Stroke 25:1099–1104, 1994

Andersen G, Vestergaard K, Riis JO, et al: Dementia of depression or depression of dementia in stroke? Acta Psychiatr Scand 94:272–278, 1996

Astrom M: Generalized anxiety disorder in stroke patients: a 3-year longitudinal study. Stroke 27:270–275, 1996

Astrom M, Adolfsson R, Asplund K: Major depression in stroke patients: a 3-year longitudinal study. Stroke 24:976–982, 1993a

Astrom M, Olsson T, Asplund K: Different linkage of depression to hypercortisolism early versus late after stroke: a 3-year longitudinal study. Stroke 24:52–57, 1993b

Babinski J: Contribution a l'etude des troubles mentaux dans l'hemiplegic organique cerebrale (anosognosie). Rev Neurol (Paris) 27:845–848, 1914

Bakchine S, Lacomblez L, Benoit N, et al: Manic-like state after orbitofrontal and right temporoparietal injury: efficacy of clonidine. Neurology 39:778–781, 1989

Bamford J, Sandercock P, Dennis M, et al: A prospective study of acute cerebrovascular disease in the community: the Oxfordshire Community Stroke Project 1981–86, 1: methodology, demography and incident cases of first-ever stroke. J Neurol Neurosurg Psychiatry 51(11):1373–1380, 1988

Bolla-Wilson K, Robinson RG, Starkstein SE, et al: Lateralization of dementia of depression in stroke patients. Am J Psychiatry 146:627–634, 1989

Bonita R: Epidemiology of stroke. Lancet 339:342–344, 1992

Bonita R, Beaglehole R, North JD: Event, incidence and case fatality rates of cerebrovascular disease in Auckland, New Zealand. Am J Epidemiol 120(2):236–243, 1984

Broderick JP, Phillips SJ, Whisnant JP, et al: Incidence rates of stroke in the eighties: the end of the decline in stroke? Stroke 20(5):577–582, 1989

Burvill PW, Johnson GA, Jamrozik KD, et al: Prevalence of depression after stroke: the Perth Community Stroke Study. Br J Psychiatry 166(3):320–327, 1995

Castillo CS, Schultz SK, Robinson RG: Clinical correlates of early onset and late-onset poststroke generalized anxiety. Am J Psychiatry 152:1174–1179, 1995

Chemerinski E, Robinson RG: The neuropsychiatry of stroke. Psychosomatics 41(1):5–14, 2000

Collin SJ, Tinson D, Lincoln NB: Depression after stroke. Clin Rehabil 1:27–32, 1987

Dennis M, O'Rourke S, Lewis S, et al: Emotional outcomes after stroke: factors associated with poor outcome. J Neurol Neurosurg Psychiatry 68(1):47–52, 2000

Denny-Brown D, Meyer JS, Horenstein S: The significance of perceptual rivalry resulting from parietal lesions. Brain 75:434–471, 1952

Eastwood MR, Rifat SL Nobbs H, et al: Mood disorder following cerebrovascular accident. Br J Psychiatry 154:195–200, 1989

Ebrahim S, Barer D, Nouri F: Affective illness after stroke. Br J Psychiatry 151:52–56, 1987

Fedoroff JP, Lipsey JR, Starkstein SE, et al: Phenomenological comparisons of major depression following stroke, myocardial infarction or spinal cord lesions. J Affect Disord 22(1–2):83–89, 1991

Feibel JH, Springer CJ: Depression and failure to resume social activities after stroke. Arch Phys Med Rehabil 63(6):276–278, 1982

Finklestein S, Benowitz LI, Baldessarini RJ, et al: Mood, vegetative disturbance, and dexamethasone suppression test after stroke. Ann Neurol 12(5):463–468, 1982

Finset A, Goffeng L, Landro NI, et al: Depressed mood and intra-hemispheric location of lesion in right hemisphere stroke patients. Scand J Rehabil Med 21(1):1–6, 1989

Folstein MF, Folstein SE, McHugh PR: Mini-Mental State: a practical method for grading the cognitive state of patients for the clinician. J Psychiatr Res 12:189–198, 1975

Folstein MF, Mairberger R, McHugh PR: Mood disorder as a specific complication of stroke. J Neurol Neurosurg Psychiatry 40(10):1018–1020, 1977

Gainotti G: Emotional behavior and hemispheric side of the brain. Cortex 8:41–55, 1972

Gainotti G, Azzoni A, Marra C: Frequency, phenomenology and anatomical-clinical correlates of major poststroke depression. Br J Psychiatry 175:163–167, 1999

Goldstein K: The Organism: A Holistic Approach to Biology Derived From Pathological Data in Man. New York, American Books, 1939

Goldstein K: After Effects of Brain Injuries in War. New York, Grune & Stratton, 1942

Granger CV, Denis LS, Peters NC, et al: Stroke rehabilitation: analysis of repeated Barthel Index measures. Arch Phys Med Rehabil 60:14–17, 1979

Haecen H, de Ajuriaguerra J, Massoner J: Les troubles visoconstructifs para lesion parieto occipitale droit. Encephale 40:122–179, 1951

Hamilton MA: A rating scale for depression. J Neurol Neurosurg Psychiatry 23:56–62, 1960.

Herrmann M, Bartles C, Wallesch C-W: Depression in acute and chronic aphasia: symptoms, pathoanatomical-clinical correlations and functional implications. J Neurol Neurosurg Psychiatry 56:672–678, 1993

Herrmann N, Black SE, Lawrence J, et al: The Sunnybrook Stroke Study: a prospective study of depressive symptoms and functional outcome. Stroke 29:618–624, 1998

Hibbard MR, Grober SE, Gordon WA, et al: Modification of cognitive psychotherapy for the treatment of poststroke depression. Behav Ther 13:15–17, 1990

House A, Dennis M, Warlow C, et al: Mood disorders after stroke and their relation to lesion location: a CT scan study. Brain 113:1113–1130, 1990a

House A, Dennis M, Warlow C, et al: The relationship between intellectual impairment and mood disorder in the first year after stroke. Psychol Med 20(4):805–814, 1990b

House A, Dennis M, Mogridge L, et al: Mood disorders in the year after first stroke. Br J Psychiatry 158:83–92, 1991

Kimura M, Robinson RG, Kosier T: Treatment of cognitive impairment after poststroke depression. Stroke 31(7):1482–1486, 2000

Kotila M, Numminen H, Waltimo O, et al: Depression after stroke: results of the FINNSTROKE Study. Stroke 29:368–372, 1998

Levine DN, Finklestein S: Delayed psychosis after right temporoparietal stroke or trauma: relation to epilepsy. Neurology 32: 267–273, 1982

Lipsey JR, Robinson RG, Pearlson GD, et al: Nortriptyline treatment of poststroke depression: a double-blind study. Lancet 2:297–300, 1984

Lipsey JR, Spencer WC, Rabins PV, et al: Phenomenological comparison of functional and poststroke depression. Am J Psychiatry 143:527–529, 1986

Mayberg HS, Robinson RG, Wong DF, et al: PET imaging of cortical S2-serotonin receptors after stroke: lateralized changes and relationship to depression. Am J Psychiatry 145:937–943, 1988

Meyer A: The anatomical facts and clinical varieties of traumatic insanity. American Journal of Insanity 60:373, 1904

Morris PLP, Robinson RG, Raphael B: Prevalence and course of depressive disorders in hospitalized stroke patients. Int J Psychiatry Med 20:349–364, 1990

Morrison JR, Molliver ME, Grzanna R: Noradrenergic innervation of the cerebral cortex: widespread effects of local cortical lesions. Science 205:313–316, 1979

Murray GB, Shea V, Conn DR: Electroconvulsive therapy for poststroke depression. J Clin Psychiatry 47:258–260, 1987

Oradei CM, Waite NS: Group psychotherapy with stroke patients during the immediate recovery phase. Am J Orthopsychiatry 44:386–395, 1974

Paradiso S, Ohkubo T, Robinson RG: Vegetative and psychological symptoms associated with depressed mood over the first two years after stroke. Int J Psychiatry Med 27:137–157, 1997

Parikh RM, Robinson RG, Lipsey JR, et al: The impact of poststroke depression on recovery in activities of daily living over two year follow-up. Arch Neurol 47:785–789, 1990

Pohjasvaara T, Leppavuori A, Siira I, et al: Frequency and clinical determinants of poststroke depression. Stroke 29(11): 2311–2317, 1998

Rabins PV, Starkstein SE, Robinson RG: Risk factors for developing atypical (schizophreniform) psychosis following stroke. J Neuropsychiatry Clin Neurosci 3:6–9, 1991

Reding MJ, Orto LA, Winter SW, et al: Antidepressant therapy after stroke: a double-blind trial. Arch Neurol 43:763–765, 1986

Robinson RG: Differential behavioral and biochemical effects of right and left hemispheric cerebral infarction in the rat. Science 105:707–710, 1979

Robinson RG: The Clinical Neuropsychiatry of Stroke. New York, Cambridge University Press, 1998

Robinson RG, Price TR: Post-stroke depressive disorders: a follow-up study of 103 patients. Stroke 13(5):635–641, 1982

Robinson RG, Szetela B: Mood change following left hemispheric brain injury. Ann Neurol 9:447–453, 1981

Robinson RG, Kubos KL, Starr LG, et al: Mood changes in stroke patients: relationship to lesion location. Compr Psychiatry 24:555–566, 1983a

Robinson RG, Starr LB, Kubos KL, et al: A two year longitudinal study of poststroke mood disorders: findings during the initial evaluation. Stroke 14:736–744, 1983b

Robinson RG, Kubos KL, Starr LB, et al: Mood disorders in stroke patients: importance of location of lesion. Brain 107:81–93, 1984

Robinson RG, Bolla-Wilson K, Kaplan E, et al: Depression influences intellectual impairment in stroke patients. Br J Psychiatry 148:541–547, 1986

Robinson RG, Boston JD, Starkstein SE, et al: Comparison of mania with depression following brain injury: causal factors. Am J Psychiatry 145:172–178, 1988

Robinson RG, Parikh RM, Lipsey JR, et al: Pathological laughing and crying following stroke: validation of measurement scale and double-blind treatment study. Am J Psychiatry 150:286–293, 1993

Robinson RG, Schultz SK, Castillo C, et al: Nortriptyline versus fluoxetine in the treatment of depression and in short term recovery after stroke: a placebo controlled, double-blind study. Am J Psychiatry 157:351–359, 2000

Ross ED, Mesulam MM: Dominant language functions of the right hemisphere: prosody and emotional gesturing. Arch Neurol 36:144–148, 1979

Ross ED, Rush AJ: Diagnosis and neuroanatomical correlates of depression in brain-damaged patients. Arch Gen Psychiatry 38:1344–1354, 1981

Schubert DS, Burns R, Paras W, et al: Increase of medical hospital length of stay by depression in stroke and amputation patients: a pilot study. Psychother Psychosom 57(1–2):61–66, 1992

Schwartz JA, Speed NM, Brunberg JA, et al: Depression in stroke rehabilitation. Biol Psychiatry 33(10):694–699, 1993

Shimoda K, Robinson RG: Effect of anxiety disorder in impairment and recovery from stroke. J Neuropsychiatry Clin Neurosci 10:34–40, 1998a

Shimoda K, Robinson RG: The relationship between social impairment and recovery from stroke. Psychiatry 61(2):101–111, 1998b

Shimoda K, Robinson RG: The relationship between poststroke depression and lesion location in long-term follow-up. Biol Psychiatry 45:187–192, 1999

Sinyor D, Jacques P, Kaloupek DG, et al: Poststroke depression and lesion location: an attempted replication. Brain 109:539–546, 1986

Spitzer RL, Endicott J, Robins E: Research diagnostic criteria: rationale and reliability. Arch Gen Psychiatry 35:773–782, 1978

Starkstein SE, Pearlson GD, Boston J, et al: Mania after brain injury: a controlled study of causative factors. Arch Neurol 44:1069–1073, 1987a

Starkstein SE, Robinson RG, Price TR: Comparison of cortical and subcortical lesions in the production of poststroke mood disorders. Brain 110:1045–1059, 1987b

Starkstein SE, Boston JD, Robinson RG: Mechanisms of mania after brain injury: 12 case reports and review of the literature. J Nerv Ment Dis 176:87–100, 1988a

Starkstein SE, Robinson RG, Price TR: Comparison of patients with and without poststroke major depression matched for size and location of lesion. Arch Gen Psychiatry 45:247–252, 1988b

Starkstein SE, Robinson RG, Price TR: Comparison of spontaneously recovered versus non-recovered patients with poststroke depression. Stroke 19:1491–1496, 1988c

Starkstein SE, Berthier PL, Lylyk A, et al: Emotional behavior after a WADA test in a patient with secondary mania. J Neuropsychiatry Clin Neurosci 1:408–412, 1989

Starkstein SE, Cohen BS, Fedoroff P, et al: Relationship between anxiety disorders and depressive disorders in patients with cerebrovascular injury. Arch Gen Psychiatry 47:785–789, 1990a

Starkstein SE, Mayberg HS, Berthier ML, et al: Secondary mania: neuroradiological and metabolic findings. Ann Neurol 27:652–659, 1990b

Starkstein SE, Fedoroff JP, Berthier MD, et al: Manic depressive and pure manic states after brain lesions. Biol Psychiatry 29:149–158, 1991

Starkstein SE, Robinson RG, Berthier ML: Post-stroke delusional and hallucinatory syndromes. J Neuropsychiatry Neuropsychol Behav Neurol 5:114–118, 1992

Starkstein SE, Fedoroff JP, Price TR, et al: Apathy following cerebrovascular lesions. Stroke 24:1625–1630, 1993a

Starkstein SE, Fedoroff JP, Price TR, et al: Catastrophic reaction after cerebrovascular lesions: frequency, correlates, and validation of a scale. J Neurol Neurosurg Psychiatry 5:189–194, 1993b

Starkstein SE, Fedoroff JP, Price TR, et al: Neuropsychological and neuroradiological correlates of emotional prosody comprehension. Neurology 44:515–522, 1994

Terent A: Increasing incidence of stroke among Swedish women. Stroke 19(5):598–603, 1988

Wade DT, Legh-Smith J, Hewer RA: Depressed mood after stroke: a community study of its frequency. Br J Psychiatry 151:200–205, 1987

Watzlawick P, Coyne JC: Depression following stroke: brief, problem-focused family treatment. Fam Process 19(1):13–18, 1980

Wolf PA, Dawber TR, Thomas HE, et al: Epidemiology of stroke, in Advances in Neurology. Edited by Thompson RA, Green JR. New York, Raven, 1977, pp 5–19

Neuropsychiatric Aspects of Brain Tumors

Trevor R. P. Price, M.D.

Kenneth L. Goetz, M.D.

Mark R. Lovell, Ph.D.

Tumors involving the central nervous system (CNS) are common. The annual incidence of primary brain tumors is 9.0 per 100,000, and that of metastatic brain tumors is 8.3 per 100,000.

Brain tumors are typically classified according to whether they are primary or metastatic, as well as according to location and histologic cell type. Seventy percent of all tumors are supratentorial, with distribution by lobe as indicated in Figure 12–1.

Metastatic disease is more frequent in the elderly and occurs with higher incidence than primary brain tumors.

It has been reported that primary brain tumors are up to 10 times more common among psychiatric patients than in psychiatrically healthy control subjects and that mental changes and behavioral symptoms, including confusion and various other neuropsychiatric symptoms, are more frequent early indicators of primary brain tumors than are classic physical manifestations such as headaches, seizures, and focal neurologic signs (Kocher et al. 1984).

Although the various tumor classifications may eventually turn out to be important in understanding the occurrence of neuropsychiatric symptoms associated with brain tumors, there have been as yet no large-scale, detailed studies carefully examining correlations between clinical phenomenology and various tumor parameters. Our knowledge of the neuropsychiatric and neuropsychological aspects of brain tumors is based on a relatively small number of clinical case reports and larger, uncontrolled case series from the older neurologic and neurosurgical literature. Much of the discussion that follows draws on this database.

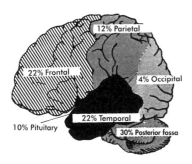

FIGURE 12–1. Relative frequency of intracranial brain tumors according to location in the adult.

Source.   Reprinted from Lohr JB, Cadet JL: "Neuropsychiatric Aspects of Brain Tumors," in *The American Psychiatric Press Textbook of Neuropsychiatry*. Edited by Talbott JA, Hales RE, Yudofsky SC. Washington, DC, American Psychiatric Press, 1987, p. 355. Used with permission.

Frequency of Neuropsychiatric Symptoms in Patients With Brain Tumors

Unfortunately, and surprisingly, there is a paucity of recent studies examining the frequency of psychiatric symptoms in patients with brain tumors. Studies that are available tend to be large autopsy studies, predominantly from the first half of the twentieth century.

For example, Keschner et al. (1938) noted psychiatric symptoms in 413 (78%) of 530 patients with brain tumors, and Schlesinger (1950) found behavioral changes in 301 (51%) of his series of 591 patients. Although tumor-associated, complex neuropsychiatric symptoms may occur along with focal neurologic signs and symptoms; often they may be the first clinical indication of a tumor, as was the case in 18% of patients examined by Keschner et al. (1938). This, of course, also suggests that with modern technologies, 82% of this population would have

had medical or surgical intervention before the advent of behavioral symptoms.

Minski (1933) studied 58 patients with cerebral tumors and, in addition to reporting that the psychiatric symptomatology of 25 of these patients simulated "functional psychoses," noted that 19 actually attributed the onset of their behavioral symptoms to a number of stresses, including financial worries and the deaths of relatives. This underscores the difficulty that clinicians face in making an appropriate diagnosis early in the course of disease: It may be impossible on purely clinical grounds to determine the organic basis of the patient's complaints until progression of the tumor has resulted in the emergence of more typical and unmistakable neurologic signs and symptoms.

Despite the high prevalence of psychiatric symptoms in patients with brain tumors, the prevalence of intracranial tumors in psychiatric patients, compiled from autopsy data from mental hospitals, was only about 3%. Some studies suggest that the risk of an occult neoplasm in patients presenting with purely psychiatric complaints may be as low as 0.1% (Hobbs 1963; Remington and Robert 1962), and two large autopsy studies (Klotz 1957; Selecki 1965) of psychiatric patients have suggested that approximately half of all tumors go undiagnosed before postmortem examination.

General Neuropsychiatric and Neuropsychological Considerations in Relation to Brain Tumors

General Neuropsychiatric Considerations

Patients with CNS tumors can present with mental symptoms that are virtually identical to those found in patients with the full range of primary psychiatric disorders. Over the years, clinicians and researchers have hypothesized a specific relationship between tumor location and neuropsychiatric phenomenology. Small series have supported the belief that depression is more common in frontal lobe tumors and psychosis with temporal lobe neoplasms (Filley and Kleinschmidt-DeMasters 1995). Older, autopsy-based studies have failed to show that behavioral changes were of localizing value (Keschner et al. 1938; Selecki 1965). Overall the literature suggests that the nature and severity of psychiatric dysfunction accompanying tumors are determined by factors other than anatomic location.

The best examples of this are behaviors mediated by tumors involving the limbic system. Tumors affecting any of these structures may produce similar psychopathology. Furthermore, lesions outside the limbic system may produce similar symptoms, attributable to limbic release, disinhibition, diaschisis, or disconnection syndromes (Malamud 1967) (see "General Neuropsychological Considerations" on next page). Limbic tumors have often been associated with depression, affective flattening, apathy, agitation, assaultive behavior, and even a variety of psychotic symptoms.

A study (Starkstein et al. 1988) of patients who developed mania after a variety of brain lesions, including tumors, also illustrates the difficulty of trying to associate specific kinds of psychiatric symptoms with the anatomic location of tumors. Although right-sided involvement was predominant, lesions occurred in frontal, temporoparietal, and temporo-occipital lobes, as well as in cerebellum, thalamus, and pituitary. The unifying aspects among these lesions was not anatomic location but rather interconnection of involved structures with orbitofrontal cortex. These clinical observations call for more sophisticated localization models combining both neuroanatomic location and connectivity.

Other factors include the following:

- Increased intracranial pressure, a nonspecific consequence of CNS tumors that has been implicated in behavioral changes such as apathy, depression, irritability, agitation, and changes in consciousness (Allen 1930).
- Premorbid level of functioning, which often has a significant impact on the nature of the clinical presentation. Tumors often cause an exaggeration of the individual's previous character traits and coping styles. The behavioral changes associated with a brain tumor usually represent a complex combination of the patient's premorbid psychiatric status, tumor-associated mental symptoms, and adaptive or maladaptive responses to the stress of a brain tumor diagnosis.
- Rate of growth. Rapidly growing tumors are often associated with acute psychiatric symptoms as well as cognitive dysfunction. Patients with slow-growing tumors often present with vague personality changes, apathy, or depression, often without associated cognitive changes (Lishman 1987).
- Multiple tumor foci produce behavioral symptoms with greater frequency than do single lesions.
- Tumor type. The relationship between tumor type and neuropsychiatric symptoms is also complex.

Whereas some studies show a correlation, many others do not. Taken together they seem to indicate that tumor type is less important than other factors in determining the nature of neuropsychiatric symptoms.

In summary, tumor-associated factors that most significantly influence symptom formation appear to be extent of involvement, rapidity of growth, and propensity to cause increased intracranial pressure. In addition, the patient's premorbid psychiatric history, level of functioning, and characteristic psychological coping mechanisms significantly influence the nature of the behavioral symptoms that occur.

Interestingly, physicians continue to search for neuropsychiatric syndromes characteristic of lesions in specific neuroanatomic regions in spite of earlier autopsy studies that generally have supported the conclusion that there is little or no specificity between the anatomic locations of brain tumors and the types of abnormal behaviors with which they are associated (Keschner et al. 1936; Schlesinger 1950; Selecki 1965).

Mental changes are twice as likely to occur among patients with supratentorial tumors as with infratentorial tumors (Keschner et al. 1938). Likewise, mental changes tend to occur early in 18% of patients with supratentorial tumors but in only 5% with infratentorial tumors. Psychiatric disturbances are also more common among patients with tumors of the frontal and temporal lobes than in those with tumors of the parietal or occipital lobes.

Psychotic symptoms tend to be particularly frequent among patients with tumors of the temporal lobes and pituitary gland and less common with occipital and cerebellar tumors (Davison and Bagley 1969).

Overall, the literature seems to support a higher frequency of behavioral changes among patients with lesions of the frontal and temporal lobes, as well as deep midline structures. Similarly, bilateral tumors and those with multifocal involvement appear to be more frequently associated with neuropsychiatric symptoms.

General Neuropsychological Considerations

Neuropsychological testing is often helpful in patients with CNS neoplasms in determining the extent of cognitive dysfunction associated with a tumor, providing a preoperative baseline measure of cognitive and memory functioning, and monitoring the efficacy and progress of cognitive rehabilitation efforts after treatment.

Histologic type and rate of growth of a tumor may affect the nature and severity of cognitive symptoms. For example, rapidly growing, invasive tumors, such as glioblastomas, have been thought to cause cognitive dysfunction, whereas slower-growing, noninvasive tumors, such as meningiomas, have not as frequently been associated with cognitive changes or focal neurologic deficits (Reitan and Wolfson 1985). However, a more recent, well-controlled study did not find significant differences between patients with glioblastomas and those without on a battery of neuropsychological tests (Scheibel et al. 1996). In patients with slower-growing tumors, the degree to which cognitive deficits will become clinically apparent is related to the individual's level of intelligence and adaptive functioning before the development of the tumor. In addition, younger patients may be less likely than older patients to manifest cognitive and behavioral deficits (Bigler 1984).

Specific patterns of cognitive deficits may reflect anatomic location (Scheibel et al. 1996), and tumors may also produce disruption of brain function in nonadjacent regions. "Distance effects" (Lezak 1995) may be important in determining the deficits found on neuropsychological testing. First, the phenomenon of diaschisis refers to impairment of neuronal activity in a functionally related though distant region of the brain (von Monakow 1914).

Second, disconnection of a given region of the brain from a distant region by a structural lesion can affect the nature and expression of symptoms.

Specific Neuropsychiatric and Neuropsychological Symptoms and Brain Tumor Location

The discussion that follows reviews the neuropsychiatric and neuropsychological signs and symptoms that have been reported to co-occur preferentially with brain tumors involving various brain regions.

Tumors of the Frontal Lobe

Neuropsychiatric and Behavioral Manifestations

Tumors of the frontal lobes may be associated with behavioral symptoms in as many as 90% of cases (Strauss and Keschner 1935), and often occur early in the course of the illness. This is not surprising when one considers that higher-level executive and cognitive functions are mediated by this region of the cortex.

Pathology in the frontal lobes has been associated with three different kinds of clinical syndromes (Cummings 1993):

- The orbitofrontal syndrome is characterized by changes in personality, irritability and lability, poor judgment, and lack of insight.
- Patients with the so-called dorsolateral prefrontal syndrome often present with apathy, indifference, and psychomotor retardation. Cognitively, such patients have difficulty initiating or persisting in activities, have problems with sustained attention and/or sequencing, and may demonstrate perseverative behavior (Goldberg 1986).

- Patients with the anterior cingulate syndrome may be akinetic with mutism and inability to respond to commands.

Most patients with tumors of the frontal lobes present with a combination of symptoms. This is probably due in part to the fact that tumors of the frontal lobe are rarely confined to a single subregion of the frontal lobes and may be causing effects on other areas, both directly and indirectly via increased pressure and edema, as well as diaschisis and disconnection.

Psychiatric and behavioral presentations of frontal lobe tumors can be quite variable. Anxiety has been described and has been noted to increase with tumor progression (Kaplan and Miner 1997). Affective symptoms are common and can include depression, irritability, apathy, and euphoria. Often psychomotor retardation with aspontaneity, hypokinesia, or akinesia occurs. In one study of 25 patients with frontal lobe tumors (Direkze et al. 1971), 5 had initially presented to psychiatric units with what appeared to be mood disturbances. In their study of 85 patients, Strauss and Keschner (1935) reported affective symptoms in 63%, of whom 30% presented with euphoria and 4% with hypomania.

Changes in personality have been found in as many as 70% of patients with frontal lobe tumors (Strauss and Keschner 1935). These changes, which have been described as "characteristic" of frontal lobe disease (Pincus and Tucker 1978), include irresponsibility, childishness, facetiousness, disinhibition, and indifference toward others, as well as inappropriate sexual behavior.

Psychotic symptoms occur with some regularity in patients with frontal lobe tumors. Strauss and Keschner (1935) reported a 10% incidence of both delusions and hallucinations in their series.

Other psychotic symptoms reported in patients with frontal lobe tumors have included paranoid ideation and ideas of reference.

The presence of leg weakness, gait abnormalities, or urinary incontinence with psychiatric and behavioral symptoms should strongly indicate the need for a thorough search for frontal lobe pathology.

Neuropsychological Manifestations

In patients with tumors of the frontal regions of the brain, previously acquired cognitive skills are often preserved, and performance on formal intelligence testing may be quite adequate. More sophisticated neuropsychological assessment of executive functioning, however, often reveals profound deficits in the individual's ability to organize, initiate, and direct personal behavior (Lezak 1995; Teuber 1972). Deficits in executive functioning are often the most devastating and disabling types of cognitive dysfunctions encountered in neurologic, neurosurgical, and psychiatric patients (Luria 1980). Such deficits disrupt the very core of an individual's drive, initiative, and ability to function effectively in many different roles, as well as the ability to carry out critical higher cognitive functions (Luria 1980).

Tumors of the frontal lobes can also result in significant deficits in attentional processes (Luria 1973). In addition, tumors of the posterior frontal lobe can lead to expressive (Broca's) aphasia, when the lesion is localized to the dominant hemisphere (Benson 1979), or aprosody, when it is localized to the anterior nondominant hemisphere (Ross 1988).

Tumors of the Temporal Lobe

Neuropsychiatric and Behavioral Manifestations

Patients with temporal lobe tumors have a high frequency of schizophrenia-like illnesses. Malamud (1967) reported that 6 of 11 patients (55%) with temporal lobe tumors were initially given a diagnosis of schizophrenia. Selecki (1965) reported that an initial diagnosis of schizophrenia had been made in 2 of his 9 patients with temporal lobe tumors, and he reported auditory hallucinations in 5. More recently, Roberts et al. (1990) reported that gangliogliomas, neoplastic hamartomatous lesions that preferentially involve the left medial temporal lobes, are frequently found in patients with delayed-onset, schizophrenia-like psychoses associated with chronic temporal lobe epilepsy.

Other studies, however, have not confirmed the apparent high frequency of psychotic syndromes in patients with temporal lobe tumors. Keschner et al. (1936) studied 110 such patients and found that only 2 had complex hallucinations. In another study (Mulder and Daly 1952), only 4 of 100 patients with temporal lobe tumors had psychotic symptoms. Strobos (1953) noted complex auditory hallucinations in only 1 (1%) of his 62 patients with temporal lobe tumors. He found complex visual hallucinations in 5 (8%) and simple olfactory or gustatory hallucinations in approximately 19 (30%), although these almost invariably immediately preceded the onset of seizures.

Regardless of how often specific psychotic symptoms may occur with temporal lobe tumors, these lesions are commonly associated with behavioral disturbances. Neuropsychiatric symptoms associated with temporal lobe tumors tend to be similar to those seen in patients with frontal lobe tumors and may include depressed mood with apathy and irritability or euphoric, expansive mood with hypomania or mania. As noted previously, this probably reflects the complex interconnections among the frontal lobes, temporal lobes, and related structures within the limbic system.

Personality changes have been described in more than 50% of patients with temporal lobe tumors and may be an early symptom thereof (Keschner et al. 1936). Research by Bear and Fedio (1977) suggests that characteristic interictal personality traits occur in patients with temporal lobe epilepsy and, furthermore, that the presence or absence of certain traits depends on whether the seizure focus is in the right or the left temporal lobe. More recent studies (Mungas 1982; Rodin and Schmaltz 1984), however, have failed to confirm these initial findings. Often temporal lobe tumor patients present with an intensification of premorbid character traits or with symptoms similar to those seen in conjunction with frontal lobe tumors. Personality changes, including affective lability, episodic behavioral dyscontrol, intermittent anger, irritability, euphoria, and facetiousness, are also commonly seen (Lishman 1987).

Anxiety symptoms are commonly associated with temporal lobe tumors. Mulder and Daly (1952) noted anxiety in 36 of their 100 patients. Two cases of panic attacks in patients with right temporal lobe tumors have been reported also (Drubach and Kelly 1989; Ghadirian et al. 1986).

Neuropsychological Manifestations

Tumors of the temporal lobes can result in verbal or nonverbal memory dysfunction, depending on the cerebral hemisphere involved. Tumors of the dominant temporal lobe may also result in receptive (Wernicke's) aphasia, whereas tumors of the nondominant lobe may lead to disruption of the discrimination of nonspeech sounds (Spreen et al. 1965).

Tumors of the Parietal Lobe

Neuropsychiatric and Behavioral Manifestations

In general, tumors of the parietal lobe are relatively "silent" with respect to psychi-

atric symptoms. Schlesinger (1950) found affective symptoms in only 5 (16%) of 31 patients with parietal lobe tumors. The affective symptoms in these patients were predominantly depression and apathy. More recently, two case studies have reported mania in patients with right parietal tumors (Khouzam et al. 1994; Salazar-Calderon Perriggo et al. 1993).

Although psychotic symptoms also appear to be less common in patients with parietal lobe tumors, Selecki (1965) reported episodes of "paranoid psychosis" in two of the seven patients with parietal lobe tumors in his series. Cotard's syndrome, involving the denial of one's own existence, has been reported in a patient with a left parietal astrocytoma (Bhatia 1993).

Neuropsychological Manifestations

Of greater significance than the psychiatric and behavioral symptoms associated with parietal lobe tumors are the complex sensory and motor abnormalities that may accompany them.

Tumors of the anterior parietal lobes may result in inability to identify objects placed in the contralateral hand (astereognosis) and difficulty in recognizing shapes, letters, and numbers drawn on the hand (agraphesthesia). Apraxias may also be present. Parietal lobe tumors may interfere with the ability to decipher visuospatial information, particularly when they are localized to the nondominant hemisphere (Warrington and Rabin 1970).

Tumors of the dominant parietal lobe may lead to dysgraphia, acalculia, finger agnosia, and right-left confusion (Gerstmann's syndrome) and often affect reading and spelling. Individuals with parietal lobe tumors often present with a marked lack of awareness or even frank denial of their neurologic and/or neuropsychiatric difficulties, even in the face of obvious dysfunctions, such as hemiparesis

(Critchley 1964a). Such phenomena are referred to as anosognosia or neglect syndromes. Because of the often bizarre neurologic complaints and atypical symptoms that may accompany parietal lobe tumors, patients with these lesions are often initially misdiagnosed as having either a conversion disorder or some other type of somatization disorder (Critchley 1964b; Jones and Barklage 1990).

Tumors of the Occipital Lobe

Neuropsychiatric and Behavioral Manifestations

Patients with tumors of the occipital lobe may present with psychiatric symptoms, but they are less likely to do so than are those with tumors of the frontal or temporal lobes (Keschner et al. 1938). In 1930, Allen found psychiatric symptoms in 55% of a large series ($N = 40$) of patients with occipital lobe tumors. In 17% of these patients, behavioral symptoms had been the presenting complaint. The most characteristic finding was visual hallucinations, which were present in 25% of the patients. These hallucinations tended to be simple and unformed and were frequently merely flashes of light. In only two patients were there complex visual hallucinations. Keschner et al. (1938) observed affective symptoms in 5 of 11 patients with occipital lobe tumors. Three of these patients were dysphoric, and 2 presented with euphoria or facetiousness.

Neuropsychological Manifestations

Tumors of the occipital lobes may cause significant difficulties in cognitive and perceptual functions. A typical finding in patients with occipital lobe neoplasms is homonymous hemianopsia, the loss of one-half of the visual field in each eye. Inability to recognize items visually (visual agnosia) may also be seen (Lezak 1995). Inability to recognize familiar faces, a con-

dition known as prosopagnosia, may also accompany tumors of the occipital lobes, particularly when they are bilateral (Meadows 1974).

Diencephalic Tumors

Neuropsychiatric and Behavioral Manifestations

Tumors of the diencephalon involve regions that are part of or contiguous to the limbic system. These lesions interrupt various cortical-striatal-pallidal-thalamic-cortical loops, which may adversely affect many frontal lobe functions (Alexander and Crutcher 1990). These lesions are often associated with psychiatric and behavioral disturbances. Thus, Malamud (1967) reported diagnoses of schizophrenia in four of seven patients with tumors involving structures near the third ventricle. Cairns and Mosberg (1951) reported "emotional instability" and psychosis in patients with colloid cysts of the third ventricle. Burkle and Lipowski (1978) also reported depression, affective flattening, and withdrawal in a patient with a colloid cyst of the third ventricle. Personality changes similar to those seen in patients with frontal lobe disease (Alpers 1937; Gutmann et al. 1990), akinetic mutism (Cairns et al. 1941), and catatonia (Neuman et al. 1996) have also been reported in patients with diencephalic or deep midline tumors.

Hypothalamic tumors have been associated with disorders of eating behavior, including hyperphagia (Coffey 1989), and with symptoms suggestive of anorexia nervosa. Chipkevitch (1994) reported on 21 cases in the literature in which patients with brain lesions presented with symptoms consistent with a diagnosis of anorexia nervosa. Eleven of these patients had tumors of the hypothalamus. In eight of these patients, surgical resection or radiation treatment led to improvement in the anorexia. Patients with lesions of the hypothalamus can also present with hypersomnia.

Neuropsychological Manifestations

Neoplasms originating in subcortical brain regions often have their most dramatic effects on memory. These lesions often result in significant impairment in the retrieval of previously learned material, whereas other aspects of neuropsychological functioning may appear to be relatively intact (Lishman 1987). Detailed neuropsychological evaluation of patients with subcortical tumors may reveal a pattern of "subcortical dementia" characterized by a general slowing of thought processes, forgetfulness, apathy, abulia, depression, and impaired ability to manipulate previously acquired knowledge (Albert et al. 1974; Cummings 1990). Tumors in this area may also lead indirectly to more diffuse, generalized cognitive dysfunction by interfering with the normal circulation of cerebrospinal fluid (CSF), causing hydrocephalus and/or increased CSF pressure.

Tumors of the Corpus Callosum

Tumors of the corpus callosum, especially of the genu and splenium, have been associated with behavioral symptoms in as many as 90% of patients (Schlesinger 1950; Selecki 1964). Affective symptoms appear to be particularly common with tumors involving this area.

Pituitary Tumors

Patients with craniopharyngiomas sometimes present with disorders of sleep, temperature regulation, or anorexia nervosa syndromes (Chipkevitch 1994).

Tumors of the pituitary also cause endocrine disturbances and neuropsychiatric symptoms. Basophilic adenomas are commonly associated with Cushing's syndrome and are frequently associated with affective lability, depression, or psychotic symptoms. Patients with acidophilic adenomas may present with acromegaly, anxiety, and depression (Avery 1973).

The entire spectrum of psychiatric symptoms, from depression and apathy to paranoia, has been reported to occur in patients with pituitary tumors. One review of 5 patients with pituitary lesions reported delusions and hallucinations in 3 (White and Cobb 1955). In a study by Russell and Pennybacker (1961), 8 (33%) of 24 patients had severe mental disturbances that dominated their clinical picture, and 3 (13%) had initially presented to psychiatric hospitals for diagnosis and treatment. The heterogeneous psychiatric and behavioral symptoms associated with pituitary tumors probably reflect the direct and indirect involvement of nearby diencephalic and hypothalamic structures, as well as the effects of various endocrine disturbances.

Tumors of the Posterior Fossa

Patients with infratentorial tumors generally present with psychiatric symptoms less often than do those with other types of tumors. A wide variety of behavioral symptoms may occur in patients with such tumors, which further underscores the difficulty of localizing lesions on the basis of the typology of associated psychiatric symptoms.

In one series, psychiatric and behavioral symptoms, including paranoid delusions and affective disorders (Wilson and Rupp 1946), were found in 76% of patients with lesions of the posterior fossa. Pollack et al. (1996) reported affective disorders, psychosis, personality changes, and somatization in their small series. Cases of mania have also been noted (e.g., Greenberg and Brown 1985). Tumors of the posterior fossa have been associated with irritability, apathy, hypersomnolence, and auditory hallucinations (Cairns 1950). Visual hallucinations have been reported in conjunction with tumors compressing the midbrain (Dunn and Weisberg 1983; Nadvi and van Dellen 1994), and manic or mixed states have been described in patients with acoustic neuromas (Kalayam et al. 1994). Over-anxious disorder of childhood with school phobia was reported in a 12-year-old boy with a fourth-ventricle tumor (Blackman and Wheler 1987). The anxiety symptoms were alleviated by surgical removal of the tumor.

Laterality of Brain Tumors and Clinical Manifestations

Despite the fact that many older studies reported no consistent differences in the psychiatric and behavioral symptoms associated with left- and right-sided tumors, more recent studies have raised questions about this. The importance of cerebral hemispheric lateralization in the causation of psychiatric symptomatology has been elegantly demonstrated by Robinson et al. (1984) in their work with stroke patients. Although there have been few reports specifically addressing laterality and psychiatric symptoms in patients with brain tumors, studies reviewing cases of mania secondary to CNS lesions, including tumors, have found a preponderance of right hemisphere lesions (Cummings and Mendez 1984; Jamieson and Wells 1979; Starkstein et al. 1988). A study of unilateral frontal tumors (Belyi 1987) reported that left-sided lesions were commonly associated with akinesia and depression, whereas right-sided lesions were more often associated with euphoria and patients' underestimating the seriousness of their illnesses. Pringle et al. (1999) also reported an overall higher incidence of psychiatric disturbances in women with left-sided lesions.

These studies suggest that lesion later-

ality may be a more important factor in symptom formation in brain tumor patients than had previously been thought. The available literature suggests the need to reevaluate tumor location and its implications for neuropsychiatric and neuropsychological symptomatology from a more topographic perspective. There is a need to consider not only regional anatomic localization but also factors such as laterality, anterior/posterior and cortical/subcortical localization, and afferent and efferent projections between the regions directly involved with the tumor and those at a distance. More important, such a perspective will provide a more clinically relevant, though necessarily more complex, theoretical framework from which to approach the study of psychopathologic symptoms and syndromes associated with brain tumors.

Clinical Diagnosis and Treatment

General Clinical Characteristics of Brain Tumors

Prompt and accurate diagnosis of brain tumors rests on awareness of their many clinical manifestations. A high index of suspicion, appropriate specialty consultations, and diagnostic studies are critical to early diagnosis.

Characteristic of CNS tumors is the occurrence of neurologic signs and symptoms and neuropsychiatric symptoms. The former are more frequent than the latter in early brain tumors and include changes in personality and affect, sensorium and cognition, and memory. The clinical picture depends on the type, size, location, and rate of growth of the tumor; whether it is benign or malignant; and whether cerebral edema, increased intracranial pressure, and/or hydrocephalus are present.

When to Suspect a Brain Tumor in a Psychiatric Patient

It may be difficult to diagnose brain tumors in patients presenting with predominantly psychiatric and behavioral symptoms. However, the occurrence of one or more of the following five signs and symptoms in patients with psychiatric symptoms should greatly heighten the clinician's index of suspicion:

1. Seizures, especially if focal or partial, with or without secondary generalization
2. Headaches, especially if generalized and dull, of increasing severity and/or frequency; or positional, nocturnal, or present immediately on awakening
3. Nausea and vomiting, especially in conjunction with headaches
4. Sensory changes: loss or diminution of vision, visual field defects, or diplopia; tinnitus or hearing loss, especially when unilateral; or vertigo
5. Other neurologic signs and symptoms, such as weakness, sensory loss, paresthesias or dysesthesias, ataxia, and incoordination (see Table 12–1)

Nausea and vomiting, visual field defects, papilledema, and other focal neurologic signs and symptoms may not be seen until very late, especially with "silent" tumors, such as meningiomas or slow-growing astrocytomas.

Diagnostic Evaluation

A detailed history of the nature, onset, and time course of both psychiatric and neurologic signs and symptoms is the cornerstone of diagnosis. This should be supplemented by careful physical and neurologic examinations, appropriate brain imaging and electrodiagnostic studies, and bedside neurocognitive assessment, including the Mini-Mental State Exam (MMSE) (Folstein et al. 1975), as well as formal neuropsychological testing as indicated.

Physical and Neurologic Examinations

All patients presenting with psychiatric and behavioral symptoms for the first time or with new symptoms should have careful physical, neurologic, and mental status examinations. Patients with brain tumors often have focal neurologic findings as well as abnormalities in cognitive functioning. Table 12–1 highlights localizing neurologic findings that may be found in association with brain tumors in various locations. Some brain tumors may not become clinically apparent until relatively late in their course. Such tumors often involve the anterior frontal lobes, corpus callosum, nondominant parietal and temporal lobes, and posterior fossa, the so-called silent regions. Thus, in patients without focal neurologic findings, other diagnostic studies are essential.

Computed Tomography (CT) Scans

In the 1970s, CT scans largely replaced plain skull films, radioisotope brain scans, electroencephalography, echoencephalography, and pneumoencephalography in the diagnosis of brain tumors. The capacity of CT scans to reveal neoplasms can be further enhanced through the use of intravenous iodinated contrast materials, such as iohexol, that highlight tumors when they are present. CT scans can also suggest the presence of tumors by revealing calcifications, cerebral edema, obstructive hydrocephalus, a shift in midline structures, or other abnormal changes in the ventricular system. CT scans may not reveal very small tumors, tumors in the posterior fossa, tumors that are isodense with respect to brain tissue or CSF, and tumors diffusely involving the meninges (i.e., carcinomatosis).

TABLE 12–1. Neurologic and neuropsychological findings with localizing value

Brain region	Neurologic and neuropsychological findings
Frontal lobes	
Prefrontal	Contralateral grasp reflex, executive functioning deficits (inability to formulate goals, to plan, and to effectively carry out these plans), decreased oral fluency (dominant hemisphere), decreased design fluency (nondominant hemisphere), motor perseveration or impersistence, and inability to hold set
Posterior	Contralateral hemiparesis; decreased motor strength, speed, and coordination; and Broca's aphasia
Temporal lobes	Partial complex seizures, contralateral homonymous inferior quadrantanopsia, Wernicke's aphasia, decreased learning and retention of verbal material (dominant hemisphere), decreased learning and retention of nonverbal material (nondominant hemisphere), amusia (nondominant hemisphere), and auditory agnosia
Parietal lobes	Partial sensory seizures, agraphesthesia, astereognosis, anosognosia, Gerstmann's syndrome (acalculia, agraphia, finger agnosia, and right-left confusion), ideomotor and ideational apraxia, constructional apraxia, agraphia with alexia, dressing apraxia, prosopagnosia, and visuospatial problems
Occipital lobes	Partial sensory seizures with visual phenomena, homonymous hemianopsia, alexia, agraphia, prosopagnosia, color agnosia, and construction apraxia
Corpus callosum	Callosal apraxia
Thalamus	Contralateral hemisensory loss and pain
Basal ganglia	Contralateral choreoathetosis, dystonia, rigidity, motor perseveration, and parkinsonian tremor
Pituitary	Bitemporal hemianopia, optic atrophy, hypopituitarism, and hypothalamus and diabetes insipidus
Pineal	Loss of upward gaze (Parinaud's syndrome)
Cerebellum	Ipsilateral hypotonia, ataxia, dysmetria, intention tremor, and nystagmus toward side of tumor
Brain stem	
Midbrain	Pupillary and extraocular muscle abnormalities and contralateral hemiparesis
Pons	Sixth and seventh nerve involvement (diplopia and ipsilateral facial paralysis)

Source. Reprinted from Lohr JB, Cadet JL: "Neuropsychiatric Aspects of Brain Tumors," in *The American Psychiatric Press Textbook of Neuropsychiatry*. Edited by Talbott JA, Hales RE, Yudofsky SC. Washington, DC, American Psychiatric Press, 1987, p. 354. Used with permission.

Magnetic Resonance Imaging Scans

In general, magnetic resonance imaging (MRI) scans are superior to CT scans in the diagnosis of brain tumors and other soft-tissue lesions in the brain because of higher degrees of resolution and greater ability to detect very small lesions. In addition, MRIs do not involve exposure to radiation. The chief drawbacks of MRIs are their cost and inability to reveal calcified lesions. They also cannot be used in patients in whom ferrometallic foreign objects are present. Enhancement of MRIs with gadolinium further enhances their diagnostic sensitivity.

Cisternography

CT cisternography, a radiographic technique for evaluating the ventricular system, subarachnoid spaces, and basilar cisterns, may be helpful in the differential diagnosis of intraventricular tumors as well as tumor-associated hydrocephalus.

Skull Films

Although plain skull films are no longer routinely used in the diagnosis of brain tumors, tomographs of the sella turcica may be helpful in the diagnosis of pituitary tumors, craniopharyngiomas, and the so-called empty sella syndrome. Plain skull films may also be helpful in the diagnosis of bone (skull) metastases, but bone scans are generally superior in this regard.

Cerebral Angiography

Cerebral angiography may be important in delineating the vascular supply to a brain tumor before surgery.

Neuropsychological Testing

Neuropsychological testing plays an important role in the management of patients with cerebral tumors. It can be very helpful in determining the extent of tumor-associated cognitive dysfunction and in providing baseline, preoperative, and/or preradiation measures of cognitive functioning. It may also be helpful in assessing the efficacy of surgery with respect to improvements in tumor-associated cognitive and neuropsychological dysfunction. It is also helpful in documenting postoperative and postradiation cognitive changes and monitoring the effectiveness of rehabilitative efforts.

Lumbar Puncture

Given the range of sensitive, specific, and less invasive diagnostic studies currently available, lumbar puncture is used less frequently than in the past in the diagnosis of brain tumors. Brain tumors may be associated with elevated CSF protein and increased intracranial pressure, but these findings are diagnostically nonspecific, and in the presence of the latter, there is a potential danger of herniation after a lumbar puncture. Therefore, before proceeding with a lumbar puncture in a patient with a brain tumor, the clinician should carefully examine the eyegrounds for indications of papilledema, and a CT or MRI scan should be done to rule out increased intracranial pressure. With certain types of neoplastic diseases of the CNS, such as meningeal carcinomatosis and leukemia, however, lumbar puncture may play an important diagnostic role when other neurodiagnostic studies have been unrevealing.

Electroencephalography

Electroencephalography in patients with brain tumors may reveal nonspecific electrical abnormalities, such as diffuse or focal spikes and slow waves, which may be paroxysmal or continuous. Frequently, however, the electroencephalogram is normal in brain tumor patients. It is not a very specific or sensitive test and thus not very helpful in differentiating brain tumors from other localized structural cerebral lesions.

Other Testing

Obtaining a chest X ray is important in evaluating brain tumors because it may reveal a primary lung neoplasm, which may be the source of brain metastases. Single photon emission computed tomography (SPECT), positron emission tomography (PET), and brain electrical activity mapping (BEAM) are quantitative, computer-based techniques for evaluating brain structure and function. At present, none of these techniques appears to have major advantages over the standard approaches discussed previously, but this may change as clinical experience with them accumulates. SPECT may have some utility in differentiating tumor recurrence from radiation necrosis in brain tumor patients who have received radiation therapy, or in the differentiation of CNS lymphoma from infectious processes such as toxoplasma encephalitis in AIDS patients (Ruiz et al. 1994).

Magnetoencephalography (MEG) is more precise than electroencephalography in localizing abnormal electrical activity in the brain and has the additional advantage of being able to be used repeatedly in assessing brain activity over time without radiation exposure. The role MEG may play in the evaluation of brain tumors is unclear at present, but it may prove useful in the assessment of tumor-associated diaschisis and disconnection syndromes.

Treatment of Psychiatric and Behavioral Symptoms Associated With Cerebral Tumors

General Considerations

Psychiatric and behavioral symptoms may be completely eliminated after removal of the cerebral tumor with which they are associated. When this does not happen, decreasing the size or interfering with the growth of the tumor through surgery, chemotherapy, or radiation therapy (alone, sequentially, or in combination) may ameliorate the severity of associated behavioral symptoms. Improvement in cognitive and behavioral symptoms may be rapid and dramatic with treatments that diminish increased intracranial pressure or relieve hydrocephalus associated with brain tumors.

In cases where neuropsychiatric or behavioral symptoms persist or worsen after optimal surgical and nonsurgical interventions, psychopharmacologic, psy-

chotherapeutic, and psychosocial interventions become a major treatment focus. These symptoms are distressing, cause functional impairment and disability, and negatively impact the patient's quality of life (Weitzner 1999).

The interventions of the consulting psychiatrist, working closely with the attending neurosurgeon, may improve the patient's level of functioning and overall quality of life (Fox 1998). Ameliorating the disabling dysphoria and anergia of severe depression, alleviating the distress caused by overwhelming anxiety, or simply providing consistent supportive contacts to fearful patients and their families may make an enormous difference to all concerned. Often such interventions also improve treatment outcomes through increased patient motivation and improved treatment compliance, which may enhance the efficacy of the surgical, radiotherapeutic, and/or chemotherapeutic treatment of the patient's brain tumor.

Although patients with brain tumors often have psychiatric and behavioral symptoms, only a portion of these reflect a mental disorder directly related to the tumor. Patients may also have persistent or recurrent symptoms of affective or anxiety disorders that were present premorbidly and have been exacerbated by the stress of living with a brain tumor. Anxiety and depressive symptoms may also arise de novo in any brain tumor patient, with or without a history of a psychiatric disorder, as a result of psychological reactions to the stress of the initial diagnosis of a brain tumor; concerns about how it will be treated; fears about the potential adverse effects of surgery, radiation therapy, and/or chemotherapy; and worries about long-term prognosis. Other psychiatric symptoms may emerge later in reaction to the difficulties of adjusting to functional disabilities or distressing life changes that may result from the tumor itself or from the side effects and complications of the various therapeutic interventions brought to bear on it. It is important for the consulting psychiatrist to differentiate as precisely as possible among symptoms that are specifically tumor related; those that result from preexisting primary psychiatric disorders; and those that are predominantly reactive in nature and secondary to acute and chronic psychological stresses. This is because the choice of optimal pharmacologic and psychotherapeutic interventions depends on which of these are the primary cause of the patient's symptoms.

Pharmacologic Management of Patients With Primary Psychiatric Disorders Who Develop Brain Tumors

The psychopharmacologic management of patients with preexisting primary psychiatric illnesses who develop cerebral tumors should follow the same general therapeutic principles that apply to tumor-free patients with similar disorders. However, it is important for the psychiatrist to be cognizant of the potential need to make downward adjustments in medication dose and to use drugs that are less likely to cause delirium in patients with brain tumors, as a result of their increased susceptibility to develop side effects when given psychotropic medications. This is especially true of patients who are in the immediate postoperative period or are receiving chemotherapy or radiation therapy. Lithium, low-potency antipsychotic drugs, tertiary amine tricyclic antidepressants (TCAs), and antiparkinsonian agents all have significant, dose-related deliriogenic potential when given individually, and even more so when given in combination with each other or other potentially deliriogenic agents. It may be necessary to substitute an atypical anti-

psychotic, carbamazepine, valproic acid, and/or a benzodiazepine, such as lorazepam or clonazepam, for lithium in patients with mania; a newer-generation heterocyclic, a selective serotonin reuptake inhibitor (SSRI), or one of the newer, novel-structured antidepressants for secondary or tertiary amine TCAs in patients with depression; or one of the atypical antipsychotics for old-line, standard neuroleptics in patients with schizophrenia.

Another significant concern is the potential for precipitating seizures, especially in patients with brain tumors in whom seizures are more likely to occur. Neuroleptics, antidepressants, and lithium all variably lower seizure threshold. Although the available data are inconclusive, older standard neuroleptics such as molindone and fluphenazine (Oliver et al. 1982), and possibly haloperidol (Mendez et al. 1984), are among the antipsychotic drugs that are believed to carry the smallest risk for seizures; whereas low-potency agents like chlorpromazine and clozapine are associated with an increased frequency of seizures (Stoudemire et al. 1993). In general, the newer atypical antipsychotics as a class are believed to have a lower likelihood of precipitating seizures and thus offer an important therapeutic advantage over the older antipsychotics. Among the antidepressants, maprotiline and bupropion appear to have the greatest seizure-inducing potential (Dubovsky 1992). Compared to TCAs, the SSRIs in general have been reported to have lower potential to precipitate seizures. In acutely manic patients with brain tumors, for whom lithium might otherwise be the drug of choice, carbamazepine, valproic acid, lorazepam, clonazepam, topiramate, and gabapentin—all of which have anticonvulsant properties—may be preferable alternatives (Massey and Folger 1984).

The psychiatrist should also bear in

mind that patients with brain tumors and seizures should be monitored carefully for the adequacy of anticonvulsant blood levels and should have their anticonvulsant doses adjusted as appropriate when psychotropic agents are given concurrently. This is because the epileptogenic effects of certain of these psychotropic medications, as well as their potential for altering anticonvulsant blood levels through drug-drug interactions resulting in changes in protein binding and/or hepatic metabolism involving the cytochrome P450 system, may lead to recrudescence of previously controlled seizures or the development of signs of anticonvulsant toxicity.

Psychotherapeutic Management of Syndromes Associated With Brain Tumors

Supportive psychotherapy geared to the patient's functional status, psychosocial situation, interpersonal and family relationships, cognitive capacities, and emotional needs is very important in the treatment of patients with brain tumors. The psychological stress of being diagnosed with a brain tumor and then having to undergo invasive, painful, and potentially debilitating treatments can trigger both recurrences of preexisting primary psychiatric disorders as well as the de novo appearance of reactive psychiatric symptoms from coping with the multiple stressors associated with the illness and its treatment. The diagnosis and treatment of a brain tumor in a loved one is also enormously stressful for families. Supportive psychotherapy for patients and psychoeducation for their families should play a major role in clinical management.

Supportive psychotherapy ideally should focus on concrete, reality-based, cognitive, and psychoeducational issues relating to diagnosis, treatment, and prognosis. Psychotherapeutic interventions should be geared to the patient's cognitive capacities, which may be diminished by the tumor itself or by one or more of the tumor treatments. Typically, the focus of psychotherapy will be on the impact of the illness on the patient's emotional and functional status, its effect on the family, the challenges of coping with functional disabilities, and the anticipatory grief related to potential losses and eventual death. Patients with brain tumors worry a great deal about decrements in cognitive and intellectual functioning, physical disability and incapacity, and ultimately, death. Patients vary widely in their capacity to cope with the consequences of brain tumors, depending on the flexibility and adequacy of their premorbid coping capacities. Some patients may appear to be little affected, whereas others may experience severe symptoms of anxiety and depression. Such patients experience greater difficulty continuing to function in their usual work and family roles and need more aggressive psychotherapeutic and psychopharmacologic interventions.

Use of denial is common and may initially be adaptive and effective in helping patients cope with their fears and anxieties, especially in the early stages of a life-threatening illness such as a brain tumor. Denial may also be maladaptive and result in the failure of patients to comply with optimal treatment recommendations or confront important legal, personal, family, and other reality-based issues and obligations that need to be addressed while the patient is still able. When denial is producing such maladaptive effects, the clinician may, in a sensitive and supportive manner, need to directly encourage the patient and family to address issues such as increasing disability, growing incapacity, and even impending death.

Although there are no clear-cut guidelines for the nature and timing of discussions of prognosis with brain tumor patients, most clinicians believe that patients and families should be given realistic prognostic information in a time frame that will allow them to make appropriate decisions and plans. Such prognostic information should, of course, be conveyed by the physician in as sensitive and supportive a fashion as possible, with ample opportunity for questions and discussion. This is another juncture where the involvement of the consulting psychiatrist is important in helping the patient and family process such information in a helpful and constructive way.

Some patients who have been completely cured of a brain tumor may nonetheless manifest significant psychiatric symptoms, including anxiety, fear, and depression. They may also benefit from psychiatric treatment. Unless the psychiatric symptoms are causing functional disability, are severe and distressing, persist over extended periods of time, or evolve into an autonomous psychiatric syndrome, psychotherapy rather than pharmacotherapy is generally the preferred treatment. Short-term, symptomatically targeted pharmacotherapy can, at times, be a useful adjunct, even if the major treatment emphasis is psychotherapeutic.

Psychodynamically focused, insight-oriented psychotherapy, which generally requires intact higher-level cognitive and abstracting capacities, may be relatively contraindicated in psychiatrically ill patients with brain tumors. Such patients often have neurocognitive impairments as a result of the effects of the tumor or of various neurosurgical, chemotherapeutic, or radiotherapeutic interventions. When cognitive impairment is present, not only will psychodynamically oriented therapies be unlikely to be beneficial, they may also cause substantial frustration and acute psychic distress as patients are confronted with psychological tasks and cognitive demands that they are unable to meet. In general, more concretely focused, "here-and-now" psychotherapeutic approaches based on a cognitive-behavioral orientation with the psychiatrist assuming an active, supportive, and educational role are likely to be most beneficial.

Somatic Treatment of Mental Disorders Due to Brain Tumors

The psychopharmacologic treatment of behavioral symptoms and syndromes caused by cerebral tumors, whether characterized by psychotic, affective, anxiety, or neurocognitive disturbances, follows the same principles as the drug treatment of phenomenologically similar symptoms due to primary psychiatric illnesses. However, in treating secondary psychiatric symptoms in patients with brain tumors, some important caveats must be borne in mind. Patients with psychiatric symptoms that are a direct consequence of a brain tumor frequently respond favorably to and will only tolerate lower doses of psychotropic medications. Side-effect profiles of psychotropic drugs being considered in the treatment of such patients need to be carefully evaluated, especially with regard to sedative, extrapyramidal, deliriogenic, and epileptogenic effects, as well as the potential for drug interactions. These five potential adverse effects are especially important for the clinician to bear in mind because they can result in additional clinical morbidity.

Drug Treatment of Psychotic Disorders Due to Brain Tumors

Standard antipsychotic medications may be beneficial in treating the hallucinations, delusions, and thought content and process disturbances that often accompany tumor-associated psychotic syndromes.

High-potency antipsychotics, which have fewer non-neurologic side effects than do the low-potency antipsychotics, are generally preferable. The former more often cause extrapyramidal symptoms, which may be more severe and persistent in patients with brain tumors. In patients with "organic" psychotic disorders, the therapeutically effective dose of an antipsychotic is often considerably lower than that required for the treatment of primary "functional" psychoses. Thus, as little as 1–5 mg, rather than 10–20 mg, of haloperidol per day (or equivalent doses with other antipsychotics) may be effective. Although there is currently a paucity of controlled research on the efficacy of the newer atypical antipsychotics in the treatment of psychotic symptoms in brain tumor patients, given their efficacy in other psychotic syndromes associated with neurologic disorders and their low side-effect profile, they may well turn out to be the treatment of choice in such patients. As per the general rule in the use of other psychotropics in patients with brain tumors, when initiating treatment with antipsychotics one should "start low and go slow." This is especially true in elderly patients, in whom effective antipsychotic doses may be lower than they are in younger patients because of aging-related pharmacokinetic and pharmacodynamic factors.

Antiparkinsonian agents, such as benztropine, trihexyphenidyl, and orphenadrine, are effective in the treatment of extrapyramidal side effects resulting from the use of neuroleptics in patients with brain tumors. However, in such patients these agents may cause or contribute to the occurrence of anticholinergic delirium. Thus, their use should be avoided unless there is a clear-cut clinical indication, and if there is, the dose minimized. Diphenhydramine or amantadine for dystonic and parkinsonian symptoms and benzodiazepines for akathisia are effective alternatives and are less deliriogenic.

Treatment of Mood Disorders Due to Brain Tumors

Antidepressant medications are often effective in the treatment of depression in patients with brain tumors. Standard TCAs may be useful, although currently the SSRIs and newer-generation heterocyclic and atypical antidepressants are used preferentially because of their lower anticholinergic activity and sedating effects and greater patient acceptance, which results in improved treatment compliance. In recent years, methylphenidate has been shown to be effective (Masand et al. 1991) and to have a rapid onset of action (Woods et al. 1986) in patients with secondary depression related to medical and neurologic disorders, including brain tumors. It is also generally well tolerated and does not lower the seizure threshold. In 30 patients with malignant gliomas with progressive neurobehavioral deficits resulting from their tumors and the radiation and chemotherapy they had received, Meyers et al. (1998) showed that methylphenidate in as low a dosage as 10 mg twice a day had significant beneficial effects. These included significant improvement in cognitive function, improved gait, increased stamina and motivation, and, in one case, improved bladder control, all of which occurred despite evidence of progressive neurologic changes on MRI during the period they were receiving methylphenidate. Untoward effects reported were minimal; there was no increase in seizure frequency, and many patients who were taking glucocorticoids were able to have their doses reduced.

Adjunctive treatment with atypical antipsychotics, which appear to have antidepressant as well as antipsychotic properties, may also be helpful.

Monoamine oxidase inhibitors may be effective when other antidepressants are not. They do not ordinarily pose an undue risk in patients with brain tumors, but, of course, the clinician must bear in mind that any cognitive impairment in such patients may interfere with their ability to maintain a tyramine-free diet.

If single antidepressant medication regimens are ineffective, various combinations may work. When pharmacologic treatments have failed, electroconvulsive therapy should be given serious consideration. Previously, brain tumors were thought to be an absolute contraindication to electroconvulsive therapy, especially when tumors were associated with increased intracranial pressure. More recent studies (Starkstein and Migliorelli 1993; Zwil et al. 1990), however, have reported cases of refractory depression associated with brain tumors without associated evidence of increased intracranial pressure that have been treated successfully and safely with electroconvulsive therapy.

Mood disorders with manic features due to brain tumors, though relatively rare, may respond to lithium in the usual therapeutic range of 0.8–1.4 mEq/L. For patients in whom seizures have been a part of the clinical picture, however, carbamazepine, valproate, lorazepam, clonazepam, topiramate, gabapentin, or electroconvulsive therapy (in cases where drug therapy has been ineffective) are alternatives, because they do not have the epileptogenic potential of lithium and have anticonvulsant properties of their own.

Newer, still largely experimental and unapproved treatment approaches, including vagal nerve stimulation and transcranial magnetic stimulation, have shown promise in early clinical trials with a variety of affective disorders, including depressions refractory to other treatments, mania (Berman et al. 2000; Grisaru et al. 1998; Rush et al. 2000), and psychotic symptoms (Hoffman et al. 1999). Clarification of their role in the treatment of brain tumor patients with depression and other neuropsychiatric syndromes awaits further research.

Treatment of Anxiety Disorders Due to Brain Tumors

Anxiety symptoms caused either directly or indirectly by brain tumors should not be treated with neuroleptics unless psychotic features are present. The benzodiazepines, particularly long-acting agents such as clonazepam, are often effective and have the added benefit of possessing anticonvulsant properties. However, benzodiazepines may induce delirium in patients with organic brain disease, including brain tumors, when used in high doses and in older age groups. This argues for the preferential use of short-acting agents in lower doses on a short-term basis, especially in older patients. Other disadvantages of benzodiazepines include their abuse potential and occasional tendency to cause paradoxical reactions, characterized by increased arousal and agitation. Buspirone, which is free of these potentially negative effects, should be considered an alternative to the benzodiazepines. Its main drawbacks are its delayed onset and only modest degree of anxiolytic action unless used in full pharmacologic doses. Hydroxyzine, SSRIs, or low doses of tertiary amine TCAs, such as doxepin or amitriptyline, may also have beneficial anxiolytic effects in some patients. Finally, panic attacks associated with temporal lobe tumors may respond to carbamazepine, valproate, or primidone, as well as to the usually effective antidepressant and antianxiety drugs.

Treatment of Delirium

Delirium in patients with brain tumors may be associated with a wide variety of psychiatric and behavioral symptoms in addition to cognitive impairments. Hallucinations, especially visual, and delusions are common in these patients and often respond to symptomatic treatment with low doses of haloperidol, other high-potency neuroleptics, or atypical antipsychotics while the underlying cause(s) of the delirium are being sought and treated.

Treatment of Personality Changes Due to Brain Tumors

Mood lability may be a manifestation of personality changes due to a brain tumor and may respond to lithium or carbamazepine. Some patients with frontal lobe syndromes associated with tumors may respond to carbamazepine, as do some patients with temporal lobe tumors who may present with associated interictal aggression and violent behavior. Patients with brain tumors who have impulse dyscontrol and rageful, explosive episodes, like patients with intermittent explosive disorders due to other medical and neurologic conditions, may respond to anticonvulsants, such as carbamazepine, valproic acid, or phenytoin; lithium; high-potency neuroleptics; and/or stimulants or β-blockers.

Cognitive, Occupational, and Functional Rehabilitation

In addition to psychopharmacologic and psychotherapeutic treatments, cognitive, occupational, and vocational rehabilitative interventions can be very helpful for patients whose tumors, or the treatments they have received for them, have produced behavioral, cognitive, or functional sequelae. Such sequelae can be identified and quantified by comparing preoperative with postoperative test results using the Halstead-Reitan Neuropsychological Test Battery (Reitan 1979) or other comprehensive neuropsychological test batteries and various functional assessment tools. Serial testing at intervals during the patient's postoperative rehabilitation allows for objective documentation of changes in neuropsychological and functional deficits and allows for objective monitoring of improvement or deterioration in them over time.

Cognitive, occupational, and vocational rehabilitative strategies can be developed that will specifically address deficits in intellectual, language, visuospatial, memory, and neurocognitive functioning, as well as vocational functioning and the ability to carry out activities of daily living resulting from a brain tumor. In addition, behavioral techniques have been successfully applied to problematic behaviors resulting from insults to the brain.

Neuropsychiatric Consequences of Treatments of Brain Tumors

A number of psychiatric and behavioral symptoms, as well as neurocognitive deficits, may result from surgical, pharmacologic, and radiation treatments of brain tumors. Intraoperative injury to normal brain tissue proximate to a brain tumor during the course of resection or debulking may result in the postoperative appearance of various behavioral or neurocognitive symptoms depending on the location and connectivity of the tissues involved. The same is true of other perioperative and postoperative complications, such as infections and bleeding. Chemotherapy of brain tumors may cause delirium and neurocognitive dysfunction as well as other neurologic complications, and the administration of steroids for secondary phenomena such as cerebral edema and/or increased intracranial pressure may cause psychotic symptoms or manic, depressive, or mixed manic and depressive affective syndromes. Radiation therapy directed at brain tumors may result in immediate or delayed neurocognitive and behavioral sequelae due to radiation-induced damage to white matter. These sequelae may be either transient (Hylton et al. 1987) or permanent (Al-Mefty et al. 1990; Burger et al. 1979) and vary considerably in severity from mild and completely reversible, presumably related to edema, to severe and permanent changes due to parenchymal necrosis. In the most severe cases, which are fortunately quite rare, progressive dementia and eventual coma and death may occur.

Conclusions

Brain tumors frequently present with a broad range of psychiatric, behavioral, and/or neurocognitive symptoms. The differential diagnosis of patients who display acute or progressive changes in behavior, personality, or cognitive function should include brain tumors, especially if there are any associated focal neurologic signs and symptoms. In addition to assessment of psychiatric and behavioral symptoms, a full neuropsychiatric evaluation should include physical, neurologic, and mental status examinations; appropriate brain imaging and other neurodiagnostic studies; and formal neuropsychological testing, particularly when there is any question of neurocognitive dysfunction on bedside mental status testing.

The nature, frequency, and severity of psychiatric symptoms observed in patients with brain tumors depend on a number of clinical factors, including the type, location, size, rate of growth, and malignancy of the tumor. In general, behavioral symptoms associated with smaller, slower-growing, less aggressive tumors are most likely to be misdiagnosed as psychiatric in origin, particularly when the tumors involve "silent" regions of the brain, which do not give rise to focal neurologic signs or symptoms.

Although tumors of the frontal and temporal lobes and the diencephalon are most commonly associated with psychiatric and behavioral symptoms, the variation in those symptoms is exceedingly broad. In general, the relationship between neuropsychiatric symptoms and specific anatomic locations of the brain tumors causing them is not very robust. A number of other tumor-associated factors appear to be at least as important in determining the type and severity of psychiatric and behavioral symptoms in brain tumor patients.

Optimal treatment of tumor-associated psychiatric, neuropsychiatric, and neuropsychological dysfunctions requires coordinated intervention by a multidisciplinary treatment team. The psychopharmacologic treatment of brain tumor-associated psychiatric and behavioral syndromes should follow the same general principles as that of corresponding primary psychiatric disorders. However, the choice of drugs and/or dosages employed may require modification, because many of the psychotropic agents may induce seizures or delirium, and patients with brain tumors are more vulnerable to these and other CNS side effects.

Adjunctive, supportive psychotherapy for both the patient and the family is very important, as are psychosocial and psychoeducational interventions. Such psychotherapeutic and psychosocial interventions must be thoughtfully integrated with psychopharmacologic; neurocognitive; physical, occupational, and vocational rehabilitative; and behavioral interventions as clinically indicated. In turn, these must be coordinated with the ongoing primary treatment of the brain tumor to optimize the patient's overall management. With well-planned integration and coordination of these complementary treatment approaches, the ability of the patient and his or her family to cope with the tumor may be strengthened, and both the quantity and quality of the patient's life may be enhanced.

References

Albert MS, Feldman RG, Willis A: The "subcortical dementia" syndrome of progressive supranuclear palsy. J Neurol Neurosurg Psychiatry 37:121–130, 1974

Alexander GE, Crutcher MD: Functional architecture of basal ganglia circuits: neural substrates of parallel processing. Trends Neurosci 13:266–271, 1990

Allen IM: A clinical study of tumors involving the occipital lobe. Brain 53:196–243, 1930

Al-Mefty O, Kersh JE, Routh A, et al: The long-term side effects of radiation therapy for benign brain tumors in adults. J Neurosurg 73:502–512, 1990

Alpers BJ: Relation of the hypothalamus to disorders of personality. Archives of Neurology and Psychiatry 38:291–303, 1937

Avery TL: A case of acromegaly and gigantism with depression. Br J Psychiatry 122:599–600, 1973

Bear DM, Fedio P: Quantitative analysis of interictal behavior in temporal lobe epilepsy. Arch Neurol 34:454–467, 1977

Belyi BI: Mental impairment in unilateral frontal tumors: role of the laterality of the lesion. Int J Neurosci 32:799–810, 1987

Benson DF: Aphasia, Alexia, and Agraphia. New York, Churchill Livingstone, 1979

Berman RM, Narasimhan M, Sanacora G, et al: A randomized clinical trial of repetitive transcranial magnetic stimulation in the treatment of major depression. Biol Psychiatry 47:332–337, 2000

Bhatia MS: Cotard's syndrome in parietal lobe tumor. Indian Pediatr 30:1019–1021, 1993

Bigler ED: Diagnostic Clinical Neuropsychology. Austin, TX, University of Texas Press, 1984

Blackman M, Wheler GH: A case of mistaken identity: a fourth ventricular tumor presenting as school phobia in a 12 year old boy. Can J Psychiatry 32:584–587, 1987

Burger PC, Mahaley MS, Dudka L, et al: The morphologic effects of radiation administered therapeutically for intracranial gliomas. Cancer 44:1256–1272, 1979

Burkle FM, Lipowski ZJ: Colloid cyst of the third ventricle presenting as psychiatric disorder. Am J Psychiatry 135:373–374, 1978

Cairns H: Mental disorders with tumors of the pons. Folia Psychiatrica Neurologica Neurochirurgica 53:193–203, 1950

Cairns H, Mosberg WH: Colloid cysts of the third ventricle. Surg Gynecol Obstet 92:545–570, 1951

Cairns H, Oldfield RC, Pennybacker JB, et al: Akinetic mutism with an epidermoid cyst of the 3rd ventricle. Brain 64: 273–290, 1941

Chipkevitch E: Brain tumors and anorexia nervosa syndrome. Brain Dev 16:175–179, 1994

Coffey RJ: Hypothalamic and basal forebrain germinoma presenting with amnesia and hyperphagia. Surg Neurol 31:228–233, 1989

Critchley M: The problem of visual agnosia. J Neurol Sci 1:274–290, 1964a

Critchley M: Psychiatric symptoms and parietal disease: differential diagnosis. Proc R Soc Med 57:422–428, 1964b

Cummings JL: Subcortical Dementia. New York, Oxford University Press, 1990

Cummings JL: Frontal-subcortical circuits and human behavior. Arch Neurol 50:873–880, 1993

Cummings JL, Mendez MF: Secondary mania with focal cerebrovascular lesions. Am J Psychiatry 141:1084–1087, 1984

Davison K, Bagley CR: Schizophrenia-like psychoses associated with organic disorders of the central nervous system: a review of the literature, in Current Problems in Neuropsychiatry: Schizophrenia, Epilepsy, the Temporal Lobe (British Journal of Psychiatry Special Publication No 4). Edited by Harrington RN. London, Headley Brothers, 1969, pp 126–130

Direkze M, Bayliss SG, Cutting JC: Primary tumors of the frontal lobe. Br J Clin Pract 25:207–213, 1971

Drubach DA, Kelly MP: Panic disorder associated with a right paralimbic lesion. Neuropsychiatry Neuropsychol Behav Neurol 2:282–289, 1989

Dubovsky SL: Psychopharmacological treatment in neuropsychiatry, in The American Psychiatric Press Textbook of Neuropsychiatry. Edited by Yudofsky SC, Hales RE. Washington, DC, American Psychiatric Press, 1992, pp 663–701

Dunn DW, Weisberg LA: Peduncular hallucinations caused by brainstem compression. Neurology 33:1360–1361, 1983

Filley CM, Kleinschmidt-DeMasters BK: Neurobehavioral presentations of brain neoplasms. West J Med 163:19–25, 1995

Folstein MF, Folstein SE, McHugh PR: Mini-Mental State: a practical method for grading the cognitive state of patients for the clinician. J Psychiatr Res 12:189–198, 1975

Fox S: Use of a quality of life instrument to improve assessment of brain tumor patients in an outpatient setting. J Neurosci Nurs 30:322–325, 1998

Ghadirian AM, Gauthier S, Bertrand S: Anxiety attacks in a patient with a right temporal lobe meningioma. J Clin Psychiatry 47:270–271, 1986

Goldberg E: Varieties of perseverations: comparison of two taxonomies. J Clin Exp Neuropsychol 6:710–726, 1986

Greenberg DB, Brown GL: Mania resulting from brain stem tumor: single case study. J Nerv Ment Dis 173:434–436, 1985

Grisaru N, Chudakov B, Yaroslavsky Y, et al: Transcranial magnetic stimulation in mania: a controlled study. Am J Psychiatry 155:1608–1610, 1998

Gutmann DH, Grossman RI, Mollman JE: Personality changes associated with thalamic infiltration. J Neurooncol 8:263–267, 1990

Hobbs GE: Brain tumors simulating psychiatric disorder. Can Med Assoc J 88:186–188, 1963

Hoffman RE, Boutros NN, Berman RM, et al: Transcranial magnetic stimulation of left temporoparietal cortex in three patients reporting hallucinated "voices." Biol Psychiatry 46:130–132, 1999

Hylton PD, Reichman OH, Palutsis R: Monitoring of transient central nervous system postirradiation effects by 133-xenon inhalation regional cerebral blood flow measurements. Neurosurgery 21:843–848, 1987

Jamieson RC, Wells CE: Manic psychosis in a patient with multiple metastatic brain tumors. J Clin Psychiatry 40:280–283, 1979

Jones JB, Barklage NE: Conversion disorder: camouflage for brain lesions in two cases. Arch Intern Med 150:1343–1345, 1990

Kalayam B, Young RC, Tsuboyama GK: Mood disorders associated with acoustic neuromas. Int J Psychiatry Med 24:31–43, 1994

Kaplan CP, Miner ME: Anxiety and depression in elderly patients receiving treatment for cerebral tumours. Brain Inj 11:129–135, 1997

Keschner M, Bender MB, Strauss I: Mental symptoms in cases of tumor of the temporal lobe. Archives of Neurology and Psychiatry 35:572–596, 1936

Keschner M, Bender MB, Strauss I: Mental symptoms associated with brain tumor: a study of 530 verified cases. J Am Med Assoc 110:714–718, 1938

Khouzam HR, Emery PE, Reaves B: Secondary mania in late life. J Am Geriatr Soc 42:85–87, 1994

Klotz M: Incidence of brain tumors in patients hospitalized for chronic mental disorders. Psychiatr Q 31:669–680, 1957

Kocher R, Linder M, Stula D: Primary brain tumors in psychiatry. Schweiz Arch Neurol Neurochir Psychiatr 135:217–227, 1984

Lezak MD: Neuropsychological Assessment, 3rd Edition. New York, Oxford University Press, 1995

Lishman WA: Organic Psychiatry: The Psychological Consequences of Cerebral Disorder. New York, Oxford University Press, 1987

Lohr JB, Cadet JL: Neuropsychiatric aspects of brain tumors, in The American Psychiatric Press Textbook of Neuropsychiatry. Edited by Talbott JA, Hales RE, Yudofsky SC. Washington, DC, American Psychiatric Press, 1987, pp 351–364

Luria AR: The Working Brain: An Introduction to Neuropsychology. New York, Basic Books, 1973

Luria AR: Higher Cortical Functions in Man. New York, Basic Books, 1980

Malamud N: Psychiatric disorder with intracranial tumors of limbic system. Arch Neurol 17:113–123, 1967

Masand P, Murray GB, Pickett P: Psychostimulants in post-stroke depression. J Neuropsychiatry Clin Neurosci 3:23–27, 1991

Massey EW, Folger WN: Seizures activated by therapeutic levels of lithium carbonate. South Med J 77:1173–1175, 1984

Meadows JC: The anatomical basis of prosopagnosia. J Neurol Neurosurg Psychiatry 37:489–501, 1974

Mendez MF, Cummings JL, Benson DF: Epilepsy: psychiatric aspects and use of psychotropics. Psychosomatics 25:883–894, 1984

Meyers CA, Weitzner MA, Valentine AD, et al: Methylphenidate therapy improves cognition, mood, and function of brain tumor patients. J Clin Oncol 16:2522–2527, 1998

Minski L: The mental symptoms associated with 58 cases of cerebral tumor. Journal of Neurology and Psychopathology 13:330–343, 1933

Mulder DW, Daly D: Psychiatric symptoms associated with lesions of temporal lobe. J Am Med Assoc 150:173–176, 1952

Mungas D: Interictal behavior abnormality in temporal lobe epilepsy: a specific syndrome or non-specific psychopathology? Arch Gen Psychiatry 39:108–111, 1982

Nadvi SS, van Dellen JR: Transient peduncular hallucinations secondary to brain stem compression by a medulloblastoma. Surg Neurol 41:250–252, 1994

Neuman E, Rancurel G, Lecrubier Y, et al: Schizophreniform catatonia in 6 cases secondary to hydrocephalus with subthalamic mesencephalic tumor associated with hypodopaminergia. Neuropsychobiology 34:76–81, 1996

Oliver AP, Luchins DJ, Wyatt RJ: Neuroleptic-induced seizures: an in vitro technique for assessing relative risk. Arch Gen Psychiatry 39:206–209, 1982

Pincus JH, Tucker GJ: Behavioral Neurology, 2nd Edition. New York, Oxford University Press, 1978

Pollack L, Klein C, Rabey JM, et al: Posterior fossa lesions associated with neuropsychiatric symptomatology. Int J Neurosci 87:119–126, 1996

Pringle AM, Taylor R, Whittle IR: Anxiety and depression in patients with an intracranial neoplasm before and after tumor surgery. Br J Neurosurg 13:46–51, 1999

Reitan RM: An investigation of the validity of Halstead's measures of biological intelligence. Archives of Neurology and Psychiatry 73:28–35, 1979

Reitan RM, Wolfson D: Neuroanatomy and Neuropathology for Neuropsychologists. Tucson, AZ, Neuropsychology Press, 1985, pp 167–192

Remington FB, Robert SL: Why patients with brain tumors come to a psychiatric hospital: a thirty-year survey. Am J Psychiatry 119:256–257, 1962

Roberts GW, Done DJ, Bruton C, et al: A "mock up" of schizophrenia: temporal lobe epilepsy and schizophrenia-like psychosis. Biol Psychiatry 28:127–143, 1990

Robinson RG, Kubos KL, Starr LB, et al: Mood disorders in stroke patients: importance of location of lesion. Brain 107:81–93, 1984

Rodin E, Schmaltz S: The Bear-Fedio personality inventory and temporal lobe epilepsy. Neurology 34:591–596, 1984

Ross E: Prosody and brain lateralization: fact vs. fancy or is it all just semantics? Arch Neurol 45:338–339, 1988

Ruiz A, Ganz WI, Donovan Post J, et al: Use of thallium-201 brain SPECT to differentiate cerebral lymphoma from toxoplasma encephalitis in AIDS patients. AJNR Am J Neuroradiol 15:1885–1894, 1994

Rush AJ, George MS, Sackheim HA, et al: Vagus nerve stimulation (VNS) for refractory depressions: a multicenter study. Biol Psychiatry 47:276–286, 2000

Russell RW, Pennybacker JB: Craniopharyngioma in the elderly. J Neurol Neurosurg Psychiatry 24:1–13, 1961

Salazar-Calderon Perriggo VH, Oommen KJ, Sobonya RE: Silent solitary right parietal chondroma resulting in secondary mania. Clin Neuropathol 12:325–329, 1993

Scheibel RS, Meyers CA, Levin VA: Cognitive dysfunction following surgery for intracerebral glioma: influence of histopathology, lesion location, and treatment. J Neurooncol 30:61–67, 1996

Schlesinger B: Mental changes in intracranial tumors and related problems. Confin Neurol 10:225–263, 1950

Selecki BR: Cerebral mid-line tumours involving the corpus callosum among mental hospital patients. Med J Aust 2:954–960, 1964

Selecki BR: Intracranial space-occupying lesions among patients admitted to mental hospitals. Med J Aust 1:383–390, 1965

Spreen O, Benton A, Fincham R: Auditory agnosia without aphasia. Arch Neurol 13:84–92, 1965

Starkstein SE, Migliorelli R: ECT in a patient with a frontal craniotomy and residual meningioma. J Neuropsychiatry Clin Neurosci 5:428–430, 1993

Starkstein SE, Boston JD, Robinson RG: Mechanisms of mania after brain injury: 12 case reports and review of the literature. J Nerv Ment Dis 176:87–100, 1988

Stoudemire A, Fogel BS, Gulley LR, et al: Psychopharmacology in the medical patient, in Psychiatric Care of the Medical Patient. Edited by Stoudemire A, Fogel BS. New York, Oxford University Press, 1993, pp 155–206

Strauss I, Keschner M: Mental symptoms in cases of tumor of the frontal lobe. Archives of Neurology and Psychiatry 33:986–1005, 1935

Strobos RRJ: Tumors of the temporal lobe. Neurology 3:752–760, 1953

Teuber HL: Unity and diversity of frontal lobe functions. Acta Neurobiol Exp 32:615–656, 1972

von Monakow C: Die Lokalisation im Grossheim und der Abbav der Funktion durch Kortikale Herde. Wiesbaden, Germany, JF Bergmann, 1914

Warrington EK, Rabin P: Perceptual matching in patients with cerebral lesions. Neuropsychologia 8:475–487, 1970

Weitzner MA: Psychosocial and neuropsychiatric aspects of patients with primary brain tumors. Cancer Invest 17:285–291, 1999

White J, Cobb S: Psychological changes associated with giant pituitary neoplasms. Archives of Neurology and Psychiatry 74:383–396, 1955

Wilson G, Rupp C: Mental symptoms associated with extramedullary posterior fossa tumors. Trans Am Neurol Assoc 71:104–107, 1946

Woods SW, Tesar GE, Murray GB, et al: Psychostimulant treatment of depressive disorders secondary to medical illness. J Clin Psychiatry 47:12–15, 1986

Zwil AS, Bowring MA, Price TRP, et al: ECT in the presence of a brain tumor: case reports and a review of the literature. Convuls Ther 6:299–307, 1990

Neuropsychiatric Aspects of Ethanol and Other Chemical Dependencies

Eric J. Nestler, M.D., Ph.D.

David W. Self, Ph.D.

Drug addiction continues to exact enormous human and financial costs on society, at a time when available treatments remain inadequately effective for most people. Given that advances in treating other medical disorders have resulted directly from research of the molecular and cellular pathophysiology of the disease process, an improved understanding of the basic neurobiology of addiction should likewise translate into more efficacious treatments.

Our knowledge of the basic neurobiology of drug addiction is leading psychiatric neuroscience in establishing the biological basis of a complex and clinically important behavioral abnormality. This is because many features of drug addiction in people can be reproduced in laboratory animals, where findings are directly referable back to the clinical situation. Earlier work on drug reinforcement mechanisms, and more recently developed animal models that target the addiction process and drug craving, have made it possible to identify regions of the brain that play important roles in distinct behavioral features of addiction. These neural substrates are now the focus of extensive research on the molecular and cellular alterations that underlie these behavioral changes.

This chapter provides an overview of recent progress made in our understanding of the neurobiological basis of drug addiction. After providing brief definitions of commonly used terminology, we summarize the anatomic and neurochemical substrates that mediate the reinforc-

---

This work was supported by grants from the National Institute on Drug Abuse.

ing effects of short-term drug exposure. We then describe how repeated drug exposure can induce gradually developing, progressive alterations in molecular and cellular signaling pathways, and how these neuroadaptive changes may ultimately contribute to addictive behavior.

Definition of Terms

From a pharmacologic perspective, drug addiction can be defined by processes such as tolerance, sensitization, dependence, and withdrawal. *Tolerance* refers to a progressive weakening of a given drug effect after repeated exposure, which may contribute to an escalation of drug intake as the addiction process proceeds. *Sensitization*, or *reverse tolerance*, refers to the opposite circumstance, whereby repeated administration of the same drug dose elicits an even stronger effect; sensitization to certain "incentive motivational" effects of drugs is believed to contribute to high relapse rates seen in addicted individuals. Thus, both tolerance and sensitization to different aspects of drug action can occur simultaneously. *Dependence* is defined as the need for continued drug exposure to avoid a withdrawal syndrome, which is characterized by physical or motivational disturbances when the drug is withdrawn. Presumably, the processes of tolerance, sensitization, dependence, and withdrawal are each caused by molecular and cellular adaptations in specific brain regions in response to repeated drug exposure. It is important to emphasize that these phenomena are not associated uniquely with drugs of abuse, as many clinically used medications that are not addicting (e.g., clonidine, propranolol, tricyclic antidepressants) can also produce similar phenomena. Rather, the manifestation of tolerance, sensitization, dependence, and withdrawal specifi-

cally in brain regions that regulate motivation is believed to underlie addiction-related changes in behavior.

Drugs of abuse are unique in terms of their reinforcing properties. A drug is defined as a reinforcer if the probability of a drug-seeking response is increased and maintained by pairing drug exposure with the response. Initially, most abused drugs function as positive reinforcers, presumably because they produce a positive affective state (e.g., euphoria). Such rapid and powerful associations between a drug reinforcer and a drug-seeking response probably reflect the drug's ability to usurp preexisting brain reinforcement mechanisms, which normally mediate the reinforcing effects of natural reinforcers such as food, sex, and social interaction.

Long-term exposure to reinforcing drugs can lead to drug addiction, which is characterized by an escalation in both the frequency and the amount of drug use and by intense drug craving during withdrawal despite grave adverse consequences. In the context of long-term drug use, a drug may serve not only as a positive reinforcer but also as a negative reinforcer by alleviating the negative consequences of drug withdrawal. The persistence of drug craving and drug seeking (relapse) despite prolonged periods of abstinence suggests that long-lasting adaptations have occurred in the neural substrates that mediate acute drug reinforcement.

Addictive disorders are often defined clinically as a state of "psychological dependence," for example, in DSM-IV-TR (American Psychiatric Association 2000). However, it is important to emphasize that in more precise pharmacologic terms, we do not yet know the relative contributions of neurobiological changes that underlie tolerance, sensitization, or dependence to the compulsive drug-seeking behavior that is the clinical hallmark of an addictive disorder. It is possible that drug craving and relapse involve dependence-related dysphoria associated with drug withdrawal. Such factors are likely to be important during the relatively early phases of abstinence. However, a major question remains regarding the types of adaptations that underlie particularly long-lived aspects of addiction, for example, the increased risk of relapse that many addicts show even after years of abstinence. As stated above, such persistent drug craving may involve adaptations that underlie sensitization to the incentive motivational properties of drugs, drug-associated (conditioned) stimuli, and stressful events. In other words, sensitization to these various stimuli would increase their ability to "reinstate"—or "prime"—drug seeking despite prolonged abstinence. Identification of long-lasting adaptations that underlie these persisting behavioral changes is paramount to the ultimate development of truly effective treatments.

The Synapse as the Immediate Target of Drugs of Abuse

The initial actions of drugs of abuse on the brain can be understood at the level of synaptic transmission. A classic view of a synapse involves a presynaptic nerve terminal releasing a neurotransmitter in response to a nerve impulse along its axon that acts on a postsynaptic receptor to elicit changes in neuronal excitability of the postsynaptic neuron. The activity of the neurotransmitter is then turned off by its reuptake into the nerve terminal, or by enzymatic degradation (for review, see Nestler et al. 2001).

All drugs of abuse initially affect the brain by influencing the amount of a neurotransmitter present at the synapse or by interacting with specific neurotransmitter receptors. Table 13–1 lists examples of such acute pharmacologic actions of some commonly used drugs of abuse. The fact that drugs of abuse initially influence different neurotransmitter and receptor systems in the brain explains the very different actions produced by these drugs acutely. For example, the presence of very high levels of opioid receptors in the brain stem and spinal cord explains why opiates can exert such profound effects on respiration, level of consciousness, and nociception. In contrast, the importance of noradrenergic mechanisms in the regulation of cardiac function explains why cocaine can exert such profound cardiotoxic effects.

In contrast to the many disparate acute actions of drugs of abuse, the drugs do appear to exert some common behavioral effects: as discussed above, they are all positively reinforcing after short-term exposure. This suggests that there are certain regions of the brain where the distinct acute pharmacologic actions of these drugs converge at the level of a common reinforcement substrate. That is, in certain regions of the brain, which are discussed below, activation of opioid receptors (by opiates), inhibition of monoamine reuptake (by cocaine), or facilitation of GABAergic and inhibition of N-methyl-D-aspartate (NMDA) glutamatergic neurotransmission (by ethanol) would appear to elicit some common neurobiological response(s) that mediates their reinforcing properties.

Molecular and Cellular Adaptations as the Long-Term Consequences of Drugs of Abuse

The acute pharmacologic actions of a drug of abuse per se do not explain the long-term effects of repeated drug exposure.

TABLE 13–1. Examples of acute pharmacologic actions of drugs of abuse

Drug	Action
Opiates	Agonist at μ, δ, and κ opioid receptors[a]
Cocaine	Inhibits monoamine reuptake transporters
Amphetamine	Stimulates monoamine release
Ethanol	Facilitates GABA$_A$ receptor function and inhibits NMDA glutamate receptor function[b]
Nicotine	Agonist at nicotinic acetylcholine receptors
Cannabinoids	Agonist at CB$_1$ cannabinoid receptors[c]
Hallucinogens	Partial agonist at 5-HT$_2$ serotonin receptors
Phencyclidine (PCP)	Antagonist at NMDA glutamate receptors

Note. GABA$_A$ = γ-aminobutyric acid type A; NMDA = N-methyl-D-aspartate; 5-HT$_2$ = 5-hydroxytryptamine (serotonin) type 2.
[a]Activity at μ and δ receptors is thought to mediate the reinforcing actions of opiates.
[b]The mechanism by which ethanol produces these effects has not been established.
[c]The endogenous ligand(s) for this receptor has not yet been definitively identified; one candidate is anandamide.
Source. See Nestler et al. 2001 for references.

To understand such long-term effects, it is necessary to move beyond the classic view of a synapse to a more sophisticated, complete view, such as that shown in Figure 13–1. Thus, we now know that neurotransmitter-receptor activation does more to influence a target neuron than simply regulate its ion channels and immediate electrical properties: virtually every process in a neuron can be affected by neurotransmitter-receptor activation (Nestler et al. 2001). Such effects are mediated by modulating the functional activity of proteins that are already present in the neuron or by regulating the

actual amount of the proteins. Neurotransmitter-receptor activation produces these diverse effects through biochemical cascades of intracellular messengers, which involve G proteins (guanosine triphosphate–binding membrane proteins that couple extracellular receptors to intracellular effector proteins), and the subsequent regulation of second messengers (such as cyclic adenosine monophosphate [cAMP], calcium, phosphatidylinositol, or nitric oxide) and protein phosphorylation (see Nestler et al. 2001). Protein phosphorylation is a process whereby phosphate groups are added to proteins by protein kinases or are removed from proteins by protein phosphatases. The addition or removal of phosphate groups dramatically alters protein function and leads to the myriad biological responses in question.

Neurotransmitter receptors function presynaptically to regulate the synthesis and storage of neurotransmitter via phosphorylation of synthetic enzymes and transporter proteins. In addition, altered phosphorylation of synaptic vesicle–associated proteins can modulate the release of neurotransmitters from presynaptic nerve terminals. Postsynaptically, altered phosphorylation of receptors and ion channels can modify the ability of neurotransmitters to regulate the physiologic responses to the same or different neurotransmitter stimuli. Neurotransmitter-mediated phosphorylation of cytoskeletal proteins can produce structural and morphologic changes in target neurons. Finally, altered phosphorylation of nuclear or ribosomal proteins can alter gene transcription and protein synthesis and hence the total amounts of these various types of proteins in the target neurons. Given the gradual development of drug addiction in most people and the persistence of drug craving for long periods after cessation of drug exposure, it is likely that repeated

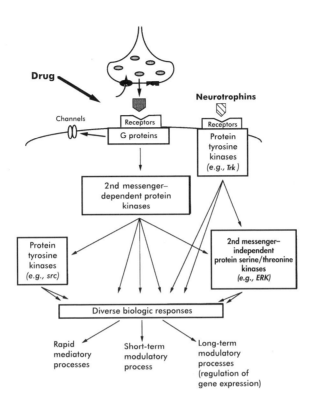

FIGURE 13–1.   A working model of synaptic transmission.

Studies in basic neuroscience have focused on the involvement of intracellular messenger systems involving coupling factors (termed G proteins), second messengers (e.g., cyclic adenosine monophosphate [cAMP], calcium, nitric oxide, and the metabolites of phosphatidylinositol), and protein phosphorylation (involving the phosphorylation of phosphoproteins by protein kinases and their dephosphorylation by protein phosphatases) in mediating multiple actions of neurotransmitters on their target neurons. Second messenger–dependent protein kinases (e.g., those activated by cAMP or calcium) are classified as protein serine/threonine kinases, because they phosphorylate substrate proteins on serine or threonine residues. Each second messenger–dependent protein kinase phosphorylates a specific array of substrate proteins (which can be considered third messengers) and thereby leads to multiple biological responses of the neurotransmitter. Brain also contains many important intracellular regulatory pathways in addition to those regulated directly by G proteins and second messengers. These include numerous protein serine/threonine kinases (e.g., the extracellular signal–regulated kinases [ERKs] or mitogen-activated protein [MAP] kinases), as well as numerous protein tyrosine kinases (which phosphorylate substrate proteins on tyrosine residues), some of which reside in the receptors for neurotrophins and most other growth factors (e.g., the Trk proteins), and others that are not associated with growth factor receptors (e.g., src kinase). Each of these various protein kinases are highly regulated by extracellular stimuli. The second messenger–dependent protein kinases are regulated by receptor–G protein–second messenger pathways as mentioned above. The receptor-associated protein tyrosine kinases are activated on growth factor binding to the receptor. The second messenger–independent protein serine/threonine kinases and the protein tyrosine kinases that are not receptor associated seem to be regulated indirectly via the second messenger–dependent and growth factor–dependent pathways as depicted in the figure. The brain also contains numerous types of protein serine/threonine and protein tyrosine phosphatases, not shown in the figure, which are also subject to regulation by extracellular and intracellular stimuli. Thus, the binding of neurotransmitter to its receptor extracellularly results in numerous short-term and long-term biological responses through the complex regulation of multiple intracellular regulatory pathways and the phosphorylation or dephosphorylation of numerous substrate proteins.

drug exposure causes altered patterns of gene expression and protein synthesis that underlie some of these long-term actions of drugs of abuse on the nervous system (Nestler 1992; Nestler et al. 1993).

Neurotransmitter regulation of G proteins and second messenger–dependent protein phosphorylation is a small part of a neuron's intracellular regulatory machinery (Figure 13–1) (Nestler et al. 2001). Neurons also express high levels of protein tyrosine kinases (e.g., Trk proteins) that mediate the actions of neurotrophins and other growth factors. Growth factors play an important role in neuronal development, but more recently they have been shown to exert powerful effects on fully differentiated adult neurons. This implies that the traditional distinction between neurotransmitters and growth factors is becoming increasingly arbitrary. In addition, neurons contain high levels of protein kinases that are not regulated directly by extracellular signals but are influenced by those signals indirectly via "crosstalk" among various intracellular pathways. Thus, each neurotransmitter-receptor system can interact with others via secondary, tertiary, etc., effects on various intracellular signaling pathways, all of which will contribute to the myriad effects of the original neurotransmitter stimulus.

This means that, despite the initial actions of a drug of abuse on the activity of a neurotransmitter or receptor system, the many actions of drugs of abuse on brain function are achieved ultimately through the complex network of intracellular messenger pathways that mediate physiologic responses to neurotransmitter-receptor interactions. Moreover, repeated exposure to drugs of abuse would be expected to produce molecular and cellular adaptations as a result of repeated perturbation of these intracellular pathways. These adaptations may be responsible for tolerance, sensitization, dependence, withdrawal, and, ultimately, the addiction process.

We will begin our discussion of specific molecular and cellular adaptations that result from long-term drug exposure by considering the locus coeruleus, where adaptations in the cAMP second messenger and protein phosphorylation systems have been implicated in the molecular, cellular, and behavioral changes associated with physical signs of opiate dependence and withdrawal. Because similar molecular adaptations to long-term drug exposure are seen in brain regions associated with drug reinforcement and craving, the locus coeruleus has served as a model system to guide investigations into the molecular mechanisms underlying motivational dependence. These studies suggest that both physical and motivational changes associated with drug addiction are caused by some similar molecular adaptations, but in distinct neural substrates that regulate these behaviors.

Role of the Locus Coeruleus in Opiate Physical Dependence

The locus coeruleus is located on the floor of the fourth ventricle in the anterior pons. It contains the major noradrenergic nucleus in the brain with widespread projections to both the brain and spinal cord. This diffuse innervation allows the locus coeruleus to regulate the animal's general state of arousal, attention, and autonomic tone. An important role for the locus coeruleus in opiate physical dependence and withdrawal has been established at both the behavioral and electrophysiological levels: overactivation of locus coeruleus neurons is both necessary and sufficient for producing many behavioral signs of opiate withdrawal (see Aghajanian 1978;

Koob et al. 1992; Maldonado and Koob 1993; Nestler 1992; Nestler and Aghajanian 1997; Rasmussen et al. 1990). Indeed, it was this knowledge of the role of the locus coeruleus in physical dependence to opiates that led to the introduction of clonidine—an α_2-adrenergic agonist that produces effects similar to those of morphine on neurons of the locus coeruleus (Aghajanian 1978)—as the first nonopiate treatment for opiate withdrawal in humans (Gold et al. 1978). Overactivation of locus coeruleus neurons during withdrawal arises from both extrinsic and intrinsic sources. The extrinsic source involves a hyperactive, excitatory glutamatergic input to the locus coeruleus from the nucleus paragigantocellularis. The intrinsic source involves intracellular adaptations in opioid receptor–coupled signal transduction pathways in locus coeruleus neurons.

Mechanisms Intrinsic to the Locus Coeruleus

Acutely, opiates inhibit locus coeruleus neurons via activation of an inward-rectifying K^+ channel and inhibition of an inward Na^+ current (e.g., Alreja and Aghajanian 1991, 1993; North et al. 1987). Both actions are mediated via pertussis toxin–sensitive G proteins (i.e., Gi and Go). Opiates directly activate the K^+ channel via Gi and Go. In contrast, inhibition of the Na^+ current appears to be indirect, through Gi-mediated inhibition of cAMP formation and reduced activation of cAMP-dependent protein kinase (protein kinase A). Biochemical studies confirm that opiates acutely inhibit adenylyl cyclase activity and cAMP-dependent protein phosphorylation in the locus coeruleus (Figure 13–2, top) (Nestler 1992).

With long-term exposure, locus coeruleus neurons develop tolerance to these acute inhibitory actions, as neuronal activity recovers toward preexposure levels

(Aghajanian 1978; Christie et al. 1987). Administration of an opioid receptor antagonist causes a rebound increase in neuronal firing rates above preexposure levels both in vivo and in isolated slice preparations (Aghajanian 1978; Kogan et al. 1992; Rasmussen et al. 1990). These electrophysiological correlates of tolerance, dependence, and withdrawal are mediated in part via upregulation of the cAMP pathway as a compensatory, or homeostatic, adaptation to long-term exposure to opiates. Long-term opiate exposure increases locus coeruleus levels of Gi and Go, adenylyl cyclase types I and VIII, catalytic and regulatory protein kinase A, and several phosphoprotein substrates for the kinase (see Lane-Ladd et al. 1997; Nestler 1992; Nestler and Aghajanian 1997). One of these substrates, tyrosine hydroxylase, is the rate-limiting enzyme in the biosynthesis of norepinephrine (and other catecholamines), which suggests that norepinephrine synthesis is increased after long-term opiate administration. Upregulation of the cAMP pathway occurs in the absence of alterations in several other intracellular signaling pathways in this brain region.

The mechanisms by which long-term opiate exposure upregulates the cAMP pathway are complex. Some of the adaptations, including induction of adenylyl cyclase type VIII and tyrosine hydroxylase, occur via increased gene expression that involves the transcription factor cAMP response element binding protein (CREB) (Boundy et al. 1998b; Lane-Ladd et al. 1997). CREB is activated when it is phosphorylated by protein kinase A or other protein kinases, and it is itself upregulated in the locus coeruleus after long-term morphine administration. A role for CREB-regulated genes in opiate physical dependence is consistent with the observation that mice lacking CREB show reduced opiate withdrawal symptoms (Maldonado et al. 1996).

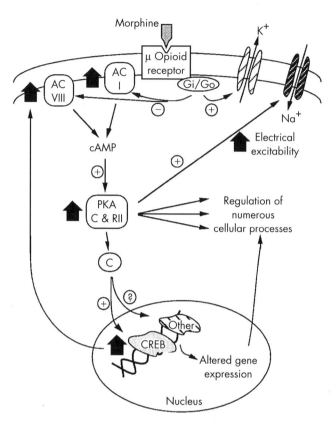

FIGURE 13–2. Schematic illustration of opiate actions in the locus coeruleus (LC).

Opiates acutely inhibit LC neurons by increasing the conductance of an inwardly rectifying K+ channel (*light crosshatch*) via coupling with subtypes of Gi and Go and by decreasing an Na+-dependent inward current (*dark crosshatch*) via coupling with Gi and Go and the consequent inhibition of adenylyl cyclase (AC). Reduced levels of cyclic adenosine monophosphate (cAMP) decrease protein kinase A (PKA) activity and the phosphorylation of the responsible channel or pump. Inhibition of the cAMP pathway also decreases phosphorylation of numerous other proteins and thereby affects many additional processes in the neuron. For example, it reduces the phosphorylation state of cAMP response element binding protein (CREB), which may initiate some of the longer-term changes in LC function. Upward bold arrows summarize effects of long-term morphine use in the LC. Long-term morphine use increases levels of AC types I and VIII, PKA catalytic (C) and regulatory type II (RII) subunits, and several phosphoproteins, including CREB. These changes contribute to the altered phenotype of the drug-addicted state. For example, the intrinsic excitability of LC neurons is increased via enhanced activity of the cAMP pathway and Na+-dependent inward current, which contributes to the tolerance, dependence, and withdrawal exhibited by these neurons. Upregulation of AC type VIII is mediated via CREB, whereas upregulation of AC type I of the PKA subunits appears to occur via a CREB-independent mechanism not yet identified.

Source. Reprinted with permission from Nestler EJ, Aghajanian GK: "Molecular and Cellular Basis of Addiction." *Science* 278:58–63, 1997. Copyright © 1997 American Association for the Advancement of Science.

Other aspects of the upregulated cAMP pathway—for example, induction of protein kinase A subunits—appear to occur at a posttranscriptional level, apparently independent of gene transcription (Boundy et al. 1998a).

The upregulated cAMP pathway is thought to contribute to the reduced ability of opiates to inhibit the activity of locus coeruleus neurons and thus accounts, at least in part, for opiate tolerance. In addition, these compensatory adaptations appear to contribute to the intrinsic hyperexcitability of locus coeruleus neurons seen during withdrawal (Kogan et al. 1992; Nestler 1992; Nestler et al. 1993) (Figure 13–2, bottom). This scheme is similar to one proposed earlier based on studies of neuroblastoma x glioma cells (Sharma et al. 1975). Although other mechanisms of opiate dependence in the locus coeruleus and elsewhere likely exist, manifestations of opiate dependence can be attributed directly to molecular and cellular adaptations in the cAMP pathway in specific neurons (Nestler and Aghajanian 1997). Related work suggests that similar types of adaptations underlie the long-term actions of opiates in other regions of the central nervous system (see, for example, Bonci and Williams 1997; Jolas et al. 2000; Terwilliger et al.1991; Tjon et al. 1994; Unterwald et al. 1993).

Role of the Mesolimbic Dopamine System in Drug Reinforcement

A substantial body of literature has established the mesolimbic dopamine system as a major neural substrate for the reinforcing effects of opiates, psychostimulants, ethanol, nicotine, and cannabinoids in animals (see Dworkin and Smith 1993; Koob 1992; Kuhar et al. 1991; Olds 1982; Wise 1998). This system consists of dopaminergic neurons in the ventral tegmental area (VTA) of the midbrain and their target neurons in forebrain regions such as the nucleus accumbens. For example, rats will self-administer dopamine, amphetamine (which releases dopamine), and cocaine and nomifensine (which elevate dopamine levels by blocking reuptake) directly into the nucleus accumbens, suggesting that dopamine

receptors in the nucleus accumbens mediate reinforcing stimuli. In contrast, opiates are self-administered directly into the dopamine cell body region of the VTA, where they activate dopamine neurons via disinhibitory mechanisms (see Johnson and North 1992) and thereby stimulate dopamine release in the nucleus accumbens. Other drugs of abuse, such as ethanol, nicotine, and cannabinoids, also cause increased dopamine release in the nucleus accumbens (Chen et al. 1990; Di Chiara and Imperato 1988), possibly through similar disinhibition of VTA dopamine neurons (Tanda et al. 1997). These findings have led some investigators to suggest that dopamine release in the nucleus accumbens is a final common mechanism in the acute reinforcing effects of opiates, psychostimulants, and other abused drugs.

However, there is evidence that opiates such as heroin and morphine can produce reinforcement independently of the dopamine system, by acting directly on opioid receptors in the nucleus accumbens and other brain regions (for review, see Bardo 1998). Dopamine antagonists and lesions of mesolimbic dopamine neurons, for example, fail to affect intravenous heroin self-administration. Animals also will self-administer opiates directly into the nucleus accumbens, where opioid receptors on nucleus accumbens neurons in essence bypass dopamine inputs. These data indicate that opiates can utilize both dopaminergic and nondopaminergic mechanisms in the nucleus accumbens to produce reinforcement of drug self-administration. Importantly, lesions of nucleus accumbens neurons attenuate both cocaine and heroin self-administration, suggesting that the nucleus accumbens is a critical neural substrate for both psychostimulant and opiate reinforcement.

Neurobiological Mechanisms of Relapse

Whereas drug self-administration is thought to provide a measure of the acute reinforcing properties of a drug, it is quite different from drug craving and drug seeking, which are the core behavioral abnormalities that define a state of addiction. Drug craving and drug seeking are cognitive states that are measured by subjective reports in humans and cannot be directly measured in laboratory animals. However, relapse is an operational event that can be measured directly when a laboratory animal reinitiates lever-press responding after abstaining from drug self-administration. To measure relapse in an experimental setting, investigators first introduce extinction conditions to animals with drug self-administration experience, thereby attenuating reinforcement of further lever-press responding. As animals learn that the drug is no longer available, their efforts to self-administer the drug quickly diminish. After a given period of abstinence, the animals are presented with specific stimuli that induce responding at the lever that previously delivered drug injections. This reinitiation of responding is interpreted as relapse to drug-seeking behavior. The level of drug-seeking behavior is measured by the amount of effort (lever-pressing) exerted by the animals to self-administer the drug. Because these efforts are no longer reinforced by drug infusions, this behavior is also referred to as nonreinforced responding. In essence, this behavioral paradigm separates the incentive motivational component of drug reinforcement (drug seeking) from the consummatory component (drug taking) and is believed to measure changes in the motivational state of the animal in the absence of drug reinforcement.

Only three types of stimuli have been shown to induce relapse to drug-seeking behavior in animals. These stimuli consist of low doses of the drug that was previously self-administered (for a review, see Self and Nestler 1998; Shaham et al. 2000), drug-associated (conditioned) cues, and stress. Because all three of these stimuli also trigger drug craving in human drug abusers, relapse to drug-seeking behavior in animals may represent a valid model of drug craving. Moreover, given that measures of drug craving can be confounded by the subjective nature of self-reports in humans (Tiffany et al. 1993), animal models of relapse may offer a more direct and objective measure of relapse to drug seeking than human reports of drug craving.

Drug-Induced Relapse to Drug-Seeking Behavior

A powerful trigger of relapse in animal models is a low "priming" injection with the drug that was self-administered by the animal on previous occasions (see Self and Nestler 1998; Shaham et al. 2000). This priming effect has been demonstrated for both opiates and psychostimulants. Interestingly, opiates such as morphine can trigger relapse to cocaine-seeking behavior (De Wit and Stewart 1981; Slikker et al. 1984), and vice versa (De Wit and Stewart 1983). Such "cross-priming" may reflect activation of a common neural substrate, perhaps the common ability of these drugs to activate the mesolimbic dopamine system.

Indeed, considerable evidence suggests that relapse triggered by priming injections of opiates and psychostimulants is mediated by the mesolimbic dopamine system. For example, microinfusion of amphetamine directly into the nucleus accumbens, where it causes local dopamine release, effectively induces relapse to heroin-seeking behavior (Stewart and Vezina 1988). Conversely, microinfusion of morphine into the VTA, which indirectly activates dopamine neurons and consequently increases dopamine release in the nucleus accumbens, induces relapse to heroin- and cocaine-seeking behavior (Stewart et al. 1984). In contrast, microinfusion of morphine into other brain regions rich in opioid receptors is ineffective at inducing relapse to drug-seeking behavior. Dopaminergic involvement in drug-induced relapse is bolstered by the fact that several directly acting dopaminergic agonists are powerful inducers of relapse to both cocaine- and heroin-seeking behavior (De Wit and Stewart 1983; Self et al. 1996; Wise et al. 1990), whereas dopamine antagonists can block the priming effects of heroin, amphetamine, and cocaine (Ettenberg 1990; Shaham and Stewart 1996; Weissenborn et al. 1996). Taken together, these studies suggest that dopamine release in the nucleus accumbens is both necessary and sufficient for inducing relapse to opiate- and psychostimulant-seeking behavior that is elicited by priming injections of the drugs (Figure 13–3).

Cue-Induced Relapse to Drug-Seeking Behavior

Cue-induced relapse to drug-seeking behavior involves the process of classical conditioning, whereby environmental stimuli, through repeated and specific association with drug exposure, acquire the ability to trigger relapse when presented in the absence of the drug (e.g., Ehrman et al. 1992; O'Brien et al. 1992; Robinson and Berridge 1993). The fact that these drug-associated cues can trigger appetitive or approach behavior has led investigators to hypothesize that these stimuli also activate the mesolimbic dopamine system (Robinson and Berridge 1993; Stewart et al. 1984; Wise 1998). At present, this hypothesis remains equivocal because the conditioned behavioral

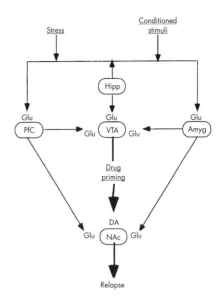

FIGURE 13–3. Schematic representation of the primary pathways through which stress, drugs of abuse, and drug-associated conditioned stimuli are hypothesized to trigger drug craving and relapse to drug seeking.

Stress and conditioned stimuli can activate excitatory glutamatergic projections (Glu) to the ventral tegmental area (VTA) from the prefrontal cortex (PfC), amygdala (Amyg), and hippocampus (Hipp), whereas priming injections of drugs directly stimulate dopamine (DA) release in the nucleus accumbens (NAc). In this sense, dopamine release in the nucleus accumbens may be a final common trigger of drug craving by all three stimuli. At the level of nucleus accumbens neurons, dopamine from the VTA modulates direct excitatory signals from the prefrontal cortex, amygdala, and hippocampus, where complex spatiotemporal integration of relapse-related information occurs. Studies showing involvement of these brain regions in relapse to drug seeking suggest that long-term changes in gene expression in these regions would alter the functionality of this circuitry and could produce profound changes in reactivity to stimuli that trigger drug craving and relapse to drug seeking.

effects of drugs such as cocaine are not necessarily associated with an increase in dopamine release in the nucleus accumbens (Brown and Fibiger 1992). However, at least two studies have reported enhanced dopamine release in the nucleus accumbens following presentation of drug-associated cues (Di Ciano et al. 1998; Fontana et al. 1993). In addition, others have found that presentation of cues associated with food rewards do in fact activate dopamine neurons in the VTA and elicit food-seeking behavior (Mirenowicz and Schultz 1996). Although elusive, the question of dopamine involvement in conditioned drug effects is crucial to our understanding of how drug-associated cues gain access to appetitive motivational systems in the brain to trigger relapse.

Growing evidence implicates the amygdala as a critical substrate for cue-induced relapse to drug-seeking behavior. For example, lesions of the amygdala attenuate the ability of drug-associated cues to induce relapse (Meil and See 1997). Cue-induced relapse is attenuated even when the lesions are produced after learned associations between cues and drugs have already formed, which suggests that conditioned cues utilize the amygdala to access and activate appetitive motivational systems. In this regard, projections from the amygdala are known to activate VTA dopamine neurons through both monosynaptic and polysynaptic pathways, presumably leading to increased dopaminergic transmission in the nucleus accumbens. Figure 13–3 illustrates this pathway whereby drug-associated cues can activate the mesolimbic dopamine system via known excitatory (glutamatergic) inputs from the amygdala. Also illustrated is an amygdala projection to the prefrontal cortex, which could form a secondary pathway whereby drug-associated cues activate VTA dopamine neurons.

Stress-Induced Relapse to Drug-Seeking Behavior

Psychological stress can also trigger drug craving in humans and relapse to drug seeking in animals. In animals, stress-induced relapse is triggered after a brief period of mild intermittent footshock. Presentation of this stress effectively induces relapse to both cocaine- and heroin-seeking behavior (Ahmed and Koob 1997; Erb et al. 1996; Shaham and Stewart 1995). Interestingly, stress-induced relapse to heroin-seeking behavior is equally effective whether animals are physically dependent on heroin or not (Shaham et al. 1996). Similar to drug- and cue-induced relapse, stress-induced relapse also may involve activation of the mesolimbic dopamine system. This idea is supported by the finding that stress-induced dopamine release in the nucleus accumbens correlates temporally with relapse to heroin-seeking behavior (Shaham and Stewart 1995). Moreover, stress-induced relapse is partially attenuated by pretreatment with dopamine antagonists (Shaham and Stewart 1996). A primary neural pathway through which stress can stimulate dopamine release in the nucleus accumbens may involve stress-induced activation of the prefrontal cortex (Karreman and Moghaddam 1996; Moghaddam 1993; Taber et al. 1995) and, consequently, activation of an excitatory projection from the prefrontal cortex to dopamine neurons in the VTA (Figure 13–3).

Another pathway by which stress can activate the mesolimbic dopamine system involves the ability of stress to stimulate release of the neuropeptide corticotropin-releasing factor (CRF). Infusion of CRF into the cerebral ventricles mimics the effects of stress in inducing relapse to heroin-seeking behavior, and similar infusions of a CRF antagonist reduce stress-induced relapse (Shaham et al. 1997). Because CRF can activate central dopamine systems (e.g., via the hypothalamic-pituitary-adrenal axis and corticosterone secretion [Overton et al. 1996; Piazza et al. 1996]), CRF-induced relapse may also involve activation of the mesolimbic dopamine system. Indeed, systemic injections of corticosterone can induce relapse to cocaine-seeking behavior (Deroche et al. 1997). However, because stress can trigger relapse in adrenalectomized animals (Shaham et al. 1997), and stress-induced relapse is associated with relatively small increases in dopamine release in the nucleus accumbens (Shaham et al. 1996), stress-induced relapse likely involves corticosterone- and dopamine-independent mechanisms as well.

Clearly, the effects of stress, cues, and drugs themselves on the mesolimbic dopamine system resemble druglike, or proponent, processes. In contrast, drug opposite or withdrawal-like processes fail to induce relapse to drug-seeking behavior in animal models. For example, precipitation of opiate withdrawal with naltrexone fails to induce relapse in animals with heroin self-administration experience, even when the animals are markedly physically dependent on the opiate (Shaham et al. 1996). Similarly, blockade of dopamine receptors with dopamine antagonists fails to induce heroin- or cocaine-seeking behavior (Shaham and Stewart 1996; Weissenborn et al. 1996), despite their ability to produce aversive consequences. Although these data contrast sharply with human studies in which drug craving is associated with negative emotionality during opiate and ethanol withdrawal, they agree with reports of druglike, and even mood-elevating, symptoms of craving in cocaine addicts (Childress et al. 1988; Robbins et al. 1997).

Even though naltrexone-precipitated withdrawal fails to trigger relapse to heroin-seeking behavior in animals, spontaneous withdrawal from heroin has been associated with relapse in the same models (Shaham et al. 1996). This finding may be relevant to factors involved in maintaining daily drug use in active drug abus-

ers. In this sense, dependence and withdrawal may play a more prominent role in drug craving during active drug use, whereas druglike processes (e.g., sensitization) may be more important in triggering drug craving and relapse after prolonged periods of abstinence, when withdrawal symptoms are no longer apparent.

Although it has not been clearly resolved, cue- and stress-induced reinstatement of drug-seeking behavior also may involve dopamine-independent neural substrates (reviewed in Self 1998). Thus, the basolateral and central nuclei of the amygdala, as well as the prefrontal cortex and hippocampus, send direct excitatory projections to the nucleus accumbens in addition to the VTA. Excitatory inputs from these regions converge with VTA dopamine inputs at the level of nucleus accumbens neurons, where excitatory transmission in the nucleus accumbens has been implicated in relapse to cocaine-seeking behavior (Cornish and Kalivas 2000). Together, these brain regions all form a complex circuit with primary sites of convergence in both the VTA and the nucleus accumbens of the mesolimbic dopamine system, as depicted in Figure 13–3. Given the central role of the nucleus accumbens in the output of these circuits, regulation of nucleus accumbens neuronal activity, whether by dopamine or glutamate, may be a critical event in triggering drug craving.

Mechanisms of Dopamine-Induced Relapse

The studies described in the preceding sections suggest that relapse to drug seeking can be triggered by activation of dopamine receptors on nucleus accumbens neurons. Dopamine receptors are divided into two general classes that are distinguishable by their structural properties and opposite modulation of adenylyl cyclase. The D_1-like receptors (D_1 and D_5) are positively coupled to adenylyl cyclase activity, whereas the D_2-like receptors (D_2, D_3, and D_4) are either negatively coupled or have no detectable effect on the enzyme. The two receptor classes also exert opposite effects on phosphatidylinositol turnover. Neurons intrinsic to the nucleus accumbens express both D_1-like and D_2-like dopamine receptors, but in somewhat different neuronal populations (Curran and Watson 1995; Meador-Woodruff et al. 1991). In most cases, these receptors produce similar, even synergistic, responses at the physiologic and behavioral levels (Hu and White 1994, Waddington and Daly 1993).

In contrast to these cooperative actions, activation of D_2-like, but not of D_1-like, dopamine receptors induces a profound and prolonged relapse to cocaine-seeking behavior in rats (De Vries et al. 1999; Self et al. 1996). These findings suggest that D_2-like receptors are primarily involved in inducing drug-seeking behavior by priming stimuli that release dopamine in the nucleus accumbens. Although selective activation of D_1-like receptors fails to markedly induce cocaine-seeking behavior, D_1 receptors may have a permissive role in the priming effects mediated by D_2 receptors, as both D_1 and D_2 receptor antagonists can block the priming effects of cocaine and heroin (Shaham and Stewart 1996; Weissenborn et al. 1996). Thus, transmission of D_2-mediated priming signals may require some minimal level of D_1 receptor activation. Interestingly, however, D_1-like receptor activation completely abolishes the ability of cocaine to induce relapse (Self et al. 1996). The opposing influence of D_1-like and D_2-like dopamine receptor activation on relapse to cocaine-seeking behavior is intriguing, because both D_1 and D_2 receptor agonists have reinforcing

properties, have similar abilities to mimic the subjective effects of cocaine, and stimulate locomotor activity. One possible explanation for these findings is that D_2-like receptors mediate the incentive to seek further drug reinforcement, whereas D_1-like receptors could mediate some aspect of drug reward related to gratification, drive reduction, or satiety.

Opposite modulation of drug-seeking behavior by D_1 and D_2 dopamine receptors could involve their opposite effects on cAMP formation. In this regard, microinfusion of a selective inhibitor of protein kinase A into the nucleus accumbens triggers relapse to cocaine-seeking behavior and potentiates cocaine-induced relapse to cocaine-seeking behavior in rats (Self et al. 1998). The effect of the protein kinase inhibitor resembles the effect of D_2 receptor stimulation, suggesting that dopamine triggers relapse by stimulating D_2 receptors that function via inhibition of protein kinase A activity. In any event, these findings suggest that protein kinase A activity in certain nucleus accumbens neurons could play a pivotal role in regulating incentive motivation during drug craving and relapse.

Adaptations in the Mesolimbic Dopamine System After Long-Term Drug Exposure

Although symptoms of physical withdrawal from opiates and other drugs typically persist for short periods of time after cessation of long-term drug exposure, drug addicts report intense drug craving long after these physical symptoms have subsided. This suggests that different brain regions mediate physical and motivational symptoms of drug dependence, a view supported by direct experimental evidence (e.g., Koob et al. 1992). The motivational symptoms, which include an escalation of drug intake (tolerance), increased drug craving (sensitization), and withdrawal-induced dysphoria (dependence), could result from drug-induced adaptations in the normal functioning of reinforcement-related brain regions, such as the VTA and nucleus accumbens. Recent studies have found that long-term drug exposure produces adaptations at the molecular and cellular levels in VTA dopamine neurons, and in their target neurons in the nucleus accumbens, that may underlie motivational aspects of tolerance, sensitization, and dependence associated with drug addiction (e.g., see Nestler and Aghajanian 1997; Self 1998; Self and Nestler 1998; White and Kalivas 1998; Wolf 1998). The results from these studies provide the basis for specific hypotheses that now guide future investigations to test, more directly, the role of specific adaptations in mediating drug craving in addicted subjects.

The ability of various drugs of abuse to produce similar types of changes in drug-taking and drug-seeking behavior after repeated administration raises the possibility that these drugs also produce similar types of molecular and cellular adaptations in specific brain regions. Support for this possibility comes from behavioral data, in which long-term exposure to stimulants, opiates, or ethanol can cross-sensitize the animal to the effects of the other drugs (e.g., Cunningham and Kelley 1992; Fahlke et al. 1994; Vezina and Stewart 1990). As demonstrated below, there is also now considerable biochemical evidence that different drugs of abuse can produce similar molecular adaptations in the VTA–nucleus accumbens pathway after long-term administration. These adaptations may be part of a common general mechanism of drug addiction and craving.

Regulation of G Proteins and the cAMP Pathway in the Ventral Tegmental Area and Nucleus Accumbens

Repeated cocaine treatment produces transient decreases in the level of inhibitory G protein subunits, Gi and Go, that couple to D_2 autoreceptors in the VTA (Nestler 1992; Striplin and Kalivas 1992). The level of these G proteins in the VTA is negatively correlated with the initial level of locomotor activation produced by cocaine (Striplin and Kalivas 1992). In addition, pertussis toxin injected directly into the VTA, which functionally inactivates these G proteins, increases the locomotor activating effects of cocaine and thereby mimics locomotor sensitization. Together, these findings support the possibility that reduced levels of Gi and Go could account for the D_2 receptor subsensitivity observed electrophysiologically after long-term cocaine exposure and may play a role in some of the long-term effects of cocaine on mesolimbic dopamine function.

Repeated cocaine treatment also decreases levels of Gi and Go in the nucleus accumbens (Nestler 1992; Striplin and Kalivas 1993) and increases levels of adenylyl cyclase and of cAMP-dependent protein kinase in this brain region (Terwilliger et al. 1991). Together, these changes would be expected to result in a concerted upregulation in the functional activity of the cAMP pathway. Because D_1 receptors are generally thought to produce their effects via activation of the cAMP pathway, these molecular adaptations could account for D_1 receptor supersensitivity observed during later withdrawal times. Long-term exposure to morphine, cocaine, heroin, or ethanol— but not to several drugs without reinforcing properties—produces similar changes in G proteins and the cAMP pathway

(Ortiz et al. 1995; Self et al. 1995; Terwilliger et al. 1991). Although the long-term effects of morphine and ethanol on the electrophysiological state of nucleus accumbens neurons have not yet been investigated, the biochemical findings suggest that an upregulated cAMP pathway may be part of a common mechanism of altered nucleus accumbens function associated with the drug-treated state. A critical question regarding these neuroadaptations is whether they contribute to changes in drug self-administration habits and to drug craving and relapse during abstinence.

We tested the former possibility by artificially upregulating the cAMP pathway in the nucleus accumbens of animals during drug self-administration tests (Self et al. 1994, 1998). In these studies, escalation of drug self-administration is produced by inactivation of inhibitory G proteins with pertussis toxin or by sustained protein kinase A activity after microinfusion of a membrane-permeable cAMP analog into the nucleus accumbens. Artificially mimicking the drug-induced neuroadaptations by sustained downregulation of inhibitory G proteins or by sustained increases in protein kinase A activity produces increases in drug self-administration. This effect is usually interpreted as a reduction in drug reward, with animals compensating by increasing their drug intake. These findings suggest that neuroadaptations in the nucleus accumbens–cAMP pathway caused by repeated drug use may represent an intracellular mechanism of tolerance to the rewarding effects of drugs, which leads to escalating drug intake during drug self-administration. One possible mechanism for such tolerance may involve protein kinase A–mediated phosphorylation, desensitization, and downregulation of D_1 receptors (see Sibley et al. 1998). On the other hand, activation of the cAMP path-

way in the nucleus accumbens was shown to produce an enhancement of conditioned reinforcement produced by cues associated with food reward (Kelley and Holahan 1997). This suggests that upregulation of the cAMP pathway in the nucleus accumbens may potentiate the incentive motivational effects of reward-associated cues, and possibly their ability to elicit craving. Further work is needed to study this latter hypothesis.

One of the important consequences of pertubation of intracellular messenger pathways is the regulation of gene expression (see Figure 13–1). Consequently, the ability of drugs of abuse to alter such signaling pathways means that they alter the expression of specific target genes within neurons, and such changes are thought to be important mediators of the stable neural and behavioral plasticity that underlies addiction. Most studies to date have focused on drug regulation of transcription factors, such as CREB and ΔFosB (Nestler 2001). There is now direct evidence that these and other transcription factors are part of the molecular mechanisms by which drugs of abuse alter the brain.

Conclusions

The availability of animal models that accurately reproduce important features of drug addiction in humans has made it possible to identify specific regions in the brain that play an important role in addictive disorders. Whereas the locus coeruleus plays an important role in physical dependence on opiates, it is the mesolimbic dopamine system as well as regions of the prefrontal cortex and amygdala that appear to be integrally involved in drug-seeking behavior, the essential clinical feature of drug addiction. Basic neurobiological investigations are now providing an increasingly complete understanding of the adaptations at the molecular and cellular levels that occur in these various brain regions and are responsible for behavioral features of drug addiction. Work to date has focused on adaptations in intracellular messenger pathways, particularly G proteins and the cAMP pathway, although many other types of adaptations will also prove to be involved. As the pathophysiological mechanisms underlying drug addiction become increasingly understood, it will be possible to develop more efficacious pharmacotherapies for the treatment of addictive disorders. Parallel studies, not covered in this chapter, of different inbred animal strains and of individual differences among large outbred populations promise to yield information concerning the specific proteins that underlie inherent differences in an individual's responsiveness to drugs of abuse. This work will lead eventually to the identification of specific genes and environmental factors that control individual variations in the susceptibility to drug addiction. Ultimately, this work could lead to the development of specific interventions that prevent drug addiction in particularly vulnerable individuals.

References

Aghajanian GK: Tolerance of locus coeruleus neurons to morphine and suppression of withdrawal response by clonidine. Nature 276:186–188, 1978

Ahmed SH, Koob GF: Cocaine- but not food-seeking behavior is reinstated by stress after prolonged extinction. Psychopharmacology (Berl) 132:289–295, 1997

Alreja M, Aghajanian GK: Pacemaker activity of locus coeruleus neurons: whole-cell recordings in brain slices show dependence on cAMP and protein kinase A. Brain Res 556:339–343, 1991

Alreja M, Aghajanian GK: Opiates suppress a resting sodium-dependent inward current in addition to activating an outward potassium current in locus coeruleus neurons. J Neurosci 13:3525–3532, 1993

American Psychiatric Association: Diagnostic and Statistical Manual of Mental Disorders, 4th Edition, Text Revision. Washington, DC, American Psychiatric Association, 2000

Bardo MT: Neuropharmacological mechanisms of drug reward: beyond dopamine in the nucleus accumbens. Crit Rev Neurobiol 12:37–67, 1998

Bonci A, Williams JT: Increased probability of GABA release during withdrawal from morphine. J Neurosci 17:796–803, 1997

Boundy VA, Chen JS, Nestler EJ: Regulation of cAMP-dependent protein kinase subunit expression in CATH.a and SH-SY5Y cells. J Pharmacol Exp Ther 286:1058–1065, 1998a

Boundy VA, Gold SJ, Messer CJ, et al: Regulation of tyrosine hydroxylase promoter activity by chronic morphine in TH9.0-LacZ transgenic mice. J Neurosci 18:9989–9995, 1998b

Brown EE, Fibiger HC: Cocaine-induced conditioned locomotion: absence of associated increases in dopamine release. Neuroscience 48:621–629, 1992

Chen J, Paredes W, Li J, et al: Delta 9-tetrahydrocannabinol produces naloxone blockable enhancement of presynaptic dopamine efflux in nucleus accumbens of conscious, freely moving rats as measured by intracerebral microdialysis. Psychopharmacology (Berl) 102:156–162, 1990

Childress AR, McLellan AT, O'Brien CP: Extinguishing conditioned responses in drug dependent persons, in Learning Factors in Drug Dependence: NIDA Research Monograph. Edited by Ray B. Washington, DC, U.S. Government Printing Office, 1988, pp 137–144

Christie MJ, Williams JT, North RA: Cellular mechanisms of opioid tolerance: studies in single brain neurons. Mol Pharmacol 32:633–638, 1987

Cornish JL, Kalivas PW: Glutamate transmission in the nucleus accumbens mediates relapse in cocaine addiction. J Neurosci 20(15):RC89, 2000

Cunningham ST, Kelley AE: Evidence for opiate-dopamine cross-sensitization in nucleus accumbens: studies of conditioned reward. Brain Res Bull 29:675–680, 1992

Curran EJ, Watson SJ: Dopamine receptor mRNA expression patterns by opioid peptide cells in the nucleus accumbens of the rat: a double in situ hybridization study. J Comp Neurol 361:57–76, 1995

Deroche V, Marinelli M, Le Moal M, et al: Glucocorticoids and behavioral effects of psychostimulants, II: cocaine intravenous self-administration and reinstatement depend on glucocorticoid levels. J Pharmacol Exp Ther 281:1401–1407, 1997

De Vries TJ, Schoffelmeer ANM, Binnekade R, et al: Dopaminergic mechanisms mediating the incentive to seek cocaine and heroin following long-term withdrawal of IV drug self-administration. Psychopharmacology (Berl) 143:254–260, 1999

De Wit H, Stewart J: Reinstatement of cocaine-reinforced responding in the rat. Psychopharmacology (Berl) 75:134–143, 1981

De Wit H, Stewart J: Drug reinstatement of heroin-reinforced responding in the rat. Psychopharmacology (Berl) 79:29–31, 1983

Di Chiara G, Imperato A: Drugs abused by humans preferentially increase synaptic dopamine concentrations in the mesolimbic system of freely moving rats. Proc Natl Acad Sci U S A 85:5274–5278, 1988

Di Ciano P, Blaha CD, Phillips AG: Conditioned changes in dopamine oxidation currents in the nucleus accumbens of rats by stimuli paired with self-administration or yoked-administration of d-amphetamine. Eur J Neurosci 10:1121–1127, 1998

Dworkin SI, Smith JE: Opiates/opioids and reinforcement, in Biological Basis of Substance Abuse. Edited by Korenman SG, Barchas JD. New York, Oxford University Press, 1993, pp 327–338

Ehrman RN, Robbins SJ, Childress AR, et al: Conditioned responses to cocaine-related stimuli in cocaine abuse patients. Psychopharmacology (Berl) 107:523–529, 1992

Erb S, Shaham Y, Stewart J: Stress reinstates cocaine-seeking behavior after prolonged extinction and a drug-free period. Psychopharmacology (Berl) 128:408–412, 1996

Ettenberg A: Haloperidol prevents the reinstatement of amphetamine-rewarded runway responding in rats. Pharmacol Biochem Behav 36:635–638, 1990

Fahlke C, Hansen S, Engel JA, et al: Effects of ventral striatal 6-OHDA lesions or amphetamine sensitization on ethanol consumption in the rat. Pharmacol Biochem Behav 47: 345–349, 1994

Fontana DJ, Post RM, Pert A: Conditioned increases in mesolimbic dopamine overflow by stimuli associated with cocaine. Brain Res 629:31–39, 1993

Gold MS, Redmond DE, Kleber HD: Clonidine in opiate withdrawal. Lancet 11: 599–602, 1978

Hu XT, White FJ: Loss of D1/D2 dopamine receptor synergisms following repeated administration of D1 or D2 receptor selective antagonists: electrophysiological and behavioral studies. Synapse 17(1):43–61, 1994

Johnson SW, North RA: Opioids excite dopamine neurons by hyperpolarization of local interneurons. J Neurosci 12: 483–488, 1992

Jolas T, Nestler EJ, Aghajanian GK: Chronic morphine increases GABA tone on serotonergic neurons of the dorsal raphe nucleus: association with an upregulation of the cyclic AMP pathway. Neuroscience 95: 433–443, 2000

Karreman M, Moghaddam B: The prefrontal cortex regulates the basal release of dopamine in the limbic striatum: an effect mediated by ventral tegmental area. J Neurochem 66:589–598, 1996

Kelley AE, Holahan MR: Enhanced reward-related responding following cholera toxin infusion into the nucleus accumbens. Synapse 26:46–54, 1997

Kogan JH, Nestler EJ, Aghajanian GK: Elevated basal firing rates and enhanced responses to 8-Br-cAMP in locus coeruleus neurons in brain slices from opiate-dependent rats. Eur J Pharmacol 211:47–53, 1992

Koob GF: Drugs of abuse: anatomy, pharmacology and function of reward pathways. Trends Pharmacol Sci 13:177–184, 1992

Koob GF, Maldonado R, Stinus L: Neural substrates of opiate withdrawal. Trends Neurosci 15:186–191, 1992

Kuhar MJ, Ritz MC, Boja JW: The dopamine hypothesis of the reinforcing properties of cocaine. Trends Neurosci 14:299–302, 1991

Lane-Ladd SB, Pineda J, Boundy V, et al: CREB in the locus coeruleus: biochemical, physiological, and behavioral evidence for a role in opiate dependence. J Neurosci 17: 7890–7901, 1997

Maldonado R, Koob GF: Destruction of the locus coeruleus decreases physical signs of opiate withdrawal. Brain Res 605: 128–138, 1993

Maldonado R, Blendy JA, Tzavara E, et al: Reduction of morphine abstinence in mice with a mutation in the gene encoding CREB. Science 273:657–659, 1996

Meador-Woodruff JH, Mansour A, Healy DJ, et al: Comparison of the distribution of D1 and D2 dopamine receptor mRNAs in rat brain. Neuropsychopharmacology 5:231–242, 1991

Meil WM, See RE: Lesions of the basolateral amygdala abolish the ability of drug associated cues to reinstate responding during withdrawal from self-administered cocaine. Behav Brain Res 87:139–148, 1997

Mirenowicz J, Schultz W: Preferential activation of midbrain dopamine neurons by appetitive rather than aversive stimuli. Nature 379:449–451, 1996

Moghaddam B: Stress preferentially increases extraneuronal levels of excitatory amino acids in the prefrontal cortex: comparison to hippocampus and basal ganglia. J Neurochem 60:1650–1657, 1993

Nestler EJ: Molecular mechanisms of drug addiction. J Neurosci 12:2439–2450, 1992

Nestler EJ: Molecular basis of long-term plasticity underlying addiction. Nat Rev Neurosci 2(2):119–128, 2001

Nestler EJ, Aghajanian GK: Molecular and cellular basis of addiction. Science 278:58–63, 1997

Nestler EJ, Hope BT, Widnell KL: Drug addiction: a model for the molecular basis of neural plasticity. Neuron 11:995–1006, 1993

Nestler EJ, Hyman SE, Malenka RC: Molecular Neuropharmacology: A Foundation for Clinical Neuroscience. New York, McGraw-Hill, 2001

North RA, Williams JT, Suprenant A, et al: Mu and delta receptors belong to a family of receptors that are coupled to potassium channels. Proc Natl Acad Sci U S A 84:5487–5491, 1987

O'Brien C, Childress A, McLellan A, et al: A learning model of addiction, in Addictive States. Edited by O'Brien CP, Jaffe JH. New York, Raven, 1992, pp 157–177

Olds ME: Reinforcing effects of morphine in the nucleus accumbens. Brain Res 237:429–440, 1982

Ortiz J, Fitzgerald LW, Charlton M, et al: Biochemical actions of chronic ethanol exposure in the mesolimbic dopamine system. Synapse 21:289–298, 1995

Overton PG, Tong ZY, Brain PF, et al: Preferential occupation of mineralocorticoid receptors by corticosterone enhances glutamate-induced burst firing in rat midbrain dopaminergic neurons. Brain Res 737:146–154, 1996

Piazza PV, Rouge-Pont F, Deroche V, et al: Glucocorticoids have state-dependent stimulant effects on the mesencephalic dopamine transmission. Proc Natl Acad Sci U S A 93: 8716–8720, 1996

Rasmussen K, Beitner-Johnson D, Krystal JH, et al: Opiate withdrawal and the rat locus coeruleus: behavioral, electrophysiological, and biochemical correlates. J Neurosci 10:2308–2317, 1990

Robbins SJ, Ehrman RN, Childress AR, et al: Relationships among physiological and self-report responses produced by cocaine-related cues. Addict Behav 22:157–167, 1997

Robinson TE, Berridge KC: The neural basis of drug craving: an incentive-sensitization theory of addiction. Brain Res Rev 18:247–291, 1993

Self DW: Neural substrates of drug craving and relapse in drug addiction. Ann Med 30:379–389, 1998

Self DW, Nestler EJ: Relapse to drug seeking: neural and molecular mechanisms. Drug Alcohol Depend 51:49–60, 1998

Self DW, Terwilliger RZ, Nestler EJ, et al: Inactivation of Gi and Go proteins in nucleus accumbens reduces both cocaine and heroin reinforcement. J Neurosci 14:6239–6247, 1994

Self DW, McClenahan AW, Beitner-Johnson D, et al: Biochemical adaptations in the mesolimbic dopamine system in response to heroin self-administration. Synapse 21:312–318, 1995

Self DW, Barnhart WJ, Lehman DA, et al: Opposite modulation of cocaine-seeking behavior by D1-like and D2-like dopamine receptor agonists. Science 271:1586–1589, 1996

Self DW, Genova LM, Hope BT, et al: Involvement of cAMP-dependent protein kinase in the nucleus accumbens in cocaine self-administration and relapse of cocaine-seeking behavior. J Neurosci 18:1848–1859, 1998

Shaham Y, Stewart J: Stress reinstates heroin-seeking in drug-free animals: an effect mimicking heroin, not withdrawal. Psychopharmacology (Berl) 119:334–341, 1995

Shaham Y, Stewart J: Effects of opioid and dopamine receptor antagonists on relapse induced by stress and re-exposure to heroin in rats. Psychopharmacology (Berl) 125:385–391, 1996

Shaham Y, Rajabi H, Stewart J: Relapse to heroin-seeking in rats under opioid maintenance: the effects of stress, heroin priming, and withdrawal. J Neurosci 16:1957–1963, 1996

Shaham Y, Funk D, Erb S, et al: Corticotropin-releasing factor in stress-induced relapse to heroin-seeking in rats. J Neurosci 17:2605–2614, 1997

Shaham Y, Erb S, Stewart J: Stress-induced relapse to heroin and cocaine seeking in rats: a review. Brain Res Brain Res Rev 33:13–33, 2000

Sharma SK, Klee WA, Nirenberg M: Dual regulation of adenylate cyclase accounts for narcotic dependence and tolerance. Proc Natl Acad Sci U S A 72:3092–3096, 1975

Sibley DR, Ventura AL, Jiang D, et al: Regulation of the D1 receptor through cAMP-mediated pathways. Adv Pharmacol 42:447–450, 1998

Slikker WJ, Brocco MJ, Killam KFJ: Reinstatement of responding maintained by cocaine or thiamylal. J Pharmacol Exp Ther 228:43–52, 1984

Stewart J, Vezina P: A comparison of the effects of intra-accumbens injections of amphetamine and morphine on reinstatement of heroin intravenous self-administration behavior. Brain Res 457:287–294, 1988

Stewart J, De Wit H, Eikelboom R: Role of unconditioned and conditioned drug effects in the self-administration of opiates and stimulants. Psychol Rev 91:251–268, 1984

Striplin CD, Kalivas PW: Correlation between behavioral sensitization to cocaine and G protein ADP-ribosylation in the ventral tegmental area. Brain Res 579:181–186, 1992

Striplin CD, Kalivas PW: Robustness of G protein changes in cocaine sensitization shown with immunoblotting. Synapse 14:10–15, 1993

Taber MT, Das S, Fibiger HC: Cortical regulation of subcortical dopamine release: mediation via the ventral tegmental area. J Neurochem 65:1407–1410, 1995

Tanda G, Pontieri FE, Di Chiara G: Cannabinoid and heroin activation of mesolimbic dopamine transmission by a common mu1 opioid receptor mechanism. Science 276:2048–2050, 1997

Terwilliger RZ, Beitner-Johnson D, Sevarino KA, et al: A general role for adaptations in G-proteins and the cyclic AMP system in mediating the chronic actions of morphine and cocaine on neuronal function. Brain Res 548:100–110, 1991

Tiffany ST, Singleton E, Haertzen CA, et al: The development of a cocaine craving questionnaire. Drug Alcohol Depend 34:19–28, 1993

Tjon GH, De Vries TJ, Ronken E, et al: Repeated and chronic morphine administration causes differential long-lasting changes in dopaminergic neurotransmission in rat striatum without changing its delta- and kappa-opioid receptor regulation. Eur J Pharmacol 252:205–212, 1994

Unterwald EM, Cox BM, Creek MJ, et al: Chronic repeated cocaine administration alters basal and opioid-regulated adenylyl cyclase activity. Synapse 15:33–38, 1993

Vezina P, Stewart J: Amphetamine administered to the ventral tegmental area but not to the nucleus accumbens sensitizes rats to systemic morphine: lack of conditioned effects. Brain Res 516:99–106, 1990

Waddington JL, Daly SA: Regulation of unconditioned motor behaviour by D1:D2 interaction, in D-1:D-2 Dopamine Receptor Interactions. Edited by Waddington JL. London, Academic Press, 1993, pp 203–233

Weissenborn R, Deroche V, Koob G, et al: Effects of dopamine agonists and antagonists on cocaine-induced operant responding for a cocaine-associated stimulus. Psychopharmacology (Berl) 126:311–322, 1996

White FJ, Kalivas PW: Neuroadaptations involved in amphetamine and cocaine addiction. Drug Alcohol Depend 51:141–153, 1998

Wise RA: Drug-activation of brain reward pathways. Drug Alcohol Depend 51:13–22, 1998

Wise RA, Murray A, Bozarth MA: Bromocriptine self-administration and bromocriptine-reinstatement of cocaine-trained and heroin-trained lever pressing in rats. Psychopharmacology (Berl) 100:355–360, 1990

Wolf ME: The role of excitatory amino acids in behavioral sensitization to psychomotor stimulants. Prog Neurobiol 54:679–720, 1998

CHAPTER 14

Neuropsychiatric Aspects of Alzheimer's Disease and Other Dementing Illnesses

Sylvia Askin-Edgar, M.D., Ph.D.

Katherine E. White, M.D.

Jeffrey L. Cummings, M.D.

Dementia is a generic term for a syndrome that has a variety of etiologies. The most common etiology is Alzheimer's disease (AD), which accounts for approximately 60%–70% of cases of late-onset dementia. In this chapter, we review the neuropsychiatric aspects of AD, dementia with Lewy bodies (DLB), frontotemporal dementia (FTD), Huntington's disease (HD), Parkinson's disease (PD), progressive supranuclear palsy (PSP), Wilson's disease (WD), corticobasal degeneration (CBD), multiple system atrophy (MSA), vascular dementia (VaD), hydrocephalic dementia, and Creutzfeldt-Jakob disease (CJD). The evaluation and treatment of dementia syndromes and their neuropsychiatric manifestations are discussed. Dementias associated with other brain diseases are described in the relevant chapters of this volume addressing head injury (Chapter 8), cerebral tumors (Chapter 12), and alcoholism and substance use disorders (Chapter 13).

DSM-IV-TR (American Psychiatric Association 2000) defines dementia as a syndrome with impairment of memory and at least one other cognitive ability that is disabling, that represents a decline from a previous higher level of intellectual functioning, and that is not present exclusively during a delirium. Dementia is dis-

Jeffrey L. Cummings is supported by National Institute on Aging Alzheimer's Disease Research Center Grant AG16570, an Alzheimer's Disease Research Center of California grant, and the Sidell-Kagan Foundation.

tinguished from acute confusional states (delirium) by intact arousal, more preserved attention, less fluctuation, and persistence of intellectual changes. The course of dementia is usually progressive, although 10%–15% of cases may be reversible (e.g., hypothyroid dementia) or treatable without reversing existing intellectual deficits (e.g., prevention of further ischemic injury in patients with VaD). Treatments of AD include those that are disease-modifying (e.g., vitamin E) or are intended to improve cognitive symptoms (e.g., cholinesterase inhibitors). Dementing diseases are often accompanied by neuropsychiatric syndromes, including personality alterations, mood changes, and psychosis.

Alzheimer's Disease

AD is the single most common dementing illness of the elderly and is a progressive degenerative disorder that affects primarily the neurons of the cerebral cortex. Neuropathological and neurotransmitter changes are two pathophysiological components of the disease process. AD starts in the mesial temporal lobe, in the entorhinal cortex. Limbic, paralimbic, and heteromodal association cortex are maximally affected, whereas primary sensory and motor areas, thalamus, basal ganglia, and cerebellum are comparatively spared (Cummings and Benson 1992). Pathologic changes include neurofibrillary tangles (NFTs), neuritic plaques (NPs), and synaptic and neuronal loss. The accumulation of amyloid in the brain leads to formation of plaques and nerve cell death. Loss of cells in the transmitter-related nuclei in turn leads to transmitter deficits, especially the loss of acetylcholine, which contribute to the cognitive deficit and the behavioral changes of AD.

AD usually begins after age 55, its greatest risk factor being increasing age. Women are at slightly increased risk of developing AD compared with men (1.2 to 1). Genetic factors also contribute to the risk for AD (having one close relative triples the risk for developing the disease).

Mutations in three genes, the amyloid precursor protein (APP) gene on chromosome 21, presenilin 1 (PS1) gene on chromosome 14, and presenilin 2 (PS2) gene on chromosome 1, produce the autosomal dominant form of AD, which can manifest as early as the fourth decade of life. The mutations, which are rare (2%–3% of all cases of AD), are highly penetrant and essentially all carriers develop AD.

A polymorphism of the apolipoprotein-E (ApoE) gene on chromosome 19 has been identified as a susceptibility marker for AD (Kamboh 1995). ApoE has three allelic forms, 2, 3, and 4. Absence of the E4 allele correlates with a risk of late-onset AD of approximately 15%; this risk increases to 30%–50% with one copy and up to 60%–90% with two copies of the E4 allele (Kamboh 1995). The presence of ApoE4 is neither necessary nor sufficient for the development of AD.

A history of head injury, especially one associated with loss of consciousness of 1 hour or more, also increases the risk for AD. The presence of the E4 variant of ApoE combined with head trauma increases risk for AD eightfold (Nemetz et al. 1999).

Clinical Diagnosis

The diagnosis of AD is stratified as definite, probable, or possible according to the available information (McKhann et al. 1984) (Table 14–1). A diagnosis of *definite AD* requires that the patient exhibit 1) a characteristic clinical syndrome meeting criteria for probable AD and 2) histologic evidence of AD pathology obtained from biopsy or autopsy. The diagnosis of *probable AD* requires that 1) the patient meets criteria for dementia based on a clinical examination, structured mental status questionnaire, and neuropsychological testing; 2) the patient has deficits in at least two areas of intellectual function—memory impairment and abnormalities in at least one other domain; 3) memory and other intellectual functions progressively worsen; 4) consciousness is not disturbed; 5) the disease begins between age 40 and 90; and 6) no systemic or other brain disorder could account for the deficits observed. Thus, accurate diagnosis depends on a combination of inclusionary clinical features as well as excluding other possible causes of dementia. AD should not be regarded as purely an exclusionary diagnosis. Neuropathological studies demonstrate that 65%–90% of patients identified as having probable AD will have the diagnosis confirmed at autopsy (Risse et al. 1990; Tierney et al. 1988).

Possible AD is diagnosed when 1) deviations from the classic pattern of AD in the onset, presentation, or course of a dementing illness are present with no alternative explanation; 2) a systemic illness or brain disease is present that is not considered to be the cause of the dementia syndrome; or 3) there is a single gradually progressive cognitive deficit in the absence of any other brain disorder. Focal neurologic signs, sudden onset, the early occurrence of a gait disorder, or seizures make the diagnosis of AD unlikely.

Neuropsychiatric Aspects

Neuropsychiatric symptoms are ubiquitous in AD, affecting nearly all patients during the course of illness, and they are the primary cause of caregiver burden and nursing home placement.

Personality alterations, apathy, mood changes, anxiety, irritability, disinhibition, disturbances of psychomotor activity,

TABLE 14–1. Criteria for definite, probable, and possible Alzheimer's disease (AD)

Definite AD
    Clinical criteria for probable AD
    Histopathologic evidence of AD (autopsy or biopsy)

Probable AD
    Dementia established by clinical examination and documented by mental status questionnaire
    Dementia confirmed by neuropsychological testing
    Deficits in two or more areas of cognition
    Progressive worsening of memory and other cognitive functions
    No disturbance of consciousness
    Onset between ages 40 and 90
    Absence of systematic disorders or other brain diseases capable of producing a dementia syndrome

Possible AD
    Presence of a systemic disorder or other brain disease capable of producing dementia but not thought to be the cause of the dementia
    Gradually progressive decline in a single intellectual function in the absence of any other identifiable cause (e.g., memory loss or aphasia)

Unlikely AD
    Sudden onset
    Focal neurologic signs
    Seizures or gait disturbance early in the course of the illness

Source. Adapted from McKhann et al. 1984.

delusions, hallucinations, and a variety of miscellaneous behavioral changes, including disturbances of sleep and appetite, altered sexual behavior, and Klüver-Bucy syndrome can be associated with AD (Mega et al. 1996).

The most common personality change is passivity or disengagement: patients exhibit diminished emotional responsiveness, decreased initiative, loss of enthusiasm, diminished energy, and decreased emotion (Petry et al. 1988; Rubin et al. 1987).

Delusions are common in patients with AD, affecting 30%–50% of patients (Cummings et al. 1987; Wragg and Jeste 1989). The most frequent delusions involve false beliefs of theft, infidelity of the spouse, abandonment, persecution, a phantom boarder, or Capgras' syndrome (Reisberg et al. 1987).

Hallucinations are not a common manifestation of AD; 9%–27% of patients have hallucinatory experiences. Visual hallucinations are most common, followed by auditory or combined auditory and visual hallucinations. Typical visual hallucinations include visions of persons from the past (e.g., deceased parents), intruders, animals, complex scenes, or inanimate objects (Mendez et al. 1990).

A variety of mood changes, including depressive symptoms, elation, and lability, have been observed in patients with AD. Few patients meet the criteria for major depressive episodes, but elements of a depressive syndrome are frequent, occurring in 20%–40% of patients with AD (Cummings et al. 1987; Mendez et al. 1990). Anxiety has been reported in approximately 40% of patients with AD. The most common manifestation is excessive anticipatory concern regarding upcoming events (Mendez et al. 1990) and marked uneasiness when separated from the caregiver.

Disturbances in psychomotor activity and troublesome behaviors are common in patients with AD and become increasingly evident as the disease progresses. Wandering and pacing are pervasive behaviors in the middle and later stages of the illness; providing safe, contained spaces for wandering is a major challenge for residential facilities (Morishita 1990). Restlessness is reported in up to 60% of patients, and assaultive behavior is observed in 60% of patients (Mega et al. 1996).

Neuroimaging and Laboratory Testing

Computed tomography (CT) and magnetic resonance imaging (MRI) provide structural information; positron emission tomography (PET) and single photon emission computed tomography (SPECT) reflect cerebral metabolism and blood flow. MRI demonstrates atrophy of the hippocampus and related structures early in the disease (de Leon et al. 1997; Jack et al. 1992, 1999). PET with fluorodeoxyglucose (FDG-PET) reveals a characteristic pattern of hypometabolism (Figure 14–1); glucose utilization is diminished in the parietal lobes; the frontal lobes are affected as the disease progresses. Subcortical structures and primary motor and sensory cortices are spared (Fazekas et al. 1989; Foster et al. 1983; Haxby et al. 1986; Jagust et al. 1988).

SPECT reveals diminished cerebral perfusion in the parietal and posterior temporal lobes of both hemispheres in most AD patients (Figure 14–2) (Johnson et al. 1987; Miller et al. 1990). Frontal lobe perfusion declines as the disease progresses.

Electroencephalography usually reveals theta and delta slowing as the disease advances, and computerized electroencephalographic studies with brain mapping demonstrate maximal abnormalities in the parietal regions of both hemispheres (Jordan et al. 1989).

Neuropsychological testing can help distinguish dementia from normal aging and provides details regarding the pattern of cognitive impairment. Lumbar puncture is an optional procedure and should be considered if one suspects central nervous system (CNS) infection, neoplasm, inflammation, or demyelination. Cerebrospinal fluid (CSF) tau is increased; CSF amyloid is decreased (Galasko et al. 1998; Van Nostrand et al. 1992; Wahlund 1996).

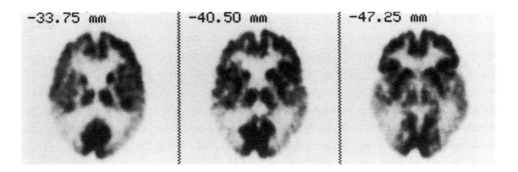

FIGURE 14–1. Transaxial positron emission tomography (PET) revealing decreased glucose metabolism bilaterally in the parietal lobes characteristic of Alzheimer's disease.

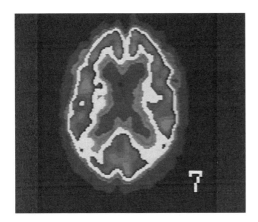

FIGURE 14–2. Transaxial single photon emission computed tomography (SPECT) of a patient with Alzheimer's disease revealing diminished cerebral perfusion in the temporoparietal regions bilaterally.

Red areas indicate normal blood flow, and yellow regions indicate diminished perfusion.

For a color version of this figure, please see the color insert at the back of this book.

Source. Image courtesy of Dr. Ismael Mena.

Neuropathology

The major pathologic alterations of AD include neuronal loss, cortical gliosis, intraneuronal cytoplasmic NFTs, NPs, granulovacuolar degeneration, and amyloid angiopathy of the cerebral vessels (Cummings and Benson 1992; Katzman 1986). NFTs are composed of the altered microtubule associated protein (MAP)

tau. Tau is hyperphosphorylated, producing a highly insoluble protein comprising paired helical filaments (PHF) (Ohtsubo et al. 1990). NPs are the other main structural change in AD. Amyloid beta protein is deposited in the center of these plaques. Neurotransmitter alterations include marked reductions of choline acetyltransferase and somatostatin as well as more modest and variable losses of serotonin, γ-aminobutyric acid (GABA), and norepinephrine (Cummings and Benson 1992; Procter et al. 1988).

Although much remains to be determined about the pathophysiology of AD, increased amyloid deposition appears to be central to the illness. Amyloid aggregation leads to the formation of NP and neuronal death. NFT may be related to the amyloid toxicity or may represent a distinct pathologic lesion. Aggregation of amyloid in the brain may be facilitated by ApoE4.

Treatment

Agents approved in the United States for the treatment of cognitive decline in AD include tacrine, donepezil, rivastigmine, and galantamine. Tacrine (Cognex) was the first of these agents to be approved but, as a result of requirements for multiple daily dosing and adverse side effects, this agent has limited use. Donepezil (Aricept) is a reversible cholinesterase inhibitor (ChE-I) that is well tolerated, is not associated with liver toxicity, and has a long half-life allowing once daily dosing. Nausea and diarrhea may occur. Galantamine (Reminyl) has similar efficacy and tolerability. It is initiated at 4 mg twice daily and increased to 8–12 mg twice daily. Rivastigmine (Exelon), a pseudoirreversible ChE-I, requires twice daily dosing and is gradually increased from 1.5 mg twice daily to 4.5–6 mg twice daily. Nausea, vomiting, and weight loss are common side effects. These agents produce a modest and temporary effect on cognitive function. They may improve behavior, delay loss of function, and defer nursing home placement. The ChE-Is are not disease-modifying agents, and effects are not sustained once the drug is discontinued (Giacobini 2000).

Vitamin E and selegiline are antioxidant compounds that have been shown to delay development of severe cognitive impairment, decline in activities of daily living, death, and nursing home placement (Sano et al. 1997). Both agents were superior to placebo, and combined administration was not more efficacious than treatment with either agent alone. Vitamin E (2,000 IU daily) or selegiline (10 mg daily) is standard therapy for AD in combination with a ChE-I.

Management of the neuropsychiatric disturbance of AD and other dementias is discussed at the end of this chapter.

Dementia With Lewy Bodies

DLB should be suspected in the presence of a dementia syndrome with the triad of fluctuating cognitive impairment, extrapyramidal symptoms, and visual hallucinations (McKeith and O'Brien 1999; McKeith et al. 1996). The extrapyramidal symptoms in DLB are preceded by dementia or can occur simultaneously with it. MRI reveals relative preservation of the temporal lobes, and SPECT demonstrates loss of presynaptic and postsynaptic dopaminergic markers. The key neuropathological feature is the Lewy body, a spherical intraneuronal cytoplasmic inclusion that had formerly been noted in brain stem nuclei in PD. In DLB, Lewy bodies are scattered throughout the subcortical nuclei, the substantia nigra, and the cortex, particularly in the paralimbic regions. Consensus guidelines for the clinical and pathologic diagnosis of DLB were established in 1996 (McKeith et al. 1996) (Table 14–2).

TABLE 14–2.　Criteria for dementia with Lewy bodies

Dementia syndrome
Two of the following three:
　Fluctuating cognitive impairment
　Visual and/or auditory hallucinations
　Parkinsonism

Source.　Adapted from McKeith et al. 1996.

Accurate diagnosis is of importance because patients with DLB are exquisitely sensitive to neuroleptics, which should be avoided. First-line therapy for DLB should be ChE-Is, which in addition to potentially improving memory and cognition may have psychotropic effects, obviating the need for antipsychotic medication in many (Cummings 2000; McKeith et al. 2000).

Frontotemporal Dementias

FTDs are a group of disorders with lobar atrophy of frontal and temporal lobes. Mutations on chromosome 17 account for 20%–40% of cases of the familial form of

FTD (Clark et al. 1998; Hutton et al. 1998; McKeith et al. 1992; Poorkaj et al. 1998). Familial FTD is inherited as an autosomal dominant condition (Chow et al. 1999). The mutations have been found to affect the gene responsible for coding tau protein (van Swieten et al. 1999).

The hallmark of FTD is personality alteration with disinhibition, emotional coarsening, loss of ability for empathy, apathy, inability to interpret social cues, lack of insight and judgment, and poor planning (Neary et al. 1998). The disease typically begins between ages 40 and 65 years. Memory and visuospatial skills are relatively preserved; language disturbances can be prominent. Three FTD syndromes are recognized: 1) a disinhibition syndrome, 2) progressive nonfluent aphasia and early mutism, and 3) semantic dementia with loss of word meaning and face and object recognition. The Lund-Manchester consensus (Lund and Manchester Groups 1994) established guidelines for the diagnosis of FTD (Table 14–3).

TABLE 14–3. Principal clinical features of frontotemporal dementia

Core diagnostic features

Behavioral disturbance

    Insidious onset and slow progression

    Early loss of personal and social awareness: poor personal hygiene, lack of social tact

    Early signs of disinhibition: excessive jocularity, inappropriate sexuality, aggression

    Stereotyped and perseverative behavior: wandering, ritualistic preoccupation

    Distractibility, impulsivity, impersistence

    Early loss of insight into altered behavioral condition

Affective disturbance

    Depression: excessive sentimentality, delusions, anxiety, or suicidal ideation

    Hypochondriasis: bizarre somatic preoccupation

    Emotional indifference and apathy

Speech disturbance

    Progressive reduction of verbal output

    Stereotypy of speech: repetition of limited-repertoire words, phrases, or themes

    Late mutism

Preserved spatial orientation and praxis: intact abilities to negotiate the environment

    Physical signs

        Early primitive reflexes

        Late akinesis, rigidity, tremor

Laboratory investigations

    EEG: normal

    MRI/CT: predominant frontal and/or anterior temporal atrophy

    SPECT/PET: predominant frontal and/or anterior temporal abnormality

    Neuropsychological testing: prominent executive dysfunction

Supportive diagnostic features

    Onset before age 65

    Positive family history of similar disorder

Note. EEG = electroencephalogram; MRI = magnetic resonance imaging; CT = computed tomography; SPECT = single photon emission computed tomography; PET = positron emission tomography.

Source. Adapted from Brun et al. 1994.

Clinical and Neuropsychiatric Features

The clinical criteria for FTD are presented in Table 14–3. Neuropsychiatric features dominate the presentation of FTD. Personality alterations with disinhibition are often florid, and depression or apathy can be prominent (Miller et al. 1991). Klüver-Bucy syndrome, or fragments of the condition, may be evident in the initial phases of the disease, and often patients gain weight as their eating habits become less discriminating (Cummings and Duchen 1981). Stereotyped behaviors with compulsive rituals and complex repetitive acts might also be observed in the course of FTD.

Neuropsychological deficits are less marked in patients with FTD than in those with AD. Memory, visuospatial skills, and mathematical abilities are relatively spared in the early and middle stages of the disease (Cummings and Benson 1992; Knopman et al. 1989). Patients have deficits in executive functioning, including difficulty with set-shifting tasks (e.g., card sorting), word list generation (e.g., number of animals named in 1 minute), divided attention, and response inhibition (Miller et al. 1991). Language may be affected relatively early in the disease. Naming deficits, impairment of auditory comprehension, and increasingly sparse verbal output are common. Speech stereotypies, echolalia, and mutism also may occur (Cummings and Benson 1992; Graff-Radford et al. 1990).

FTD can usually be distinguished from AD on the basis of contrasting clinical characteristics (Table 14–4).

Laboratory Investigations and Neuroimaging

Routine studies of serum, urine, and CSF are normal in patients with FTD. In cases of FTD associated with amyotrophic lateral sclerosis, electromyography reveals findings consistent with motor neuron disease. Frontal atrophy and enlargement of the Sylvian fissures are evident on CT and MRI; frontotemporal deficits are observed on SPECT and PET (Duara et al. 1999) (Figure 14–3).

Neuropathology

Three pathologic variants of FTD are recognized: 1) Pick's disease, 2) frontal and temporal lobar degeneration without distinctive histopathologic changes, and 3) FTD with motor neuron disease (Lund and Manchester Groups 1994). The macroscopic pathology of Pick's disease includes marked atrophy of the frontal lobe anterior to the precentral sulcus and of the anterior temporal lobe (Cummings and Benson 1992). Neurons are atrophic, and there is intense astrocytic gliosis involving all cortical layers in affected regions (Brun et al. 1994). Some of the remaining neurons contain intracytoplasmic argyrophilic Pick bodies. Ultrastructurally, the Pick bodies are composed of straight filaments (Murayama et al. 1990).

FTD patients without Pick's-type pathology have nonspecific neuronal loss and astrocytic gliosis in a similar lobar distribution. The gliosis is less severe and more circumscribed than that observed in patients with Pick's disease, involving primarily the outer (I–III) cortical layers. Spongiform change (microvacuolation) is observed in affected regions, and Pick bodies and ballooned cells are absent. As many as 15% of patients with amyotrophic lateral sclerosis develop clinical symptoms consistent with FTD (Miller et al. 1994). These patients demonstrate combined frontotemporal and motor neuron degeneration at autopsy, and their disease represents a third category of FTD, the motor neuron disease type.

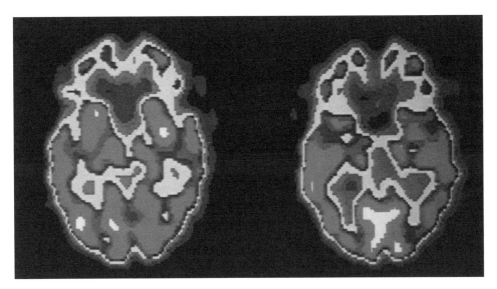

FIGURE 14–3. Transaxial single photon emission computed tomography (SPECT) of a patient with frontal lobe degeneration demonstrating decreased cerebral blood flow in the frontal lobes.

Red areas indicate normal blood flow, and yellow regions indicate diminished perfusion.

For a color version of this figure, please see the color insert at the back of this book.

TABLE 14–4. Features that distinguish Alzheimer's disease and frontotemporal dementia

Feature	Alzheimer's disease	Frontotemporal dementia
Clinical		
Personality changes	Disengagement	Disinhibition or apathy
Social skills	Late deterioration	Early deterioration
Klüver-Bucy syndrome	Late onset	Early onset
Memory deficits	Early onset	Late onset
Executive function	Spared early	Prominent early
Speech-language disturbances	Fluent aphasia	Stereotyped speech; terminal mutism
Anomia	Lexical anomia	Semantic anomia
Visuospatial disturbances	Early onset	Late onset
Neuroimaging studies		
CT and MRI	Generalized atrophy	Atrophy more prominent in frontotemporal regions
SPECT	Posterior temporal and parietal hypoperfusion	Anterior frontal and/or temporal hypoperfusion
PET	Parietal hypometabolism	Frontal and/or temporal hypometabolism

Note. MRI = magnetic resonance imaging; CT = computed tomography; SPECT = single photon emission computed tomography; PET = positron emission tomography.

Huntington's Disease

HD is a genetically transmitted, progressive, neurodegenerative disorder affecting primarily the striatum. It is a paradigmatic neuropsychiatric disorder exhibiting the triadic syndrome of dyskinesia, dementia, and behavioral abnormalities. An array of psychiatric disturbances such as depression, mania, psychosis, obsessive-compulsive disorders, aggression, irritability, apathy, and sexual disorders occur in HD (Rosenblatt and Leroi 2000).

HD is inherited in an autosomal dominant fashion with complete penetrance. The HD gene has been localized to the short arm of chromosome 4 (specifically at the IT15 gene locus); the mutation consists of an expanded and unstable CAG trinucleotide repeat (Huntington's Disease Collaborative Research Group 1993).

HD typically has its onset between ages 35 and 50, and average life expectancy after onset is 15 years (Cummings and Benson 1992; Folstein 1989). Although the peak period of onset is in the fourth and fifth decades of life, juvenile and late-onset forms also occur. Men and women are equally likely to have the disease. Death often occurs secondary to pneumonia, trauma, or suicide.

The most striking neurologic features of HD are abnormal involuntary choreiform movements, dysarthria, dystonia, and rigidity. These involuntary movements are a defining feature of HD and are characterized by irregular, arrhythmic, and purposeless movements of the face, limbs, and trunk that occur at rest or in concert with purposeful activity such as walking or eating. Parkinsonian features are common in patients with juvenile-onset HD (Folstein et al. 1990).

Cognitive and Neuropsychiatric Aspects

All HD patients develop progressive subcortical dementia with initial impairment in cognitive speed, mental flexibility, concentration, verbal learning, executive function, and memory (Cummings and Benson 1992). Neuropsychological testing reveals deficits in recent and remote memory, visuospatial function, set shifting, strategy, and planning. Language skills, including naming, comprehension, and repetition, are typically spared until late in the disease. Deficits in sustained attention are apparent early in the course of HD (Folstein et al. 1990), and impaired memory retrieval, characterized by poor spontaneous recall with preserved recognition of acquired information, is typical. The ability to synthesize information and produce flexible strategies for problem solving is markedly impaired in patients with HD, and patients consistently demonstrate deficits in the organization, planning, and sequencing of material necessary to perform complex tasks (Caine et al. 1978).

Psychiatric symptoms are ubiquitous and present in up to 80% of patients; they may herald the onset of the disorder. Personality changes occur before the onset of chorea in many cases, and depression, when present, antedates the movement disorder in approximately two-thirds of patients (Cummings 1995). Personality changes can occur early or even prodromally in the disease and are almost universal with its progression (Cummings 1995). Apathy and aggression are more prominent in HD than in AD (Burns et al. 1990).

Approximately one-third of patients with HD meet the criteria for major depression or dysthymic disorder, and many more exhibit intermittent dysphoria (Cummings 1995). When present, depression frequently antedates the onset of both chorea and dementia by several years. In addition, approximately 10% of patients with HD experience episodes of mania or hypomania characterized by mood elevation with concurrent symptoms of undue optimism, pressured speech, increased energy, grandiose ideation, or disturbed sleep.

The prevalence of mood disturbance among patients with HD is evidenced in the high frequency of suicide in this population. Suicide accounts for 5.7% of deaths in patients with HD, and up to 25% of HD patients attempt suicide at least once (Farrer 1986).

Anxiety disorders are present in 10%–15% of HD patients, and anxiety may be a prodromal psychiatric symptom. Obsessive-compulsive disorder may also be observed (Cummings and Cunningham 1992). In addition to mood disturbances and anxiety disorders, a schizophrenia-like psychosis characterized by auditory hallucinations and persecutory delusions can occur in patients with HD. Psychoses occur in approximately 10% of HD patients.

Laboratory Investigations and Neuroimaging

Results of routine serum, urine, and CSF studies are unremarkable in patients with HD. The electroencephalogram (EEG) reveals low voltage and poorly developed or absent alpha activity in symptomatic patients (Cummings and Benson 1992). Structural neuroimaging (CT or MRI) demonstrates atrophy of the caudate and putamen, most readily appreciated as enlargement of the frontal horns of the lateral ventricles (Figure 14–4). PET shows reduction in caudate glucose metabolism; SPECT demonstrates decreased caudate blood flow even before clear evidence of structural changes.

Neuropathology

The most striking pathology in patients with HD occurs in the basal ganglia. On gross inspection, atrophy of the caudate

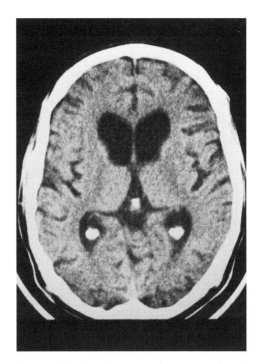

FIGURE 14–4. Computed tomography of a patient with Huntington's disease demonstrating marked atrophy of the caudate nucleus and putamen, evidenced by enlargement of the frontal horns of the lateral ventricles.

nucleus and, less dramatically, the putamen is visible. The globus pallidus may be affected (Folstein 1989). Microscopically, these structures reveal degenerative changes, with preferential loss of the small spiny neurons of the striatum accompanied by gliosis. Neurochemical alterations are numerous in patients with HD, but GABA and its synthesizing enzyme, glutamic acid decarboxylase, are markedly reduced in striatal regions. Acetylcholine transferase, cysteic acid decarboxylase, dopamine, and several neurokinins are reduced to a lesser extent (Cummings and Benson 1992).

Treatment

Pharmacologically the choreiform movements of HD are treated with antipsychotic medication, which reduces their severity. Conventional antipsychotics such as haloperidol or fluphenazine carry the risk of tardive dyskinesia with long-term treatment. No specific treatments exist for the cognitive disorders of HD. Sertraline and propranolol may curb aggression (Ranen et al. 1996; Stewart 1993). Major depression responds to serotonergic or tricyclic antidepressants. Carbamazepine is the preferred agent for the treatment of mania in patients with HD (Cummings 1995); lithium, valproic acid, and clonazepam can also be effective.

Parkinson's Disease

PD is a degenerative disorder of unknown etiology that affects mainly the pigmented brain stem nuclei and basal ganglia and produces a characteristic triad of bradykinesia, rigidity, and resting tremor. The prevalence of the disease is approximately 1 per 1,000. Onset generally occurs between the ages of 50 and 70 years, and the disease reaches its highest prevalence in the eighth decade (Martilla 1987). The disease is more common among men than women. The mean duration of the illness is 12.8 years, and a range of 2–30 years has been described (Hughes et al. 1992). Death results from a variety of causes, including aspiration pneumonia, urinary tract infection, and unrelated medical conditions.

Clinical Features

Bradykinesia, expressed as slowness in initiation and execution of movement, is a primary symptom of PD and accounts for many of its clinical manifestations. Decreased facial expression, prolonged response latencies, slowed gait with diminished arm swing, sialorrhea, hypophonic speech, and micrographia are all common bradykinetic features of PD.

Rigidity is present in the trunk and limb musculature, and superimposed tremor gives rise to cogwheel rigidity. The typical tremor of PD consists of alternating flexion and extension movements of the fingers and wrists that occur when the patient is alert but resting; the tremor disappears with action. Rigidity and tremor are often unilateral at the onset of the disease and can show asymmetry throughout its course. The clinical diagnostic criteria for PD are presented in Table 14–5.

Cognitive and Neuropsychiatric Aspects

Approximately 40% of patients with PD demonstrate overt dementia, and most exhibit more subtle neuropsychological deficits (Cummings and Benson 1992; Pirozzolo et al. 1982). The subcortical dementia of PD is characterized by memory impairment, visuospatial disturbances, executive dysfunction, and bradyphrenia. Spontaneous recall and skill acquisition (procedural memory) are impaired, whereas recognition memory is largely spared (Cummings and Benson 1992). Visuospatial deficits are apparent on both motor-dependent and motor-free tasks (Boller et al. 1984; Villardita et al. 1982), and disturbances of executive function, including poor concept formation, strategy formulation, and difficulties with set shifting, are consistently observed (Cummings 1988a).

Neuropsychiatric manifestations are common in patients with PD and can arise as an integral feature of the disorder or in association with antiparkinsonian treatment. Depression occurs in 40%–60% of PD patients (Cummings and Benson 1992).

Approximately 10%–20% of patients with PD meet the criteria for major depressive episodes; an additional 30%–40% have milder symptoms consistent with dysthymia (Cummings 1992).

TABLE 14–5. Clinical diagnostic criteria for Parkinson's disease

Step 1: Diagnosis of parkinsonian syndrome
  Bradykinesia and at least one of the
    following:
  Muscular rigidity
  4–6 Hz rest tremor
  Postural instability not caused by primary
    visual, vestibular, cerebellar, or
    proprioceptive dysfunction
**Step 2: Exclusion criteria for Parkinson's
disease**
  History of repeated strokes with stepwise
    progression of parkinsonian features
  History of repeated head injury
  History of definite encephalitis
  Oculogyric crisis
  Neuroleptic treatment at onset of
    symptoms
  More than one affected relative
  Sustained remission
  Strictly unilateral features after 3 years
  Supranuclear gaze palsy
  Cerebellar signs
  Early severe autonomic involvement
  Early severe dementia with disturbances
  Babinski's sign
  Presence of cerebral tumor or
    communicating hydrocephalus on
    neuroimaging
  Negative responses to large doses of
    levodopa
  1-Methyl-4-phenyl-1,2,3,6-
    tetrahydropyridine (MPTP) exposure
**Step 3: Supportive prospective criteria for
Parkinson's disease**[a]
  Unilateral onset
  Resting tremor present
  Progressive disorder
  Persistent asymmetry affecting side of
    onset most
  Excellent response (70%–100%) to
    levodopa
  Severe levodopa-induced chorea
  Levodopa response for 5 years or more
  Clinical course of 10 years or more

[a]Three or more of these criteria are required for the diagnosis of definite Parkinson's disease.
Source. Adapted from Hughes et al. 1992.

Patients with PD evidence dysphoria, pessimism about the future, sadness, irritability, and suicidal ideation, and only limited endorsement of guilt, self-blame, or feelings of failure (R.G.Brown et al. 1988). Other distinctive features of the depression seen in PD patients include high rates of associated anxiety, a low incidence of psychotic symptomatology, and low rates of completed suicide despite frequent suicidal ideation (Cummings 1992).

Anxiety disorders occur in patients with PD. Stein et al. (1990) reported generalized anxiety disorders in 38% of PD patients studied. Panic disorder, obsessive-compulsive disorder, and discrete phobias also have been observed in patients with PD.

Drug-Associated Psychiatric Disorders

Neuropharmacologic agents, including anticholinergic drugs, amantadine, levodopa, selegiline, catechol-O-methyltransferase inhibitors, and dopamine receptor agonists, used in the treatment of PD directly affect central neurotransmitter function, and their administration can precipitate adverse behavioral side effects. Behavioral complications of antiparkinsonian therapy include hallucinations, delusions, attentional impairment, mood disorders, anxiety, and alterations in sexual behavior.

Hallucinations

Visual hallucinations are the most common neuropsychiatric side effects associated with PD treatment. Approximately 30% of treated patients experience visual hallucinations, whereas other types of hallucinations (auditory or tactile) are comparatively rare (Cummings 1991). Visual hallucinations can be induced by any antiparkinsonian agent and typically occur at night, may be preceded by sleep disturbances, and usually consist of fully formed visions of human or animal figures (Mosko-vitz et al. 1978; Shaw et al. 1980). Dementia, older age, a history of multiple drug therapy, longer duration of treatment, and the use of anticholinergic medications have all been found to be risk factors for visual hallucinosis (Tanner et al. 1983).

Delusions

Delusions are notably rare in patients with untreated PD and usually indicate an adverse response to treatment. Like hallucinations, delusions can occur with all types of antiparkinsonian therapy. The frequency of delusions is 3%–17% (Cummings 1991). Delusions can be antedated by vivid dreams or visual hallucinations and are typically persecutory in content (Cummings 1991). Older patients and those with preexisting dementia syndromes are at increased risk for the development of delusions.

Management of delusions should begin with discontinuation of anticholinergic agents, selegiline, and amantadine. This should be followed by reductions in levodopa and other dopaminergic agents. Persistent delusional syndromes can require the administration of antipsychotic agents. Clozapine, an atypical antipsychotic that produces few extrapyramidal side effects, has been shown to be effective in the treatment of delusions in PD patients (Friedman and Lannon 1989; Roberts et al. 1989) and appears to be well tolerated in low doses (12.5–75 mg) (Factor et al. 1994). Clozapine may cause bone marrow suppression, and weekly hematologic monitoring is required. Quetiapine may be an effective alternative to clozapine.

Alterations in Mood

Dopaminergic agents have been associated with mood elevation in some patients. Behavioral manifestations range from a feeling of unusual well-being to fully developed manic episodes with elation, grandiosity, pressured speech, diminished need for sleep, and increased libido. These symptoms typically subside with dose reduction.

Anxiety

Levodopa therapy can initiate the onset of anxiety in patients not previously predisposed to this disorder. Symptoms include apprehension, irritability, nervousness, palpitations, hyperventilation, and insomnia. In addition, levodopa can exacerbate anxiety in PD patients with a history of prior symptomatology. These symptoms usually improve with dose adjustments, although anxiolytic agents might be required in some cases.

Altered Sexual Behavior

PD patients may experience a renewal of sexual interest and potency in conjunction with antiparkinsonian therapy. This leads to the return of normal sexual activity in many individuals. In rare cases, however, increased libido reaches pathologic proportions with hypersexuality. Hypersexuality is reported more often in men than in women, and levodopa is the most common causative agent (Cummings 1991; Koller and Megaffin 1994). Paraphilic behavior has occasionally been reported in conjunction with dopaminergic therapy. Treatment involves reduction of drug dose.

Laboratory Investigations and Neuroimaging

PD is a clinical diagnosis, and routine laboratory studies are uninformative. CT scans are normal or show findings consistent with cortical atrophy, and MRI has demonstrated reductions in the size of the substantia nigra in advanced cases of PD (Duguid et al. 1986). FDG-PET investigations reveal posteriorly predominant reductions in cerebral glucose metabolism (Cummings and Benson 1992), and PET studies with fluorodopa reveal markedly diminished uptake in the striatum (Leenders et al. 1986).

Neuropathology

Loss of pigmented cells in the substantia nigra and other pigmented nuclei (locus coeruleus, dorsal motor nucleus of the vagus) is the most consistently observed finding in patients with PD. Prominent depigmentation of the substantia nigra is grossly apparent, and microscopic inspection reveals reactive gliosis in the areas of cell loss (Cummings and Benson 1992). The remaining neurons of the involved nuclei contain distinctive eosinophilic cytoplasmic inclusions called Lewy bodies. On microscopic examination, Lewy bodies appear as round intracellular hyaline bodies with a pale peripheral halo and have been observed in the nucleus basalis of Meynert and in the hypothalamus of patients with PD as well as in the substantia nigra (Cummings and Benson 1992; Whitehouse et al. 1983). Alpha-synuclein is the main protein found in Lewy bodies. Lewy body formation is common in cortical regions in patients manifesting dementia syndromes.

Neurochemical analysis of the basal ganglia reveals that the dopamine content of this region is markedly diminished. Norepinephrine, GABA, and serotonin and its metabolite 5-hydroxyindoleacetic acid also are decreased in PD patients, although these reductions are less severe (Cummings and Benson 1992). Atrophy of the nucleus basalis and concomitant reduction in cortical choline acetyltransferase is present in some patients with PD, particularly those with dementia (Whitehouse et al. 1983; Wikkelso et al. 1982).

Treatment

The movement disorder of PD responds to levodopa or dopamine agonists (Cum-mings and Benson 1992). Unfortunately, the benefits of levodopa therapy last only 5–10 years, and disabling symptoms (progressive rigidity, tremor, and bradykinesia) eventually reemerge (Dogali et al. 1995). Selegiline can slow the progression of the disorder and thus can defer the need for dopaminergic therapy (Cummings and Benson 1992). Amantadine and dopamine receptor agonists (bromocriptine, pergolide, pramipexole, ropinirole) are useful adjuncts in the therapy of PD and form the mainstay of treatment in patients who are unable to tolerate levodopa. Dopamine agonists may be used as initial therapy and are less likely to be associated with adverse long-term motor consequences. The affinity of pramipexole and ropinirole for the D_3 receptor subtype can allow those agents to treat motor as well as psychiatric symptoms, particularly depression (Bennet and Piercey 1999; Hall et al. 1996; Parkinson's Study Group 1997). In patients whose condition is refractory to medical therapy, surgical procedures such as stereotactic ventral pallidotomy or deep brain stimulation can significantly reduce parkinsonian symptoms (Dogali et al. 1995).

Progressive Supranuclear Palsy

PSP is an idiopathic neurodegenerative disorder that affects the brain stem and basal ganglia and is characterized by supranuclear gaze paresis, pseudobulbar palsy, axial rigidity, and dementia. Onset usually occurs in the sixth or seventh decade, and the average course from onset to death is 5–10 years. The disease is sporadic and affects men more commonly than women (Steele 1972; Steele et al. 1964). Its prevalence is estimated to be 1.4 per 100,000 population.

Movement Disorder

The characteristic motor features of PSP include bradykinesia, axial rigidity, pseudobulbar palsy, and supranuclear gaze paresis. Rigidity affects truncal and neck tone more than limb tone, resulting in axial dystonia with nuchal rigidity as the disease progresses. The posture is typically one of extension (contrasting with the flexed posture of PD). Pseudobulbar palsy is manifested by dysphagia, sialorrhea, and dysarthria. Supranuclear ophthalmoplegia is the hallmark of the disorder and presents with marked restrictions in volitional gaze that are more prominent in the vertical than the horizontal plane. The clinical criteria for PSP are presented in Table 14–6.

Cognitive and Neuropsychiatric Features

The cognitive alterations in patients with PSP are similar to those seen in patients with other extrapyramidal syndromes and include slowing of thought processes, difficulties with set shifting and abstraction, memory retrieval disturbances, and personality alterations. Disorders reflecting primary cortical involvement, such as agnosia, apraxia, and aphasia, are typically absent in patients with PSP (Albert et al. 1974). PSP patients are impaired on tasks measuring frontal lobe function (Litvan et al. 1996).

Personality and mood disturbances occur in patients with PSP. The most commonly reported disturbances are apathy, emotional indifference, and depression. Irritability, disinhibition, inappropriate crying or laughing, and episodic outbursts of rage can emerge (Albert et al. 1974). PSP has been associated with obsessive-compulsive behaviors (Destee et al. 1990).

Laboratory Investigations and Neuroimaging

Results of blood, serum, urine, and CSF studies are all within normal limits in patients with PSP. CT and MRI reveal diminished midbrain size; cortical atrophy involving the frontotemporal regions may be seen (Lees 1990). PET studies of glucose metabolism reveal marked metabolic reductions in the frontal lobes (Foster et al. 1988), and SPECT reveals bilateral frontal lobe hypoperfusion (Lees 1990). Fluorodopa PET demonstrates diminished striatal dopamine formation and storage (Leenders et al. 1988).

Neuropathology

Postmortem examinations of patients with PSP disclose cell loss, gliosis, and NFTs involving primarily the structures of

TABLE 14–6. Clinical diagnostic criteria for progressive supranuclear palsy (PSP)

Essential for diagnosis
  Onset after age 40
  Progressive course
  Bilateral supranuclear disorder of ocular
    motility
  Rigidity with axial predominance
  Bradykinesia
Confirmatory manifestations
  Poor or absent response to levodopa
    therapy
  Severe bradyphrenia with frontal lobe
    features (e.g., grasping, perseveration,
    utilization behavior)
  Axial dystonia with cervical
    hyperextension
  Onset with gait impairment, frequent
    falls, and postural instability
  Dysarthria with dysphagia
  Ocular fixation instability
  Apraxia of eyelid opening and/or closing;
    infrequency of eye blink
Features inconsistent with diagnosis of PSP
  Early or prominent cerebellar signs
  Unexplained polyneuropathy
  Aphasia or agnosia
  Sensory deficits
  Seizures

Source. Adapted from Duvoisin 1992.

the mesencephalic-diencephalic junction. The NFTs in patients with PSP are composed of straight filaments, unlike the twisted filaments seen in AD patients (Cummings and Benson 1992). The structures maximally affected are the subthalamic nucleus, globus pallidus, red nucleus, substantia nigra, superior colliculi, dentate nuclei, and the nuclei of cranial nerves IV, VI, and VIII. The thalamus and hypothalamus are minimally affected, and the cerebral cortex is relatively spared (Steele 1972). Neurochemical alterations include marked nigrostriatal dopamine deficiency with less pronounced cholinergic system impairment. Cortical nicotinic cholinergic receptors and subcortical dopamine, subtype 2 (D_2), receptors are reduced (Cummings and Benson 1992).

Treatment

PSP has no cure; supportive therapy is critical in this relentlessly progressive disease. Contact with patient and family support groups should be recommended. Dopaminergic medication is generally not useful, although a few patients respond at least transiently. Tricyclic antidepressants may be of some benefit in improving depressive symptoms in patients with PSP (Kvale 1982; Newman 1985), and violent outbursts have been treated effectively with serotonergic agents (Schneider et al. 1989).

Wilson's Disease (Hepatolenticular Degeneration)

WD, also called hepatolenticular degeneration, is an autosomal recessive disorder of copper metabolism leading to abnormal deposition of copper, primarily in the basal ganglia of the brain, liver, and cor-

nea. WD was first described by Westphal in 1883 and later by Wilson in 1912. The gene for WD has been localized to chromosome 13, and the disorder occurs with an estimated frequency of 1 in 40,000 births (Akil and Brewer 1995). The worldwide incidence of WD approximates 12–30 per million, with higher prevalences reported in Japan. Age at onset ranges from 5 to 35, with mean age 17; onset and initial manifestations vary among families. Males and females are affected with equal frequency. Neurologic and psychiatric symptoms are the most prominent features of WD, however, liver disease can be the presenting manifestation. The presenting features of WD can be divided approximately into thirds, with one-third each evidencing predominantly with hepatic, neurologic, or psychiatric symptomatology.

Clinical Features

The neurologic manifestations of WD include tremor, rigidity, dystonia, poor coordination, and abnormalities of gait and posture. Dysarthria, dysphagia, and hypophonia may be present. Chronic hepatitis and hemolytic anemia may be detected on laboratory assessment, and slit-lamp examination reveals the presence of corneal copper deposits (Kayser-Fleischer rings) in most patients with neurologic disturbances (Akil and Brewer 1995). CT reveals ventricular enlargement, and MRI demonstrates increased signal on T2-weighted images as a result of copper deposition in the lenticular, caudate, thalamic, and dentate nuclei (Hier and Cummings 1990). The diagnosis of WD is confirmed by decreased blood ceruloplasmin level (<20 mg/dL), increased 24-hour urine copper excretion (>100 mg), or the presence of excessive hepatic copper in needle biopsy tissue (Akil and Brewer 1995).

Patients with WD demonstrate mild

impairment in memory retrieval and executive functions (abstraction and set shifting). Psychiatric disturbances can be prominent and precede other manifestations of the disorder in 20% of patients (Akil and Brewer 1995). Common personality alterations include increased irritability, impulsivity, and lability. Aggressive, reckless, disinhibited, and criminal behavior may be observed (Dening and Berrios 1989). Depression is reported in 20%–30% of patients, and other mood disorders, such as hypomania or overt mania, can occur. Rarely, a schizophrenia-like psychosis can occur (Akil and Brewer 1995). Psychiatric manifestations correlate with the presence of neurologic symptoms (dystonic and bulbar disorders) rather than with hepatic dysfunction (Dening and Berrios 1989).

Neuropathology

The major pathologic finding in patients with WD is cavitary necrosis of the putamen. Atrophy of the brain stem and dentate nuclei of the cerebellum also may be marked. Histologic findings include neuronal loss, liquefaction, reactive gliosis, and the presence of Opalski cells (large oval cells with a finely granular cytoplasm) in affected regions (Cummings and Benson 1992).

Treatment

Early treatment with penicillamine, a copper-chelating agent, and maintenance of a copper-deficient diet can lead to significant improvement in both the neurologic and neuropsychiatric manifestations of WD (Akil and Brewer 1995; Hier and Cummings 1990). However, penicillamine therapy can lead to further neurologic disability, seizures, movement disorders, and psychosis in some cases. These reactions can be irreversible and can occur in previously asymptomatic

patients (Glass et al. 1990; McDonald and Lake 1995).

Tetrathiomolybdate has received support for the initial treatment of WD and has been suggested as first-line treatment; exacerbations generally did not occur but more data are needed (Brewer and Cummings 1995). Dramatic improvements as evidenced by neurologic examination and near complete T2 signal resolution in putamen, thalamus, and brain stem were demonstrated in patients undergoing zinc treatment, though neurologic exacerbations are possible with this agent (Heckmann et al. 1994; Lang et al. 1993).

Corticobasal Degeneration

CBD is a rare neurodegenerative disorder characterized by parkinsonism, supranuclear gaze palsy, "alien hand" phenomenon, myoclonus, and dementia. Aphasia, apraxia, and marked visuospatial deficits are common in patients with this condition. Impaired recall, acalculia, right-left disorientation, attentional deficits, and personality alterations also have been reported (Cohen and Freedman 1995). Neuropsychiatric syndromes include depression, frontal lobe–type behavioral abnormalities, and obsessive-compulsive behaviors (Cummings and Litvan 2000). Pathologically, neuronal loss and gliosis are seen in the substantia nigra, and round, faintly fibrillar, inclusion bodies are apparent in the remaining pigmented cells. Focal cortical degeneration is seen in the frontal and parietal lobes bilaterally and can be associated with sparse Pick cell formation. Subcortical white-matter gliosis exists in proportion to the degree of overlying cortical cell loss (Gibb 1992). Table 14–7 summarizes the diagnostic criteria for CBD.

TABLE 14–7. Diagnostic criteria for corticobasal degeneration (CBD)

Inclusion criteria
> Rigidity plus one cortical sign (apraxia, cortical sensory loss, or alien limb phenomenon); or
> Asymmetric rigidity, dystonia, and focal reflex myoclonus

Qualifications of clinical features
> Rigidity: easily detectable without reinforcement
> Apraxia: more than simple use of limb as object; clear absence of cognitive or motor deficit sufficient to explain disturbance
> Cortical sensory loss: preserved primary sensation; asymmetrical
> Alien limb phenomenon: more than simple levitation
> Dystonia: focal in limb; present at rest at onset
> Myoclonus: reflex myoclonus spreads beyond stimulated digits

Exclusion criteria
> Early dementia (this will exclude some patients who have CBD but whose illness cannot be clinically distinguished from other primary dementing diseases)
> Early vertical gaze palsy
> Rest tremor
> Severe autonomic disturbances
> Sustained responsiveness to levodopa
> Lesions on imaging studies indicating another pathologic process is responsible

Multiple System Atrophies

The multiple system atrophies (MSAs) are a diverse group of disorders with pathology that demonstrates various degrees of combined striatonigral and olivopontocerebellar degeneration. The four domains of clinical features are autonomic failure/urinary dysfunction, parkinsonism, cerebellar ataxia, and corticospinal dysfunction. The diagnosis of possible MSA requires one criterion plus features from two other domains (Table 14–8). The diagnosis of probable MSA requires the criterion for autonomic failure/urinary dysfunction plus either a) parkinsonism with a poor response to levodopa or b) cerebellar ataxia. The diagnosis of definite MSA is a postmortem diagnosis (Table 14–8) (Gilman et al. 1999). The disease affects both genders, usually starting in middle age with a median survival of 9.3 years from time of first symptoms (Wenning et al. 1994). These disorders can present with a wide array of neurologic disturbances, including ataxia, limb incoordination, parkinsonism, dysautonomia, choreoathetosis, and hyperreflexia. Dementia with prominent frontal deficits occurs in some but not all cases of MSA (Cohen and Freedman 1995), and neuropsychiatric manifestations, including mood lability, depression, and a schizophrenia-like psychosis have been reported (Cohen and Freedman 1995; Cummings and Benson 1992). The parkinsonian features usually respond poorly to levodopa, but therapy should be tried because up to 30% of patients improve at least transiently.

Vascular Dementia

VaD is a dementing condition produced by ischemic or hemorrhagic brain injury. In its classic form, it is characterized by an abrupt onset, stepwise deterioration, a patchy pattern of intellectual deficits, focal neurologic symptoms (transient ischemic attacks), focal neurologic signs, a history of hypertension, and evidence of associated cardiovascular disease (American Psychiatric Association 2000; Hachinski et al. 1975). Most cases of VaD are produced by hypertensive cerebrovascular disease and thrombo-occlusive disease, but the condition can also occur with mul-

TABLE 14–8.   Diagnostic categories of multiple system atrophy (MSA)

Possible MSA

One criterion plus two factors (one each) from two other domains. When the criterion is parkinsonism, a poor levodopa response qualifies as one feature (one additional feature required).

Criterion for autonomic features of urinary dysfunction: orthostatic fall in blood pressure (by 30 mm Hg systolic or 15 mm Hg diastolic) or urinary incontinence.

Criterion for parkinsonism: bradykinesia plus one of rigidity, postural instability, tremor.

Criterion for cerebellar dysfunction: gait ataxia plus one of ataxia dysarthria, limb ataxia, sustained gaze-evoked nystagmus.

Probable MSA

Criterion for autonomic failure/urinary dysfunction plus either a) parkinsonism poorly responsive to levodopa or b) cerebellar dysfunction.

Definite MSA

Pathologically confirmed by the presence of a high density of glial cytoplasmic inclusions in association with a combination of degenerative changes in the nigrostriatal and olivopontocerebellar pathways.

tiple cerebral emboli, systemic hypotension, intracerebral hemorrhage, and inflammatory and infectious vascular disease (Cummings and Benson 1992; Roman et al. 1993). Symptoms generally appear when a certain volume of infarcted tissue is present or if small strokes are strategically placed. Deep white matter ischemia and subcortical lacunar infarcts are common in VaD.

VaD is most common after the age of 50 and affects men more often than it affects women. Patients commonly survive for 6–8 years after onset, and death usually results from cardiovascular disease or stroke.

Clinical Diagnosis

The National Institute for Neurologic Disorders and Stroke–Association Internationale pour la Recherche et l'Enseignement en Neurosciences (NINDS-AIREN) criteria for the diagnosis of definite, probable, and possible VaD are presented in Table 14–9 (Roman et al. 1993). The diagnosis of *definite VaD* requires that the patient meet the clinical criteria for probable VaD and that there be histologic confirmation of ischemic brain injury obtained at autopsy.

The diagnosis of *probable VaD* requires the presence of dementia, evidence of cerebrovascular disease, and a relationship between the onset or course of the dementia and the cerebrovascular disease. Cerebrovascular disease is established by focal neurologic signs consistent with stroke (e.g., hemiparesis, sensory deficit, Babinski's sign) and neuroimaging (CT or MRI) evidence of vascular lesions. A relationship between dementia and cerebrovascular disease must be demonstrated by at least one of the following: 1) onset of dementia within 3 months after a known stroke, 2) abrupt deterioration in cognitive ability, or 3) fluctuation in or stepwise progression of cognitive impairment.

Possible VaD is diagnosed in the presence of dementia and neurologic signs when neuroimaging confirmation of cerebrovascular disease is lacking; when the temporal relationship between dementia and stroke is unclear; or when there are variations in the onset, course, or presentation of cognitive deficits despite evidence of relevant cerebrovascular disease.

On examination, patients with VaD exhibit a combination of motor abnormalities, neuropsychological deficits, and neuropsychiatric symptoms. Motor find-

TABLE 14–9. Diagnostic criteria for definite, probable, and possible vascular dementia (VaD)

Definite VaD

    Clinical criteria for probable VaD

    Autopsy demonstration of appropriate ischemic brain injury and no other cause of dementia

Probable VaD

  Dementia

      Decline from a previous higher level of cognitive functioning

      Impairment of two or more cognitive domains

      Deficits severe enough to interfere with activities of daily living and not due to physical effects of stroke alone

      Absence of delirium; absence of psychosis, aphasia, or sensorimotor impairment that precludes neuropsychological testing; and absence of any other disorder capable of producing a dementia syndrome

  Cerebrovascular disease

      Focal neurologic signs consistent with stroke

      Neuroimaging evidence of extensive vascular lesions

  Relationship between dementia and cerebrovascular disease, as evidenced by one or more of the following:

      Onset of dementia within 3 months of a recognized stroke

      Abrupt deterioration or fluctuating or stepwise progression of the cognitive deficit

Supporting features

  Subtle onset and variable course of cognitive deficits

  Early presence of gait disturbance

  History of unsteadiness, frequent and unprovoked falls

  Early urinary frequency, urgency, and other urinary symptoms not explained by urologic disease

  Pseudobulbar palsy

  Personality and mood changes, abulia, depression, emotional incontinence, and subcortical deficits, including psychomotor retardation and abnormal executive function

Possible VaD

  Dementia with focal neurologic signs but without neuroimaging confirmation of definite cerebrovascular disease

  Dementia with focal signs but without a clear temporal relationship between dementia and stroke

  Dementia and focal signs but with subtle onset and variable course of cognitive deficits

Source. Adapted from Roman et al. 1993.

ings may include weakness, spasticity, hyperreflexia, extensor plantar responses, bradykinesia, parkinsonism, and pseudobulbar palsy (Ishii et al. 1986). Gait abnormalities are common and can appear early in the course of the disorder.

The pattern of neuropsychological abnormalities in patients with VaD is characterized by "patchiness," with pres-ervation of some abilities and mild to severe compromise of others. Slowing of cognitive function and impairment of executive function are common elements of the dementia syndrome.

Neuropsychiatric Aspects

Neuropsychiatric abnormalities are common in patients with VaD: personality changes, depression, lability of mood, and delusions occur regularly. Personality changes are the most common neuropsychiatric alterations in patients with VaD. Apathy, abulia, and aspontaneity dominate the clinical syndrome; interpersonal relatedness and affect, however, are more preserved in patients with VaD than in those with AD (Dian et al. 1990; Ishii et al. 1986).

Major depressive disorders occur in 25%–50% of patients with VaD, and up to 60% show symptoms of a depressive syndrome (Cummings 1988b; Cummings et al. 1987; Erkinjuntti 1987). Sadness, anxiety, psychomotor retardation, and somatic complaints are the most commonly reported depressive symptoms. Little relationship exists between the severity of depression and the degree of dementia (Cummings et al. 1987). Lability of mood and affect are common in patients with VaD.

Psychosis with delusional ideation occurs in approximately 50% of VaD patients (Cummings et al. 1987).

Laboratory Investigations

Serum studies of VaD patients should routinely include complete blood count, erythrocyte sedimentation rate, and serum cholesterol and triglyceride levels. In young patients or those without risk factors for stroke, the potential etiologic contribution of inflammatory vasculitis should be investigated. These circumstances require more extensive laboratory studies, including antinuclear antibodies, antiphospholipid antibodies, and lupus anticoagulant levels (Briley et al. 1989; Cummings and Benson 1992; Young et al. 1989).

Neuroimaging studies provide support for the clinical diagnosis of VaD. CT can reveal cortical infarctions or evidence of periventricular ischemic changes (Aharon-Peretz et al. 1988; Erkinjuntti 1987; Loeb

and Gandolfo 1983). MRI is more revealing than is CT and demonstrates small subcortical infarctions and ischemic white-matter changes that are invisible on CT (J.J. Brown et al. 1988; Hershey et al. 1987). MRI is the technique of choice for the identification of structural changes in VaD (Figure 14–5). FDG-PET and SPECT show multiple irregular areas of hypometabolism or hypoperfusion that are consistent with focal regions of tissue infarction (Benson et al. 1983; Gemmell et al. 1987).

Classification and Neuropathology

Several subtypes of VaD, based on the mechanism of cerebrovascular injury and size of the affected vessel, have been described (Roman et al. 1993) (Table 14–10). Multi-infarct dementia results from the cumulative effect of multiple large- and small-vessel occlusions. Both cortical and subcortical regions can be affected, and infarction can result from atherosclerotic or arteriosclerotic disease or cardiac embolization.

Strategically placed, solitary infarcts can result in well-defined dementia syndromes (Roman et al. 1993). Small lesions involving the left angular gyrus or medial thalamic nuclei can disrupt multiple cognitive faculties and result in the abrupt onset of dementia. These lesions can be a product of atherosclerotic disease, cardiac embolization, or sustained hypertension with hyaline necrosis of arterioles.

Subcortical small-vessel disease can result in dementia. Sustained hypertension leads to fibrinoid necrosis of small arteries and arterioles. These vessels supply the deep gray-matter nuclei, including the striatum and thalamus, as well as the hemispheric white matter. Multiple small lacunar infarctions of the basal ganglia and thalamus produce the syndrome of lacunar state. Binswanger's disease is a use of ChE-Is. Nonaspirin antiaggregants are appropriate alternatives in patients who are resistant to or intolerant of aspirin's effects. In rare circumstances, the use of anticoagulants or steroids might be warranted. Administration of baclofen can assist with spasticity in the poststroke patient. Supportive measures such as gait retraining, prophylaxis against limb contractures, and speech therapy are indicated in selected patients. Pseudobulbar affect has been successfully treated with nortriptyline and selective serotonin reuptake inhibitors, and patients with depression or psychosis typically respond to antidepressant or antipsychotic therapy (Starkstein and Robinson 1994). ChE-Is improve cognition temporarily and may reduce the rate of loss of function and improve behavior (Erkinjuntti et al. 2002).

Hydrocephalic Dementia

Hydrocephalus refers to enlargement of the cerebral ventricles with an increased amount of intraventricular CSF. Ventricular enlargement can be on an *ex vacuo* basis (from loss of cerebral tissue) or as a result of interruption of CSF flow (obstructive hydrocephalus).

The two types of obstructive hydrocephalus are noncommunicating and communicating. Noncommunicating hydrocephalus arises from obstruction of CSF flow within the ventricular system or between the ventricles and the subarachnoid space. Communicating hydrocephalus occurs with obstruction of CSF flow within the subarachnoid space, preventing absorption of the CSF into the superior sagittal sinus. Noncommunicating hydrocephalus is usually an acute process accompanied by headache, confusion, and ophthalmoplegia; intracranial pressure is typically elevated. Communicating hydrocephalus presents as

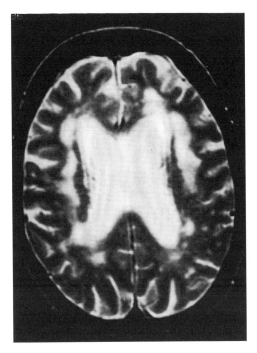

FIGURE 14–5. T2-weighted magnetic resonance imaging (MRI) scan of a patient with vascular dementia

Notice irregular periventricular lesions and confluent high signal areas in the hemispheric white matter, consistent with ischemic cerebral injury.

syndrome characterized by extensive ischemic injury of white matter.

Reduced cerebral perfusion as a result of cardiac arrest, loss of blood volume, or profound hypotension can lead to border zone infarction. Border zone regions (or "watershed areas") lie between the territories served by the three principal intracranial vessels and are thus particularly vulnerable to ischemic insult.

Mixed AD and cerebrovascular disease is commonly found at autopsy in VaD patients.

Treatment

Treatment of VaD consists of control of blood pressure in the upper normal range, administration of aspirin or other platelet antiaggregants (Meyer et al. 1986), and

TABLE 14–10. Subtypes of ischemic vascular dementia

Syndrome	Specific vessels	Common etiologies	Anatomic region of involvement
Multi-infarct	Large and small arteries	Atherosclerosis, hypertension	Cortical and subcortical regions
Strategic single infarct	Major intracranial arteries and branches, arterioles of the thalamus and caudate	Atherosclerosis, cardiac emboli, hypertension	Small, localized ischemic damage in functionally important regions (e.g., angular gyrus, caudate, medial nuclei of the thalamus)
Small-vessel disease (lacunar state and Binswanger's disease)	Arterioles of the deep gray nuclei, arterioles of white matter	Hypertension	Basal ganglia, periventricular white matter
Hypoperfusion (border zone infarction)	Distal segments of the major intracranial arteries	Cardiac arrest, hypotension, loss of blood volume	Border zone ischemia involving frontal and/or parietal regions, including periventricular white matter

a dementia syndrome with normal intracranial pressure, hence the alternate name "normal-pressure hydrocephalus" (NPH). NPH accounts for approximately 2%–5% of dementia syndromes in adults (Cummings and Benson 1992).

Clinical and Neuropsychiatric Features

The classic syndrome of NPH consists of dementia, gait disturbance, and incontinence. The dementia of NPH has prominent features of frontal-subcortical dysfunction, including impaired attention and mental control, poor learning, visuospatial disturbances, and impaired abstraction and judgment (Cummings and Benson 1992; Gustafson and Hagberg 1978; Thomsen et al. 1986). Aphasia, apraxia, and agnosia are absent or mild. The gait abnormalities of NPH are variable but commonly include shortened stride, diminished step height, and slow speed (Sudarsky and Simon 1987). Urinary incontinence is more common than loss of bowel control.

A variety of neuropsychiatric syndromes have been described in patients with NPH, including personality alterations, anxiety, mood changes, and (rarely) psychosis. Apathy, inertia, and indifference are the typical personality alterations; aggressive outbursts have also been reported (Crowell et al. 1973; Gustafson and Hagberg 1978). A wide range of mood disturbances have been described in patients with NPH. Patients may manifest euphoria, mania, or depression (Gustafson and Hagberg 1978; Kwentus and Hart 1987).

Etiologies

NPH results from obstruction of CSF flow over the cerebral convexities and impaired absorption of fluid into the superior sagittal sinus (Cummings and Benson 1992). Classic NPH follows subarachnoid hemorrhage, head trauma, encephalitis, or meningitis. Less common causes include carcinomatous meningitis and partial aqueductal stenosis. Many cases have no identified etiology.

Diagnosis

Although the syndrome's classic triad of ataxia, dementia, and urinary incontinence is a hallmark of NPH, the diagnosis remains a challenge. Many patients with gait disorder, bladder dysfunction, and mental deterioration have other diseases; many have subcortical arteriosclerotic encephalopathy or VaD (Gallassi et al. 1991). Many patients do not display the classic symptoms, and MRI is often equivocal.

The diagnosis of NPH depends on a combination of neuroimaging, CSF flow, and CSF pressure observations. CT studies reveal markedly enlarged ventricles and periventricular lucencies. Ventriculomegaly is most evident anteriorly, with enlarged frontal and temporal horns. MRI demonstrates the same pattern of ventricular enlargement, increased periventricular signal on T2-weighted images, and an aqueductal flow void (Cummings and Benson 1992). Routine lumbar puncture reveals normal CSF pressure, and 24-hour pressure monitoring demonstrates increased B waves (Graff-Radford et al. 1989). Cisternography provides a means of assessing the pattern of CSF flow. After injection of radionuclide tracer into the lumbar subarachnoid space, there is reflux into the enlarged ventricular system and an absence of expected flow over the convexities to the superior sagittal sinus. Isotope cisternography has limited utility in predicting shunt responsiveness (Larsson et al. 1994).

Treatment

NPH is treated with ventriculoperitoneal shunting and diversion of CSF from the ventricles into the peritoneum. Lumboperitoneal shunts, diverting CSF from the lumbar subarachnoid space into the peritoneum, also can be employed. The mean rate of improvement is 30%–50% in idiopathic and 50%–70% in secondary NPH.

Subacute Spongiform Encephalopathies

The human subacute spongiform encephalopathies (SSEs) are divided into sporadic CJD, acquired SSE (kuru, iatrogenic CJD, new variant CJD [nvCJD]), and familial SSEs. Most cases of SSE are sporadic, but about 10% have an inherited mode of transmission of the autosomal dominant type. These are familial CJD, Gerstmann-Straussler-Scheinker disease (GSS), and fatal familial insomnia (FFI) (Weihl and Roos 1999). The term *prion* was coined in 1982 by Prusiner and colleagues, who showed that the cause of scrapie was not a virus but a novel proteinaceous infectious agent (Prusiner 1982). The hallmark of all prion diseases is the aberrant metabolism of the prion protein (PrP).

Creutzfeldt-Jakob Disease

CJD is the most common SSE in humans, with an incidence of 1 per million worldwide. Usually the affected persons are 50–70 years of age, although cases in teenagers and in those older than 80 years have been reported (Ironside 1996).

Often there is a prodrome with nonspecific complaints of asthenia, anxiety, sleep disturbance, decreased appetite, and weight loss. Cognitive or other neurologic dysfunction (such as cerebellar ataxia, pyramidal or extrapyramidal signs, and visual impairment) is common, as are behavioral abnormalities. Most patients develop myoclonic jerks. The EEG typi-cally shows periodic or pseudoperiodic paroxysms of sharp waves or spikes against background slowing. Neuroimaging, CT or T2-weighted MRI, is useful primarily to exclude other disorders. Increased signal on the T2-weighted image is common in the basal ganglia. Spinal fluid is normal except for mild protein and neuron-specific enolase elevation caused by neuronal loss. Protein 14–3–3, if present, supports the diagnosis (Hsich et al. 1996). The average duration of illness is limited to 4–5 months. On autopsy the brain contains numerous amyloid plaques as well as spongiform changes (Josephson 1998).

nvCJD represents the communication to humans of bovine spongiform encephalopathy (BSE) in the United Kingdom and some other European countries. The average age at onset for nvCJD is 29 years. Illness is of longer duration (9–38 months) than classic CJD, and behavioral changes are prominent, often prompting psychiatric consultation. Ataxia follows psychiatric changes and, unlike CJD, typical electroencephalographic abnormalities are often absent. MRI can show increased signal in the pulvinar on T2-weighted images (Will et al. 2000). Cases of nvCJD have a distinctive neuropathological profile. Findings include large PrP immunoreactive amyloid plaques with eosinophilic cores and a pale periphery surrounded by spongiform change, known as florid plaques. These features were present in addition to the typical spongiform changes, astrogliosis, and neuronal loss in the basal ganglia and thalamus, typical of classic CJD (Will et al. 1996, 2000).

Treatment

SSEs are fatal diseases for which there is no current treatment. CJD patients can be treated symptomatically by addressing target symptoms such as extrapyramidal signs and epileptiform discharges.

Evaluation of Neuropsychiatric Alterations in Patients With Dementia

Evaluation of the patient with dementia should include a careful history, mental status testing, and general physical and neurologic examination. An assessment of past and current neuropsychiatric alterations (e.g., personality changes, anxiety, depression, mania, psychosis, and hallucinations) should be included (Cummings et al. 1994).

Laboratory Investigations

Five to fifteen percent of all dementias have potentially reversible causes when treated early enough (Clarfield 1988; Larson et al. 1986). Routine tests include a complete blood count, electrolytes, serum glucose, blood urea nitrogen, vitamin B_{12}, and thyroid-stimulating hormone. Tests for human immunodeficiency virus, Lyme disease, heavy metal intoxication, urinary tract infection, and syphilis are optional (Knopman et al. 2001).

Neuroimaging procedures are an important part of the evaluation of the patient with dementia (Knopman et al. 2001). CT is adequate for identifying intracranial tumors, hydrocephalus, larger strokes, abscesses, or subdural hematomas. Contrast enhancement can increase the detection of acute ischemic and demyelinating lesions. MRI is more sensitive to detection of ischemic injury and demyelination and is capable of revealing more intracranial pathology than CT can reveal.

In the degenerative disorders, where structural imaging techniques such as CT and MRI reveal only nonspecific atrophy, PET and SPECT reveal characteristic topographies of brain dysfunction that can be helpful in differential diagnosis (Benson et al. 1983; Cummings and Benson 1992; Gemmell et al. 1987).

Management

The treatment of dementia involves halting the progression of disease (when possible) and minimizing disability. AD has no curative therapy, but ChE-Is can improve or temporarily stabilize cognitive deficits in some patients. Vitamin E delays the progression of AD. Likewise, ChE-Is have been shown to be beneficial in VaD. VaD patients also receive treatment with antihypertensive agents and platelet anti-aggregants (Meyer et al. 1986). Pharmacologic intervention in patients with FTD is limited to the behavioral manifestations of the disorder. Dopaminergic agents improve motor performance in selected patients with extrapyramidal disorders, but these agents have little effect on cognition. Hydrocephalic patients have ventriculoperitoneal shunts placed.

Late medical complications of dementia include seizures, pneumonia, urinary tract infections, and pressure ulcers. Patients with AD and VaD can develop seizures; management involves treatment with phenytoin or other anticonvulsants. Appropriate preventive measures (position rotation, ambulation) can reduce pressure ulcer formation; respiratory and urinary tract infections require antibiotic therapy. Early recognition and management of the medical complications of dementia lead to improved quality of life in these patients.

Most treatment of patients with dementia is directed at control of associated behavioral disturbances rather than the underlying dementing illness. Table 14–11 lists neuropsychiatric disorders that occur in dementia syndromes and the pharmacologic agents most commonly used in their treatment. Conventional neuroleptics traditionally have been the agents of choice for the control of delusions and agitation in patients with

TABLE 14–11. Neuropsychiatric alterations of dementia syndromes and the pharmacologic agents commonly used in their treatment

Symptom	Available agents	Usual daily oral dose (range)
Psychosis	Olanzapine	5 mg (5–10 mg)
	Quetiapine	100 mg (25–300 mg)
	Clozapine	25 mg (12.5–75.0 mg)
	Risperidone	1 mg (0.5–2.0 mg)
	Haloperidol	1 mg (0.5–3.0 mg)
Agitation	Antipsychotic agents	
	Olanzapine	5 mg (5–10 mg)
	Quetiapine	100 mg (25–300 mg)
	Risperidone	1 mg (0.5–2.0 mg)
	Haloperidol	1 mg (0.5–3.0 mg)
	Other agents	
	Trazodone	100 mg (100–300 mg)
	Carbamazepine	600 mg (200–1,200 mg)
	Buspirone	15 mg (15–30 mg)
	Divalproex	1,000 mg (250–2,000 mg)
	Lorazepam	1 mg (0.5–6.0 mg)
	Propranolol	120 mg (80–240 mg)
Depression	Citalopram	20 mg (10–30 mg)
	Sertraline	100 mg (50–150 mg)
	Paroxetine	20 mg (20–40 mg)
	Fluoxetine	20 mg (10–40 mg)
	Nortriptyline	50 mg (50–100 mg)
	Desipramine	50 mg (50–150 mg)
	Bupropion	300 mg (200–450 mg)
	Venlafaxine	150 mg (75–350 mg)
	Nefazodone	300 mg (300–600 mg)
Mania	Carbamazepine	600 mg (200–1,200 mg)
	Divalproex	1,000 mg (250–2,000 mg)
	Clonazepam	4 mg (0.5–15.0 mg)
	Lithium	300 mg (150–1,200 mg)
Anxiety	Buspirone	15 mg (15–30 mg)
	Oxazepam	30 mg (20–60 mg)
	Lorazepam	1 mg (0.5–6.0 mg)
	Propranolol	120 mg (80–240 mg)
Insomnia	Temazepam	15 mg (15–30 mg)
	Nortriptyline	25 mg (20–75 mg)
	Trazodone	50 mg (25–150 mg)
	Zolpidem	5 mg (5–10 mg)
	Zaleplon	5 mg (5–10 mg)
Sexual aggression (males)	Medroxyprogesterone	300 mg/week intramuscularly
	Leuprolide	7.5 mg/month intramuscularly

dementia (Devanand et al. 1988; Helms 1985; Raskind and Risse 1986), but novel antipsychotic agents such as olanzapine, risperidone, quetiapine, and clozapine have proven antipsychotic and antiagitation efficacy and the advantage of fewer adverse extrapyramidal effects (De Deyn et al. 1999; Street et al. 2000). The potential for agranulocytosis and the need for weekly hematologic monitoring can preclude the use of clozapine in some patients. Agitated patients who are unresponsive or unable to tolerate antipsychotic drugs might respond to treatment with trazodone, carbamazepine, valproate, buspirone, lorazepam, fluoxetine, or propranolol. Depression is treated with nortriptyline, desipramine, trazodone, nefazodone, sertraline, paroxetine, fluoxetine, bupropion, or venlafaxine (Cummings and Benson 1992). Agents used in the treatment of mania include carbamazepine, valproic acid, clonazepam, and lithium; anxiety can be managed with buspirone, oxazepam, lorazepam, or propranolol. Temazepam, lorazepam, nortriptyline, trazodone, zaleplon, and zolpidem can afford relief of insomnia. Men with sexually aggressive behavior can improve with administration of medroxyprogesterone or leuprolide (Cooper 1987; Rich and Ovsiew 1994).

A variety of nonpharmacologic interventions can be employed in patients with dementia in different phases of their illness. These include cognitive therapy, family therapy, supportive therapy, reminiscent therapy, and behavioral modification (Maletta 1988). Other valuable adjuncts are memory training, physical activity, and nutrition. Memory training can be helpful in the earlier stages of dementias.

Care of dementia patients is delivered primarily by family members, and the educational, psychological, social, and legal needs of caregivers must be addressed. Education regarding the diagnosis, nature, and prognosis of the particular dementia syndrome is essential to the caregiver's understanding and care of the patient with dementia. Reading materials such as *The 36-Hour Day* (Mace and Rabins 1991) can complement physician instruction. The Alzheimer's Association, a lay organization devoted to helping patients and families of patients with dementia, can provide significant support and is an excellent source of information regarding available community resources.

References

Aharon-Peretz J, Cummings JL, Hill MA: Vascular dementia and dementia of the Alzheimer type: cognition, ventricular size, and leuko-araiosis. Arch Neurol 45:719–721, 1988

Akil M, Brewer GJ: Psychiatric and behavioral abnormalities in Wilson's disease, in Behavioral Neurology of Movement Disorders (Advances in Neurology, Vol 65). Edited by Weiner WJ, Lang AE. New York, Raven, 1995, pp 171–178

Albert ML, Feldman RG, Willis AL: The "subcortical dementia" of progressive supranuclear palsy. J Neurol Neurosurg Psychiatry 37:121–130, 1974

American Psychiatric Association: Diagnostic and Statistical Manual of Mental Disorders, 4th Edition, Text Revision. Washington, DC, American Psychiatric Association, 2000

Bennet JP, Piercey MF: Pramipexole—a new dopamine agonist for the treatment of Parkinson's disease. J Neurol Sci 63(1): 25–31, 1999

Benson DF, Kuhl DE, Hawkins RA, et al: The fluorodeoxyglucose 18F scan in Alzheimer's disease and multi-infarct dementia. Arch Neurol 40:711–714, 1983

Boller F, Passafiume D, Keefe NC, et al: Visuospatial impairment in Parkinson's disease. Role of perceptual and motor factors. Arch Neurol 41:485–490, 1984

Brewer M, Cummings JL: Interactions of zinc and molybdenum with copper in therapy of Wilson's disease. Nutrition 11 (suppl 1): 114–116, 1995

Briley DP, Coull BM, Goodnight SH Jr: Neurological disease associated with antiphospholipid antibodies. Ann Neurol 25:221–227, 1989

Brown JJ, Hesselink JR, Rothrock JF: MR and CT of lacunar infarcts. American Journal of Radiology 151:367–372, 1988

Brown RG, MacCarthy B, Gotham AM, et al: Depression and disability in Parkinson's disease: a follow-up study of 132 cases. Psychol Med 18:49–55, 1988

Brun A, Englund B, Gustafson L, et al: Clinical and neuropathological criteria for frontotemporal dementia. J Neurol Neurosurg Psychiatry 57:416–418, 1994

Burns A, Folstein S, Brandt J, et al: Clinical assessment of irritability, aggression, and apathy in Huntington and Alzheimer disease. J Nerv Ment Dis 178(1):20–26, 1990

Caine ED, Hunt RD, Weingartner H, et al: Huntington's dementia. Arch Gen Psychiatry 35:377–384, 1978

Chow TW, Miller BL, Hayashi VN, et al: Inheritance of frontotemporal dementia. Arch Neurol 56(7):817–822, 1999

Clarfield AM: The reversible dementias: do they reverse? Ann Intern Med 109(6): 476–486, 1988

Clark LN, Poorkaj P, Wszolek Z, et al: Pathogenic implications of mutations in the tau gene in pallido-ponto-nigral degeneration and related neurodegenerative disorders linked to chromosome 17. Proc Natl Acad Sci U S A 95(22):13103–13107, 1998

Cohen S, Freedman M: Cognitive and behavioral changes in the Parkinson-plus syndromes, in Behavioral Neurology of Movement Disorders (Advances in Neurology, Vol 65). Edited by Weiner WJ, Lang AE. New York, Raven, 1995, pp 139–157

Cooper AJ: Medroxyprogesterone acetate (MPA) treatment of sexual acting out in men suffering from dementia. J Clin Psychiatry 48:368–370, 1987

Crowell RM, Tew JM Jr, Mark VH: Aggressive dementia associated with normal pressure hydrocephalus. Neurology 23:461–464, 1973

Cummings JL: The dementias of Parkinson's disease: prevalence, characteristics, neurobiology, and comparison with dementia of the Alzheimer type. Eur Neurol 28 (suppl 1):15–23, 1988a

Cummings JL: Depression in vascular dementia. Hillside J Clin Psychiatry 10:209–231, 1988b

Cummings JL: Behavioral complications of drug treatment of Parkinson's disease. J Am Geriatr Soc 39:708–716, 1991

Cummings JL: Depression and Parkinson's disease: a review. Am J Psychiatry 149:443–454, 1992

Cummings JL: Behavioral and psychiatric symptoms associated with Huntington's disease, in Behavioral Neurology of Movement Disorders (Advances in Neurology, Vol 65). Edited by Weiner WJ, Lang AE. New York, Raven, 1995, pp 179–186

Cummings JL: Cholinesterase inhibitors: a new class of psychotropic compounds. Am J Psychiatry 157:4–15, 2000

Cummings JL, Benson DF: Dementia: A Clinical Approach. Boston, MA, Butterworth, 1992

Cummings JL, Cunningham K: Obsessive-compulsive disorder in Huntington's disease. Biol Psychiatry 31(3):263–270, 1992

Cummings JL, Duchen LW: Klüver-Bucy syndrome in Pick disease: clinical and pathologic correlations. Neurology 31:1415–1422, 1981

Cummings JL, Litvan I: Neuropsychiatric aspects of corticobasal degeneration. Adv Neurol 82:147–152, 2000

Cummings JL, Miller B, Hill MA, et al: Neuropsychiatric aspects of multi-infarct dementia and dementia of the Alzheimer type. Arch Neurol 44(4):389–393, 1987

Cummings JL, Mega M, Gray K, et al: The Neuropsychiatric Inventory: comprehensive assessment of psychopathology in dementia. Neurology 44:2308–2314, 1994

De Deyn PP, Rabheru K, Rasmussen A, et al: A randomized trial of risperidone, placebo, and haloperidol for behavioral symptoms of dementia. Neurology 53:946–955, 1999

de Leon MJ, George AE, Golomb J, et al: Frequency of hippocampal formation atrophy in normal aging and Alzheimer's disease. Neurobiol Aging 18(1):1–11, 1997

Dening TR, Berrios GE: Wilson's disease: psychiatric symptoms in 195 cases. Arch Gen Psychiatry 46:1126–1134, 1989

Destee A, Gray F, Parent M, et al: Obsessive-compulsive behavior and progressive supranuclear palsy. Rev Neurol 146:12–18, 1990

Devanand DP, Sackeim HA, Mayeux R: Psychosis, behavioral disturbance, and the use of neuroleptics in dementia. Compr Psychiatry 29:387–401, 1988

Dian L, Cummings JL, Petry S, et al: Personality alterations in vascular dementia. Psychosomatics 31:415–419, 1990

Dogali M, Fazzini DO, Kolodny E, et al: Stereotactic ventral pallidotomy for Parkinson's disease. Neurology 45:753–761, 1995

Duara R, Barker W, Luis CA, et al: Frontotemporal dementia and Alzheimer's disease: differential diagnosis. Dement Geriatr Cogn Disord 10 (suppl 1):37–42, 1999

Duguid JR, De La Paz R, DeGroot J: Magnetic resonance imaging of the midbrain in Parkinson's disease. Ann Neurol 20:744–747, 1986

Duvoisin RC: Clinical diagnosis, in Progressive Supranuclear Palsy: Clinical and Research Approaches. Edited by Litvan I, Agid Y. New York, Oxford University Press, 1992, pp 17–33

Erkinjuntti T: Types of multi-infarct dementia. Acta Neurol Scand 75:391–399, 1987

Erkinjuntti T, Kurz A, Gauthier S, et al: Efficacy of galantamine in probable vascular dementia and Alzheimer's disease combined with cerebrovascular disease: a randomised trial. Lancet 359:1283–1290, 2002

Factor SA, Brown D, Molho ES, et al: Clozapine: a two year open trial in Parkinson's disease patients with psychosis. Neurology 44:544–546, 1994

Farrer LA: Suicide and attempted suicide in Huntington's disease: implications for preclinical testing of persons at risk. Am J Med Genet 24:305–311, 1986

Fazekas F, Alavi A, Chawluk JB, et al: Comparison of CT, MR, and PET in Alzheimer's dementia and normal aging. J Nucl Med 30(10):1607–1615, 1989

Folstein SE: Huntington's Disease: A Disorder of Families. Baltimore, MD, Johns Hopkins University Press, 1989

Folstein SE, Brandt J, Folstein MF: Huntington's disease, in Subcortical Dementia. Edited by Cummings JL. New York, Oxford University Press, 1990, pp 87–107

Foster NL, Chase TN, Fedio P, et al: Alzheimer's disease: focal cortical changes shown by positron emission tomography. Neurology 33:961–965, 1983

Foster NL, Gilman S, Berent S, et al: Cerebral hypometabolism in progressive supranuclear palsy studied with positron emission tomography. Ann Neurol 24:399–406, 1988

Friedman JH, Lannon MC: Clozapine in the treatment of psychosis in Parkinson's disease. Neurology 39:1219–1221, 1989

Galasko DL, Chang L, Motter R, et al: High cerebrospinal fluid tau and low amyloid B42 levels in the clinical diagnosis of Alzheimer disease and relation to apolipoprotein E genotype. Arch Neurol 55:937–945, 1998

Gallassi R, Morreale A, Montagna P, et al: Binswanger's disease and normal-pressure hydrocephalus: clinical and neuropsychological comparison. Arch Neurol 48(11):1156–1159, 1991

Gemmell HG, Sharp PF, Besson JAO, et al: Differential diagnosis in dementia using the cerebral blood flow agent 99mTc HM-PAO: a SPECT study. J Comput Assist Tomogr 11:398–402, 1987

Giacobini E: Cholinesterase inhibitors: from the calabar bean to Alzheimer therapy, in Cholinesterases and Cholinesterase Inhibitors. Edited by Giacobini E. London, Martin Dunitz, 2000, pp 181–226

Gibb WRG: Neuropathology of Parkinson's disease and related syndromes. Neurol Clin 10:361–376, 1992

Gilman S, Low PA, Quinn N, et al: Consensus statement on the diagnosis of multiple system atrophy. J Neurol Sci 163(1): 94–98, 1999

Glass JD, Reich SG, De Long MR: Wilson's disease. Development of neurological disease after beginning penicillamine therapy. Arch Neurol 47(5):595–596, 1990

Graff-Radford NR, Godersky JC, Jones MP: Variables predicting surgical outcome in symptomatic hydrocephalus in the elderly. Neurology 36:1601–1604, 1989

Graff-Radford NR, Damasio AR, Hyman BT, et al: Progressive aphasia in a patient with Pick's disease: a neuropsychological, radiologic, and anatomic study. Neurology 40:620–626, 1990

Gustafson L, Hagberg B: Recovery of hydrocephalic dementia after shunt operation. J Neurol Neurosurg Psychiatry 41: 940–947, 1978

Hachinski VC, Iliff LD, Zilhka E, et al: Cerebral blood flow in dementia. Arch Neurol 32:632–637, 1975

Hall PK, Andrus JA, Oostveen JA, et al: Neuroprotective effects of the dopamine D2/D3 agonist pramipexole against postischemic or methamphetamine-induced degeneration of nigrostriatal neurons. Brain Res 742:80–88, 1996

Haxby JV, Grady CL, Duara R, et al: Neocortical metabolic abnormalities precede nonmemory cognitive defects in early Alzheimer's-type dementia. Arch Neurol 43:882–885, 1986

Heckmann JM, Eastman RW, De Villiers JC, et al: Wilson's disease: neurological and magnetic resonance imaging improvement on zinc treatment. J Neurol Neurosurg Psychiatry 57(10):1273–1274, 1994

Helms PM: Efficacy of antipsychotics in the treatment of behavioral complications of dementia: a review of the literature. J Am Geriatr Soc 33:206–209, 1985

Hershey LA, Modic MT, Greenough G, et al: Magnetic resonance imaging in vascular dementia. Neurology 37:29–36, 1987

Hier DB, Cummings JL: Rare acquired and degenerative dementias, in Subcortical Dementia. Edited by Cummings JL. New York, Oxford University Press, 1990, pp 199–217

Hsich G, Kenney K, Gibbs CJ, et al: The 14–3–3 brain protein in cerebrospinal fluid as a marker for transmissible spongiform encephalopathies. N Engl J Med 335:924–930, 1996

Hughes AJ, Daniel SE, Kilford L, et al: Accuracy of clinical diagnosis of idiopathic Parkinson's disease: a clinico-pathological study of 100 cases. J Neurol Neurosurg Psychiatry 55:181–184, 1992

Huntington's Disease Collaborative Research Group: A novel gene containing a trinucleotide repeat that is expanded and unstable on Huntington's disease chromosomes. Cell 72:971–983, 1993

Hutton M, Lendon CL, Rizzu P, et al: Association of missense and 5´-splice-site mutations in tau with the inherited dementia FTDP-17. Nature 393:702–705, 1998

Ironside JW: Review: Creutzfeldt-Jakob disease. Brain Pathol 6:527–530, 1996

Ishii N, Nishihara Y, Imamura T: Why do frontal lobe symptoms predominate in vascular dementia with lacunes? Neurology 36:340–345, 1986

Jack CR Jr, Petersen RC, O'Brien PC, et al: MR-based hippocampal volumetry in the diagnosis of Alzheimer's disease. Neurology 42(1):183–188, 1992

Jack CR Jr, Petersen RC, Xu YC, et al: Prediction of AD with MRI-based hippocampal volume in mild cognitive impairment. Neurology 52(7):1397–1403, 1999

Jagust WJ, Friedland RP, Budinger TF, et al: Longitudinal studies of regional cerebral metabolism in Alzheimer's disease. Neurology 38(6):909–912, 1988

Johnson KA, Mueller ST, Walsh TM, et al: Cerebral perfusion imaging in Alzheimer's disease. Arch Neurol 44:165–168, 1987

Jordan SE, Nowacki R, Nuwer M: Computerized electroencephalography in the evaluation of early dementia. Brain Topogr 1:271–274, 1989

Josephson J: Focus: cows for fear. Environ Health Perspect 106:A137–A138, 1998

Kamboh MI: Apolipoprotein E polymorphism and susceptibility to Alzheimer's disease. Hum Biol 67:195–215, 1995

Katzman R: Alzheimer's disease. N Engl J Med 314:964–973, 1986

Knopman DS, Christensen KJ, Schut LJ, et al: The spectrum of imaging and neuropsychological findings in Pick's disease. Neurology 39:362–368, 1989

Knopman DS, DeKosky ST, Cummings JL, et al: Practice parameter: diagnosis of dementia (an evidence-based review). Report of the Quality Standards Subcommittee of the American Academy of Neurology. Neurology 56:1143–1153, 2001

Koller WC, Megaffin BB: Parkinson's disease and parkinsonism, in Textbook of Geriatric Neuropsychiatry. Edited by Coffey CE, Cummings JL. Washington, DC, American Psychiatric Press, 1994, pp 434–456

Kvale JN: Amitriptyline in the management of progressive supranuclear palsy. Arch Neurol 39:387–388, 1982

Kwentus JA, Hart RP: Normal pressure hydrocephalus presenting as mania. J Nerv Ment Dis 175:500–502, 1987

Lang CJ, Rabas-Kolominsky P, Engelhardt A, et al: Fatal deterioration of Wilson's disease after institution of oral zinc therapy. Arch Neurol 50(10):1007–1008, 1993

Larson EB, Reifler BV, Sumi SM, et al: Diagnostic tests in the evaluation of dementia. A prospective study of 200 elderly outpatients. Arch Intern Med 146(10):1917–1922, 1986

Larsson A, Arlig A, Bergh AC, et al: Quantitative SPECT cisternography in normal pressure hydrocephalus. Acta Neurol Scand 90(3):190–196, 1994

Leenders KL, Palmer AJ, Quinn N, et al: Brain dopamine metabolism in patients with Parkinson's disease measured with positron emission tomography. J Neurol Neurosurg Psychiatry 49:853–860, 1986

Leenders KL, Frackowiak RSJ, Lees AJ: Steele-Richardson-Olszewski syndrome: brain energy metabolism, blood flow, and fluorodopa uptake measured by positron emission tomography. Brain 111:615–630, 1988

Lees AJ: Progressive supranuclear palsy (Steele-Richardson-Olszewski syndrome), in Subcortical Dementia. Edited by Cummings JL. New York, Oxford University Press, 1990, pp 121–131

Litvan I, Mega MS, Cummings JL, et al: Neuropsychiatric aspects of progressive supranuclear palsy. Neurology 47(5):1184–1189, 1996

Loeb C, Gandolfo C: Diagnostic evaluation of degenerative and vascular dementia. Stroke 14:390–401, 1983

Lund and Manchester Groups: Consensus statement: clinical and neuropathological criteria for frontotemporal dementia. J Neurol Neurosurg Psychiatry 57:416–418, 1994

Mace N, Rabins P: The 36-Hour Day: A Family Guide to Caring for Persons with Alzheimer's Disease, Related Dementing Illnesses, and Memory Loss Later in Life. Baltimore, MD, Johns Hopkins University Press, 1991

Maletta GJ: Management of behavior problems in elderly patients with Alzheimer's disease and other dementias. Clin Geriatr Med 4:719–747, 1988

Martilla RJ: Epidemiology, in Handbook of Parkinson's Disease. Edited by Koller WC. New York, Marcel Dekker, 1987, pp 35–50

McDonald LV, Lake CR: Psychosis in an adolescent patient with Wilson's disease: effects of chelation therapy. Psychosom Med 57(2):202–204, 1995

McKeith I, O'Brien J: Dementia with Lewy bodies. Aust N Z J Psychiatry 33(6):800–808, 1999

McKeith IG, Perry RH, Fairbairn SJ, et al: Operational criteria for senile dementia of Lewy body type (SDLT). Psychol Med 22:911–922, 1992

McKeith IG, Galasko D, Kosaka K, et al: Consensus guidelines for the clinical and pathologic diagnosis of dementia with Lewy bodies (DLB): report of the consortium on DLB international workshop. Neurology 47:1113–1124, 1996

McKeith I, Del Ser T, Spano P, et al: Efficacy of rivastigmine in dementia with Lewy bodies: a randomised, double-blind, placebo-controlled international study. Lancet 356:2031–2036, 2000

McKhann G, Drachman D, Folstein M, et al: Clinical diagnosis of Alzheimer's disease: report of the NINCDS-ADRDA Work Group under the auspices of Department of Health and Human Services Task Force on Alzheimer's Disease. Neurology 34(7):939–944, 1984

Mega MS, Cummings JL, Fiorello T, et al: The spectrum of behavioral changes in Alzheimer's disease. Neurology 46(1):130–135, 1996

Mendez MF, Martin RJ, Smyth KA, et al: Psychiatric symptoms associated with Alzheimer's disease. J Neuropsychiatry Clin Neurosci 2:28–33, 1990

Meyer JS, Judd BW, Tawakina T, et al: Improved cognition after control of risk factors for multi-infarct dementia. JAMA 256:2203–2209, 1986

Miller BL, Mena I, Daly J, et al: Temporal-parietal hypoperfusion with single-photon emission computerized tomography in conditions other than Alzheimer's disease. Dementia 1:41–45, 1990

Miller BL, Cummings JL, Villanueva-Mayer J, et al: Frontal lobe degeneration: clinical, neuropsychological, and SPECT characteristics. Neurology 41(9):1374–1382, 1991

Miller BL, Chang L, Oropilla G, et al: Alzheimer's disease and frontal lobe dementias, in Textbook of Geriatric Neuropsychiatry. Edited by Coffey CE Cummings JL. Washington, DC, American Psychiatric Press, 1994, pp 390–404

Morishita L: Wandering behavior, in Alzheimer's Disease: Treatment and Long-Term Management. Edited by Cummings JL, Miller BL. New York, Marcel Dekker, 1990 pp 157–176

Moskovitz C, Moses H III, Klawans HL: Levodopa induced psychosis: a kindling phenomenon. Am J Psychiatry 135:669–675, 1978

Murayama S, Mori H, Ihara Y, et al: Immunocytochemical and ultrastructural studies of Pick's disease. Ann Neurol 27:394–405, 1990

Neary D, Snowden JS, Gustafson L, et al: Frontotemporal lobar degeneration: a consensus on clinical diagnostic criteria. Neurology 51(6):1546–1554, 1998

Nemetz PN, Leibson C, Naessens JM, et al: Traumatic brain injury and time to onset of Alzheimer's disease: a population-based study. Am J Epidemiol 149(1):32–40, 1999

Newman GC: Treatment of progressive supranuclear palsy with tricyclic antidepressants. Neurology 35:1189–1193, 1985

Ohtsubo K, Isumiyama N, Shimada H, et al: Three-dimensional structure of Alzheimer's neurofibrillary tangles of the aged human brain revealed by the quick-freeze, deep-etch and replica method. Acta Neuropathol (Berl) 79:480–485, 1990

Parkinson's Study Group: Safety and efficacy of pramipexole in early Parkinson disease: a randomized dose-ranging study. JAMA 278:125–130, 1997

Petry S, Cummings JL, Hill MA, et al: Personality alterations in dementia of the Alzheimer type. Arch Neurol 45(11):1187–1190, 1988

Pirozzolo FJ, Hansch EC, Mortimer JA, et al: Dementia in Parkinson's disease: a neuropsychological analysis. Brain Cogn 1:71–83, 1982

Poorkaj P, Bird TD, Wijsman E, et al: Tau is a candidate gene for chromosome 17 frontotemporal dementia. Ann Neurol 43:815–825, 1998

Procter A, Lowe SL, Palmer AM, et al: Topographical distribution of neurochemical changes in Alzheimer's disease. J Neurol Sci 84:125–140, 1988

Prusiner SB: Novel proteinaceous infectious particles cause scrapie. Science 216:136–144, 1982

Ranen NG, Lipsey JR, Treisman G, et al: Sertraline in the treatment of severe aggressiveness in Huntington's disease. J Neuropsychiatry Clin Neurosci 8(3):338–340, 1996

Raskind MA, Risse SC: Antipsychotic drugs and the elderly. J Clin Psychiatry 45:17–22, 1986

Reisberg B, Borenstein J, Salob SP, et al: Behavioral symptoms in Alzheimer's disease: phenomenology and treatment. J Clin Psychiatry 48 (5 suppl):9–15, 1987

Rich SS, Ovsiew F: Leuprolide acetate for exhibitionism in Huntington's disease. Mov Disord 9:353–357, 1994

Risse SC, Raskind MA, Nochlin D, et al: Neuropathological findings in patients with clinical diagnoses of probable Alzheimer's disease. Am J Psychiatry 147(2):168–172, 1990

Roberts HE, Dean RC, Stoudemire A: Clozapine treatment of psychosis in Parkinson's disease. J Neuropsychiatry Clin Neurosci 1:190–192, 1989

Roman GC, Tatemichi TK, Erkinjuntti T, et al: Vascular dementia: diagnostic criteria for research studies. Report of the NINDS-AIREN International Workshop. Neurology 43: 250–260, 1993

Rosenblatt A, Leroi I: Neuropsychiatry of Huntington's disease and other basal ganglia disorders. Psychosomatics 41(1): 24–30, 2000

Rubin EH, Morris JC, Storandt M, et al: Behavioral changes in patients with mild senile dementia of the Alzheimer's type. Psychiatry Res 21:55–62, 1987

Sano M, Ernesto C, Thomas RG, et al: A controlled trial of selegiline, alpha-tocopherol, or both as treatment for Alzheimer's disease. The Alzheimer's Disease Cooperative Study. N Engl J Med 336: 1216–1222, 1997

Schneider LS, Gleason RP, Chui HC: Progressive supranuclear palsy with agitation: response to trazodone but not to thiothixene or carbamazepine. J Geriatr Psychiatry Neurol 2:109–112, 1989

Shaw KM, Lees AJ, Stern GM: The impact of treatment with levodopa on Parkinson's disease. QJM 49:283–293, 1980

Starkstein SE, Robinson RG: Neuropsychiatric aspects of stroke, in Textbook of Geriatric Neuropsychiatry. Edited by Coffey CE, Cummings JL. Washington, DC, American Psychiatric Press, 1994, pp 457–475

Steele JC: Progressive supranuclear palsy. Brain 95:693–704, 1972

Steele JC, Richardson JC, Olszewski J: Progressive supranuclear palsy. Arch Neurol 10:333–359, 1964

Stein MB, Heuser IJ, Juncos JL, et al: Anxiety disorders in patients with Parkinson's disease. Am J Psychiatry 147:217–220, 1990

Stewart JT: Huntington's disease and propranolol. Am J Psychiatry 150(1):166–167, 1993

Street JS, Clark WS, Gannon KS, et al: Olanzapine treatment of psychotic and behavioral symptoms in patients with Alzheimer disease in nursing care facilities: a double-blind, randomized, placebo-controlled trial. The HGEU Study Group. Arch Gen Psychiatry 57:968–976, 2000

Sudarsky L, Simon S: Gait disturbances in late-life hydrocephalus. Arch Neurol 44:263–267, 1987

Tanner CM, Vogel C, Goetz CG, et al: Hallucinations in Parkinson's disease: a population study (abstract). Ann Neurol 14:136, 1983

Thomsen AM, Borgesen SE, Bruhn P, et al: Prognosis of dementia in normal-pressure hydrocephalus after a shunt operation. Ann Neurol 20:304–310, 1986

Tierney MC, Fisher RH, Lewis AJ, et al: The NINCDS-ADRDA Work Group criteria for the clinical diagnosis of probable Alzheimer's disease: a clinicopathologic study of 57 cases. Neurology 38(3):359–364, 1988

Van Nostrand WE, Wagner SL, Shankle WR, et al: Decreased levels of soluble amyloid beta-protein precursor in cerebrospinal fluid of live Alzheimer disease patients. Proc Natl Acad Sci U S A 89:2551–2555, 1992

van Swieten JC, Stevens M, Rosso SM, et al: Phenotypic variation in hereditary fronto-temporal dementia with tau mutations. Ann Neurol 46:617–626, 1999

Villardita C, Smirni P, Le Pira F, et al: Mental deterioration, visuoperceptive disabilities, and constructional apraxia in Parkinson's disease. Acta Neurol Scand 66:112–120, 1982

Wahlund LO: Biological markers and diagnostic investigations in Alzheimer's disease. Acta Neurol Scand Suppl 165:85–91, 1996

Weihl CC, Roos RP: Creutzfeldt-Jakob disease, new variant Creutzfeldt-Jakob disease, and bovine spongiform encephalopathy. Neurol Clin 17:835–855, 1999

Wenning GK, Ben Shlomo Y, Magalhaes M, et al: Clinical features and natural history of multiple system atrophy. An analysis of 100 cases. Brain 117(4):835–845, 1994

Westphal KFO: Über eine dem Bilde der cerebrospinalen grauen Degeneration ähnliche Erkrankung des centralen Nervensystems ohne anatomischen Befund, nebst einigen Bemerkungen über paradoxe Contraktion. Archiv für Psychiatrie und Nervenkrankheiten 14:87–134, 767–769, 1883

Whitehouse PJ, Hedreen JC, White CL III, et al: Basal forebrain neurons in the dementia of Parkinson's disease. Ann Neurol 1:243–248, 1983

Wikkelso C, Andersson H, Blomstrand C, et al: The clinical effect of lumbar puncture in normal pressure hydrocephalus. J Neurol Neurosurg Psychiatry 45:64–69, 1982

Will RG, Ironside JW, Zeidler M, et al: A new variant of Creutzfeldt-Jakob disease in the UK. Lancet 347:921–925, 1996

Will RG, Zeidler M, Stewart GE, et al: Diagnosis of new variant Creutzfeldt-Jakob disease. Ann Neurol 47:575–582, 2000

Wilson SAK: Progressive lenticular degeneration. A familial nervous disease associated with cirrhosis of the liver. Brain 34:295–507, 1912

Wragg RE, Jeste DV: Overview of depression and psychosis in Alzheimer's disease. Am J Psychiatry 146(5):577–587, 1989

Young SM, Fisher M, Sigsbee A, et al: Cardiogenic brain embolism and lupus anticoagulant. Ann Neurol 26:390–392, 1989

CHAPTER 15

Neuropsychiatric Aspects of Schizophrenia

Carol A. Tamminga, M.D.

Gunvant K. Thaker, M.D.

Deborah R. Medoff, Ph.D.

Despite centuries of curiosity and study focused on schizophrenia, its pathophysiology remains unknown. We know that schizophrenia is a psychiatric illness with well-established diagnostic criteria, clear signs and symptoms, and variably effective symptomatic treatments (Andreasen 1995; Carpenter and Buchanan 1994). Soon, relevant information will expand, both in quantity and in quality, because of the increased sensitivity of newer human research techniques—from rating precision to diagnostic specificity to functional imaging resolution—and because of the exponential increase in basic neuroscience knowledge, and now the completed human genome.

Clinical Characteristics

Diagnosis

Adequately distinguishing schizophrenia from other psychotic disorders was problematic but became clearer as etiologies and treatments of some of the other psychotic disorders were developed. For example, it was discovered that niacin was an effective treatment for pellagra, and penicillin for central nervous system

Support for this chapter was generated by a National Institute of Mental Health (NIMH) grant for dopaminergic treatments (MH49667), GABAergic treatments for tardive dyskinesia (MH37073), and ketamine and cerebral blood flow (DA-94–03), as well as an NIMH CRC Center Grant (MH40279). Several scientific collaborators contributed data, advice, and critique: X.-M. Gao, H.H. Holcomb, A.C. Lahti, R.C. Lahti, and R. Roberts. Patients and staff of the Maryland Psychiatric Research Center Residential Treatment Unit invested their time and energy to many of these scientific projects.

(CNS) syphilis—both of which are diseases that can manifest themselves with psychotic conditions. The DSM-IV-TR criteria (American Psychiatric Association 2000) and the tenth revision of the International Classification of Diseases and Related Health Problems (ICD-10) (World Health Organization 1992) are the world's two major diagnostic systems for schizophrenia, and with the current editions they have reconciled their major differences. Such structured diagnostic criteria have led to observation that incidence and the symptomatic expression are similar between countries and across cultures (Sartorius 1974).

Schizophrenia may well be the tip of an iceberg of schizophrenia-related diagnoses, augmented by the related personality disorders (Tsuang et al. 2000). Schizophrenia-related personality disorders evidence mild symptoms and signs similar to schizophrenia, especially in some nonpsychotic first-degree relatives (Faraone et al. 2000). Moreover, antipsychotic treatment may improve functioning in persons with certain personality disorders (Tsuang et al. 1999).

Symptoms

The list of the most frequently reported symptoms developed by the International Pilot Study of Schizophrenia conducted by the World Health Organization (Sartorius 1974) is entirely descriptive of the disease we see today.

Although the use of DSM-IV-TR clearly identifies a syndrome, investigators remain unsure that schizophrenia is a unitary illness with a single etiology and pathophysiology as opposed to a group of diseases or a collection of interrelated conditions (Carpenter and Buchanan 1994). Therefore, various attempts have been made to delineate testable subtypes of the illness on the basis of clinical characteristics, which then can be evaluated

for distinguishing brain characteristics (Carpenter et al. 1993). These analyses have consistently revealed three distinct symptom domains in schizophrenia: 1) hallucinations, delusions, and paranoia; 2) thought disorder and bizarre behavior; and 3) negative symptoms of anhedonia, social withdrawal, and thought poverty (Andreasen et al. 1995; Arndt et al. 1991; Barnes and Liddle 1990; Carpenter and Buchanan 1989; Kay and Sevy 1990; Lenzenweger et al. 1991; Liddle 1987). Although these symptom clusters characteristically occur together, and one cluster may predominate in some patients, one domain is not exclusive of another.

Course

The diagnosis of schizophrenia usually implies a lifelong course of psychotic illness. Occasionally, the illness is of fast onset and episodic, with symptoms first occurring in late teen and early adult years, and showing satisfactory recovery between episodes. However, more often other patterns of illness occur characterized by an insidious onset, partial recovery, or a remarkable lack of recovery between episodes (Bleuler 1978; Ciompi and Müller 1976). In most schizophrenic patients, a profound deterioration in mental and social functioning occurs within the first few years of the illness. After the initial deteriorating years, the further course of illness settles at a low, but flat, plateau. Surprisingly, symptoms may improve in later life after age 50 (Harding et al. 1987a, 1987b). Specifically, in this study of 269 patients (with a 97% follow-up rate), more than half of the individuals had no psychotic symptoms after 10 years of study (after approximately 15–20 years of illness), and most had a "good" level of functioning in their later life (Bleuler 1978; Ciompi and Müller 1976; Huber et al. 1979; Tsuang et al. 1979). That the disease course is generally flat in its middle years distinguishes schizophrenia from traditional neurodegenerative disorders in which the course is progressively downhill (such as Parkinson's disease or Alzheimer's dementia) and from traditional neurodevelopmental disorders (such as mental retardation) in which the course is steady and low from the beginning of life.

Risk Factors

Although the etiology of schizophrenia is not known, certain factors have been associated with a propensity toward the illness. These risk factors suggest the importance of very early life events in the onset of an illness whose florid symptoms appear much later in life.

Genetics

The evidence is currently clear and consistent across many methodologically sound studies that schizophrenia aggregates in families. First-degree relatives of schizophrenic individuals have a lifetime risk of 3%–7% for manifesting schizophrenia compared with a 0.5%–1% lifetime risk of relatives of control subjects (Kendler and Diehl 1995). Twin studies have been pivotal in identifying the familial factor as a genetic rather than an environmental risk (Gottesman and Shields 1982; Kety 1987). The monozygotic twin of a person with schizophrenia has a 31%–78% chance of contracting the illness, compared with a 0%–28% chance for a dizygotic twin. Although schizophrenia is firmly believed to be genetic, the genetic mechanism of transmission has not been defined despite significant efforts in both association and linkage studies (Kendler and Diehl 1993).

Perinatal Factors

Pregnancy and birth complications are associated with schizophrenia (Lewis and Murray 1987). The overall effect is small,

increasing risk of disease by only 1% or so. The markers used to indicate these perinatal insults include low birth weight, prematurity, preeclampsia, prolonged labor, hypoxia, and fetal distress (McGrath and Murray 1995). However, any evidence of causality is lacking in these studies; the only available evidence is for an association between the two. As such, these pregnancy and birth complications, even if actually more frequent in schizophrenia than in the general population, could be an epiphenomena of the schizophrenia genotype without any causal relationship to the illness.

Winter Birth

A consistently found epidemiologic characteristic of schizophrenia is the excess of winter births over spring births among schizophrenic individuals (Bradbury and Miller 1985). Again, the effect is small but highly replicable. The reason for the association remains obscure. Seasonal variations in birth complications, temperature, lifestyle, diet, and rates of infections are the possibilities that have been most discussed.

Anatomic Features

In Vivo Brain Structure Using Magnetic Resonance Imaging

The first magentic resonance imaging (MRI) studies revealed a reduction in overall brain size, an increase in ventricular size, and variable cortical wasting in schizophrenia (Shelton and Weinberger 1987). The studies confirmed and extended older literature describing the examination of schizophrenic patients with computed axial tomography (CAT), which demonstrated the ventricular enlargement with the lower resolution (CAT) technique (Johnstone et al. 1976).

More recently, MRI studies have frequently revealed a volume decrease in the medial temporal cortical structures, hippocampus, amygdala, and parahippocampal gyrus, especially in the studies with dense sampling (Barta et al. 1990; Bogerts et al. 1990; Breier et al. 1992; Suddath et al. 1990). New analytic techniques allowing shape analysis of the hippocampus have revealed striking regional shape differences of the hippocampus in schizophrenia (Csernansky et al. 1998). Not only has the volume of the superior temporal gyrus been reported to be reduced in schizophrenia, but the magnitude of the reduction has been correlated with the presence of hallucinations (Menon et al. 1995; Shenton et al. 1992) and with electrophysiological changes in the patients (McCarley et al. 1993). Neocortical volume reduction may be present in only some symptomatic subgroups of schizophrenic subjects, for example, middle frontal cortex volume reduction in negative-symptom schizophrenia (Andreasen et al. 1992). The thalamus may have a reduced volume in schizophrenia, particularly the posterior portion (Andreasen et al. 1994); this is an observation that should direct future interest to this structure. However, these changes as a consequence of drug action have not been ruled out.

The extent to which the overall volume of a brain structure reflects any internal pathology, especially if the pathology is subtle, is necessarily limited. Although positive MRI data can identify a brain area for further study, negative results do not rule out areas as pathologic; moreover, MRI as a technique does not provide critical knowledge to differentiate functional relevance. Thus it is important to follow up the identification of structural abnormalities with functional, pharmacologic, and electrophysiological techniques.

Microscopic Analysis of Postmortem CNS Tissue

It is widely accepted that no obvious, currently identifiable neuropathologic lesion is present in schizophrenia as occurs in Parkinson's disease or Alzheimer's dementia. Of universal caution in reviewing any schizophrenia neuropathologic studies are careful attention to the possible confounds of tissue artifacts, long-term neuroleptic treatment, lifelong altered mental state, and relevant demographic factors.

The technical range of measures performed on CNS tissue represents a great breadth of anatomic expertise. However, the application of these multiple techniques in the face of incomplete guiding hypotheses has left the postmortem literature of schizophrenia very broad and sometimes fragmented (Bogerts 1993; Harrison 1999). The changes that have most consistently been found suggest a common localization for a neural defect in the illness (that is, in limbic and prefrontal cortices) but not necessarily a common neuropathologic feature. The primary limbic structures in the brain (namely, hippocampus, cingulate cortex, anterior thalamus, and mammillary bodies) and their intimately associated cortical areas (entorhinal cortex) have been found to regularly display pathologic abnormalities. These are abnormalities of cell size (Jeste and Lohr 1989), cell number (Falkai and Bogerts 1986), area (Suddath et al. 1989), neuronal organization (Scheibel and Kovelman 1981), and gross structure (Colter et al. 1987). Moreover, the entorhinal cortex has been observed to show abnormalities of cellular organization in layer 2 neurons (Arnold et al. 1991a). It is interesting to recall that both structural changes on MRI (Suddath et al. 1989) and (as will be described shortly) functional changes in positron emission tomography (PET) (Tamminga et al. 1992) have targeted these same areas for interest in schizophrenia pathophysiology.

Even though they are consistently altered, limbic structures are not the only ones affected in the postmortem schizophrenic brain. The neocortex (especially frontal cortex) has been more recently studied, with varying reports of cell or tissue loss: one study reported volume reductions in gray matter (Pakkenberg 1987), two did not (Heckers et al. 1991; Rosenthal and Bigelow 1972), and one reported increased neuronal packing in frontal cortex (Goldman-Rakic 1995). The thalamus, because of its pivotal position in relationship to afferent sensory information and as a station in the cortical-subcortical circuits, has been the occasional object of study with inconsistent but not negative results. Several studies report cell loss and reduced tissue volume in thalamus (Pakkenberg 1990; Treff and Hempel 1958), whereas another study reports none of this (Lesch and Bogerts 1984). Additional study in both the frontal cortex and thalamus must be done before firm conclusions can be made. Moreover, it is possible that variability might be reduced (and the answer made clearer) by seeking neuropathologic changes within symptom domains.

The interesting neuropathologic finding of basal ganglia enlargement in schizophrenia (in both caudate nucleus and putamen) was subsequently confirmed using in vivo MRI techniques (Chakos et al. 1994). These studies showed a small but clear increase in the size of both caudate nucleus and putamen in schizophrenic patients treated with neuroleptics. That this volume increase occurs only after long-term neuroleptic treatment but not before (Chakos et al. 1994) suggests that it is an effect of long-term treatment with neuroleptics. It has also been observed that long-term neuroleptic

treatment in laboratory rats increases striatal mitochondrial size, increases the size of some axon terminals, and causes a trend toward an increase in the size of dendrites (Roberts et al. 1995); these findings are consistent with a striatal volume increase with neuroleptic treatment in schizophrenic patients. This finding is a good example of a postmortem finding in schizophrenia that is associated not with the illness but probably with its treatment (Figure 15–1).

Anatomic Markers of Brain Development

Regional studies of postmortem cortical tissue from schizophrenic individuals have generated several persuasive observations consistent with the idea that developmental mistakes in migratory pattern may be associated with schizophrenia. This evidence consists of cortical neurons appearing incorrectly in cortical layers lower (more inferior) than expected. Akbarian et al. (1993) reported a reduction in nicotinamide adenine dinucleotide phosphate (NADPH)–diaphorase staining neurons in the higher cortical layers of the schizophrenic dorsolateral prefrontal cortex and an increase ("trailing") of these neurons in underlying white-matter layers. The researchers interpreted these findings as being consistent with an impairment of neuronal migration of these particular cells into upper layers of frontal cortex during their critical developmental period (second trimester) in schizophrenia. Earlier studies reported alterations in superficial cellular organization (for example, in layer 2 entorhinal cortex), with layer 2 cell reduced in the neuronal islands, again consistent with a neuronal migratory failure in this area of cortex (Arnold et al. 1991a; Jakob and Beckman 1986). Another study found cingulate and middle frontal cortices to have more neurons present in lower rather than in superficial

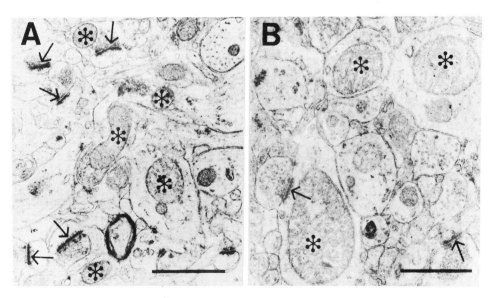

FIGURE 15–1. Electron micrographs of striatal neurophils in control (*Panel A*) and high-VCM (*Panel B*) groups.

Note the decreased synaptic density and hypertrophied mitochondria in the high-VCM group compared with the control group. Arrows indicate synapses; asterisks indicate mitochondrial profiles.

Scale bars = 1 μm. VCM = vacuous chewing movements.

Source. Micrograph contributed by Dr. Rosalinda Roberts.

layers, again consistent with a concept of migratory failure (Benes 1993). Other kinds of developmental studies have focused on changes in structural and/or growth-related elements in the neurons themselves that would disturb normal development. The early observations of hippocampal neuronal disarray in schizophrenia are consistent with the reported selective loss of two microtubule-associated proteins (MAP2 and MAP5) in schizophrenic postmortem hippocampal tissue (Arnold et al. 1991b). Another study found that the protein GAP-43 is increased in frontal and lingual gyral tissue of schizophrenic persons (Sower et al. 1995). GAP-43, a synaptic marker associated with the establishment and remodeling of synaptic connections, is normally enriched in associational cortex and hippocampus. This finding suggests the possibility of unusual synaptic remodeling in frontal and hippocampal cortices in

schizophrenia and is consistent with altered neuronal activity in these areas, possibly secondary to failed or incomplete neuronal projection systems to or within these regions.

Akbarian and colleagues (1995) and Volk et al. (2000) reported decreased expression of glutamic acid decarboxylase (GAD) mRNA in prefrontal cortex of schizophrenic persons without significant cell loss. It is thought that only one of the multiple types of γ-aminobutyric acid (GABA)–containing cortical neurons may be reduced in schizophrenia, the chandelier cell (D.A. Lewis 2000). These alterations in GABA system activity may be the basis of the already observed frontal hypometabolism repeatedly reported in functional imaging studies of the illness. In the excitatory glutamatergic system, alteration in the composition of the *N*-methyl-D-aspartate (NMDA)–sensitive glutamate receptor in hippocampus has been reported (Gao et al. 2000), possibly reflecting disruption of limbic system function.

Biochemical Studies

Dopamine

Concentrations of dopamine in the CNS were originally identified in the 1950s, and its function was defined as a neurotransmitter in the CNS. Dopamine neuronal cell bodies in the brain have a highly localized distribution in the mesencephalon, limited here to the substantia nigra pars compacta (SNC) and to the ventral tegmental area (VTA); projection fibers from the SNC travel predominantly to the caudate nucleus and putamen, and less dense fibers from the VTA largely project to frontal and cingulate cortices. Release of dopamine into the synapse is characteristically phasic, not tonic, although some studies tend to suggest that both may occur (Grace 1991). Considerable basic pharmacology about the dopamine system has been described in the last three decades. This has provided a rich opportunity for study in schizophrenia and in other related diseases of the brain.

In schizophrenia studies, measurement of the dopamine metabolite homovanillic acid (HVA) in plasma has provided interesting results in its correlation with good treatment outcome (Bowers et al. 1984; Davidson and Davis 1988; Pickar et al. 1986). Although it is tempting to take this peripheral metabolite measure as an indicator of brain dopamine metabolism, both common sense and data tend to discourage this (Elsworth et al. 1987). Activation and stress have been proposed as potentially critical primary factors in altering plasma HVA in schizophrenia. The use of plasma HVA as a marker of a disease characteristic rather than a measure of

regional brain biochemistry is still being pursued with positive results.

The measurement of transmitters and metabolites in lumbar cerebrospinal fluid (CSF) as a reflection of neurotransmitter activity in the brain has not critically contributed to our understanding of schizophrenia pathophysiology even though the CSF is in direct contact with brain tissue; moreover, its sampling and analysis are beset with potential confounds. Significant influences on study outcome include subject size, diet, seasonal and circadian variability, and sample dilution by CSF from nontarget areas. HVA is the CSF metabolite most studied (Bowers et al. 1969). Not surprisingly, results of these CSF studies of HVA are conflicting, with most studies reporting no change (reviewed in Issa et al. 1994a, 1994b) but with two studies reporting an HVA decrease in schizophrenia (Bjerkenstedt et al. 1985; Lindström et al. 1985). Postmortem tissue has provided the most valuable specimen source for biochemical studies. Several investigators have found regional increases in dopamine and/or its major metabolite HVA in schizophrenic brain in postmortem studies of tissue from schizophrenic individuals (Bacopoulos et al. 1979; Mackay et al. 1982; Owen et al. 1978; Reynolds 1983; Toru et al. 1988). These results can be expected to be regularly confounded by the ubiquitous use of neuroleptic medication in life in these patients, even when the analytic techniques are adequate and tissue collection is consistent. However, in at least one case a regional change in HVA was reported that is not likely to have been caused by neuroleptic treatment due to its localized nature (Reynolds 1983). Likewise, in the measurement of dopamine receptor density, studies have regularly reported increased dopamine type 2 (D_2)–family receptor density in caudate nucleus and putamen of schizophrenic individuals (Cross et al. 1981; Mackay et al. 1982; Reynolds and Mason 1995; Seeman et al. 1984). This latter change is almost always taken to be a consequence of long-term neuroleptic treatment and can be similarly demonstrated in rats (Clow et al. 1980; Shirakawa et al. 1994), monkeys (Lidow and Goldman-Rakic 1994), and neuroleptic-treated nonschizophrenic humans. The work comparing individual D_2-family receptors (D_2, D_3, and D_4) in tissue from neuroleptic-free schizophrenic persons with caudate nucleus or putamen tissue from healthy control subjects is currently being done in several laboratories and so far shows no differences in density of the D_2-family subtypes in striatum (R.A. Lahti et al. 1995; Reynolds and Mason 1995) (Figure 15–2).

Human brain imaging studies performed in vivo have been carried out with dopamine receptor ligands to look for dopamine receptor defects in schizophrenia. Although an initial study reported increases in D_2-family receptors in neuroleptic-naive and neuroleptic-free schizophrenic patients (Wong et al. 1986) and a later report suggested similar increases in psychotic nonschizophrenic individuals (Pearlson et al. 1995), subsequent studies using various other D_2 ligands and replications with the initial ligand have been unable to replicate this finding (Farde et al. 1990; Hietala et al. 1991; Martinot et al. 1990, 1991).

Laruelle et al. (1996) studied schizophrenia using single photon emission computed tomography (SPECT) or PET imaging of low-affinity dopamine receptor ligands to measure the quantity of dopamine released into the synapse under certain circumstances. These researchers reported that persons with schizophrenia, during the acute phases of their illness, have an increased release of dopamine

into the synapse in response to amphetamine challenge relative to healthy control subjects (Abi-Dargham et al. 1998). This increased release does not appear to be secondary to chronic antipsychotic treatment, as augmented release also occurs in first-episode patients (Laruelle et al. 1999). Persons with other psychiatric illnesses do not show increased release. This is one of the first replicated findings of dopaminergic dysfunction in schizophrenia.

Other Monoamines

Norepinephrine levels have consistently been found to be elevated in several studies of CSF in schizophrenia (Beckmann et al. 1983; Lake et al. 1980), even if only to a slight degree. Complementary studies looking for changes in noradrenergic receptors have been predominantly negative. Moreover, noradrenergic antagonist drugs do not reduce psychotic symptoms in schizophrenia. It has been suggested that the norepinephrine increases in CSF in schizophrenic individuals may be related to stress (van Kammen et al. 1990), but the increases have not been linked with psychosis.

Serotonin has recently been revisited for its potential role in schizophrenia because of the strong antiserotonergic action of clozapine. The unique antipsychotic clozapine is a potent 5-hydroxytryptamine type 2 (5-HT$_2$) receptor antagonist, suggesting a possible positive role (even if not primary) of this neurotransmitter system in psychosis response. The inconsistency of changes in serotonin levels in CSF or brain tissue or in its metabolite levels, or even in serotonin receptor binding in vivo, is apparent in this literature, discouraging a formulation of serotonin pathology as primary in schizophrenia. Also, the potential confound of long-term neuroleptic treatment in schizophrenia altering this measure in

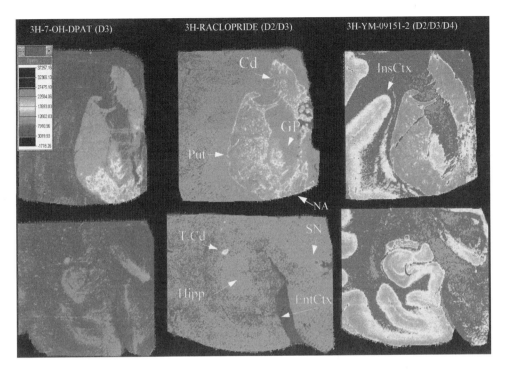

FIGURE 15–2. Binding of three different dopamine receptor ligands in human brain tissue to illustrate the localization of the dopamine type 2 (D$_2$) family receptors.

The top row includes three contiguous slices taken from a midstriatal coronal brain section; the bottom row includes three contiguous slices taken from an inferior midhippocampal coronal brain section. The left column shows binding of [^{3}H]7-OH DPAT, a ligand that labels dopamine type 3 (D$_3$) receptors, in both of these areas. D$_3$ receptors are localized chiefly in the inferior striatum nucleus accumbens (NA) and substantia nigra pars compacta (SN). The middle column shows binding of ^{3}H-raclopride, a ligand labeling D$_2$ and D$_3$ receptors. D$_2$ receptors are densely represented in the caudate nucleus (Cd) and putamen (Put) and are even apparent in the tail of the caudate nucleus (T.Cd); D$_2$ and D$_3$ receptors are intermingled in the nucleus accumbens and substantia nigra. The right column shows binding of [^{3}H]YM-09151-2, a ligand labeling D$_2$, D$_3$, and dopamine type 4 (D$_4$) receptors, in the two regions. A "mental" subtraction of the middle from the right autoradiograph suggests the D$_4$ localization to be predominantly in neocortex (InsCtx), hippocampus (Hipp), and entorhinal cortex (EntCtx). This illustration suggests that the D$_2$ receptor is predominantly localized in the caudate nucleus and putamen; the D$_2$ and D$_3$ receptors are localized in the nucleus accumbens and substantia nigra; and the D$_4$ receptor is predominant in the neocortex and in the hippocampal and parahippocampal cortices.

For a color version of this figure, please see the color insert at the back of this book.

Source. Autoradiograph contributed by Dr. Robert Lahti.

CSF or in postmortem brain tissue must again be recognized (Elkashef et al. 1995). However, the possibility that modifying serotonin transmission may be important to an optimal antipsychotic response in schizophrenia is interesting.

On the rather timely assumption that neurotransmitter interactions may be important in schizophrenia, one study compared the levels of 17 neurotransmit-

ters and their related metabolites in the CSF of untreated schizophrenic patients with those in healthy control subjects. While the levels of metabolites of dopamine, serotonin, or norepinephrine were found not to discriminate groups, a multivariate analysis of the entire data set found that the combination of tryptophan, tryptophol, and epinephrine discriminated the schizophrenic group from the control group. Although they do not identify anything specific about biochemistry in schizophrenia, these results— along with reports of kynurenic acid abnormalities in postmortem cortex from schizophrenic individuals (Schwarcz et al. 2001)—focus attention on the potential importance of the kynurenine pathway of tryptophan metabolism in schizophrenia (Issa et al. 1994a, 1994b). The identification of this association does not imply causality, especially knowing that it is reasonable to consider changes in excitatory neural transmission as a consequence, as well as a possible cause, of schizophrenia. Biochemical evidence of monoamine involvement in schizophrenia mechanisms is not strong, but the potential involvement of these systems in therapeutics remains an active possibility.

Glutamate

More than a decade ago, the report of reduced glutamate levels in CSF of schizophrenic patients was interpreted to suggest neuronal hypoglutamatergic function in the illness (Kim et al. 1980). This report was not consistently replicated (Gattaz et al. 1985; Korpi et al. 1987; Macciardi et al. 1990). Because the fraction of CSF glutamate considered to come from the transmitter pool is so small (<5%), this CSF method was not considered sensitive enough to uncover potential changes. However, Kornhuber's idea (Kim et al. 1980) of reduced glutamatergic transmission in schizophrenia has continued to capture the interest of the field. This has been the case in part because of the demonstration of the antiglutamatergic action of phencyclidine (PCP) (Anis et al. 1983), a drug with psychotomimetic (perhaps schizophrenia-like) properties at the NMDA receptor (Domino and Luby 1981). This demonstration allowed the hypothesis that PCP has its psychotomimetic properties secondary to its anti-

glutamatergic actions and that perhaps this is the mechanism of endogenous psychosis (Deutsch et al. 1989; Olney and Farber 1995). This hypothesis continues to be actively explored.

Ulas and Cotman (1993) looked carefully at NMDA, α-amino-3-hydroxy-5-methyl-4-isoxalone propionic acid (AMPA), and kainate receptors in schizophrenic hippocampus, albeit in a limited number of patients ($N = 4$), without identifying definite group changes. These researchers commented on striking individual changes, however, leading to their suggestion of deafferentation of the hippocampus in some schizophrenic subjects. More recent studies of NMDA-sensitive receptor subunits suggest the possibility of a change in NMDA receptor composition in schizophrenia, which could alter glutamatergic transmission (Gao et al. 2000).

Overall, the literature on the involvement of glutamate in schizophrenia is suggestive, but the findings have not been entirely consistent in pointing out a particular defect (Tamminga 1998). It is important to note that many assessments for the glutamate system in mammalian brain are early and lack sensitivity and selectivity. Moreover, our understanding of the processes involved in glutamatergic transmission is yet incomplete.

Functional Processing: Psychological and Electrophysiological

Psychological assessment of brain activity in schizophrenia might be expected to provide the most relevant clues to abnormalities in the illness, because the core symptoms of schizophrenia are of a cognitive variety. Even though it is difficult to distinguish the brain of a schizophrenic person from the brain of a healthy person by traditional anatomic or biochemical features, several psychological and physiologic measures are clearly able to provide distinguishing features between the two groups. Any ability to account for these differences with a compelling biological explanation would certainly enable advances in our concepts of mechanisms in the illness.

Psychological Characteristics

Specific neuropsychological deficits in schizophrenia are broad; they include memory, executive function, and motor performance (Braff et al. 1991; Gold et al. 1992; Goldberg et al. 1990; Gruzelier et al. 1988; R.C. Gur et al. 1991; Liddle and Morris 1991). No cognitive domains are entirely spared, and deficits in performance are highly intercorrelated within persons (Sullivan et al. 1994). Schizophrenic subjects in many of the studies show a pattern of deficits, ruling out a complete lack of motivation as a factor in performance. In schizophrenic persons, memory deficits occur (as shown, for example, in the recurring digit span test) that are consistent with temporohippocampal dysfunction (Gruzelier et al. 1988). Tests of frontal cortical function are also abnormal (e.g., verbal fluency, spatial performance, pattern recognition), and long-term memory deficits have been documented (Gruzelier et al. 1988). The study of identical twins discordant for schizophrenia has been a highly productive technique in providing a genetically matched control group, circumventing critical comparison confounds. In such a study, Goldberg and colleagues found that almost all schizophrenic twins performed more poorly than their unaffected identical co-twin on all performance measures. Specifically, the schizophrenic twin performed significantly worse on assessments of intelligence, memory, attention, verbal fluency, and pattern recognition than their

identical twin control subject. The performance of nonschizophrenic twins did not differ from that of unrelated healthy control subjects except for reduced performance in "logical memory" (Wechsler Adult Intelligence Scale [WAIS]) and in Trails A; in both of these cognitive areas, performance was still considerably different between the schizophrenic and nonschizophrenic twins (Goldberg et al. 1990).

Similarly, persons with schizophrenia consistently perform poorly on tasks that require sustained attention or vigilance (Nuechterlein et al. 1992). Other studies document deficits in memory, including explicit memory and verbal memory (Gold et al. 1994; Saykin et al. 1991). Working memory, which permits task-relevant information to be kept active for brief periods, has received much attention in the schizophrenia literature. Individuals with schizophrenia have difficulties maintaining working memory (Goldman-Rakic 1994; Park and Holzman 1992). Deficits in working memory may explain serious disorganization and functional deterioration observed in the schizophrenia spectrum. This is because the ability to hold information "online" is critical for organizing future thoughts and actions in the context of the recent past (Goldman-Rakic 1994).

Several studies have observed that the first-degree relatives of schizophrenic probands demonstrate many of the cognitive deficits observed in schizophrenia, even though these individuals do not experience overt psychosis (Asarnow et al. 1991; Balogh and Merritt 1985; Braff 1981; Cornblatt et al. 1989; Green et al. 1997; Park et al. 1995). These deficits include impairments in different dimensions of attention, language comprehension, verbal fluency, verbal memory, and spatial working memory. This pattern of findings has been documented by two of the most comprehensive studies of relatives of schizophrenic patients (Cannon et al. 1994; Faraone et al. 1995). These studies show that even after adjusting for IQ, measures of auditory attention, abstraction, and verbal memory differentiated relatives of patients with schizophrenia from the comparison groups.

These data on neuropsychological function in schizophrenia are consistent with an overall brain disturbance in cognitive ability. Complicating these considerations further are the observations that the cognitive defects are not present in every person at all times and that the pattern of defects can change over time within an individual. This makes it hard to propose permanent changes in connectivity in the illness and forces a concept of flexible or reversible functional changes.

Neurophysiological Deficits

From the beginning of the twentieth century, studies have suggested an abnormality in the smooth-pursuit eye movements in schizophrenia (Clementz and Sweeney 1990; Holzman 1987). Extensive work carried out by Holzman and others in schizophrenic patients has shown that the measure is stable, and the findings in schizophrenia cannot be explained by disease-related factors or overt psychotic symptoms (Clementz and Sweeney 1990; Holzman 1987). Many of the nonpsychotic family members of schizophrenic patients also show poor pursuit as measured globally (Keefe et al. 1997; Thaker et al. 1996, 1998), by pursuit gain (Clementz et al. 1990), or by other measures (Clementz and Sweeney 1990; Whicker et al. 1985). Most studies note that abnormalities in smooth-pursuit eye movements occur mostly in relatives with schizophrenia-spectrum personality symptoms (Arolt et al. 1996a; Clementz et al. 1990; Thaker et al. 1996); one study did not find such an association (Keefe et

al. 1997). Studies that examined eye movements in individuals with schizophrenia-spectrum personality with and without a known family history of schizophrenia noted smooth-pursuit deficits only in subjects who had a positive family history of schizophrenia (Thaker et al. 1996, 1998). A preliminary report found linkage of the smooth-pursuit eye movement abnormality to chromosome 6p21 in relatives of patients with schizophrenia (Arolt et al. 1996b). Based on psychophysical motion perception experiments, some investigators have argued that there is a deficit in motion processing in schizophrenia, thus explaining the smooth-pursuit eye movement abnormality (Chen et al. 1999). Based on the findings of normal saccadic eye movements to a moving target, others have argued that the underlying deficit occurs subsequent to the motion processing, during either the integration of the motion signal into a smooth-pursuit response (Sweeney et al. 1994) or the holding of the motion signal "online" for the smooth-pursuit maintenance (Thaker et al. 1998, 1999). The latter hypothesis would implicate lesions in posterior parietal and/or frontal cortical ocular motor regions associated with the smooth-pursuit abnormality in schizophrenia. This assertion is supported by the findings from two functional imaging studies in schizophrenia-spectrum disorders (O'Driscoll et al. 1999; Ross et al. 1995).

In addition to the smooth-pursuit abnormality, recent studies note subtle abnormalities in saccadic measures in schizophrenic patients (Crawford et al. 1998; Fukushima et al. 1988; Thaker et al. 1996). These studies examined performance in an antisaccade task in which subjects were instructed to look in the opposite direction of a target jump. Patients with schizophrenia made more errors (i.e., made saccades to the target rather than away from the target) than the comparison groups. Nonpsychotic relatives, akin to the findings in schizophrenia, also show an inability to inhibit an inappropriate saccade toward the target (Clementz et al. 1994; Crawford et al. 1998; Katsanis et al. 1997; McDowell et al. 1999; Thaker et al. 1996, 2000). This deficit is modestly correlated with the smooth-pursuit abnormality in the relatives of schizophrenic patients (Thaker et al. 2000). The saccadic findings also implicate frontal cortical regions in schizophrenia (Berman et al. 1999).

Evoked Potentials and Sensory Gating

In contrast to the neuropsychological and eye-movement studies, neurophysiological studies have identified abnormalities in information processing that can often be elicited in the absence of a behavioral response. P300 has increased latency and decreased amplitude in persons with schizophrenia. Although these electroencephalographic measures may vary with changes in symptoms, the P300 amplitude is consistently small in schizophrenia even during relative remission of psychotic symptoms (Blackwood et al. 1991; Pfefferbaum et al. 1984). Other components of evoked potential are observed to be abnormal in schizophrenia. Mismatched negativity response that occurs earlier than P300 is observed to have smaller amplitude in schizophrenia, which suggests an abnormality in the early response to stimulus novelty (Javitt et al. 1995).

In contrast to a healthy comparison group, persons with schizophrenia show poor prepulse inhibition. Braff and others have proposed that schizophrenia is associated with an inability to gate sensory information, leading to sensory overload (Braff 1993). According to this hypothesis, positive symptoms develop due to

misinterpretation or misidentification of unfiltered sensory information. Negative symptoms may occur due to the withdrawal from the sensory overload.

Sensory gating is also evaluated by using positive change in the evoked potentials 50 msec (P50) after each of two auditory stimuli presented about 500 msec apart (Freedman et al. 1987). Normally, subjects show a much muted evoked potential response to the second stimulus compared with the first stimulus. In contrast, the P50 evoked potential response in schizophrenia is of similar amplitude as the response to the preceding stimulus. The ratio of amplitude of P50 response to the second (test) stimulus to the amplitude of the first (conditioning) stimulus is generally used as a measure of gating. Using a ratio of 0.4 or lower as normal and 0.5 or higher as abnormal gating, a segregation analysis in the families of patients with schizophrenia suggested that P50 gating deficit is a result of an autosomal dominant effect of a single gene. Subsequent linkage analysis showed evidence for linkage of the gating deficit in families of schizophrenic patients with markers of location in the chromosome 15q14 region (Freedman et al. 1997). This region has been shown to be the locus of the α-7 nicotinic cholinergic receptor subunit gene, although no molecular abnormality has yet been found in this region of linkage (Freedman et al. 1999).

Functional Studies Using In Vivo Imaging Techniques

Positron Emission Tomography With Fluorodeoxyglucose

PET with fluorodeoxyglucose (FDG) was the first high-resolution functional imaging modality used in schizophrenia. Local uptake of FDG correlates with synaptic neuronal activity under physiologic condi-

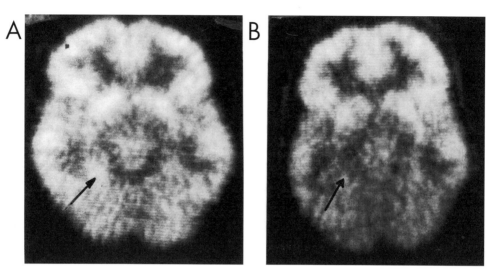

FIGURE 15–3. Positron emission tomographic images with fluorodeoxyglucose.

Both images are at the same axial level and show, among other areas, the medial temporal structures. *Panel A* is an image from a healthy control subject; the general area of parahippocampal gyrus/hippocampus is indicated by the arrow. In the schizophrenic individual (*Panel B*) there is a remarkable reduction in glucose metabolism in the medial temporal structures (arrow). This reduction in parahippocampal gyrus metabolism is representative of differences in the entire schizophrenic group.

tions (Kadekaro 1987). Detecting evidence of disease requires careful control of test conditions and a robust primary effect.

First, studies reported relative hypometabolism in frontal cortex, a finding consistent with earlier blood flow studies (Buchsbaum et al. 1982; Ingvar and Franzen 1971). Subsequent FDG PET studies in schizophrenia produced inconsistent detection of frontal cortex hypometabolism, with some studies continuing to find it (Buchsbaum et al. 1984), others reporting no change in the measure (Tamminga et al. 1992), and still others finding frontal hypermetabolism (Cleghorn et al. 1989). These controversies now can be partially explained by two potential confounds: a neuroleptic effect and a skewed target population effect. Neuroleptics reduce cerebral metabolism in frontal cortex (Holcomb et al. 1996a), thus likely producing a confound in those early studies that compared neuroleptic-treated schizophrenic persons with

healthy control subjects. We also know that frontal cortical dysfunction is associated with deficit (negative)–type schizophrenia, seemingly selectively. The composition of a patient group with neuroleptic-treated, deficit-type schizophrenic persons (who are often available for study) will skew the results. Other results at first associated with the disease (for example, increased metabolism in the caudate nucleus and putamen) are now known to be a neuroleptic effect (Holcomb et al. 1996a; Szechtman et al. 1988).

Our own studies detected metabolic differences in schizophrenia in limbic structures (anterior cingulate and hippocampal cortices), with both areas showing reduced metabolism (Figure 15–3). Within the schizophrenic group, primary negative-symptom patients showed the additional abnormalities of reduced metabolism in frontal and parietal cortices and thalamus compared with the non-negative-symptom group. Both of these findings (limbic changes overall in schizophrenia, and frontal cortex reductions in negative symptoms) are consistent with considerable other literature in their regional localization (Andreasen et al. 1992; Tamminga et al. 1992). Reflecting the pathology found in postmortem tissue studies of schizophrenia, these results are consistent with limbic cortical dysfunction associated with the illness, particularly with its positive symptoms.

Regional Cerebral Blood Flow Studies

Regional cerebral blood flow (rCBF) studies were originally done using xenon 133 with individual cortical detectors.

More recently, blood flow studies using contemporary scanning and analytic techniques to examine normal and schizophrenic persons during performance of hierarchical tasks within a single task modality (Raichle 1994) have begun to reveal fascinating aspects of CNS function. The use of a variable error-rate task with all subjects fixed to the same performance level has been an innovation in this area, allowing comparisons without a prominent performance confound (Holcomb et al. 1996b, 2000). We have generated an rCBF comparison between schizophrenic patients and matched nonschizophrenic control subjects, conducted while both groups are performing a practiced auditory recognition task at a similar performance level (for example, with task difficulty set to an 80% error level). The schizophrenic subjects had considerably more activation in extent and magnitude of response in the control task, showing activation not only in the superior temporal auditory cortex (left > right) but also in the left premotor cortex, left parietal cortex, right insula, and cingulate cortex. In the decision task (in which control subjects demonstrated considerable activation in these regions) the schizophrenic

subjects showed very little incremental increase in activation except for a mild flow increase in right frontal cortex (Figure 15–4). Overall, in comparing the "decision minus rest" subtraction between groups, the schizophrenic patients showed activation of approximately the same areas as control subjects. Significantly more of this activation (which accompanied the decision task in nonschizophrenic subjects) was recruited for the relatively easy control (sensorimotor) task in the schizophrenic subjects. Moreover, when the patients increased their performance in the decision task (demonstrated by reduced accuracy and slower response times), no additional flow changes were apparent. Patients were performing this task at a similar accuracy level as nonschizophrenic subjects.

Other scientists have used this method to understand the localization and type of functional defects in schizophrenia as well. Liddle and colleagues (1992) studied the correlation between well-delineated symptom clusters in schizophrenia (negative symptoms, hallucinations/delusions, and disorganization) and rCBF. Most interesting was the demonstration in this study, as well as elsewhere, that in vivo functional manifestations associated with schizophrenia are diverse. In overview, Liddle reported that negative symptoms were negatively associated with rCBF in left frontal cortex and left parietal areas. Hallucinations and delusions were positively associated with flow in the left parahippocampal gyrus and the left ventral striatum. Disorganization was associated with flow in anterior cingulate cortex and mediodorsal thalamus. This study shows that different brain areas are differently involved in symptom manifestations in schizophrenia, perhaps either as a cause or an effect of the disorder. A $H_2^{15}O$ PET study of hallucinating schizophrenic persons revealed several CNS

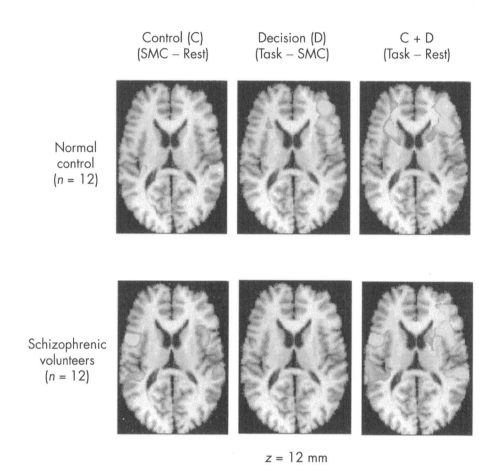

Control (C)   Decision (D)   C + D
(SMC – Rest)   (Task – SMC)   (Task – Rest)

Normal
control
(*n* = 12)

Schizophrenic
volunteers
(*n* = 12)

z = 12 mm

FIGURE 15–4.   Regional cerebral blood flow elevations seen at an axial level 12 mm above the anterior commissure–posterior commissure (ACPC) line in healthy control (*top row*) and schizophrenic (*bottom row*) subjects, each in a sensorimotor control (SMC) (*left column*) and a decision performance (*middle column*) condition.

Control subjects merely activate the auditory cortex bilaterally (*upper left scan*) and the left motor cortex (data not shown) in the sensorimotor task, whereas the schizophrenic subjects activate those more and in more areas than control subjects (*bottom left scan*). During the decision task, the control subjects activate middle and inferior frontal cortex (*upper middle scan*) and anterior cingulate gyrus (data not shown); however the schizophrenic subjects do not recruit any additional areas or increase flow at all in their decision condition (*lower middle scan*). Overall, the schizophrenic subjects resemble the control subjects in the "task minus rest" analysis (*upper and lower right scans*), even though that activation occurred primarily in the control, not the decision, scan.

For a color version of this figure, please see the color insert at the back of this book.

Source.   Images contributed by Dr. Henry Holcomb and Dr. Adrienne Lahti.

regions that activated in the subjects in association with hallucinations; these were the left and right thalamus, right putamen, left and right parahippocampal areas, and right anterior cingulate cortex. Cortical activations were present, but their cortical localizations were highly variable between the subjects and not significant in group analysis (Silbersweig et al. 1995). Further work from this group has shown that apomorphine (which is antipsychotic in schizophrenia, despite being a dopamine agonist) improves (i.e., "normalizes") the anterior cingulate cortical blood flow of schizophrenic persons during verbal fluency task performance (Dolan et al. 1995).

Other studies have also found evidence for limbic abnormalities in schizophrenia both at rest (Taylor et al. 1999) and with cognitive challenge (Artiges et al. 2000; Heckers et al. 1998; Spence et al. 1997). Heckers et al. (1998) found reduced hippocampal activation in schizophrenic subjects during a memory-retrieval task of previously studied words. These findings complement other postmortem and structural imaging studies of abnormalities in medial temporal lobe structures of schizophrenic individuals (Gao et al. 2000). Spence et al. (1997) studied schizophrenic subjects performing a complex motor task during an acute exacerbation of their illness and 4–6 weeks later, after their symptoms had improved. Although the subjects were acutely ill, they showed signs of prefrontal hypometabolism. When the schizophrenic volunteers' symptoms improved, the prefrontal regions were normal. However, when the schizophrenics were less symptomatic, rCBF in the anterior cingulate and bilateral parietal regions was still found to be decreased. These limbic region abnormalities are probably the result of a dysfunctional network of regions and not a series of separate lesions.

Functional Magnetic Resonance Imaging Studies

Several functional magnetic resonance imaging (fMRI) studies have explored whether rCBF changes in response to simple motor tasks are normal in schizophrenic volunteers. Braus et al. (1999) found no rCBF differences between first-episode, never-medicated schizophrenic volunteers and nonschizophrenic volunteers while they were performing a sequential finger-thumb opposition task. In the same study, these researchers found a decrease in the blood oxygen level dependent response in the sensorimotor cortices of schizophrenic volunteers medicated with traditional neuroleptics. Other studies of this task found no differences (Buckley et al. 1997), increased rCBF in the sensorimotor cortices of the schizophrenic subjects (Mattay et al. 1997), and decreases in those regions (Schroder et al. 1999). In these studies, the schizophrenic volunteers were medicated with a mixture of traditional and atypical neuroleptics. These results suggest that previous exposure to neuroleptics can have an interactive effect with task performance.

In more cognitively demanding tasks, such as working memory tasks, the fMRI results are also inconsistent. Manoach et al. (1999, 2000) used the Sternberg Item Recognition working memory paradigm, which required the subjects to remember either two or five digits. Unlike in many PET studies of working memory, these researchers found an increase instead of a decrease in prefrontal rCBF in the schizophrenic volunteers compared with the nonschizophrenic control subjects. Callicott et al. (1998), using the N-Back task, and Stevens et al. (1998), using the word and tone serial position tasks, found decreases in rCBF in inferior frontal regions of schizophrenic subjects. The task performance of the schizophrenic subjects was significantly worse on the N-Back and word serial position tasks but was matched on the tone task. Research has shown that although rCBF increases in prefrontal regions with greater working memory demands, if working memory capacity is exceeded, the activation decreases (Callicott et al. 1999). Manoach suggests that the discrepant findings in schizophrenia may be explained by an overload of working memory in schizophrenic subjects for some tasks.

These kinds of rCBF studies provide us with information now about brain mechanisms and schizophrenia, and they indicate the extent to which in vivo imaging techniques can teach us about schizophrenia brain mechanisms.

Clinical Therapeutics

Antipsychotic Drug Pharmacology

Drug development in the area of schizophrenia therapeutics has focused on dopamine receptor blockade and has been highly productive, even though empirical. Many potent, broadly active, and selective dopamine receptor antagonists were developed during the first 15 years after the discovery of chlorpromazine; these have become widely available for clinical use and have been universally applied. The drugs are all similar in their primary actions but distinctive in side-effect profile (reviewed in Klein and Davis 1969). Clozapine has a unique antipsychotic action in neuroleptic nonresponding schizophrenics compared with chlorpromazine (Kane et al. 1988). Also, clozapine produces few if any motor side effects (despite its other serious side effects), thus increasing patient comfort, social adjustment, and medication compliance. Since the clinical actions of clozapine have been clarified, several clozapine-like new neuroleptic compounds with fewer side effects have been developed and are becoming available. The pharmacologic characteristics speculatively identified as important in these new antipsychotic drugs include 1) a restricted action on dopamine neurons, as reflected in a limited expression of depolarization inactivation in A10 but not A9 dopamine cell body areas; 2) multiple monoamine receptor blockade; and 3) lower dopamine receptor affinity.

We have studied the localization of haloperidol action in the brain in schizophrenia using PET with FDG (Holcomb et al. 1996a). Previous reports documented an increase in glucose metabolism in the caudate nucleus and putamen with typical neuroleptics (R.E. Gur et al. 1987; Szechtman et al. 1988). Our study confirms that finding. In addition, we found hypermetabolism in the anterior thalamus and decreased metabolism in the frontal cortex (middle and inferior gyri) and anterior cingulate areas (Figure 15–5). Based on the known anatomic connections and their primary transmitters between basal ganglia structures and neocortex, we have hypothesized a primary drug action of haloperidol in the basal ganglia (caudate nucleus and putamen) with secondary and tertiary effects being propagated to other related brain areas over the parallel distributed neuronal circuits.

Glutamate System Pharmacology

Although there is no current evidence that glutamatergic drugs are therapeutic in schizophrenia, there are several reasons to be interested in the pharmacology of this system. First, the excitatory amino acid (EAA) system, the chief transmitter of which is glutamate, is ubiquitous in the brain; nearly every CNS cell bears EAA-sensitive receptors, indicating the extent of this system's influence. It is a complex system that has at least two major transmitters (glutamate and aspartate) and probably several minor ones; it has at least four families of receptors, three ionotropic (NMDA-sensitive, AMPA, and kainate) and one metabotropic, with each individual receptor having its own unique distribution, pharmacology, and probably distinctive functions. EAAs are the chief excitatory transmitters in the brain. They mediate not only everyday information transmission functions but are also

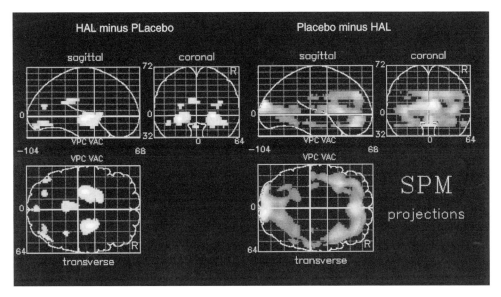

FIGURE 15–5.   Projection images showing significant areas of haloperidol (HAL)–induced increases (*left*) and decreases (*right*) in regional cerebral metabolic rate for glucose (rCMRglu) from group subtraction Statistical Parametric Mapping (SPM) analyses, in within-subject comparisons.

On the left, rCMRglu increases are apparent in the caudate nucleus, putamen, and anterior thalamus; on the right, rCMRglu decreases are apparent in anterior cingulate gyrus, occipital area, and frontal cortex (middle and inferior gyri).

VAC = vertical anterior commissure line; VPC = vertical posterior commissure line.

For a color version of this figure, please see the color insert at the back of this book.

Source.   Images contributed by Dr. Henry Holcomb.

thought to be involved in other kinds of brain activity, such as developmental pruning, learning and memory, and neuronal plasticity. Certainly the EAAs must mediate some aspects of psychosis due to their ubiquitous involvement in the CNS. Whether they are involved in schizophrenia in a more primary way is an interesting speculation.

The reason to suspect a connection between one part of the glutamate system, the NMDA-sensitive glutamate receptor system, and schizophrenia is based on the actions of PCP and its congener ketamine on human cognition. PCP produces a complex array of behaviors in humans. It can induce a psychotic state in nonschizophrenic persons (without delirium) that is characterized by many of the signs and symptoms often found in schizophrenia.

Moreover, PCP (Luby et al. 1959) and ketamine (A.C. Lahti et al. 1995b) can both selectively exacerbate a patient's psychotic symptoms in schizophrenia, suggesting an action on (or near) the site of schizophrenia pathophysiology. Associated with the NMDA-sensitive glutamate receptor is a PCP recognition site located inside of the NMDA-gated ion channel; the PCP site antagonizes ionic flow through the channel. This is a complex receptor site where NMDA, glycine, and polyamines positively gate ion flow into the cell and PCP, Zn^{2+}, and Mg^{2+} inhibit flow. It is presumed, based on a number of different observations, that PCP and ketamine both exert several of their important behavior actions through effects at the NMDA receptor (Javitt and Zukin 1991; A.C. Lahti et al. 1995b).

Not only does ketamine cause psychosis-like experiences in nonschizophrenic persons and exacerbate psychosis in schizophrenia, it also functionally affects rCBF directly in the brain areas in which postmortem tissue and in vivo imaging studies indicate dysfunction in schizophrenic persons—specifically, in hippocampal and anterior cingulate cortices. Behaviorally, ketamine increases psychosis at subanesthetic doses in both neuroleptic-treated and neuroleptic-free schizophrenic patients to the same degree. Ketamine stimulates positive, not negative, symptoms in schizophrenia, and its action is not blocked by dopamine receptor antagonism (A.C. Lahti et al. 1995b). Symptoms that are stimulated by ketamine are that person's characteristic set of schizophrenic hallucinations, delusions, and/or thought disorder. This is unlike other psychotomimetics (for example, amphetamine or muscimol), which stimulate psychotomimetic symptoms typical of the drug. This action of ketamine would be most parsimoniously explained by assuming that the drug stimulates a brain system that is already active in mediating the psychosis.

We studied the localization and time course of ketamine action in brain using $H_2^{15}O$ and PET, measuring rCBF (Figure 15–6). Schizophrenic subjects, at a dose of ketamine active in exacerbating psychosis (0.3 mg/kg), showed increased rCBF in the anterior cingulate gyrus and decreased rCBF in hippocampus and lingual gyrus (A.C. Lahti et al. 1995a). The brain areas that showed a change had different time course patterns of rCBF over the 60 minutes after ketamine administration. This suggests that each area of brain has its own sensitivity to ketamine (which might be predicted on the basis of receptor localization and anatomic connections) and its own unique time course of response. Because other drugs have not been studied this way in humans, it is impossible to know whether this phenomenon is common, unusual, or unique. It does mean that ketamine at a behaviorally active (not anesthetic) dose produces rCBF actions in specific brain regions (more restricted than its receptor distribution would predict) and that the response of various cerebral regions appears independent. Questions of how this ketamine-induced psychosis stimulation might be related to schizophrenia still need to be answered.

Synthesis

Clinical Observations Important for Formulating Pathophysiology

Several characteristics of schizophrenic illness are strikingly consistent across clinics, laboratories, and cultures, such that any theory of the illness must take them into account. These include but are not limited to the following: schizophrenic symptoms are clear and their clustering is common although not exclusive; symptoms fluctuate during the course of illness and may disappear entirely between episodes but then reappear; the illness is most often lifelong, with the most flagrant symptoms and psychosocial deterioration appearing early in the illness, showing a plateau during middle years, and frequently ending with some degree of symptom resolution in later years. The illness has a genetic component but is by no means fully genetically determined. Although no traditional anatomic or biochemical change has come to be pathognomonic of the illness, the limbic system (especially hippocampus and entorhinal and cingulate cortices) is the cerebral location where anatomic and functional changes are highly concentrated, albeit changes of a varied pathologic nature.

SPM, p<0.01, N=5,6 minutes

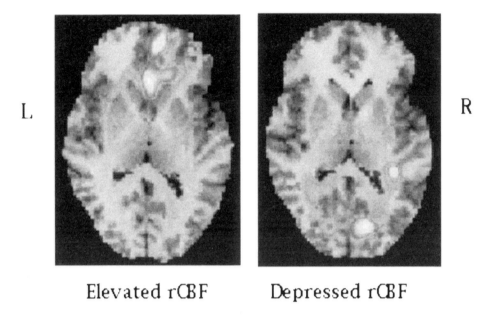

L   R

Elevated rCBF   Depressed rCBF

FIGURE 15–6.   Regional cerebral blood flow (rCBF) localization of ketamine action in schizophrenic brain.

rCBF increases occurred in anterior cingulate gyrus, extending to medial frontal areas (*left scan*); rCBF decreases are apparent in hippocampus and in the lingual gyrus (*right scan*). The colored areas indicating significant flow change are plotted onto a magnetic resonance imaging template for ease of localization.

SPM = Statistical Parametric Mapping.

For a color version of this figure, please see the color insert at the back of this book.

Source.   Images contributed by Dr. Henry Holcomb and Dr. Adrienne Lahti.

Pharmacologically, only the antagonism of dopamine-mediated transmission with neuroleptics has been therapeutic. Other pharmacologic approaches have so far resulted in negative outcomes. On the other hand, several pharmacologic strategies are psychotomimetic, including such drugs as amphetamine, lysergic acid diethylamide (LSD), mescaline, muscimol, and PCP/ketamine. Of these, PCP/ketamine is the drug class that most faithfully mimics schizophrenia in normal persons and most potently and validly exacerbates schizophrenia symptoms in affected patients even while inducing minimal primary drug symptoms. In addition, ketamine alters rCBF in cingulate cortex,

hippocampus, and lingual gyrus, the first two areas being those previously related to schizophrenia using other functional imaging techniques.

People with schizophrenia have pervasive, patterned, but interrelated cognitive dysfunction, suggesting a failure of an interactive connective function. Schizophrenic subjects, even when they are performing a task equivalent to healthy control subjects, utilize similar brain areas but activate them prematurely and not in relationship to difficulty, as is the case in nonschizophrenic individuals. The anterior cingulate cortex especially demonstrates these differences. Moreover, whereas limbic areas might be broadly affected in all or most schizophrenic sub-jects, the frontal cortex and other neocor-tical areas seem to be associated with other discrete manifestations of illness, such as negative symptoms or deficit syn-drome. Evidence of consistent, highly rep-licable biochemical change in the brain in schizophrenia has yet evaded the study of this illness. This does not mean that these parameters should not be studied, but it might suggest that only a composite bio-chemical change will give a clue (see, for example, Issa et al. 1994a and 1994b) or that an entirely new (perhaps functional) approach is needed.

References

Abi-Dargham A, Gil R, Krystal J, et al: In-creased striatal dopamine transmission in schizophrenia: confirmation in a second cohort. Am J Psychiatry 155:761–767, 1998

Akbarian S, Bunney WE, Potkin SG, et al: Altered distribution of nicotinamide-adenine dinucleotide phosphate-diapho-rase cells in frontal lobe of schizophrenics implies disturbances of cortical develop-ment. Arch Gen Psychiatry 50:169–177, 1993

Akbarian S, Kim JJ, Potkin SG, et al: Gene ex-pression for glutamic acid decarboxylase is reduced without loss of neurons in pre-frontal cortex of schizophrenics. Arch Gen Psychiatry 52:258–266, 1995

American Psychiatric Association: Diagnostic and Statistical Manual of Mental Disor-ders, 4th Edition, Text Revision. Washing-ton, DC, American Psychiatric Associa-tion, 2000

Andreasen NC: Symptoms, signs, and diagno-sis of schizophrenia. Lancet 346:477–481, 1995

Andreasen NC, Rezai K, Alliger R, et al: Hypo-frontality in neuroleptic-naive patients and in patients with chronic schizophre-nia. Arch Gen Psychiatry 49:943–958, 1992

Andreasen NC, Arndt S, Swayze V II, et al: Thalamic abnormalities in schizophrenia visualized through magnetic resonance image averaging. Science 266:294–298, 1994

Andreasen NC, Arndt S, Alliger R, et al: Symptoms of schizophrenia. Methods, meanings, and mechanisms. Arch Gen Psychiatry 52:341–351, 1995

Anis NA, Berry SC, Burton NR, et al: The dis-sociative anesthetics ketamine and phen-cyclidine selectively reduce excitation of central mammalian neurons by N-methyl-aspartate. Br J Pharmacol 79:5654–5675, 1983

Arndt S, Alliger RJ, Andreasen NC: The dis-tinction of positive and negative symp-toms: the failure of a two-dimensional model. Br J Psychiatry 158:317–322, 1991

Arnold SE, Hyman BT, Van Hoesen GW, et al: Some cytoarchitectural abnormalities of the entorhinal cortex in schizophrenia. Arch Gen Psychiatry 48:625–632, 1991a

Arnold SE, Lee VM-Y, Gur RE, et al: Abnormal expression of two microtubule-associated proteins (MAP2 and MAP5) in specific subfields of the hippocampal formation in schizophrenia. Proc Natl Acad Sci U S A 88:10850–10854, 1991b

Arolt V, Lencer R, Nolte A, et al: Eye tracking dysfunction in families with multiple cases of schizophrenia. Eur Arch Psychia-try Clin Neurosci 246(4):175–181, 1996a

Arolt V, Lencer R, Nolte A, et al: Eye tracking dysfunction is a putative phenotypic sus-ceptibility marker of schizophrenia and maps to a locus on chromosome 6p in families with multiple occurrence of the disease. Am J Med Genet 67(6):564–579, 1996b

Artiges E, Salame P, Recasens C, et al: Working memory control in patients with schizo-phrenia: a PET study during a random number generation task. Am J Psychiatry 157:1517–1519, 2000

Asarnow RF, Granholm E, Sherman T: Span of Apprehension in schizophrenia, in Handbook of Schizophrenia, Vol 5: Neuropsychology, Psychophysiology and Information Processing. Edited by Steinhauer SR, Gruzelier JH, Zubin J. Amsterdam, Elsevier, 1991, pp 335–370

Bacopoulos NG, Spokes EG, Bird ED, et al: Antipsychotic drug action in schizophrenic patients: effect on cortical dopamine metabolism after long-term treatment. Science 205: 1405–1407, 1979

Balogh DW, Merritt RD: Susceptibility to type A backward pattern masking among hypothetically psychosis-prone college students. J Abnorm Psychol 94(3):377–383, 1985

Barnes TR, Liddle PF: Evidence for the validity of negative symptoms. Mod Probl Pharmacopsychiatry 24:43–72, 1990

Barta PE, Pearlson GD, Powers RE, et al: Auditory hallucinations and smaller superior temporal gyral volume in schizophrenia. Am J Psychiatry 146:1457–1462, 1990

Beckmann H, Waldmeier P, Lauber J, et al: Phenylethylamine and monoamine metabolites in CSF of schizophrenics: effects of neuroleptic treatment. J Neural Transm 57:103–110, 1983

Benes FM: Neurobiological investigations in cingulate cortex of schizophrenic brain. Schizophr Bull 19(3):537–549, 1993

Berman RA, Colby CL, Genovese CR, et al: Cortical networks subserving pursuit and saccadic eye movements in humans: an fMRI study. Hum Brain Mapp 8:209–225, 1999

Bjerkenstedt I, Edman G, Hagenfeldt I, et al: Plasma amino acids in relation to cerebrospinal fluid monoamine metabolites in schizophrenic patients and healthy controls. Br J Psychiatry 147:276–282, 1985

Blackwood DH, St Clair DM, Muir WJ, et al: Auditory P300 and eye tracking dysfunction in schizophrenic pedigrees. Arch Gen Psychiatry 48(10):899–909, 1991

Bleuler M: The Schizophrenic Disorders: Long-Term Patient and Family Studies. Translated by Clemens SM. New Haven, CT, Yale University Press, 1978

Bogerts B: Recent advances in the neuropathology of schizophrenia. Schizophr Bull 19(2):431–445, 1993

Bogerts B, Ashtari M, Degreef G, et al: Reduced temporal limbic structure volumes on magnetic resonance images in first episode schizophrenia. Psychiatry Res 35:1–13, 1990

Bowers MB Jr, Heninger GR, Gerbode FA: Cerebrospinal fluid, 5-hydroxyindoleacetic acid and homovanillic acid in psychiatric patients. Int J Neuropharmacol 8:255–262, 1969

Bowers MB Jr, Swigar ME, Jatlow PI, et al: Plasma catecholamine metabolites and early response to haloperidol. J Clin Psychiatry 45:248–251, 1984

Bradbury TN, Miller GA: Season of birth in schizophrenia: a review of evidence, methodology, and etiology. Psychol Bull 98:569–594, 1985

Braff DL: Impaired speed of information processing in nonmedicated schizotypal patients. Schizophr Bull 7(3):499–508, 1981

Braff DL: Information processing and attention dysfunctions in schizophrenia. Schizophr Bull 19(2):233–259, 1993

Braff DL, Heaton R, Kuck J, et al: The generalized pattern of neuropsychological deficits in outpatients with chronic schizophrenia with heterogeneous Wisconsin Card Sorting Test results. Arch Gen Psychiatry 48:891–898, 1991

Braus DF, Ende G, Weber-Fahr W, et al: Antipsychotic drug effects on motor activation measured by functional magnetic resonance imaging in schizophrenic patients. Schizophr Res 39:19–29, 1999

Breier A, Buchanan RW, Elkashef A, et al: Brain morphology and schizophrenia: a magnetic resonance imaging study of limbic, prefrontal cortex, and caudate structures. Arch Gen Psychiatry 49:921–926, 1992

Buchsbaum MS, Ingvar DH, Kessler R, et al: Cerebral glucography with positron tomography. Arch Gen Psychiatry 39:251–259, 1982

Buchsbaum MS, DeLisi LE, Holcomb HH, et al: Anteroposterior gradients in cerebral glucose use in schizophrenia and affective disorders. Arch Gen Psychiatry 41:1159–1166, 1984

Buckley PF, Friedman L, Wu D, et al: Functional magnetic resonance imaging in schizophrenia: initial methodology and evaluation of the motor cortex. Psychiatry Res 74:13–23, 1997

Callicott JH, Ramsey NF, Tallent K, et al: Functional magnetic resonance imaging brain mapping in psychiatry: methodological issues illustrated in a study of working memory in schizophrenia. Neuropsychopharmacology 18:186–196, 1998

Callicott JH, Mattay VS, Bertolino A, et al: Physiological characteristics of capacity constraints in working memory as revealed by functional MRI. Cereb Cortex 9:20–26, 1999

Cannon TD, Mednick SA, Parnas J, et al: Developmental brain abnormalities in the offspring of schizophrenic mothers, II: structural brain characteristics of schizophrenia and schizotypal personality disorder. Arch Gen Psychiatry 51(12): 955–962, 1994

Carpenter WT Jr, Buchanan RW: Domains of psychopathology relevant to the study of etiology and treatment in schizophrenia, in Schizophrenia: Scientific Progress. Edited by Schulz SC, Tamminga CA. New York, Oxford University Press, 1989, pp 13–22

Carpenter WT Jr, Buchanan RW: Schizophrenia. N Engl J Med 330:681–690, 1994

Carpenter WT Jr, Buchanan RW, Kirkpatrick B, et al: Strong inference, theory testing and the neuroanatomy of schizophrenia. Arch Gen Psychiatry 50:825–831, 1993

Chakos MH, Lieberman JA, Bilder RM, et al: Increase in caudate nuclei volumes of first-episode schizophrenic patients taking antipsychotic drugs. Am J Psychiatry 151:1430–1436, 1994

Chen Y, Nakayama K, Levy DL, et al: Psychophysical isolation of a motion-processing deficit in schizophrenics and their relatives and its association with impaired smooth pursuit. Proc Natl Acad Sci U S A 96(8):4724–4729, 1999

Ciompi L, Müller C: Lebensweg und alter der schizophrenen. Eine katamnestische lonzeitstudies bis ins senium. Berlin, Springer-Verlag, 1976

Cleghorn JM, Kaplan RD, Nahmias C, et al: Inferior parietal region implicated in neurocognitive impairment in schizophrenia. Arch Gen Psychiatry 46:758–760, 1989

Clementz BA, Sweeney JA: Is eye movement dysfunction a biological marker for schizophrenia? A methodological review. Psychol Bull 108(1):77–92, 1990

Clementz BA, Sweeney JA, Hirt M, et al: Pursuit gain and saccadic intrusions in first-degree relatives of probands with schizophrenia. J Abnorm Psychol 99(4):327–335, 1990

Clementz BA, McDowell JE, Zisook S: Saccadic system functioning among schizophrenia patients and their first-degree biological relatives. J Abnorm Psychol 103(2):277–287, 1994

Clow A, Theodorou A, Jenner P, et al: Changes in cerebral dopamine function induced by a year's administration of trifluoperazine or thioridazine and their subsequent withdrawal. Adv Biochem Psychopharmacol 24:335–340, 1980

Colter N, Battal S, Crow TJ: White matter reduction in the parahippocampal gyrus of patients with schizophrenia. Arch Gen Psychiatry 44:1023–1026, 1987

Cornblatt BA, Winters L, Erlenmeyer-Kimling L: Attentional markers of schizophrenia: evidence from the New York high-risk study, in Schizophrenia: Scientific Progress. Edited by Schulz S, Tamminga C. New York, Oxford University Press, 1989, pp 83–92

Crawford TJ, Sharma T, Puri BK, et al: Saccadic eye movements in families multiply affected with schizophrenia: the Maudsley Family Study. Am J Psychiatry 155(12):1703–1710, 1998

Cross AJ, Crow TJ, Owen F: 3H-Flupenthixol binding in post-mortem brains of schizophrenics: evidence for a selective increase in dopamine D2 receptors. Psychopharmacology 74:122–124, 1981

Csernansky JG, Joshi S, Wang L, et al: Hippocampal morphometry in schizophrenia by high dimensional brain mapping. Proc Natl Acad Sci U S A 95(19):11406–11411, 1998

Davidson M, Davis KL: A comparison of plasma homovanillic acid concentrations in schizophrenics and normal controls. Arch Gen Psychiatry 45:561–563, 1988

Deutsch SI, Mastropaolo J, Schwartz B, et al: A "glutamatergic hypothesis" of schizophrenia. Rationale for pharmacotherapy with glycine. Clin Neuropharmacol 12:1–13, 1989

Dolan RJ, Fletcher P, Frith CD, et al: Dopaminergic modulation of impaired cognitive activation in the anterior cingulate cortex in schizophrenia. Nature 378:180–182, 1995

Domino EF, Luby E: Abnormal mental states induced by phencyclidine as a model of schizophrenia, in PCP (Phencyclidine): Historical and Current Perspectives. Edited by Domino EF. Ann Arbor, MI, NPP Books, 1981, pp 123–128

Elkashef AM, Issa F, Wyatt RJ: The biochemical basis of schizophrenia, in Contemporary Issues in the Treatment of Schizophrenia. Edited by Shriqui CL, Nasrallah HA. Washington, DC, American Psychiatric Press, 1995, pp 3–41

Elsworth JD, Leahy DJ, Roth RH, et al: Homovanillic acid concentrations in brain, CSF and plasma as indicators of central dopamine function in primates. J Neural Transm 68:51–62, 1987

Falkai P, Bogerts B: Cell loss in the hippocampus of schizophrenics. Eur Arch Psychiatry Neurol Sci 236:154–161, 1986

Faraone SV, Seidman LJ, Kremen WS, et al: Neuropsychological functioning among the nonpsychotic relatives of schizophrenic patients: a diagnostic efficiency analysis. J Abnorm Psychol 104:286–304, 1995

Faraone SV, Seidman LJ, Kremen WS, et al: Neuropsychologic functioning among the nonpsychotic relatives of schizophrenic patients: the effect of genetic loading. Biol Psychiatry 48(2):120–126, 2000

Farde L, Wiesel F-A, Hall H, et al: D2 dopamine receptors in neuroleptic-naive schizophrenic patients: a positron emission tomography study with [11C]raclopride. Arch Gen Psychiatry 47:213–219, 1990

Freedman R, Adler LE, Gerhardt GA, et al: Neurobiological studies of sensory gating in schizophrenia. Schizophr Bull 13(4): 669–678, 1987

Freedman R, Coon H, Myles-Worsley M, et al: Linkage of a neurophysiological deficit in schizophrenia to a chromosome 15 locus. Proc Natl Acad Sci U S A 94(2):587–592, 1997

Freedman R, Adler LE, Leonard S: Alternative phenotypes for the complex genetics of schizophrenia. Biol Psychiatry 45:551–558, 1999

Fukushima J, Fukushima K., Chiba T, et al: Disturbances of voluntary control of saccadic eye movements in schizophrenic patients. Biol Psychiatry 23(7):670–677, 1988

Gao X-M, Sakai K, Roberts RC, et al: Ionotropic glutamate receptors and expression of N-methyl-D-aspartate receptor subunits in subregions of human hippocampus: effects of schizophrenia. Am J Psychiatry 157:1141–1149, 2000

Gattaz WF, Gasser T, Beckmann H: Multidimensional analysis of the concentrations of 17 substances in the CSF of schizophrenics and controls. Biol Psychiatry 20:360–366, 1985

Gold J, Goldberg T, Weinberger D: Prefrontal function and schizophrenic symptoms. Neuropsychiatry Neuropsychol Behav Neurol 5:253–261, 1992

Gold JM, Hermann BP, Randolph C, et al: Schizophrenia and temporal lobe epilepsy. A neuropsychological analysis. Arch Gen Psychiatry 51:265–272, 1994

Goldberg TE, Ragland JD, Torrey EF, et al: Neuropsychological assessment of monozygotic twins discordant for schizophrenia. Arch Gen Psychiatry 47:1066–1072, 1990

Goldman-Rakic PS: Working memory dysfunction in schizophrenia. J Neuropsychiatry Clin Neurosci 6:348–357, 1994

Goldman-Rakic PS: Psychopathology and neuropathology of prefrontal cortex in schizophrenia, in Schizophrenia: An Integrated View. Alfred Benzon Symposium 38. Edited by Fog R, Gerlach J, Hemmingsen R. Copenhagen, Denmark, Munksgaard, 1995, pp 126–138

Gottesman II, Shields J: Schizophrenia: The Epigenetic Puzzle. New York, Cambridge University Press, 1982

Grace AA: Phasic versus tonic dopamine release and the modulation of dopamine system responsivity: a hypothesis for the etiology of schizophrenia. Neuroscience 41(1):1–24, 1991

Green MF, Nuechterlein KH, Breitmeyer B: Backward masking performance in unaffected siblings of schizophrenic patients. Evidence for a vulnerability indicator. Arch Gen Psychiatry 54:465–472, 1997

Gruzelier J, Seymour K, Wilson L: Impairments on neuropsychotic tests of temporohippocampal and frontohippocampal functions and word fluency in remitting schizophrenia and affective disorders. Arch Gen Psychiatry 45:623–629, 1988

Gur RC, Saykin AJ, Gur RE: Neuropsychological study of schizophrenia. Schizophr Res 1:153–162, 1991

Gur RE, Resnick SM, Alavi A, et al: Regional brain function in schizophrenia. Arch Gen Psychiatry 44:119–125, 1987

Harding CM, Brooks GW, Takamaru A, et al: The Vermont longitudinal study of persons with severe mental illness, I: methodology, study sample, and overall status 32 years later. Am J Psychiatry 144:718–726, 1987a

Harding CM, Brooks GW, Takamaru A, et al: The Vermont longitudinal study of persons with severe mental illness, II: long-term outcome of subjects who retrospectively met DSM-III criteria for schizophrenia. Am J Psychiatry 144(6):727–735, 1987b

Harrison PJ: The neuropathology of schizophrenia. A critical review of the data and their interpretation. Brain 122:593–624, 1999

Heckers S, Heinsen H, Heinsen YC, et al: Cortex, white matter, and basal ganglia in schizophrenia: a volumetric postmortem study. Biol Psychiatry 29:556–566, 1991

Heckers S, Rauch SL, Goff D, et al: Impaired recruitment of the hippocampus during conscious recollection in schizophrenia. Nat Neurosci 1:318–323, 1998

Hietala J, Syvälahti E, Vuorio K: Striatal dopamine D2 receptor density in neuroleptic-naive schizophrenics studied with positron emission tomography, in Biological Psychiatry, Vol 2. Edited by Racagni G, Brunello N, Fukuda T. Amsterdam, The Netherlands, Excerpta Medica, 1991, pp 386–387

Holcomb HH, Cascella NG, Thaker GK, et al: Functional sites of neuroleptic drug action in human brain: PET/FDG studies with and without haloperidol. Am J Psychiatry 153:41–49, 1996a

Holcomb HH, Gordon B, Loats HL, et al: Brain metabolism patterns are sensitive to attentional effort associated with a tone recognition task. Biol Psychiatry 39:1013–1022, 1996b

Holcomb HH, Lahti AC, Medoff DR, et al: Brain activation patterns in schizophrenic and comparison volunteers during a matched-performance auditory recognition task. Am J Psychiatry 157:1634–1645, 2000

Holzman PS: Recent studies of psychophysiology in schizophrenia. Schizophr Bull 13:49–75, 1987

Huber G, Gross G, Schüttler R: Schizophrenie: Verlaufs und socialpsychiatrische langzeit unter suchungen an den 1945 bis 1959 in Bonn hospitalisierten schizophrenen Kranken. Monogr Gesamtgeb Psychiatr Psychiatry Ser 21:1–399, 1979

Ingvar DH, Franzen G: Abnormalities of cerebral blood flow distribution in patients with chronic schizophrenia. Acta Psychiatr Scand 50:425–462, 1971

Issa F, Gerhardt GA, Bartko JJ, et al: A multidimensional approach to analysis of cerebrospinal fluid biogenic amines in schizophrenia, I: comparisons with healthy control subjects and neuroleptic-treated/unmedicated pairs analyses. Psychiatry Res 52:237–249, 1994a

Issa F, Kirch DG, Gerhardt GA, et al: A multidimensional approach to analysis of cerebrospinal fluid biogenic amines in schizophrenia, II: correlations with psychopathology. Psychiatry Res 52:251–258, 1994b

Jakob H, Beckmann H: Prenatal development disturbances in the limbic allocortex in schizophrenics. J Neural Transm 65:303–326, 1986

Javitt DC, Zukin SR: Recent advances in the phencyclidine model of schizophrenia. Am J Psychiatry 148 (10):1301–1308, 1991

Javitt DC, Doneshka P, Grochowski S, et al: Impaired mismatch negativity generation reflects widespread dysfunction of working memory in schizophrenia. Arch Gen Psychiatry 52(7):550–558, 1995

Jeste DV, Lohr JB: Hippocampal pathologic findings in schizophrenia. Arch Gen Psychiatry 46:1019–1026, 1989

Johnstone EC, Crow TJ, Frith DC, et al: Cerebral ventricular size and cognitive impairment in schizophrenia. Lancet 2:924–926, 1976

Kadekaro M, Vance WH, Terrell ML, et al: Effects of antidromic stimulation of the ventral root on glucose utilization in the ventral horn of the spinal cord in the rat. Proc Natl Acad Sci U S A 84:5492–5495, 1987

Kane JM, Honigfeld G, Singer J, et al, and the Clozapine Study Group: Clozapine for the treatment-resistant schizophrenic: a double-blind comparison with chlorpromazine. Arch Gen Psychiatry 45:789–796, 1988

Katsanis J, Kortenkamp S, Iacono WG, et al: Antisaccade performance in patients with schizophrenia and affective disorder. J Abnorm Psychol 106(3):468–472, 1997

Kay SR, Sevy S: Pyramidical model of schizophrenia. Schizophr Bull 16:537–545, 1990

Keefe RS, Silverman JM, Mohs RC, et al: Eye tracking, attention, and schizotypal symptoms in nonpsychotic relatives of patients with schizophrenia. Arch Gen Psychiatry 54(2):169–176, 1997

Kendler KS, Diehl SR: The genetics of schizophrenia: a current genetic-epidemiologic perspective. Schizophr Bull 192: 261–279, 1993

Kendler KS, Diehl SR: Schizophrenia: genetics, in Comprehensive Textbook of Psychiatry/VI. Edited by Kaplan HI, Sadock BJ. Baltimore, MD, Williams & Wilkins, 1995, pp 942–957

Kety SS: The significance of genetic factors in the etiology of schizophrenia: results from the national study of adoptees in Denmark. J Psychiatr Res 21:423–429, 1987

Kim JS, Kornhuber HH, Schmid-Burgk W, et al: Low cerebrospinal fluid glutamate in schizophrenic patients and a new hypothesis on schizophrenia. Neurosci Lett 20:379–382, 1980

Klein DF, Davis JM: Diagnosis and Drug Treatment of Psychiatric Disorders. Baltimore, MD, Williams & Wilkins, 1969

Korpi ER, Kaufmann CA, Marnela KM, et al: Cerebrospinal fluid amino acid concentrations in chronic schizophrenia. Psychiatry Res 20:337–345, 1987

Lahti AC, Holcomb HH, Medoff DR, et al: Ketamine activates psychosis and alters limbic blood flow in schizophrenia. Neuroreport 6(6):869–872, 1995a

Lahti AC, Koffel B, LaPorte D, et al: Subanesthetic doses of ketamine stimulate psychosis in schizophrenia. Neuropsychopharmacology 13:9–19, 1995b

Lahti RA, Lahti AC, Tamminga CA: D2-family receptors in schizophrenia: distribution and implications for treatment. Clin Neuropharmacol 18(1):S110–S120, 1995

Lake CR, Sternberg DE, van Kammen DP, et al: Schizophrenia: elevated cerebrospinal fluid norepinephrine. Science 207:331–333, 1980

Laruelle M, Abi-Dargham A, van Dyck CH, et al: Single photon emission computerized tomography imaging of amphetamine-induced dopamine release in drug-free schizophrenic subjects. Proc Natl Acad Sci U S A 93:9235–9240, 1996

Laruelle M, Abi-Dargham A, Gil R, et al: Increased dopamine transmission in schizophrenia: relationship to illness phases. Biol Psychiatry 46:56–72, 1999

Lenzenweger MF, Dworkin RH, Wethington E: Examining the underlying structure of schizophrenic phenomenology: evidence for a three-process model. Schizophr Bull 17:515–524, 1991

Lesch A, Bogerts B: The diencephalon in schizophrenia: evidence for reduced thickness of the periventricular grey matter. Eur Arch Psychiatry Neurol Sci 234:212–219, 1984

Lewis DA: GABAergic local circuit neurons and prefrontal cortical dysfunction in schizophrenia. Brain Res 31:270–276, 2000

Lewis SW, Murray RM: Obstetrical complications, neurodevelopmental deviance, and risk of schizophrenia. J Psychiatr Res 21:413–421, 1987

Liddle PF: The symptoms of chronic schizophrenia: a re-examination of the positive-negative dichotomy. Br J Psychiatry 151:145–151, 1987

Liddle PF, Morris DL: Schizophrenic syndromes and frontal lobe performance. Br J Psychiatry 158:340–345, 1991

Liddle PF, Friston KJ, Frith CD, et al: Patterns of cerebral blood flow in schizophrenia. Br J Psychiatry 160:179–186, 1992

Lidow MS, Goldman-Rakic PS: A common action of clozapine, haloperidol and remoxipride on D1- and D2-dopaminergic receptors in the primate cerebral cortex. Proc Natl Acad Sci U S A 91:4353–4356, 1994

Lindström LH: Low HVA and normal 5-HIAA CSF levels in drug-free schizophrenic patients compared to healthy volunteers: correlations to symptomatology and family history. Psychiatry Res 14:265–273, 1985

Luby ED, Cohen BD, Rosenbaum G, et al: Study of a new schizophrenomimetic drug—Sernyl. Arch Gen Psychiatry 81:363–369, 1959

Macciardi F, Lucca A, Catalano M, et al: Amino acid patterns in schizophrenia: some new findings. Psychiatry Res 32:63–70, 1990

Mackay AVP, Iversen LL, Rossor M, et al: Increased brain dopamine and dopamine receptors in schizophrenia. Arch Gen Psychiatry 39:991–997, 1982

Manoach DS, Press DZ, Thangaraj V, et al: Schizophrenic subjects activate dorsolateral prefrontal cortex during a working memory task, as measured by fMRI. Biol Psychiatry 45:1128–1137, 1999

Manoach DS, Gollub RL, Benson ES, et al: Schizophrenic subjects show aberrant fMRI activation of dorsolateral prefrontal cortex and basal ganglia during working memory performance. Biol Psychiatry 48:99–109, 2000

Martinot JL, Peron-Magnan P, Huret JD, et al: Striatal D2 dopaminergic receptors assessed with positron emission tomography and [76Br]bromospiperone in untreated schizophrenic patients. Am J Psychiatry 147:44–50, 1990

Martinot JL, Paillère-Martinot ML, Loch C, et al: The estimated density of D2 striatal receptors in schizophrenia: a study with positron emission tomography and 76Br-bromolisuride. Br J Psychiatry 158:346–350, 1991

Mattay VS, Callicott JH, Bertolino A, et al: Abnormal functional lateralization of the sensorimotor cortex in patients with schizophrenia. Neuroreport 8:2977–2984, 1997

McCarley RW, Shenton ME, O'Donnell, et al: Auditory P300 abnormalities and left posterior superior temporal gyrus volume reduction in schizophrenia. Arch Gen Psychiatry 50:190–197, 1993

McDowell JE, Myles-Worsley M, Coon H, et al: Measuring liability for schizophrenia using optimized antisaccade stimulus parameters. Psychophysiology 36(1):138–141, 1999

McGrath J, Murray RM: Risk factors for schizophrenia: from conception to birth, in Schizophrenia. Edited by Hirsch SR, Weinberger DR. Oxford, UK, Blackwell Science, 1995, pp 187–205

Menon RR, Barta PE, Aylward EH, et al: Posterior superior temporal gyrus in schizophrenia: grey matter changes and clinical correlates. Schizophr Res 16:127–135, 1995

Nuechterlein KH, Dawson ME, Gitlin M, et al: Developmental processes in schizophrenic disorders: longitudinal studies of vulnerability and stress. Schizophr Bull 18:387–425, 1992

O'Driscoll GA, Benkelfat C, Florencio PS, et al: Neural correlates of eye tracking deficits in first-degree relatives of schizophrenic patients: a positron emission tomography study. Arch Gen Psychiatry 56:1127–1134, 1999

Olney JW, Farber NB: Glutamate receptor dysfunction in schizophrenia. Arch Gen Psychiatry 52:998–1007, 1995

Owen F, Cross AJ, Crow TJ: Increased dopamine-receptor sensitivity in schizophrenia. Lancet 2:223–226, 1978

Pakkenberg B: Postmortem study of chronic schizophrenic brains. Br J Psychiatry 151:744–752, 1987

Pakkenberg B: Pronounced reduction of total neuron number in mediodorsal thalamic nucleus and nucleus accumbens in schizophrenics. Arch Gen Psychiatry 47:1023–1028, 1990

Park S, Holzman PS: Schizophrenics show spatial working memory deficits. Arch Gen Psychiatry 49:975–982, 1992

Park S, Holzman PS, Goldman-Rakic PS: Spatial working memory deficits in the relatives of schizophrenic patients. Arch Gen Psychiatry 52:821–828, 1995

Pearlson GD, Wong DF, Tune LE, et al: In vivo D2 dopamine receptor density in psychotic and nonpsychotic patients with bipolar disorder. Arch Gen Psychiatry 52 (6):471–477, 1995

Pfefferbaum A, Wenegrat BG, Ford JM, et al: Clinical application of the P3 component of event-related potentials, II: dementia, depression and schizophrenia. Electroencephalogr Clin Neurophysiol 59(2):104–124, 1984

Pickar D, Labarca R, Doran AR: Longitudinal measurement of plasma homovanillic acid levels in schizophrenic patients. Arch Gen Psychiatry 43:669–676, 1986

Raichle ME: Images of the mind: studies with modern imaging techniques. Annu Rev Psychol 45:333–356, 1994

Reynolds GP: Increased concentrations and lateral asymmetry of amygdala dopamine in schizophrenia. Nature 305:527–529, 1983

Reynolds GP, Mason SL: Absence of detectable striatal dopamine D4 receptors in drug-treated schizophrenia. Eur J Pharmacol 281:R5–R6, 1995

Roberts RC, Gaither LA, Gao X-M, et al: Ultrastructural correlates of haloperidol-induced oral dyskinesias in rat striatum. Synapse 20:234–243, 1995

Rosenthal R, Bigelow LB: Quantitative brain measurements in chronic schizophrenia. Br J Psychiatry 121:259–264, 1972

Ross DE, Thaker GK, Holcomb HH, et al: Abnormal smooth pursuit eye movements in schizophrenic patients are associated with cerebral glucose metabolism in oculomotor regions. Psychiatry Res 58:53–67, 1995

Sartorius N: The International Pilot Study of Schizophrenia. Schizophr Bull (Winter):21–34, 1974

Saykin AJ, Gur RC, Gur RE, et al: Neuropsychological function in schizophrenia. Selective impairment in memory and learning. Arch Gen Psychiatry 48:618–624, 1991

Scheibel AB, Kovelman JA: Disorientation of the hippocampal pyramidal cell and its processes in schizophrenia patients. Biol Psychiatry 16:101–102, 1981

Schroder J, Essig M, Baudendistel K, et al: Motor dysfunction and sensorimotor cortex activation changes in schizophrenia: a study with functional magnetic resonance imaging. Neuroimage 9:81–87, 1999

Schwarcz R, Rassoulpour A, Wu H, et al: Increased cortical kynurenate content in schizophrenia. Biol Psychiatry 50: 521–530, 2001

Seeman P, Ulpian C, Bergeron C, et al: Bimodal distribution of dopamine receptor densities in brains of schizophrenics. Science 225:728–731, 1984

Shelton RC, Weinberger DR: Brain morphology in schizophrenia, in Psychopharmacology: The Third Generation of Progress. Edited by Meltzer HY. New York, Raven, 1987, pp 773–781

Shenton ME, Kikinis R, Jolesz FA, et al: Abnormalities of the left temporal lobe and thought disorder in schizophrenia: a quantitative magnetic resonance imaging study. N Engl J Med 327:604–612, 1992

Shirakawa O, Tamminga CA: Basal ganglia GABA$_A$ and dopamine D1 binding site correlates of haloperidol-induced oral dyskinesias in rat. Exp Neurol 127:62–69, 1994

Silbersweig DA, Stern E, Frith C, et al: A functional neuroanatomy of hallucinations in schizophrenia. Nature 378:176–179, 1995

Sower AC, Bird ED, Perrone-Bizzozero NI: Increased levels of GAP-43 protein in schizophrenic brain tissues demonstrated by a novel immunodetection method. Mol Chem Neuropathol 23:1–30, 1995

Spence SA, Brooks DJ, Hirsch SR, et al: A PET study of voluntary movement in schizophrenic patients experiencing passivity phenomena (delusions of alien control). Brain 120:1997–2011, 1997

Stevens AA, Goldman-Rakic PS, Gore JC, et al: Cortical dysfunction in schizophrenia during auditory word and tone working memory demonstrated by functional magnetic resonance imaging. Arch Gen Psychiatry 55:1097–1103, 1998

Suddath RL, Casanova MF, Goldberg TE: Temporal lobe pathology in schizophrenia: a quantitative magnetic resonance imaging study. Am J Psychiatry 146:464–472, 1989

Suddath RL, Christison GW, Torrey EF, et al: Anatomical abnormalities in the brains of monozygotic twins discordant for schizophrenia. N Engl J Med 322(12):789–794, 1990

Sullivan EV, Shear PK, Zipursky RB, et al: A deficit profile of executive, memory, and motor functions in schizophrenia. Biol Psychiatry 36:641–653, 1994

Sweeney JA, Clementz BA, Haas GL, et al: Eye tracking dysfunction in schizophrenia: characterization of component eye movement abnormalities, diagnostic specificity, and the role of attention. J Abnorm Psychol 103(2):222–230, 1994

Szechtman H, Nahmias C, Garnett S, et al: Effect of neuroleptics on altered cerebral glucose metabolism in schizophrenia. Arch Gen Psychiatry 145:251–253, 1988

Tamminga CA: Schizophrenia and glutamatergic transmission. Crit Rev Neurobiol 12: 21–36, 1998

Tamminga CA, Thaker GK, Buchanan R, et al: Limbic system abnormalities identified in schizophrenia using positron emission tomography with fluorodeoxyglucose and neocortical alterations with deficit syndrome. Arch Gen Psychiatry 49:522–530, 1992

Taylor SF, Tandon R, Koeppe RA: Global cerebral blood flow increase reveals focal hypoperfusion in schizophrenia. Neuropsychopharmacology 21:368–371, 1999

Thaker GK, Cassady S, Adami H, et al: Eye movements in spectrum personality disorders: comparison of community subjects and relatives of schizophrenic patients. Am J Psychiatry 153(3):362–368, 1996

Thaker GK, Ross DE, Cassady SL, et al: Smooth pursuit eye movements to extraretinal motion signals: deficits in relatives of patients with schizophrenia. Arch Gen Psychiatry 55(9):830–836, 1998

Thaker GK, Ross DE, Buchanan RW, et al: Smooth pursuit eye movements to extraretinal motion signals: deficits in patients with schizophrenia. Psychiatry Res 88:209–219, 1999

Thaker GK, Ross DE, Cassady SL, et al: Saccadic eye movement abnormalities in relatives of patients with schizophrenia. Schizophr Res 45:235–244, 2000

Toru M, Watanabe S, Shibuya H, et al: Neurotransmitters, receptors and neuropeptides in post-mortem brains of chronic schizophrenic patients. Acta Psychiatr Scand 78: 121–137, 1988

Treff WM, Hempel KJ: Die Zelidichte bei Schizophrenen und klinisch Gesunden. J Hirnforsch 4:314–369, 1958

Tsuang MT, Woolson RD, Fleming JA: Longterm outcome of major psychoses, I: schizophrenia and affective disorders compared with psychiatrically symptomfree surgical conditions. Arch Gen Psychiatry 36:1295–1301, 1979

Tsuang MT, Stone WS, Seidman LJ, et al: Treatment of nonpsychotic relatives of patients with schizophrenia: four case studies. Biol Psychiatry 1(45):1412–1418, 1999

Tsuang MT, Stone WS, Faraone SV: Toward reformulating the diagnosis of schizophrenia. Am J Psychiatry 157:1041–1050, 2000

Ulas J, Cotman CW: Excitatory amino acid receptors in schizophrenia. Schizophr Bull 19:105–117, 1993

van Kammen DP, Peters J, Yao J, et al: Norepinephrine and relapse in chronic schizophrenia: negative symptoms revisited. Arch Gen Psychiatry 47:161–168, 1990

Volk DW, Austin MC, Pierri JN, et al: Decreased glutamic acid decarboxylase67 messenger RNA expression in a subset of prefrontal cortical gamma-aminobutyric acid neurons in subjects with schizophrenia. Arch Gen Psychiatry 57:237–245, 2000

Whicker L, Abel LA, Dell'Osso LF: Smooth pursuit eye movements in the parents of schizophrenics. Neuroophthalmology 5:1–8, 1985

Wong D, Wagner HN Jr, Tune LE, et al: Positron emission tomography reveals elevated D2 dopamine receptors in drug-naive schizophrenics. Science 234:1558–1563, 1986

World Health Organization: International Statistical Classification of Diseases and Related Health Problems, 10th Revision. Geneva, World Health Organization, 1992

Neuropsychiatric Aspects of Mood and Affective Disorders

Helen S. Mayberg, M.D.

Michelle Keightley, M.A.

Roderick K. Mahurin, Ph.D.

Stephen K. Brannan, M.D.

Disturbances of mood and affect are among the most prevalent of all behavioral disorders. Depression is especially common and is a prominent feature of many neurological conditions. Diagnosis is generally straightforward, and a wide range of treatments are available that alleviate symptoms in most patients. Although definitive mechanisms for depression have yet to be identified, theories implicating specific neurochemical and neuropeptide systems, focal lesions in specific brain regions, and selective dysfunction of known neural pathways have been proposed, supported by a growing number of clinical and basic studies demonstrating anatomic, neurochemical, genetic, endocrine, sleep, and cognitive abnormalities in depressed patients. In this chapter, we review the clinical, biochemical, neuropsychological, and imaging markers of depression. Changes in these parameters are discussed in the context of a neurobiological model of depression and mood regulation.

Clinical Features

Diagnostic Criteria

The diagnosis of primary major depression is based on the presence of a persistent

Research described in this chapter was supported by National Institute of Mental Health Grant MH49553, the National Alliance for Research on Schizophrenia and Depression, the Charles A. Dana Foundation, the Theodore and Vada Stanley Foundation, and Eli Lilly.

negative mood state in association with disturbances in attention, motivation, motor and mental speed, sleep, appetite, and libido, as well as anhedonia, anxiety, excessive or inappropriate guilt, recurrent thoughts of death with suicidal ideations, and, in some cases, suicide attempts (Table 16–1) (Spitzer et al. 1988). This diversity of clinical symptoms argues against an etiology associated with a single brain location, lesion type, or neurochemical system. Rather, the associated impairment of cognitive, motor, somatic, and circadian functions in patients with dysphoria suggests that depression is a composite disorder affecting discrete but functionally interconnected limbic, paralimbic, and neocortical circuits (Mayberg 1994, 1997).

Demographics and Epidemiology

The average lifetime prevalence of depression is about 15% and is twofold greater in women than in men (Blazer et al. 1994; Fava and Kendler 2000). That depression has a biologic etiology is suggested by family, adoption, and twin studies in which a high degree of heritability is reported (Golden and Gershon 1988; Kendler et al. 1995, 1999). Major depressive disorder generally begins after age 20 and before age 50. A later age at onset is associated with a higher incidence of structural brain lesions, including strokes and subcortical and periventricular white-matter changes (reviewed in Sheline 2000; Soares and Mann 1997). Biologic mechanisms for the increased vulnerability of women or the relative constancy of age at onset are unknown.

The influence of environmental factors in the etiology of depression is equally complex (Kessler 1997). No correlations between depression and socioeconomic status, education, or specific lifestyle have been demonstrated. Although stress is

often seen as a precipitant (Kendler et al. 1995; Robins et al. 1984), the causal relationship between stress and vulnerability to, or precipitation of, a depressive disorder is far from clear. Recent studies provide new evidence that early life trauma and stress may contribute to an increased vulnerability to develop various types of affective disorders (Heim et al. 2000; Kaufman et al. 2000; Lopez et al. 1999; Lyons et al. 2000; McEwen 2000; Meany et al. 1988; Shively et al. 1997).

TABLE 16–1. Clinical features of depression

Symptom domain	Specific symptom
Mood	Dysphoria
	Anhedonia
	Pessimism and hopelessness
	Excessive or inappropriate guilt
	Low self-esteem
	Crying spells
	Suicidality
	Anxiety
Motor	Motor slowing
	Restlessness, agitation
Somatic/ circadian	Sleep disturbance
	Abnormal appetite
	Weight change
	Decreased libido
	Easy fatigability, low energy
	Apathy, decreased drive
Cognitive	Impaired attention and short-term memory
	Poor executive functioning
	Psychomotor retardation
	Poor motivation
	Ruminations

The association of stress-provoking events with the onset of a major depressive episode appears to be stronger for the first episode than for subsequent episodes (Kessler 1997). Although not everyone who has a single episode of depression has another episode, recurrent episodes are more the rule than the exception. Furthermore, the natural course of major depressive disorder, although punctuated by periods of normality, appears to follow a recurrent pattern, and episodes occur more frequently and with greater intensity in the absence of successful intervention (Frank and Thase 1999; Keller et al. 1983).

Treatment Considerations

An untreated major depressive episode generally lasts 6–13 months, although treatment can significantly reduce this period. Options for the treatment of major depression include pharmacologic as well as nonpharmacologic strategies (American Psychiatric Association 2000; Elkin et al. 1989). For patients with mild to moderate depression, medication and cognitive therapies have been shown to be equal in their efficacy to treat depressive symptoms (DeRubeis et al. 1999; Hickie et al. 1999; Hollon et al. 1992). Empirically, it is well recognized that patients with a poor or incomplete response to one form of treatment often respond well to another. Others will respond to treatment augmentation or combination strategies using drugs with complementary pharmacologic actions, combined drug and cognitive-behavioral therapy, or, in medication-resistant patients, electroconvulsive therapy (Bourgon and Kellner 2000; Nemeroff 1996–1997; Nurnberg et al. 1999; Schatzberg 1998; Thase and Rush 1995). Such resistance to treatment is reported to occur in 20%–40% of cases (Keller et al. 1983; Thase and Rush 1995). In rare cases, patients with refractory depression are treated surgically with subcaudate tractotomy, anterior capsulotomy, or cingulotomy (Cosgrove and Rauch 1995; Fulton 1951). Patient subtyping for the purpose of treatment selection has been attempted, but at present, few reliable clinical algorithms exist to guide treatment selection at any stage of illness. Neither are there clinical, neurochemical, or imaging markers that can identify which patients will have a protracted disease course (Coryell et al. 1990; Frank and Thase 1999; Keller et al. 1983; Maj et al. 1992).

Differential Diagnosis

Depression may accompany a variety of neurological, psychiatric, and medical illnesses, and recognition of these comorbid conditions can influence the approach to treatment as well as affect outcome (Table 16–2).

In evaluating a patient who may have an affective disorder, drug-induced mood changes, comorbid general medical illnesses, and substance abuse should always be considered, particularly in patients whose symptoms are atypical or of uncharacteristic onset. In some patients the diagnosis of depression can be obscured by other neurological or psychiatric conditions, delaying appropriate treatment (Starkstein and Robinson 1993; Starkstein et al. 1990d). Certain neurological findings, such as pseudobulbar palsy (Langworthy and Hesser 1940), apathy (Marin 1990), or bradyphrenia (Rogers et al. 1987), in the absence of a true mood disturbance can superficially mimic depressive illness, potentially delaying more appropriate diagnostic or treatment interventions.

Biological Markers

Neurochemical Abnormalities

No single neurotransmitter abnormality has been identified that fully explains the pathophysiology of the depressive disorders or the associated constellation of mood, motor, cognitive, and somatic manifestations (Bauer and Frazer 1994).

TABLE 16–2.   Disorders associated with depression

Neurological disorders	*Eating disorders*
Focal lesions	Anorexia nervosa
Stroke (frontal, basal ganglia)	Bulimia nervosa
Tumor	*Substance abuse*
Surgical ablation	Alcohol and sedatives/hypnotics
Epilepsy (temporal, frontal, cingulate)	Cocaine, amphetamines, and other
Regional degenerative diseases	stimulants
Parkinson's disease	**Systemic disorders**
Huntington's disease	*Endocrine disorders*
Pick's disease	Hypothyroidism and hyperthyroidism
Fahr's disease	Adrenal diseases (Cushing's disease,
Progressive supranuclear palsy	Addison's disease)
Carbon monoxide exposure	Parathyroid disorders
Wilson's disease	*Inflammatory/infectious diseases*
Diffuse diseases	Systemic lupus erythematosus
Alzheimer's disease	Neurosyphilis
AIDS dementia	Acquired immunodeficiency syndrome
Multiple sclerosis	(AIDS)
Miscellaneous disorders	Tuberculosis
Migraine	Mononucleosis
Paraneoplastic syndromes	Sjögren's syndrome
(limbic encephalitis)	Chronic fatigue syndrome
Psychiatric disorders	*Metabolic disorders*
Mood disorders	Uremia
Major depressive disorder	Porphyria
Bipolar disorder	Vitamin deficiencies
Schizoaffective disorder	*Miscellaneous disorders*
Anxiety disorders	Medication side effects
Panic disorder	Chronic pain syndromes
Obsessive-compulsive disorder	Sleep apnea
Posttraumatic stress disorder	Cancer
Generalized anxiety disorder	Heart disease

Changes in norepinephrine, serotonin, dopamine, acetylcholine, opiates, and γ-aminobutyric acid (GABA) (Arango et al. 1997; Caldecott-Hazzard et al. 1991; Klimek et al. 1997; Stancer and Cooke 1988) have all been reported, with new studies additionally focused on dysregulation of second messenger systems, gene transcription and neurotrophic factors, and cell turnover (Duman et al. 2000; Jacobs et al. 2000; Manji et al. 2000; Reiach et al. 1999).

Postulated disturbances in serotonergic (5-HT) and noradrenergic mechanisms have dominated the neurochemical literature on depression for more than 30 years, based in large part on the consistent observations that most antidepressant drugs affect synaptic concentrations of these two transmitters (Bunney and Davis 1965; Charney 1998; Ressler and Nemeroff 1999; Schildkraut 1965; Vetulani and Sulser 1975). Serotonergic and noradrenergic metabolite abnormalities have been identified in spinal fluid, blood, and urine in subsets of depressed patients (Roy et al. 1988), but the relationship of these peripheral measures to changes in brain stem nuclei or their cortical projections is unknown (Langer and Schoemaker 1988; Maas et al. 1984). Postmortem brain studies of depressed people who committed suicide report changes in a number of additional serotonin markers including regional transmitter and metabolite levels, transporter and postsynaptic receptor density, and second messenger and transcription proteins (Arango et al. 1995, 1997; Mann et al. 2000). Involved regions include brain stem, hypothalamus, hippocampus, anterior cingulate, and frontal cortex.

In further support of a biogenic amine etiology, dietary restriction of tryptophan, resulting in an acute decrease in brain serotonin (the tryptophan depletion challenge), and catecholamines (the α-methyl-para-tyrosine challenge) are selectively associated with an abrupt transient relapse in patients whose depression was in remission (Delgado et al.1990; Leyton et al. 2000), suggesting a critical role for serotonergic tone in maintaining a euthymic state.

Although a primary dopaminergic mechanism for depression is generally considered unlikely, a role for dopamine in some aspects of the depressive syndrome is supported by several experimental observations (Cantello et al. 1989; Fibiger 1984; Kestler et al. 2000; Rogers et al. 1987; Zacharko and Anisman 1991). The mood-enhancing properties and clinical utility of methylphenidate in treating some depressed patients are well documented (Martin et al. 1971), although dopaminergic stimulation alone does not generally alleviate all depressive symptoms. Dopaminergic projections from the ventral tegmental area show regional specificity for the orbital/ventral prefrontal cortex, striatum, and anterior cingulate—areas repeatedly identified in functional imaging studies of primary and secondary depression (see later in this chapter).

Degeneration of neurons or their projections from the ventral tegmental area, however, has not been demonstrated in patients with primary unipolar depression.

Opioid, cholinergic, GABA, and corticotropin-releasing factor (CRF) changes have also been reported but have been investigated less (Gross-Isseroff et al. 1990; Janowsky et al. 1988; Nemeroff et al. 1984; Petty et al. 1992).

Endocrine Changes

Studies of endocrine function in patients with depression have identified dysregulation of the hypothalamic-pituitary-adrenal (HPA) axis. The most reproducible finding is a disturbance in the normal pattern of cortisol secretion (Carroll et al. 1976; Nemeroff et al. 1984). The dexamethasone suppression test, previously considered a specific marker of depressive illness, is abnormal in subsets of depressed patients and additionally may identify patients with a more selective abnormality of the HPA axis (Arana et al. 1987; Carroll et al. 1981; Posener et al. 2000). Recent reports of alterations in cortisol regulation associated with transient stress in patients with a history of early life trauma or abuse further suggest that HPA axis dysregulation may be an important marker of vulnerability to various types of affective disorders in later life (Heim et al. 2000; Kaufman et al. 2000; Lopez et al. 1999). Other recent studies further emphasize the role of CRF in modulating serotonergic and noradrenergic activity (Isogawa et al. 2000).

Thyroid markers also have been examined in patients with affective disorder. Even with normal levels of circulating thyroid hormone, elevated levels of thyroid antibodies have been demonstrated in patients with depression but without overt thyroid dysfunction (Nemeroff et al. 1985). A blunted response of thyroid-stimulating hormone to exogenous thyroid-releasing hormone (thyroid stimulation test) also has been described (Loosen 1985).

Sleep Disturbance

Abnormal sleep is a core symptom of major depressive disorder. Electroencephalography abnormalities in depressed patients include prolonged sleep latency, decreased slow-wave sleep, and reduced rapid eye movement (REM) latency with disturbances in the relative time spent in both REM and non-REM sleep (Benca et al. 1992).

Reduced REM latency probably is the best studied and most reproducible sleep-related electroencephalography finding in depressed patients, and this abnormality is reversed by most antidepressants (Sharpley and Cowen 1995). Sleep deprivation, particularly if instituted in the second half of the night, has an effect similar to medication, although the rapid, dramatic improvement in depressive symptoms is short-lived (Wu and Bunney 1990). Changes in nocturnal body temperature and attenuation of the normal fluctuations in core body temperature during sleep further suggest a more generalized dysregulation of normal circadian rhythms in patients with depression (Benca 1994). To date, however, none of these markers have proven to be specific to depression.

Behavioral and Performance Deficits

Motor Performance

Motor and psychomotor deficits in depression involve a range of behaviors including changes in motility, mental activity, and speech (Caligiuri and Ellwanger 2000; Dantchev and Widlocher 1998; Flint et al. 1993; Sobin and Sack-

eim 1997). Depressed patients often perceive these signs as motor slowness, difficulty translating thought to action, lack of interest, or fatigue. Motor signs appear to be well correlated with both the severity of depression and treatment outcome (Lemke et al. 1999). Spontaneous motor activity is significantly lower when patients are depressed compared with when they are in the euthymic state in which a progressive increase in activity levels is seen (Dantchev and Widlocher 1998; Royant-Parola et al. 1986). Also, evidence suggests that significantly long speech-pause times in acutely depressed patients are shortened after successful antidepressant treatment (Szabadi et al. 1976).

Cognitive Dysfunction

Cognitive deficits are a common and potentially debilitating feature of major depression. Impairment is most often encountered in the cognitive domains of attention, memory, and psychomotor speed. In contrast to deficits associated with many structural neurological disorders, specific impairments in language, perception, and spatial abilities usually are not seen except as a secondary consequence of poor attention, motivation, or organizational abilities (Blaney 1986; Brown et al. 1994; Calev et al. 1986; Elliott 1998; Weingartner et al. 1981). Cognitive deficits usually are of moderate intensity but can become severe in prolonged or intractable depression, adding to everyday functional disability. Clinically significant anxiety, which further impairs cognitive efficiency, occurs in many patients with depression (Nutt 1999; Rathus and Reber 1994).

Several authors have proposed a model of depression-related cognitive deficits based on reduced cognitive capacity or impaired ability to efficiently allocate cognitive resources to meet specific task demands (Ellis and Ashbrook 1991; Hasher and Zacks 1979; Roy-Byrne et al. 1986). These theories posit the presence of a diffuse "energetic" impairment, rather than domain-specific cognitive deficits, in patients with depression. This generalized impairment involves either an inability to increase the "gain" of the system sufficiently to handle complex cognitive material or an inability to sustain cognitive effort across memory and learning (visual and verbal, short-term and long-term) tasks (Cohen et al. 1982), as well as tests of executive function (e.g., Tower of London and Wisconsin Card Sort) (Elliott et al. 1997a).

An alternative model for cognitive impairment involves the assumption of correlations between specific deficits and localizable neuroanatomic structures. From this perspective, the pattern of memory deficits seen in patients with major depression has been found to be similar to that in prefrontal-subcortical disorders (such as Parkinson's disease and Huntington's disease), in contrast to a "cortical" pattern of memory performance seen in patients with Alzheimer's disease (Massman et al. 1992). Deficits in concentration, working memory, and psychomotor speed, planning, strategic searching, and flexibility of goal-directed mental activity are well described (Flint et al. 1993; Rogers et al. 1987). More recently, studies have focused on motivation deficits in response to performance feedback, an observation implicating orbitofrontal and ventral-striatal pathways (Elliott et al. 1997b, 1997c). State-trait factors contributing to these findings are not yet defined; however, studies of cognitive bias suggest persistent deficits even in patients whose depression was in remission (Segal et al. 1999; Teasdale 1999). The relationships between deficits in verbal memory, cortisol dysregulation, and hippocampal atrophy are another area of active research (Lyons et al. 2000; McEwen 2000; Sapolsky 2000; Sheline 2000).

The Dementia of Depression

Age in general is an influential factor with respect to cognitive deficits of depression (Lyness et al. 1994). Patients older than 40 generally demonstrate more focal deficits in tests of attention, information-processing speed, and executive function, whereas those over 50 often show more widespread abnormalities in memory and executive function (Elliott 1998; Lockwood et al. 2000). First onset of depression after age 70 is associated with an increased risk of subsequent dementia (King et al. 1995; Raskin 1986; van Reekum et al. 1999).

Depressive dementia, also referred to as pseudodementia, is encountered in a subset of depressed patients, especially in the elderly (Emery and Oxman 1992; Stoudemire et al. 1989). Estimates of the occurrence of depressive dementia range up to 15% in this clinical population (Bulbena and Berrios 1986; Reifler et al. 1982). The differentiation of depression from dementia usually is not difficult. Most elderly patients with depression perform better overall on neuropsychological tests than do age-matched subjects with primary dementia. Elderly depressed patients also show a pattern of cognitive deficits (e.g., poor memory and attention but intact language and visuospatial abilities) that is different from that seen in subjects with dementia, as well as a number of clinical features that are specific to depression (e.g., sadness, poor self-esteem, somatic symptoms) (Jones et al. 1992; LaRue 1982). In these cases, a trial of antidepressant medication is often warranted. The general finding is a return to normal levels of cognitive function in patients with depression, but not those with dementia, after an adequate course of treatment (Abas et al. 1990; Stoudemire et al. 1993). However, more recent studies more strongly suggest that comorbid depression and cognitive impairment can be an early sign of Alzheimer's disease (van Reekum et al. 1999).

Brain Imaging Studies

Modern theories regarding the neurolocalization of depressive illness have evolved from several complementary sources. The early observations of Kleist (1937) on mood and emotional sensations after direct stimulation of the ventral frontal lobes (Brodmann's areas 47 and 11) focused attention on paralimbic brain regions. Studies by Broca (1878) and, later, Papez (1937) and MacLean (1990) elaborated many of the anatomic details of these cytoarchitecturally primitive regions of the cortex, as well as adjacent limbic structures, including the cingulate gyrus, amygdala, and hippocampus. These studies were among the first to suggest a role for these regions in reward, motivation, and affective behaviors. Additional clinical observations in depressed patients have similarly identified a prominent role for the frontal and temporal lobes and the striatum in the expression and modulation of mood and affect (Bear 1983; Damasio and Van Hoesen 1983; Mesulam 1985; Robinson 1998; Stuss and Benson 1986).

Depression in Neurological Disease

Anatomic Studies

Neurological diseases associated with depression can be categorized into three main groups: 1) focal lesions, 2) degenerative disorders with regionally confined pathology, and 3) degenerative diseases with diffuse or random pathology (see Table 16–2). Computed tomography and magnetic resonance imaging (MRI) studies in stroke patients with and without mood disorders have demonstrated a high association of mood changes with infarctions of the frontal lobe and basal ganglia, particularly those occurring in close proximity to the frontal pole or involving the caudate nucleus (Robinson et al. 1984; Starkstein et al. 1987). Studies of patients with head trauma or brain tumors or who have undergone neurosurgery (Damasio and Van Hoesen 1983; Grafman et al. 1986; Stuss and Benson 1986) further suggest that dorsolateral rather than ventral-frontal lesions are more commonly associated with depression and depressive-like symptoms such as apathy and psychomotor slowing. More precise localization is hampered by the heterogeneity of these types of lesions.

Studies of systemic disorders, such as lupus erythematosus (Omdal et al. 1988), Sjögren's syndrome (Hietaharju et al. 1990), thyroid and adrenal disease (Nemeroff 1989), acquired immunodeficiency syndrome (AIDS) (Krikorian and Wrobel 1991), and cancer (Meyers and Scheibel 1990), describe mood symptoms in subsets of patients. As with the more diffuse neurodegenerative diseases, such as Alzheimer's disease (Cummings and Victoroff 1990; Reed et al. 1993; Zubenko and Moossy 1988), a classic lesion-deficit approach is generally difficult because consistent focal abnormalities are uncommon. Studies of plaque loci in patients with multiple sclerosis suggest an association of depression with lesions in the temporal lobes, although it is not yet clear whether this effect is lateralized (Honer et al. 1987).

These limitations shifted focus to those diseases in which the neurochemical or neurodegenerative changes are reasonably well localized, as in Parkinson's disease (Mayberg and Solomon 1995) or Huntington's disease (Folstein et al. 1983). In these disorders, consistent evidence shows direct or indirect involvement of the basal ganglia and associated pathways. These observations directly complement the findings described in studies of discrete brain lesions and further support the importance of cortical-striatal pathways in the development of affective disorders (Alexander et al. 1990). A paradox remains in that both depression and mania can occur as part of a given illness. With the exception of stroke, no localizing or regional differences can be offered to explain this phenomenon.

Lateralization

No consensus has been reached as to whether the left or the right hemisphere is dominant in the expression of depressive symptoms. Reports of patients with traumatic frontal lobe injury indicate a high correlation between affective disturbances and right hemisphere pathology (Grafman et al. 1986). Secondary mania, although rare, is most consistently seen with right-sided basal frontal-temporal or subcortical damage (Starkstein et al. 1990b). Some studies in patients who have experienced stroke suggest that left-sided lesions of both the frontal cortex and the basal ganglia are more likely to result in depressive symptoms than are right-sided lesions, where displays of euphoria or indifference predominate. Considerable debate continues on this issue (Carson et al. 2000; Gainotti 1972; Robinson et al. 1984; Ross and Rush 1981; Sinyor et al. 1986; Starkstein et al. 1987).

Similar contradictions are seen in studies of patients with temporal lobe epilepsy, in which an association between affective symptoms (both mania and depression) and left, right, and nonlateralized foci has been described (Altshuler et al. 1990; Flor-Henry 1969). Anatomic studies have yet to define the critical sites

within the temporal lobe that are most closely associated with mood changes.

Functional Imaging Studies

Despite the many similarities among different neurological conditions, the location of identified lesions by anatomic methods is quite variable. Functional imaging can provide complementary information in that the consequences of anatomic or chemical lesions on global and regional brain function can also be assessed. These methods provide an alternative strategy to test both how similar mood symptoms occur with anatomically or neurochemically distinct disease states and why comparable lesions do not always result in comparable behavioral phenomena. Using this approach, one can examine disease-specific control subjects, such as nondepressed patients with matched demographic and neurological characteristics. Parallel studies of patients with primary affective disorder and patients with neurological depressions provide complementary perspectives (Figure 16–1).

Studies of depression in basal ganglia disorders are such examples: Parkinson's disease, Huntington's disease, and lacunar strokes (Mayberg et al. 1990, 1991, 1992, 1994; Starkstein et al. 1990b). These disorders allow functional confirmation of lesion-deficit observations, as well as characterization of functional changes remote from the site of primary injury or degeneration (Baron 1989). These disorders have known or identifiable neurochemical, neurodegenerative, or focal changes, and the primary pathology spares frontal cortex (the region repeatedly implicated in the lesion-deficit literature). Not only do clinical signs and symptoms in these depressed groups mirror those seen in patients with idiopathic depression, but several plausible biochemical mechanisms for mood symptoms had already been postulated (Mayeux et al. 1988; Peyser and

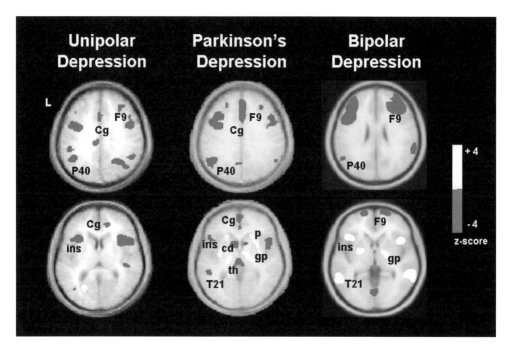

FIGURE 16–1. Positron emission tomographic imaging with fluorodeoxyglucose showing the metabolic changes common to unipolar depression, bipolar depression, and depression with Parkinson's disease (PD).

Symmetrical dorsal and ventral prefrontal (F9), inferior parietal (P40), and anterior cingulate gyrus (Cg) hypometabolism (negative z values, shown in black) characterizes the depressive syndrome, independent of underlying disease etiology. Additional disease-specific changes are seen in insula and the striatum. Striatal hypermetabolism (positive z values, shown in white) is seen in those with bipolar disorder and PD but not in unipolar patients. Insula hypometabolism is seen in unipolar and PD patients in contrast to the hypermetabolism seen in bipolar patients. Insula activity may reflect pretreatment compensatory changes, as further reductions in this region are seen with antidepressant treatment. Resting hyperactivity in bipolar patients may reflect an altered threshold for switches in mood state—a defining feature of bipolar disorder. Striatal hypermetabolism, common to bipolar disorder and PD, may contribute to mood lability, characteristic of bipolar disorder but also seen in many PD patients.

F = frontal; cd = caudate nucleus; gp = globus pallidus; th = thalamus; ins = anterior insula; T = temporal; P = parietal. Numbers are Brodmann designations.

Source. Data from Mayberg et al. 1996, 1997, and Krueger et al. 2000.

Folstein 1993; Robinson 1998). The additional observation that motor and cognitive features present in these patients often obscured recognition of mood symptoms further suggested testable anatomic hypotheses. These clinical findings in combination with published animal and human studies of regional connectivity (Alexander et al. 1990; Goldman-Rakic and Selemon 1984) provided additional foundation to postulate that regional dysfunction of specific frontal-subcortical pathways would discriminate depressed from nondepressed patients, independent of the underlying neurological disorder (Mayberg 1994).

Parkinson's Disease

Depression in patients with Parkinson's disease is common (Cummings 1992; Mayberg and Solomon 1995; Starkstein et al. 1990a, 1990c). A serotonergic etiology is supported by reduced serotonin and serotonin metabolites in the spinal fluid of depressed, but not nondepressed, patients with Parkinson's disease (Mayeux et al. 1988). A dopaminergic etiology, with differential involvement of the mesolimbic and mesocortical dopamine system, has also been proposed (Cantello et al. 1989; Fibiger 1984), supported by identification of selective cell loss in the ventral tegmental area of patients with Parkinson's disease who have prominent mood and cognitive features (Torack and Morris 1988). These findings suggest that patients with Parkinson's disease who have preferential degeneration of neurons of the ventral tegmental area may be more likely to develop depression than are those without involvement of this area.

Functional imaging studies using positron emission tomography (PET) with fluorodeoxyglucose provide support for both hypotheses. As a group, patients with Parkinson's disease without dementia or depression show relatively normal cortical metabolism. A comparison of depressed and nondepressed patients, however, shows that depressed patients have selective hypometabolism involving the caudate nucleus and prefrontal and orbitofrontal cortices (Jagust et al. 1992; Mayberg et al. 1990; Ring et al. 1994), areas with specific dopaminergic and serotonergic innervations. As described in patients with primary depression, prefrontal metabolism inversely correlates with depressive symptom severity. Although frontal changes distinguish depressed from nondepressed patients, mood and cognitive performance are not easily dissociated, suggesting a more complicated relationship between regional hypometabolic changes, depression, and cognitive-behavioral deficits in patients with Parkinson's disease (see Figure 16–1, center).

Huntington's Disease

Depression is the most prevalent mood disorder seen in patients with Huntington's disease, affecting about half of all patients (Peyser and Folstein 1993). Mania also occurs in these patients, and impulsivity and suicide are common. Depression in these patients is not merely a reaction to a terminal disease diagnosis. Rather, as in patients with Parkinson's disease, the mood disorder often precedes the motor abnormalities, even in people who may not recognize that they are genetically at risk. Pathologically, there is degeneration of the basal ganglia. Although the gene for Huntington's disease is now known, it is still unclear how this defect translates into progressive loss of cells in the caudate nucleus and putamen, with the eventual development of chorea, depression, and dementia. Neurochemical mechanisms are more obscure (Peyser and Folstein 1993).

Functional imaging studies readily identify basal ganglia dysfunction—hypometabolism and hypoperfusion of the caudate nucleus and putamen—in both symptomatic patients and genetically at-risk subjects before the emergence of symptoms (Grafton et al. 1990). Analogous to the regional abnormalities identified in depressed Parkinson's patients, depressed patients with Huntington's disease show similar decreases in paralimbic orbitofrontal and inferior prefrontal cortices. The relationship between this paralimbic frontal hypometabolism and degeneration of the basal ganglia is unclear, although disruption of the frontolimbic–basal ganglia–thalamic pathways has been proposed (Mayberg et al. 1992).

Strokes Involving the Basal Ganglia

Clinical signs and symptoms seen with strokes generally correlate with the site of direct brain injury. However, anatomically uninjured brain regions that are functionally connected but anatomically removed from the stroke lesion may also be affected (Baron 1989). This phenomenon, termed remote diaschisis, likely explains the occurrence of frontal lobe deficits in patients with subcortical strokes, for example. Therefore, to best localize both the anatomic and physiologic "lesions" that occur with strokes, structural and functional imaging methods are best used in combination. With this approach, one can determine what pattern of cortical or subcortical dysfunction is common in patients with similar clinical findings and different brain lesions, or, alternatively, what is different about patients with seemingly similar lesions but with discordant clinical symptoms.

This strategy has been used to identify the pattern of cortical hypometabolism specific to patients with secondary mood changes after unilateral lacunar subcortical strokes (Grasso et al. 1994; Mayberg 1994; Mayberg et al. 1991; Starkstein et al. 1990b). Although precise localization of the anatomic lesion in these studies was limited by the resolution of the available computed tomography images, the pattern of cortical metabolic changes nonetheless differentiated depressed from euthymic patients. Temporal lobe rather than frontal lobe changes distinguished the two groups, with bilateral hypometabolism characterizing the depressed patients. In contrast to the findings in Parkinson's disease and Huntington's disease, frontal metabolism did not identify the patients with mood changes because both depressed and nondepressed stroke patients showed bilateral frontal decreases (Mayberg 1994; Mayberg et al. 1991). These remote effects in orbitoinferior frontal cortex may be lesion specific, disrupting orbitofrontal-striatal-thalamic circuits in all patient subgroups, including a group of patients with similar lesions and secondary mania (Starkstein et al. 1990b).

Temporal lobe changes, however, appear to be mood-state specific, implicating selective disruption of basotemporal limbic pathways in the patients with mood changes (Fulton 1951; Nauta 1971, 1986).

Common Findings Across Studies

In summary, lesion-deficit and functional imaging studies of depressed neurological patients have consistently identified involvement of frontal and temporal cortices and the striatum. These common abnormalities have been interpreted as evidence of disease-specific disruption of known neurochemical pathways involving frontal-striatal-thalamic and basotemporal limbic circuits (Alexander et al. 1990; Mesulam 1985; Nauta 1971). This theory is consistent with known neurochemical and degenerative abnormalities previously characterized in patients with these disorders, as well as with known anatomic projections described in human and primate studies (Goldman-Rakic and Selemon 1984; MacLean 1990; Nauta 1971, 1986). The role of limbic regions such as the amygdala, hippocampus, and hypothalamus is less clear, despite evidence that these structures are fundamentally involved in critical aspects of motivational, affective, and emotional behaviors (Damasio 1994; Kleist 1937; LeDoux 1996; MacLean 1990; Mesulam 1985; Papez 1937; Rolls 1985, 2000) and appear to be important targets of various antidepressant treatments (Blier and de Montigny 1999; Duman et al. 1999; Hyman and Nestler 1996). Systematic comparisons of frontosubcortical and corticolimbic patterns in neurological patients to those identified in patients with primary affective disorders are needed to fully characterize common functional markers of the depressive syndrome. Divergent patterns may additionally provide explanations for subtle and not-so-subtle clinical differences across different depressed patient groups (see Figure 16–1).

Primary Affective Disorder

Anatomic Studies

Anatomic studies of patients with primary affective disorders have been less consistent than those of depressed patients with neurological disorders (reviewed in Soares and Mann 1997). Brain anatomy is grossly normal, and focal neocortical abnormalities have not been identified using imaging. Focal volume loss in subgenual medial frontal cortex has been described using both MRI and postmortem anatomic measurements (Drevets et al. 1997; Harrison 2002; Ongur et al. 1998; Rajkowska 2000). Reduced hippocampal and amygdala volumes have also been reported in patients with recurrent major depression (Sheline 2000; Sheline et al. 1996, 1998), with a postulated mechanism of glucocorticoid neurotoxicity, consistent with both animal models (Sapolsky 1994, 2000) and studies of patients with posttraumatic stress disorder (Bremner et al. 1995). Nonspecific changes in ventricular size, and T_2-weighted MRI changes in subcortical gray and periventricular white matter, have also been reported in some patient subgroups, most notably elderly depressed patients (Coffey et al. 1993; Dupont et al. 1995; Greenwald et al. 1996; Hickie et al. 1997; Steffens et al. 1998; Zubenko et al. 1990). The parallels, if any, of these observations to the regional abnormalities described in neurological patients with depression are unclear. Studies of patients with new onset of depression or preclinical at-risk subjects are needed to clarify whether these changes reflect disease pathophysiology or are the consequence of chronic illness or treatment.

Functional Imaging Studies

Resting-state PET and single photon emission computed tomography (SPECT) studies in patients with primary depression also report frontal and cingulate abnormalities, in general agreement with the pattern seen in neurological depressions. Across studies, the most robust and consistent finding is decreased frontal lobe function (Baxter et al. 1989; Bench et al. 1992; Buchsbaum et al. 1986; Drevets et al. 1997; Ebert and Ebmeier 1996; George et al. 1994c; Ketter et al. 1996; Lesser et al. 1994; Mayberg et al. 1994, 1997). The anatomic localization of frontal changes involves both dorsolateral prefrontal cortex (Brodmann areas 9, 10, 46) and ventral prefrontal and orbitofrontal cortices (Brodmann areas 10, 11, 47). Findings are generally bilateral, although asymmetries have been reported. Other limbic-paralimbic (amygdala anterior temporal, insula) and subcortical (basal ganglia, thalamus) abnormalities have also been identified, but the findings are more variable (Bonne et al. 1996; Buchsbaum et al. 1986; Drevets et al. 1992; Hornig et al. 1997; Mayberg et al. 1994, 1997; Post et al. 1987). Differences among patient subgroups (familial, bipolar, unipolar), as well as heterogeneous expression of clinical symptoms, are thought to contribute to this variance, but a consensus has not yet been reached. Use of different analytic strategies (voxelwise vs. region-of-interest) likely also accounts for some of these apparent inconsistencies.

Several neurochemical markers have also been examined in depressed patients using imaging, but findings are quite variable. Decreases in serotonin transporter binding has been reported in brain stem (Malison et al. 1998), but not in any of the other regions identified in postmortem studies of depressed people who committed suicide, for example, ventral prefrontal cortex or anterior cingulate (Arango et al. 1997, 1999). $5-HT_{1A}$ and $5-HT_{2A}$ receptor densities have also been examined, but with inconsistent findings in the drug-free state (Drevets et al. 1999; Mayberg et al. 1988; Meyer et al. 1999; Sargent et al. 2000). Parallel studies of other markers of interest are limited by available imaging ligands. Relationships between receptor and transporter markers or between neurochemical and regional metabolic changes have not been explored.

Clinical Correlates

Despite the general consensus as to the regional localization of functional change patterns, some variability exists (e.g., Baxter 1989; Drevets et al. 1992; Mayberg et al. 1997). A critical unresolved question is how these different patterns might reflect specific symptoms, such as apathy, anxiety, psychomotor slowing, and executive cognitive dysfunction, present in varying combinations with dysphoric mood in individual depressed patients.

Many studies have demonstrated an inverse relationship between prefrontal activity and depression severity (reviewed by Ketter et al. 1996). Significant correlations have also been shown for psychomotor speed (negative correlation with prefrontal and angular gyrus, Bench et al. 1993; negative correlation with ventral frontal, Mayberg et al. 1994), anxiety (positive correlation with inferior parietal lobule, Bench et al. 1993; and with parahippocampal gyrus, Osuch et al. 2000), and cognitive performance (positive correlation with medial frontal/cingulate, Bench et al. 1993; Dolan et al. 1992).

Direct mapping of these behaviors is an alternative approach, allowing head-to-head comparisons of patients and nondepressed control subjects (Dolan et al. 1993; Elliot et al. 1997a; George et al. 1994a, 1994b, 1997). With this type of design, one can quantify the neural correlates of the performance decrement as well as identify potential disease-specific sites of task reorganization. These types of studies can be performed with any of the available functional methods, including PET, functional magnetic resonance imaging (fMRI), and event-related potentials (ERPs).

For example, using this strategy, George et al. (1994a, 1997) demonstrated blunting of an expected left anterior cingulate increase during performance of a Stroop task. A shift to the left dorsolateral prefrontal cortex, a region not normally recruited for this task in healthy subjects, was also observed. Elliott et al. (1997a), using the Tower of London test, described similar attenuation of an expected increase in dorsolateral prefrontal cortex and failure to activate anterior cingulate and caudate—regions recruited in control subjects.

Provocation of transient sadness has also been used to identify putative pathways mediating sustained dysphoria in depressed patients. Pardo et al. (1993) first described blood flow increases using PET in superior and inferior prefrontal cortex during spontaneous recollection of previous sad events. Subsequent studies by George et al. (1995), Schneider et al. (1995), Gemar et al. (1996), Lane et al. (1997), Mayberg et al. (1999), Liotti et al. (2000a), and Damasio et al. (2000), using a variety of provocation methods, identified additional changes involving varying combinations of regions including insula, hypothalamus, cerebellum, and amygdala. Across studies, increases in regional activity were most prominent. Frontal decreases reminiscent of resting-state findings in clinically depressed patients were also seen, but not consistently (Damasio et al. 2000; Gemar et al. 1996; Liotti et al. 2000b; Mayberg et al. 1999). Timing of scans and the specific instructions appear to have a critical impact on both patterns and direction of regional changes.

Brain Changes With Antidepressant Treatments

Functional changes in cortical (dorsal/ventral prefrontal, parietal), limbic-paralimbic (cingulate, insula), and subcortical (caudate, thalamus) regions have been described after various types of treatments (medication, sleep deprivation, electroconvulsive therapy, repetitive transcranial magnetic stimulation [rTMS], ablative surgery). Normalization of frontal hypometabolism is the best replicated finding, seen mainly with medication, suggesting that frontal abnormalities may be state markers of the illness (Baxter et al. 1989; Bench et al. 1995; Buchsbaum et al. 1997; Ebert and Ebmeier 1996; Goodwin et al. 1993; Martinot et al. 1990; Mayberg et al. 1999, 2000). Changes in associated limbic, paralimbic, and subcortical regions are more variable (Bonne and Krausz 1997; Brody et al. 1999; Malizia 1997; Mayberg et al. 2000; Nobler et al. 2001; Smith et al. 1999; Teneback et al. 1999). Whereas certain change patterns (prefrontal, anterior cingulate increases; ventral medial frontal decreases) appear to occur more often than others, a consistent and reliable pattern has not been demonstrated.

Relation to Clinical Response

A critical issue in better understanding the reported variability in location and direction of regional changes with treatment is to consider that drug-induced effects may be different in patients who respond compared to those who do not. Metabolic changes associated with 6 weeks of fluoxetine treatment demonstrate distinct patterns of change at 1 and 6 weeks of treatment, with the time course of metabolic changes reflecting the temporal delay in clinical response (Mayberg et al. 2000). Clinical improvement was associated with limbic-paralimbic and striatal decreases and brain stem and dorsal cortical increases. Failed response to fluoxetine was associated with a persistent 1-week pattern and absence of either subgenual cingulate or prefrontal changes. These findings suggest not only an interaction between limbic-paralimbic and neocortical pathways in depression but also differences among patients in adaptation of specific target regions to chronic serotonergic modulation. Failure to induce the requisite adaptive changes might be seen as a contributing cause of treatment nonresponse. Although specific neurochemical mechanisms for these limbic, paralimbic, and neocortical metabolic changes remain speculative, preclinical studies implicated a series of receptor second messenger and molecular events (Blier and de Montigny 1999; Duman et al. 2000; Hyman and Nestler 1996; Vaidya et al. 1997). As placebo responders show comparable changes in neocortex and subgenual cingulate (but not brain stem or hippocampus) to those seen with active drug, it is further hypothesized that clinical response, regardless of treatment mode, requires specific changes in critical target brain regions and pathways (Mayberg et al. 1999, 2000), a focus of ongoing research.

Baseline Predictors of Treatment Response

Pretreatment rostral (pregenual) cingulate metabolism has been reported to predict response to pharmacotherapy (Brannan et al. 2000; Mayberg et al. 1997). Hypermetabolism was seen in eventual treatment responders; hypometabolism, in nonresponders. A similar hypermetabolic pattern in a nearby region of the dorsal anterior cingulate has also been shown to predict good response to one night of sleep deprivation (Wu et al. 1999). Differential patterns predictive of response to one treatment over another have not yet been characterized. Nonetheless, these data provide preliminary evidence that physiologic differences among patient subgroups may be critical to understanding brain plasticity and adaptation to illness, including propensity to respond to treatment. Evidence of persistent hypermetabolism in patients in full remission on maintenance selective serotonin reuptake inhibitor (SSRI) treatment for more than a year further suggests a critical compensatory or adaptive role for rostral cingulate in facilitating and maintaining clinical response (Liotti et al. 2002).

A Working Depression Model: Emphasis on Functional Neurocircuitry

Data presented in this chapter strongly support a critical role for frontal-subcortical circuits, and more specifically frontal-limbic pathways, in the mediation of clinical symptoms in patients with primary and secondary depression. The overall pattern of cortical, subcortical, and limbic changes suggests the involvement of several well-characterized pathways, schematically organized as an interactive network (Mayberg 1997; Mayberg et al. 2000) (Figure 16–2).

Brain regions with known anatomic interconnections that also show consistent and synchronized changes using PET in various behavioral states—transient sadness, baseline depressed, and pretreatment and posttreatment—have been grouped into three general compartments: dorsal, ventral, and subcortical. The dorsal-ventral segregation additionally defines those brain regions in which an inverse relationship is seen across experiments.

The dorsal compartment (Figure 16–2, attention-cognition) includes both neocortical and superior limbic elements and is postulated to mediate cognitive aspects of negative emotion such as apathy, psychomotor slowing, and impaired attention and executive function, based on complementary structural and functional lesion-deficit correlational studies (Bench et al. 1992; Devinsky et al. 1995; Dolan et al. 1993; Mayberg et al. 1994; Stuss and Benson 1986), symptom-specific treatment effects in depressed patients (Bench et al. 1993; Buchsbaum et al. 1997; Mayberg et al. 2000), activation studies designed to explicitly map these behaviors in healthy volunteers (George et al. 1995; Pardo et al. 1991), and connectivity patterns in primates (Morecraft et al. 1993; Petrides and Pandya 1984).

The ventral compartment (Figure 16–2, somatic-circadian) is composed predominantly of limbic and paralimbic regions known to mediate circadian, somatic, and vegetative aspects of depression, including sleep, appetite, libidinal, and endocrine disturbances, based on clinical and related animal studies (Augustine 1996; MacLean 1990; Mesulam and Mufson 1992; Neafsey 1990; Rolls 2000).

The rostral cingulate (Figure 16–2, rCg24a) is isolated from both the ventral and dorsal compartments based on its cytoarchitectural characteristics and reciprocal connections to both dorsal and ventral anterior cingulate (Vogt and Pandya 1987; Vogt et al. 1995). Contributing to this position in the model are the observations that metabolism in this region uniquely predicts antidepressant response in acutely depressed patients (Mayberg et al. 1997) and is also the principal site of aberrant response during mood induction in patients whose depression is in remission (Liotti et al. 2002). These anatomic and clinical distinctions suggest that the rostral anterior cingulate

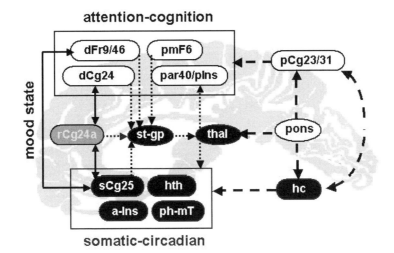

FIGURE 16–2. Depression model.

Regions with known anatomic interconnections that also show synchronized changes using positron emission tomography (PET) in three behavioral states—normal transient sadness (control subjects), baseline depression (patients), and posttreatment state (patients)—are grouped into three main compartments: dorsal (*upper box*), ventral (*lower box*), and subcortical. The dorsal-ventral segregation additionally identifies the brain regions where an inverse relationship is seen across the different PET paradigms. Sadness and depressive illness are both associated with decreases in dorsal limbic and neocortical regions (*white areas*) and relative increases in ventral paralimbic areas (*black areas*). The model, in turn, proposes that illness remission occurs when there is inhibition of the overactive ventral regions and activation of the previously hypofunctioning dorsal areas, an effect facilitated by antidepressant action in the brain stem, hippocampus, and posterior cingulate gyrus (*black dashed arrows*). Normal or abnormal functioning of the rostral cingulate gyrus (rCg24a in gray) with its bidirectional connections to both dorsal anterior cingulate gyrus (dCg24) and subgenual cingulate gyrus (sCg25) is postulated to facilitate interactions between dorsal cortical and more ventral paralimbic systems and to strategically influence pharmacologically mediated changes across the network. *Solid black arrows* identify known reciprocal corticolimbic, limbic-paralimbic, and cingulate-cingulate connections. *Dotted small black arrows* indicate known cortical-striatal-thalamic pathways.

dFr=dorsolateral prefrontal; pmF=premotor; dCg=dorsal anterior cingulate; par=parietal; pIns=posterior insula; pCg=posterior cingulate; rCg24a=rostral anterior cingulate; st-gp=striatum-globus pallidus; thal=thalamus; sCg=subgenual cingulate; hth=hypothalamus; hc=hippocampus; a-Ins=anterior insula; ph-mT=parahippocampus-medial temporal. Numbers are Brodmann designations.

Source. Adapted from Mayberg 1997 and Mayberg et al. 2000.

may serve an important regulatory role in the overall network by facilitating the interactions between the dorsal and ventral compartments (Crino et al. 1993; Pandya and Yeterian 1996; Petrides and Pandya 1984). As such, dysfunction in this area could have significant impact on remote brain regions regulating a variety of behaviors, including the interaction between mood and cognitive, somatic, and circadian responses that characterize an emotional state.

Strategic modulation of specific subcortical (brain stem, hypothalamus, hippocampus, posterior cingulate, striatal) "nodes" is seen as a primary mechanism for the observed widespread, reciprocal effects in ventral and dorsal cortical-limbic regions seen with antidepressant drug treatment (Mayberg et al. 1999, 2000). Although additional experimental studies are clearly needed, it is postulated that illness remission, whether facilitated by medication, psychotherapy, electroconvulsive therapy, or surgery, requires the reconfiguration of these reciprocally interactive pathways initiated through either top-down (cortical-limbic) or bottom-up (limbic-cortical) interventional strategies. If one assumes that both of these approaches are equally efficacious, the question shifts away from whether suppression of ventral limbic regions allows the normalization of dorsal cortical hypometabolism or whether normalization of cortical activity causes a decrease in ventral limbic regions to a focus on patterns and mechanisms underlying successful and failed responses to different forms of treatment. This will be an important area of research in coming years.

References

Abas MA, Sahakian BJ, Levy R: Neuropsychological deficits and CT scan changes in elderly depressives. Psychol Med 20:507–520, 1990

Alexander GE, Crutcher MD, De Long MR: Basal ganglia-thalamocortical circuits: parallel substrates for motor, oculomotor, "prefrontal" and "limbic" functions. Prog Brain Res 85:119–146, 1990

Altshuler LL, Devinsky O, Post RM, et al: Depression, anxiety, and temporal lobe epilepsy: laterality of focus and symptoms. Arch Neurol 47:284–288, 1990

American Psychiatric Association: Practice Guideline for the Treatment of Patients With Major Depressive Disorder (revision). Am J Psychiatry 157:1–45, 2000

Arana GW, Baldessarini RJ, Brown WA, et al: The dexamethasone suppression test: an overview of its current status in psychiatry. Task Force Report for the American Psychiatric Association. Washington, DC, American Psychiatric Association, 1987

Arango V, Underwood MD, Gubbi AV, et al: Localized alterations in pre- and postsynaptic serotonin binding sites in the ventrolateral prefrontal cortex of suicide victims. Brain Res 688(1–2):121–133, 1995

Arango V, Underwood MD, Mann JJ: Postmortem findings in suicide victims. Implications for in vivo imaging studies. Ann N Y Acad Sci 836:269–287, 1997

Arango V, Underwood MD, Kassir SA, et al: Reduction in SERT binding in prefrontal cortex in depression and suicide. Abstract and poster presentation, 38th Annual Meeting of the American College of Neuropsychopharmacology, Acapulco, Mexico, December 12–16, 1999, p 158

Augustine JR: Circuitry and functional aspects of the insular lobe in primates including humans. Brain Res Brain Res Rev 22:229–244, 1996

Baron JC: Depression of energy metabolism in distant brain structures: studies with positron emission tomography in stroke patients. Semin Neurol 9:281–285, 1989

Bauer M, Frazer A: Mood disorders, in Biological Bases of Brain Function and Disease, 2nd Edition. Edited by Frazer A, Molinoff P, Winokur A. New York, Raven, 1994, pp 303–323

Baxter LR, Schwartz JM, Phelps ME, et al: Reduction of prefrontal cortex glucose metabolism common to three types of depression. Arch Gen Psychiatry 46:243–250, 1989

Bear DM: Hemispheric specialization and the neurology of emotion. Arch Neurol 40:195–202, 1983

Benca RM: Mood disorders, in Principles and Practice of Sleep Medicine. Edited by Kryger MH, Roth T, Dement WC. Philadelphia, WB Saunders, 1994, pp 899–913

Benca RM, Obermeyer WH, Thisted RA, et al: Sleep and psychiatric disorders: a meta-analysis. Arch Gen Psychiatry 49:651–668, 1992

Bench CJ, Friston KJ, Brown RG, et al: The anatomy of melancholia—focal abnormalities of cerebral blood flow in major depression. Psychol Med 22:607–615, 1992

Bench CJ, Friston KJ, Brown RG, et al: Regional cerebral blood flow in depression measured by positron emission tomography: the relationship with clinical dimensions. Psychol Med 23:579–590, 1993

Bench CJ, Frackowiak RSJ, Dolan RJ: Changes in regional cerebral blood flow on recovery from depression. Psychol Med 25:247–251, 1995

Blaney PH: Affect and memory: a review. Psychol Bull 99:229–246, 1986

Blazer DG, Kessler RC, McGonagle KA, et al: The prevalence and distribution of major depression in a national community sample: the National Comorbidity Survey. Am J Psychiatry 151:979–986, 1994

Blier P, de Montigny C: Serotonin and drug-induced therapeutic responses in major depression, obsessive compulsive and panic disorders. Neuropsychopharmacology 21:170–178, 1999

Bonne O, Krausz Y: Pathophysiological significance of cerebral perfusion abnormalities in major depression: trait or state marker? Eur Neuropsychopharmacol 7:225–233, 1997

Bonne O, Krausz Y, Gorfine M, et al: Cerebral hypoperfusion in medication resistant, depressed patients assessed by Tc99m-HMPAO SPECT. J Affect Disord 41:163–171, 1996

Bourgon LN, Kellner CH: Relapse of depression after ECT: a review. J ECT 16:19–31, 2000

Brannan SK, Mayberg HS, McGinnis S, et al: Cingulate metabolism predicts treatment response: a replication (abstract). Biol Psychiatry 47(107S):355, 2000

Bremner JD, Randall P, Scott TM, et al: MRI-based measurement of hippocampal volume in post-traumatic stress disorder. Am J Psychiatry 152:973–981, 1995

Broca P: Anatomie comparée des circonvolutions cérébrales. le grant lobe limbique et la scissure limbique dans la série des mammifères. Revue Anthropologie 1:385–498, 1878

Brody AL, Saxena S, Silverman DH, et al: Brain metabolic changes in major depressive disorder from pre- to post-treatment with paroxetine. Psychiatry Res 91:127–139, 1999

Brown RG, Scott LC, Bench CJ, et al: Cognitive function in depression: its relationship to the presence and severity of intellectual decline. Psychol Med 24:829–847, 1994

Buchsbaum MS, Wu J, DeLisi LE, et al: Frontal cortex and basal ganglia metabolic rates assessed by positron emission tomography with 18F-2-deoxyglucose in affective illness. J Affect Disord 10:137–152, 1986

Buchsbaum MS, Wu J, Siegel BV, et al: Effect of sertraline on regional metabolic rate in patients with affective disorder. Biol Psychiatry 41:15–22, 1997

Bulbena A, Berrios G: Pseudodementia: facts and figures. Br J Psychiatry 148:87–94, 1986

Bunney WEJ, Davis JM: Norepinephrine in depressive reactions. Arch Gen Psychiatry 13:438–493, 1965

Caldecott-Hazzard S, Morgan DG, Delison-Jones F, et al: Clinical and biochemical aspects of depressive disorders, II: transmitter/receptor theories. Synapse 9:251–301, 1991

Calev A, Korin Y, Shapira B, et al: Verbal and non-verbal recall by depressed and euthymic affective patients. Psychol Med 16:789–794, 1986

Caligiuri MP, Ellwanger J: Motor and cognitive aspects of motor retardation in depression. J Affect Disord 57(1–3):83–93, 2000

Cantello R, Aguaggia M, Gilli M, et al: Major depression in Parkinson's disease and the mood response to intravenous methylphenidate: possible role of the "hedonic" dopamine synapse. J Neurol Neurosurg Psychiatry 52:724–731, 1989

Carroll BJ, Curtis GC, Mendels J: Neuroendocrine regulation in depression. Arch Gen Psychiatry 33:1039–1044, 1976

Carroll BJ, Feinberg M, Greden J: The dexamethasone suppression test, a specific laboratory test for the diagnosis of melancholia: standardization, validation and clinical utility. Arch Gen Psychiatry 38:15–22, 1981

Carson AJ, MacHale S, Allen K, et al: Depression after stroke and lesion location: a systematic review. Lancet 356 (9224):122–126, 2000

Charney DS: Monoamine dysfunction and the pathophysiology and treatment of depression. J Clin Psychiatry 59 (suppl 14):11–14, 1998

Coffey CE, Wilkinson WE, Weiner RD, et al: Quantitative cerebral anatomy in depression: a controlled magnetic resonance imaging study. Arch Gen Psychiatry 50:7–16, 1993

Cohen RM, Weingartner H, Smallberg SA, et al: Effort and cognition in depression. Arch Gen Psychiatry 39:593–597, 1982

Coryell W, Endicott J, Keller MB: Outcome of patients with chronic affective disorders: a five year follow-up. Am J Psychiatry 147:1627–1633, 1990

Cosgrove GR, Rauch SL: Psychosurgery. Neurosurg Clin N Am 6:167–176, 1995

Crino PB, Morrison JH, Hof PR: Monoamine innervation of cingulate cortex, in The Neurobiology of Cingulate Cortex and Limbic Thalamus: A Comprehensive Handbook. Edited by Vogt BA, Gabriel M. Boston, MA, Birkhauser, 1993, pp 285–310

Cummings JL: Depression and Parkinson's disease: a review. Am J Psychiatry 149:443–454, 1992

Cummings JL, Victoroff JI: Noncognitive neuropsychiatric syndromes in Alzheimer's disease. Neuropsychiatry Neuropsychol Behav Neurol 2:140–158, 1990

Damasio AR: Descartes' Error. New York, GP Putnam's Sons, 1994

Damasio AR, Van Hoesen GW: Emotional disturbances associated with focal lesions of the limbic frontal lobe, in Neuropsychology of Human Emotion. Edited by Heilman KM, Satz P. New York, Guilford, 1983, pp 85–110

Damasio AR, Grabowsky TJ, Bechara A, et al: Subcortical and cortical brain activity during the feeling of self-generated emotions. Nat Neurosci 3:1049–1056, 2000

Dantchev N, Widlocher DJ: The measurement of retardation in depression. J Clin Psychiatry 59 (suppl 14):19–25, 1998

Delgado PL, Charney DS, Price LH, et al: Serotonin function and the mechanism of antidepressant action: reversal of antidepressant-induced remission by rapid depletion of plasma tryptophan. Arch Gen Psychiatry 47:411–418, 1990

DeRubeis RJ, Gelfand LA, Tang TZ, et al: Medications versus cognitive behavioral therapy for severely depressed outpatients: mega-analysis of four randomized comparisons. Am J Psychiatry 156:1007–1013, 1999

Devinsky O, Morrell MJ, Vogt BA: Contributions of anterior cingulate cortex to behavior. Brain 118:279–306, 1995

Dolan RJ, Bench CJ, Brown RG, et al: Regional cerebral blood flow abnormalities in depressed patients with cognitive impairment. J Neurol Neurosurg Psychiatry 55:768–773, 1992

Dolan RJ, Bench CJ, Liddle PF, et al: Dorsolateral prefrontal cortex dysfunction in the major psychoses: symptom or disease specificity? J Neurol Neurosurg Psychiatry 56: 1290–1294, 1993

Drevets WC, Videen TO, Price JL, et al: A functional anatomical study of unipolar depression. J Neurosci 12:3628–3641, 1992

Drevets WC, Price JL, Simpson JR Jr, et al: Subgenual prefrontal cortex abnormalities in mood disorders. Nature 386:824–827, 1997

Drevets WC, Frank E, Price JC, et al: PET imaging of serotonin 1A receptor binding in depression. Biol Psychiatry 46:1375–1387, 1999

Duman RS, Malberg J, Thome J: Neural plasticity to stress and antidepressant treatment. Biol Psychiatry 46:1181–1191, 1999

Duman RS, Malberg J, Nakagawa S, et al: Neuronal plasticity and survival in mood disorders. Biol Psychiatry 48:732–739, 2000

Dupont RM, Jernigan TL, Heindel W, et al: Magnetic resonance imaging and mood disorders. Localization of white matter and other subcortical abnormalities. Arch Gen Psychiatry 52:747–755, 1995

Ebert D, Ebmeier K: Role of the cingulate gyrus in depression: from functional anatomy to depression. Biol Psychiatry 39:1044–1050, 1996

Elkin I, Shea MT, Watkins JT, et al: NIMH Treatment of Depression Collaborative Research Program. General effectiveness of treatments. Arch Gen Psychiatry 46:971–982, 1989

Elliott R: The neuropsychological profile in unipolar depression. Trends Cogn Sci 2:449–454, 1998

Elliott R, Baker SC, Rogers RD, et al: Prefrontal dysfunction in depressed patients performing a complex planning task: a study using positron emission tomography. Psychol Med 27(4):931–942, 1997a

Elliott R, Frith CD, Dolan RJ: Differential neural response to positive and negative feedback in planning and guessing tasks. Neuropsychologia 35:1395–1404, 1997b

Elliott R, Sahakian BJ, Herrod JJ: Abnormal response to negative feedback in unipolar depression: evidence for a diagnosis specific impairment. J Neurol Neurosurg Psychiatry 63(1):74–82, 1997c

Ellis HC, Ashbrook PW: The "state" of mood and memory research, in Mood and Memory: Theory, Research, and Applications. Edited by Kuiken D. Newbury Park, CA, Sage, 1991, pp 1–21

Emery VO, Oxman TE: Update on the dementia spectrum of depression. Am J Psychiatry 149:305–317, 1992

Fava M, Kendler KS: Major depressive disorder. Neuron 28: 335–341, 2000

Fibiger HC: The neurobiological substrates of depression in Parkinson's disease: a hypothesis. Can J Neurol Sci 11:105–107, 1984

Flint AJ, Black SE, Campbell-Taylor I, et al: Abnormal speech articulation, psychomotor retardation, and subcortical dysfunction in major depression. J Psychiatr Res 27:285–287, 1993

Flor-Henry P: Psychosis and temporal lobe epilepsy. Epilepsia 10:363–395, 1969

Folstein SE, Abbott MH, Chase GA, et al: The association of affective disorder with Huntington's disease in a case series and in families. Psychol Med 13:537–542, 1983

Frank E, Thase ME: Natural history and preventative treatment of recurrent mood disorders. Annu Rev Med 50:453–468, 1999

Fulton JF: Frontal Lobotomy and Affective Behavior: A Neurophysiological Analysis. London, Chapman & Hall, 1951

Gainotti G: Emotional behavior and hemispheric side of the lesion. Cortex 8:41–55, 1972

Gemar MC, Kapur S, Segal ZV, et al: Effects of self-generated sad mood on regional cerebral activity: a PET study in normal subjects. Depression 4:81–88, 1996

George MS, Ketter TA, Parekh PI, et al: Regional brain activity when selecting a response despite interference: an H215O PET study of the Stroop and an emotional Stroop. Hum Brain Mapp 1:194–209, 1994a

George MS, Ketter TA, Parekh PI, et al: Spatial ability in affective illness: differences in regional brain activation during a spatial matching task (H215O PET). Neuropsychiatry Neuropsychol Behav Neurol 7:143–153, 1994b

George MS, Ketter TA, Post RM: Prefrontal cortex dysfunction in clinical depression. Depression 2:59–72, 1994c

George MS, Ketter TA, Parekh PI, et al: Brain activity during transient sadness and happiness in healthy women. Am J Psychiatry 152:341–351, 1995

George MS, Ketter TA, Parekh PI, et al: Blunted left cingulate activation in mood disorder subjects during a response interference task (the Stroop). J Neuropsychiatry Clin Neurosci 9:55–63, 1997

Golden LR, Gershon ES: The genetic epidemiology of major depressive illness, in Review of Psychiatry, Vol 7. Edited by Frances AJ, Hales RE. Washington, DC, American Psychiatric Press, 1988, pp 148–168

Goldman-Rakic PS, Selemon LD: Topography of corticostriatal projections in nonhuman primates and implications for functional parcellation of the neostriatum, in Cerebral Cortex. Edited by Jones EG, Peters A. New York, Plenum, 1984, pp 447–466

Goodwin GM, Austin MP, Dougall N, et al: State changes in brain activity shown by the uptake of 99mTc-exametazime with single photon emission tomography in major depression before and after treatment. J Affect Disord 29:243–253, 1993

Grafman J, Vance SC, Weingartner H, et al: The effects of lateralized frontal lesions on mood regulation. Brain 109: 1127–1148, 1986

Grafton ST, Mazziotta JC, Pahl JJ, et al: A comparison of neurological, metabolic, structural and genetic evaluations in persons at risk for Huntington's disease. Ann Neurol 28:614–621, 1990

Grasso MG, Pantano P, Ricci M, et al: Mesial temporal cortex hypoperfusion is associated with depression in subcortical stroke. Stroke 25:980–985, 1994

Greenwald BS, Kramer-Ginsberg E, Krishnan RR: MRI signal hyperintensities in geriatric depression. Am J Psychiatry 153: 1212–1215, 1996

Gross-Isseroff R, Dollon KA, Israeli M, et al: Regionally selective increases in mu opioid receptor density in the brains of suicide victims. Brain Res 530:312–316, 1990

Harrison P: The neuropathology of primary mood disorder. Brain 125:1428–1449, 2002

Hasher L, Zacks RT: Automatic and effortful processes in memory. J Exp Psychol Gen 108:356–388, 1979

Heim C, Newport DJ, Miller AH, et al: Long-term neuroendocrine effects of childhood maltreatment (letter). JAMA 284(18): 2321, 2000

Hickie I, Scott E, Wilhelm K, et al: Subcortical hyperintensities on magnetic resonance imaging in patients with severe depression—a longitudinal evaluation. Biol Psychiatry 42(5): 367–374, 1997

Hickie IB, Scott EM, Davenport TA: Are antidepressants all the same? surveying the opinions of Australian psychiatrists. Aust N Z J Psychiatry 33:642–649, 1999

Hietaharju A, Yli-Kerttula U, Hakkinen V, et al: Nervous system manifestations in Sjogren's syndrome. Acta Neurol Scand 81:144–152, 1990

Hollon SD, DeRubeis RJ, Evans MD, et al: Cognitive therapy and pharmacotherapy for depression. Singly and in combination. Arch Gen Psychiatry 49:774–781, 1992

Honer WG, Hurwitz T, Li DKB, et al: Temporal lobe involvement in multiple sclerosis patients with psychiatric disorders. Arch Neurol 44:187–190, 1987

Hornig M, Mozley PD, Amsterdam JD: HMPAO SPECT brain imaging in treatment-resistant depression. Prog Neuropsychopharmacol Biol Psychiatry 21:1097–1114, 1997

Hyman SE, Nestler EJ: Initiation and adaptation: a paradigm for understanding psychotropic drug action. Am J Psychiatry 153:151–162, 1996

Isogawa K, Akiyoshi J, Hikichi T, et al: Effect of corticotropin releasing factor receptor 1 antagonist on extracellular norepinephrine, dopamine and serotonin in hippocampus and prefrontal cortex of rats in vivo. Neuropeptides 34:234–239, 2000

Jacobs BL, vanPraag H, Gage FH: Depression and the birth and death of cells. Am Sci 88:340–345, 2000

Jagust WJ, Reed BR, Martin EM, et al: Cognitive function and regional cerebral blood flow in Parkinson's disease. Brain 115: 521–537, 1992

Janowsky DS, Risch SC, Gillin JC: Cholinergic involvement in affective illness, in Receptors and Ligands in Psychiatry. Edited by Sen AK, Lee T. New York, Cambridge University Press, 1988, pp 228–244

Jones RD, Tranel D, Benton A, et al: Differentiating dementia from "pseudodementia" early in the clinical course: utility of neuropsychological tests. Neuropsychology 6:13–21, 1992

Kaufman J, Plotsky P, Nemeroff CB, et al: Effects of early adverse experiences on brain structure and function: clinical implications. Biol Psychiatry 48:778–790, 2000

Keller MB, Lavori PW, Klerman GL: Predictors of relapse in major depressive disorder. JAMA 250:3299–3304, 1983

Kendler KS, Kessler RC, Walters EE, et al: Stressful life events, genetic liability, and onset of an episode of major depression in women. Am J Psychiatry 152:833–842, 1995

Kendler KS, Gardner CO, Prescott CA: Clinical characteristics of major depression that predict risk of depression in relatives. Arch Gen Psychiatry 56:322–327, 1999

Kessler RC: The effects of stressful life events on depression. Annu Rev Psychol 48:191–214, 1997

Kestler LP, Malhotra AK, Finch C, et al: The relation between dopamine D2 receptor density and personality: preliminary evidence from the NEO personality inventory–revised. Neuropsychiatry Neuropsychol Behav Neurol 13(1):48–52, 2000

Ketter TA, George MS, Kimbrell TA, et al: Functional brain imaging, limbic function, and affective disorders. Neuroscientist 2:55–65, 1996

King DA, Cox C, Lyness JM, et al: Neuropsychological effects of depression and age in an elderly sample: a confirmatory study. Neuropsychology 9:399–408, 1995

Kleist K: Bericht über die Gehirnpathologie in ihrer Bedeutung für Neurologie und Psychiatrie. Zeitschrift fur des Gesamte Neurologie und Psychiatrie 158:159–193, 1937

Klimek V, Stockmeier C, Overholser J, et al: Reduced levels of NE transporters in the LC in major depression. J Neurosci 17:8451–8458, 1997

Krikorian R, Wrobel AJ: Cognitive impairment in HIV infection. AIDS 5:1501–1507, 1991

Krueger S, Goldapple K, Liotti M, et al: Regional changes in cerebral blood flow following transient sadness in bipolar affective disorder. Abstr Soc Neurosci 26 (program 866.2), 2000

Lane RD, Reiman EM, Ahern GL, et al: Neuroanatomical correlates of happiness, sadness and disgust. Am J Psychiatry 154:926–933, 1997

Langer SZ, Schoemaker H: Platelet imipramine binding in depression, in Receptors and Ligands in Psychiatry. Edited by Sen AK, Lee T. New York, Cambridge University Press, 1988, pp 327–346

Langworthy OR, Hesser FH: Syndrome of pseudobulbar palsy: an anatomic and physiologic analysis. Arch Intern Med 65:106–121, 1940

LaRue A: Memory loss and aging: distinguishing dementia from benign senescent forgetfulness and depressive pseudodementia. Psychiatr Clin North Am 5:89–103, 1982

LeDoux J: The Emotional Brain. New York, Simon & Schuster, 1996

Lemke MR, Puhl P, Koethe N, et al: Psychomotor retardation and anhedonia in depression. Acta Psychiatr Scand 99: 252–256, 1999

Lesser I, Mena I, Boone KB, et al: Reduction of cerebral blood flow in older depressed patients. Arch Gen Psychiatry 51:677–686, 1994

Leyton M, Young SN, Pihl RO, et al: Effects on mood of acute phenylalanine/tyrosine depletion in healthy women. Neuropsychopharmacology 22(1):52–63, 2000

Liotti M, Mayberg HS, Brannan SK, et al: Differential neural correlates of sadness and fear in healthy subjects: implications for affective disorders. Biol Psychiatry 48(1): 30–42, 2000a

Liotti M, Woldorff MG, Perez R, et al: An ERP study of the temporal course of the Stroop color-word interference effect. Neuropsychologia 38(5):706–716, 2000b

Liotti M, Mayberg HS, McGinnis S, et al: Mood challenge in remitted unipolar depression unmasks disease-specific cerebral blood flow abnormalities. Am J Psychiatry 159:1830–1840, 2002

Lockwood KA, Alexopoulos GS, Kakuma T, et al: Subtypes of cognitive impairment in depressed older adults. Am J Geriatr Psychiatry 8(3):201–208, 2000

Loosen PT: The TRH-induced TSH response in psychiatric patients: a possible neuroendocrine marker. Psychoneuroendocrinology 10:237–260, 1985

Lopez JF, Akil H, Watson SJ: Neural circuits mediating stress. Biol Psychiatry 46: 1461–1471, 1999

Lyness SA, Eaton EM, Schneider LS: Cognitive performance in older and middle-aged depressed outpatients and controls. J Gerontol 49(3):P129–P136, 1994

Lyons DM, Yang C, Mobley BW, et al: Early environmental regulation of glucocorticoid feedback sensitivity in young adult monkeys. J Neuroendocrinol 12(8):723–728, 2000

Maas JW, Koslow SH, Katz MM, et al: Pretreatment neurotransmitter metabolite levels and response to tricyclic antidepressant drugs. Am J Psychiatry 141:1159–1171, 1984

MacLean PD: The Triune Brain in Evolution: Role in Paleocerebral Function. New York, Plenum, 1990

Maj M, Veltro F, Pirozzi R, et al: Patterns of recurrence of illness after recovery from an episode of major depression: a prospective study. Am J Psychiatry 149:795–800, 1992

Malison RT, Price LH, Berman RM, et al: Reduced midbrain serotonin transporter availability in major depression as measured by [^{123}I]-2beta-carbomethoxy-3beta-(4-iodophenyl)tropane and single photon emission computed tomography. Biol Psychiatry 44:1090–1098, 1998

Malizia AL: The frontal lobes and neurosurgery for psychiatric disorders. J Psychopharmacol 11(2):179–187, 1997

Manji HK, Moore GJ, Chen G: Clinical and preclinical evidence for the neurotrophic effects of mood stabilizers: implications for the pathophysiology and treatment of manic-depressive illness. Biol Psychiatry 48:740–754, 2000

Mann JJ, Huang Y, Underwood MD, et al: A serotonin transporter gene promoter polymorphism (5-HTTLPR) and prefrontal cortical binding in major depression and suicide. Arch Gen Psychiatry 57:729–738, 2000

Marin RS: Differential diagnosis and classification of apathy. Am J Psychiatry 147:22–30, 1990

Martin WR, Sloan JW, Sapira JD, et al: Physiologic, subjective, and behavioural effects of amphetamine, methamphetamine, ephedrine, phenmetrazine, and methylphenidate in man. Clin Pharmacol Ther 32:632–637, 1971

Martinot JL, Hardy P, Feline A, et al: Left prefrontal glucose hypometabolism in the depressed state: a confirmation. Am J Psychiatry 147:1313–1317, 1990

Massman PJ, Delis DC, Butters N, et al: The subcortical dysfunction hypothesis of memory deficits in depression: neuropsychological validation in a subgroup of patients. J Clin Exp Neuropsychol 14:687–706, 1992

Mayberg HS: Frontal lobe dysfunction in secondary depression. J Neuropsychiatry Clin Neurosci 6:428–442, 1994

Mayberg HS: Limbic-cortical dysregulation: a proposed model of depression. J Neuropsychiatry Clin Neurosci 9:471–481, 1997

Mayberg HS, Solomon DH: Depression in PD: a biochemical and organic viewpoint, in Behavioral Neurology of Movement Disorders: Advances in Neurology Series, Vol 65. Edited by Weiner WJ, Lang AE. New York, Raven, 1995, pp 49–60

Mayberg HS, Robinson RG, Wong DF, et al: PET imaging of cortical S2-serotonin receptors after stroke: lateralized changes and relationship to depression. Am J Psychiatry 145:937–943, 1988

Mayberg HS, Starkstein SE, Sadzot B, et al: Selective hypometabolism in the inferior frontal lobe in depressed patients with Parkinson's disease. Ann Neurol 28:57–64, 1990

Mayberg HS, Starkstein SE, Morris PL, et al: Remote cortical hypometabolism following focal basal ganglia injury: relationship to secondary changes in mood (abstract). Neurology 41 (suppl):266, 1991

Mayberg HS, Starkstein SE, Peyser CE, et al: Paralimbic frontal lobe hypometabolism in depression associated with Huntington's disease. Neurology 42:1791–1797, 1992

Mayberg HS, Lewis PJ, Regenold W, et al: Paralimbic hypoperfusion in unipolar depression. J Nucl Med 35:929–934, 1994

Mayberg HS, Brannan SK, Mahurin RK, et al: Anterior cingulate function and mood: evidence from FDG PET studies of primary and secondary depression (abstract). Neurology 46:A327, 1996

Mayberg HS, Brannan SK, Mahurin RK, et al: Cingulate function in depression: a potential predictor of treatment response. Neuroreport 8:1057–1061, 1997

Mayberg HS, Liotti M, Brannan SK, et al: Reciprocal limbic-cortical function and negative mood: converging PET findings in depression and normal sadness. Am J Psychiatry 156(5):675–682, 1999

Mayberg HS, Brannan SK, Mahurin RK, et al: Regional metabolic effects of fluoxetine in major depression: serial changes and relationship to clinical response. Biol Psychiatry 48:830–843, 2000

Mayeux R, Stern Y, Sano M, et al: The relationship of serotonin to depression in Parkinson's disease. Mov Disord 3:237–244, 1988

McEwen BS: Effects of adverse experiences for brain structure and function. Biol Psychiatry 48:721–731, 2000

Meany M, Aitken D, Berkel H, et al: Effects of neonatal handling of age-related impairments associated with the hippocampus. Science 239:766–768, 1998

Mesulam MM: Patterns in behavioral neuroanatomy: association areas, the limbic system, and hemispheric specialization, in Principles of Behavioral Neurology. Edited by Mesulam MM. Philadelphia, PA, FA Davis, 1985, pp 1–70

Mesulam MM, Mufson EJ: Insula of the old world monkey I, II, III. J Comp Neurol 212:1–52, 1992

Meyer JH, Kapur S, Houle S, et al: Prefrontal cortex 5-HT2 receptors in depression: a [18F]setoperone PET imaging study. Am J Psychiatry 156:1029–1034, 1999

Meyers CA, Scheibel RS: Early detection and diagnosis of neurobehavioral disorders associated with cancer and its treatment. Oncology (Huntingt) 4:115–130, 1990

Morecraft RJ, Geula C, Mesulam MM: Architecture of connectivity within a cingulo-fronto-parietal neurocognitive network for directed attention. Arch Neurol 50:279–284, 1993

Nauta WJH: The problem of the frontal lobe: a reinterpretation. Journal of Psychology Research 8:167–187, 1971

Nauta WJH: Circuitous connections linking cerebral cortex, limbic system, and corpus striatum, in The Limbic System: Functional Organization and Clinical Disorders. Edited by Doane BK, Livingston KE. New York, Raven, 1986, pp 43–54

Neafsey EJ: Prefrontal cortical control of the autonomic nervous system: anatomical and physiological observations. Prog Brain Res 85:147–166, 1990

Nemeroff CB: Clinical significance of psychoneuroendocrinology in psychiatry: focus on the thyroid and adrenal. J Clin Psychiatry 50 (suppl):13–22, 1989

Nemeroff CB: Augmentation strategies in patients with refractory depression. Depress Anxiety 4:169–181, 1996–1997

Nemeroff CB, Widerlov E, Bissette G, et al: Elevated concentrations of CSF corticotropin-releasing factor–like immunoreactivity in depressed patients. Science 226:1342–1343, 1984

Nemeroff CB, Simon JS, Haggerty JJ, et al: Antithyroid antibodies in depressed patients. Am J Psychiatry 142:840–843, 1985

Nobler MS, Oquendo M, Kegeles LS, et al: Decreased regional brain metabolism after ECT. Am J Psychiatry 158:305–308, 2001

Nurnberg HG, Thompson PM, Hensley PL: Antidepressant medication change in a clinical treatment setting: a comparison of the effectiveness of SSRI. J Clin Psychiatry 60:574–579, 1999

Nutt DJ: Care of depressed patients with anxiety symptoms. J Clin Psychiatry 60 (suppl 17):23–27, 1999

Omdal R, Mellgren SI, Husby G: Clinical neuropsychiatric and neuromuscular manifestations in systemic lupus erythematosus. Scand J Rheumatol 17:113–117, 1988

Ongur D, Drevets WC, Price JL: Glial reduction in the subgenual prefrontal cortex in mood disorders. Proc Natl Acad Sci U S A 95:13290–13295, 1998

Osuch EA, Ketter TA, Kimbrell TA, et al: Regional cerebral metabolism associated with anxiety symptoms in affective disorder patients. Biol Psychiatry 48(10): 1020–1023, 2000

Pandya DN, Yeterian EH: Comparison of prefrontal architecture and connections. Philos Trans R Soc Lond B Biol Sci 351:1423–1432, 1996

Papez JW: A proposed mechanism of emotion. Archives of Neurology and Psychiatry 38:725–743, 1937

Pardo JV, Raichle ME, Fox PT: Localization of a human system for sustained attention by positron emission tomography. Nature 349:61–63, 1991

Pardo JV, Pardo PJ, Raichel ME: Neural correlates of self-induced dysphoria. Am J Psychiatry 150:713–719, 1993

Petrides M, Pandya DN: Projections to the frontal cortex from the posterior parietal region in the rhesus monkey. J Comp Neurol 228:105–116, 1984

Petty F, Kramer GL, Gullion CM, et al: Low plasma gamma-aminobutyric acid levels in male patients with depression. Biol Psychiatry 32:354–363, 1992

Peyser CE, Folstein SE: Depression in Huntington's disease, in Depression in Neurologic Diseases. Edited by Starkstein SE, Robinson RG. Baltimore, MD, Johns Hopkins University Press, 1993, pp 117–138

Posener JA, DeBattista C, Williams GH, et al: 24-Hour monitoring of cortisol and corticotropin secretion in psychotic and nonpsychotic major depression Arch Gen Psychiatry 57(8):755–760, 2000

Post RM, DeLisi LE, Holcomb HH, et al: Glucose utilization in the temporal cortex of affectively ill patients: positron emission tomography. Biol Psychiatry 22:545–553, 1987

Rajkowska G: Postmortem studies in mood disorders indicate altered numbers of neurons and glial cells. Biol Psychiatry 48:766–777, 2000

Raskin A: Partialing out the effects of depression and age on cognitive functions: experimental data and methodological issues, in Handbook for Clinical Memory Assessment of Older Adults. Edited by Poon LW. Washington, DC, American Psychological Association, 1986, pp 244–256

Rathus JH, Reber AS: Implicit and explicit learning: differential effects of affective states. Percept Mot Skills 79:163–184, 1994

Reed BR, Jagust WJ, Coulter L: Anosognosia in Alzheimer's disease: relationships to depression, cognitive function and cerebral perfusion. J Clin Exp Neuropsychol 15:231–244, 1993

Reiach JS, Li PP, Warsh JJ, et al: Reduced adenyl cyclase immunolabeling and activity in post-mortem temporal cortex of depressed suicide victims. J Affect Disord 56:141–151, 1999

Reifler BV, Larson E, Hanley R: Coexistence of cognitive impairment and depression in geriatric outpatients. Am J Psychiatry 139:623–626, 1982

Ressler KJ, Nemeroff CB: Role of norepinephrine in the pathophysiology and treatment of mood disorders. Biol Psychiatry 46:1219–1233, 1999

Ring HA, Bench CJ, Trimble MR, et al: Depression in Parkinson's disease: a positron emission study. Br J Psychiatry 165:333–339, 1994

Robins LN, Helzer JE, Weissman MM, et al: Lifetime prevalence of specific psychiatric disorders in three sites. Arch Gen Psychiatry 41:949–958, 1984

Robinson RG: The Clinical Neuropsychiatry of Stroke. Cambridge, UK, Cambridge University Press, 1998

Robinson RG, Kubos KL, Starr LB, et al: Mood disorders in stroke patients: importance of location of lesion. Brain 107:81–93, 1984

Rogers D, Lees AJ, Smith E, et al: Bradyphrenia in Parkinson's disease and psychomotor retardation in depressive illness: an experimental study. Brain 110:761–776, 1987

Rolls E: Connections, functions and dysfunctions of limbic structures, the prefrontal cortex and hypothalamus, in The Scientific Basis of Clinical Neurology. Edited by Swash M, Kennard C. London, Churchill Livingstone, 1985, pp 201–213

Rolls ET: The orbitofrontal cortex and reward. Cereb Cortex 10:284–294, 2000

Ross ED, Rush AJ: Diagnosis and neuroanatomical correlates of depression in brain-damaged patients. Arch Gen Psychiatry 39:1344–1354, 1981

Roy A, Pickar D, De Jong J, et al: Norepinephrine and its metabolites in cerebrospinal fluid, plasma, and urine. Arch Gen Psychiatry 45:849–857, 1988

Royant-Parola S, Borbely AA, Tobler I, et al: Monitoring of long-term motor activity in depressed patients. Br J Psychiatry 149:288–293, 1986

Roy-Byrne PP, Weingartner H, Bierer LM, et al: Effortful and automatic cognitive processes in depression. Arch Gen Psychiatry 43:265–267, 1986

Sapolsky RM: The physiological relevance of glucocorticoid endangerment of the hippocampus. Ann N Y Acad Sci 746:294–304, 1994

Sapolsky RM: The possibility of neurotoxicity in the hippocampus in major depression: a primer on neuron death. Biol Psychiatry 48:755–765, 2000

Sargent PA, Kjaer KH, Bench CJ, et al: Brain serotonin-1A receptor binding measured by PET with 11C-Way-100635. Arch Gen Psychiatry 57:174–180, 2000

Schatzberg AF: NE vs 5-HT antidepressants: predictors of treatment response. J Clin Psychiatry 59 (suppl 14):15–18, 1998

Schildkraut JJ: The catecholamine hypothesis of affective disorders: a review of supporting evidence. Am J Psychiatry 122:509–522, 1965

Schneider F, Gur RE, Mozley LH, et al: Mood effects on limbic blood flow correlate with emotional self-rating: a PET study with O-15 labeled water. Psychiatry Res 61:265–283, 1995

Segal ZV, Gemar M, Williams S: Differential cognitive response to a mood challenge following successful cognitive therapy or pharmacotherapy for unipolar depression. J Abnorm Psychol 108(1):3–10, 1999

Sharpley AL, Cowen PJ: Effect of pharmacologic treatments on the sleep of depressed patients. Biol Psychiatry 37:85–98, 1995

Sheline YI: 3D MRI studies of neuroanatomic changes in unipolar major depression: the role of stress and medical comorbidity. Biol Psychiatry 48:791–800, 2000

Sheline YI, Wang PW, Gado MH, et al: Hippocampal atrophy in recurrent major depression. Proc Natl Acad Sci U S A 93:3908–3913, 1996

Sheline YI, Gado MH, Price JL: Amygdala core nuclei volumes are decreased in recurrent major depression. Neuroreport 22:2023–2028, 1998

Shively CA, Laber-Laird K, Anton RF: Behavior and physiology of social stress and depression in female cynomolgus monkeys. Biol Psychiatry 41:871–882, 1997

Sinyor D, Jacques P, Kaloupek DG, et al: Post stroke depression and lesion location: an attempted replication. Brain 109:537–546, 1986

Smith GS, Reynolds CF, Pollock B, et al: Cerebral glucose metabolic response to combined total sleep deprivation and antidepressant Rx in geriatric depression. Am J Psychiatry 156:683–689, 1999

Soares JC, Mann JJ: The anatomy of mood disorders—review of structural neuroimaging studies. Biol Psychiatry 41:86–106, 1997

Sobin C, Sackeim HA: Psychomotor symptoms of depression. Am J Psychiatry 154:4–17, 1997

Spitzer RL, Williams JBW, Gibbon M, et al: Manual for the Structured Clinical Interview for DSM-III-R (SCID). New York, NY State Psychiatric Institute, Biometrics Research, 1988

Stancer HC, Cooke RG: Receptors in affective illness, in Receptors and Ligands in Psychiatry. Edited by Sen AK, Lee T. New York, Cambridge University Press, 1988, pp 303–326

Starkstein SE, Robinson RG (eds): Depression in Neurologic Diseases. Baltimore, MD, Johns Hopkins University Press, 1993

Starkstein SE, Robinson RG, Price TR: Comparison of cortical and subcortical lesions in the production of post-stroke mood disorders. Brain 110:1045–1059, 1987

Starkstein SE, Bolduc PL, Mayberg HS, et al: Cognitive impairments and depression in Parkinson's disease: a follow-up study. J Neurol Neurosurg Psychiatry 53:597–602, 1990a

Starkstein SE, Mayberg HS, Berthier ML, et al: Mania after brain injury: neuroradiological and metabolic findings. Ann Neurol 27:652–659, 1990b

Starkstein SE, Preziosi TJ, Bolduc PL, et al: Depression in Parkinson's disease. J Nerv Ment Dis 178:27–31, 1990c

Starkstein SE, Preziosi TJ, Forrester AW, et al: Specificity of affective and autonomic symptoms of depression in Parkinson's disease. J Neurol Neurosurg Psychiatry 53:869–873, 1990d

Steffens DC, Tupler LA, Ranga K, et al: Magnetic resonance imaging signal hypointensity and iron content of putamen nuclei in elderly depressed patients. Psychiatry Res 83:95–103, 1998

Stoudemire A, Hill CD, Gulley LR: Neuropsychological and biomedical assessment of depression-dementia syndromes. J Neuropsychiatry Clin Neurosci 1:347–361, 1989

Stoudemire A, Hill CD, Morris R, et al: Long-term affective and cognitive outcome in depressed older adults. Am J Psychiatry 150:896–900, 1993

Stuss DT, Benson DF: The Frontal Lobes. New York, Raven, 1986

Szabadi E, Bradshaw CM, Besson JA: Elongation of pause-time in speech: a simple, objective measure of motor retardation in depression. Br J Psychiatry 129:592–597, 1976

Teasdale JD: Emotional processing, three modes of mind and the prevention of relapse in depression. Behav Res Ther 37:S53–S77, 1999

Teneback CC, Nahas Z, Speer AM, et al: Changes in prefrontal cortex and paralimbic activity in depression following two weeks of daily left prefrontal TMS. J Neuropsychiatry Clin Neurosci 11(4):426–435, 1999

Thase ME, Rush AJ: Treatment-Resistant Depression: Psychopharmacology: The Fourth Generation of Progress. Edited by Bloom FE, Kupfer DJ. New York, Raven, 1995, pp 1081–1097

Torack RM, Morris JC: The association of ventral tegmental area histopathology with adult dementia. Arch Neurol 45:211–218, 1988

Vaidya VA, Marek GJ, Aghajanian GK, et al: 5-HT2A receptor-mediated regulation of brain-derived neurotrophic factor mRNA in the hippocampus and the neocortex. J Neurosci 17:2785–2795, 1997

van Reekum R, Simard M, Clarke D, et al: Late-life depression as a possible predictor of dementia: cross-sectional and short-term follow-up results. Am J Geriatr Psychiatry 7(2):151–159, 1999

Vetulani J, Sulser F: Actions of various antidepressant treatments reduces reactivity of noradrenergic cyclic AMP-generating system in limbic forebrain. Nature 257:455–456, 1975

Vogt BA, Pandya DN: Cingulate cortex of the rhesus monkey: II, cortical afferents. J Comp Neurol 262:271–289, 1987

Vogt BA, Nimchinsky EA, Vogt LJ, et al: Human cingulate cortex: surface features, flat maps, and cytoarchitecture. J Comp Neurol 359:490–506, 1995

Weingartner H, Cohen RM, Murphy DL, et al: Cognitive processes in depression. Arch Gen Psychiatry 38:42–47, 1981

Wu JC, Bunney WE: The biological basis of an antidepressant response to sleep deprivation and relapse: review and hypothesis. Am J Psychiatry 147:14–21, 1990

Wu J, Buchsbaum MS, Gillin JC, et al: Prediction of antidepressant effects of sleep deprivation on metabolic rates in the ventral anterior cingulate and medial prefrontal cortex. Am J Psychiatry 156:1149–1158, 1999

Zacharko RM, Anisman H: Stressor-induced anhedonia in the mesocorticolimbic system. Neurosci Biobehav Rev 15: 391–405, 1991

Zubenko GS, Moossy J: Major depression in primary dementia. Arch Neurol 45:1182–1186, 1988

Zubenko GS, Sullivan P, Nelson JP, et al: Brain imaging abnormalities in mental disorders of late life. Arch Neurol 47:1107–1111, 1990

Neuropsychiatric Aspects of Anxiety Disorders

Dan J. Stein, M.D., Ph.D.

Frans J. Hugo, M.B.Ch.B., M.Med.(Psych.)

It has only recently been appreciated that the anxiety disorders are among the most prevalent of the psychiatric disorders (Kessler et al. 1994) and that they account for perhaps a third of all costs of mental illness (Dupont et al. 1996). Furthermore, only in the past several years have advances in research allowed particular neuroanatomic hypotheses to be put forward about each of the different anxiety disorders. In this chapter, we review these developments in the understanding of the anxiety disorders from the perspective of neuropsychiatry. We begin by reviewing neurological disorders that may present with anxiety symptoms and then outline neuroanatomic models of each of the main anxiety disorders.

Neurological Disorders With Anxiety Symptoms

Neurological conditions that affect a range of different neuroanatomic structures may be associated with anxiety symptoms or disorders (Wise and Rundell 1999). Given that temporolimbic regions, striatum, and prefrontal cortex all likely play an important role in the pathogenesis of certain anxiety disorders, we begin by reviewing the association between lesions in these areas and subsequent anxiety symptoms. This literature not only is clinically relevant but also raises valuable questions for further research.

Various lesions of the temporolimbic

The authors are supported by the Medical Research Council of South Africa.

regions have been associated with the subsequent development of panic disorder. Temporal lobe seizures, tumors, arteriovenous malformation, lobectomy, and parahippocampal infarction all have been reported to present with panic attacks. The association seems particularly strong with right-sided lesions. (Conversely, removal of the amygdala results in placidity toward previously feared objects [Klüver and Bucy 1939] and in deficits in fear conditioning.)

This literature, taken together with clinical observations that panic disorder may be accompanied by dissociation and depersonalization and possibly by electroencephalographic abnormalities and temporal disturbances (see the section "Panic Disorder" later in this chapter), as well as preliminary data that panic disorder may respond to anticonvulsants, raises the question of whether partially overlapping mechanisms may be at work in both temporal lobe seizure disorder and panic disorder. It has been suggested that electroencephalography and anticonvulsant trials may be appropriate in panic disorder patients refractory to conventional treatment.

Lesions of the basal ganglia have been associated with obsessions and compulsions, a finding that has been crucial to the development of a "cortico-striatal-thalamic-cortical" (CSTC) hypothesis of obsessive-compulsive disorder (OCD).

Obsessions and compulsions may be seen in Huntington's disease, Parkinson's disease, spasmodic torticollis, and basal ganglia lesions of a range of etiologies, including calcification, infarction, intoxication, and trauma (Cummings and Cunningham 1992). In this context, it is noteworthy that the basal ganglia may be particularly sensitive to prenatal and perinatal hypoxic-ischemic injury (in twins with Tourette's disorder, for example, an association exists between lower birthweight and increased severity of Tourette's disorder).

Furthermore, early studies suggested a link between Sydenham's chorea and OCD symptoms, and a study by Swedo et al. (1989) reported that rheumatic fever patients with Sydenham's chorea had significantly more OCD symptoms than did those without chorea. This work has had exciting implications, insofar as it has formed the basis for an autoimmune theory of at least some cases of OCD. Swedo and colleagues (1998) coined the term *PANDAS*, or pediatric autoimmune neuropsychiatric disorders associated with streptococcal infections, to describe patients who present with acute obsessive-compulsive or tic symptoms, hypothetically after developing antistriatal antibodies in response to infection.

Some of the most promising research on the association between OCD and a movement disorder has focused on the relation of OCD to Tourette's disorder. Gilles de la Tourette's initial description of the disorder included a patient with tics, vocalizations, and perhaps obsessions. Increasing evidence suggests that a subgroup of patients with Tourette's disorder also has OCD. Conversely, a subgroup of OCD patients has tics. Furthermore, family studies have shown a high rate of OCD and/or tics in relatives of Tourette's disorder patients and a high rate of Tourette's disorder and/or tics in relatives of OCD patients. Anxiety symptoms other than OCD may, however, also be seen in striatal disorders (Lauterbach et al. 1998).

Lesions of the frontal cortex may be associated with a range of perseverative symptoms. In the classic case of Phineas Gage, in addition to impairment in executive functions, the patient also had perseverative symptoms and hoarding behaviors. Similarly, more recent cases of OCD after frontal lobe involvement have been documented.

Anxiety symptoms and disorders also can be seen in a range of neurological disorders that affect multiple brain regions, including frontal cortex. In multiple sclerosis, for example, anxiety symptoms may be found in up to 37% of subjects, and anxiety disorders are also not uncommon. Such symptoms may reflect the deposition of demyelinating plaques, and their treatment should not be ignored.

Similarly, anxiety symptoms have been noted to be common in Alzheimer's disease, particularly in moderate Alzheimer's disease. The relation between regional pathology and anxiety symptoms in Alzheimer's disease deserves further attention. Although anxiety symptoms are also present in frontotemporal dementias, they appear less common in patients with supranuclear palsy, suggesting that there is some specificity to their pathogenesis.

Although the prevalence of depression after stroke has been well studied, less research has focused on anxiety after stroke. In one study of 309 admissions to a stroke unit, generalized anxiety disorder (GAD) was present in 27% of the patients. The authors reported that anxiety plus depression was associated with left cortical lesions, whereas anxiety alone was associated with right hemisphere lesions. Also, worry was associated with anterior and GAD with right posterior lesions.

Anxiety disorders also have been reported in the aftermath of traumatic brain injury. Of interest is the finding that posttraumatic stress disorder (PTSD) can develop even when the patient has neurogenic amnesia for the traumatic event; this finding suggests that implicit memories of trauma may be sufficient for later PTSD to emerge, although subsequent appraisal processes also may be relevant. In either event, PTSD in such patients may be unusual insofar as reexperiencing symptoms are absent.

Neuroanatomy of Anxiety Disorders

In the following sections, we consider the neuropsychiatry of each of the major anxiety disorders. Each section begins by sketching a simplistic neuroanatomic model of the relevant anxiety disorder. This sketch is then used as a framework for attempting a more complex integration of animal data, clinical biological research (e.g., pharmacological probe studies), and brain imaging studies. Although much remains to be learned about the neurobiology of the anxiety disorders, there is a growing consolidation of different avenues of information, with increasingly specific models now existing for each of the major anxiety disorders.

Generalized Anxiety Disorder

The term *generalized anxiety disorder* (GAD) was first introduced in DSM-III (American Psychiatric Association 1980), where it represented a refinement of the earlier concept of *anxiety neurosis*. More recent editions of DSM have emphasized the cognitive symptoms of GAD and have also emphasized that GAD is an independent entity that may be found alone or comorbidly with other anxiety and mood conditions. GAD is the least common anxiety disorder in specialty anxiety clinics but the most common anxiety disorder in primary care practice.

Neuroanatomic models of GAD have not been well delineated to date. However, it may be speculated that GAD involves 1) a general "limbic circuit," including paralimbic cortex (e.g., anterior temporal cortex, posterior medial orbitofrontal cortex) and related subcortical structures, which may be activated across a range of different anxiety disorders; and perhaps 2) some degree of prefrontal hyperactivity, which may represent an

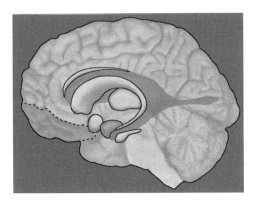

FIGURE 17–1. Neuroanatomic model of generalized anxiety disorder.

Note the increased activity in temporolimbic areas as well as in prefrontal areas.

For a color version of this figure, please see the color insert at the back of this book.

Source. Reprinted from Stein DJ: *False Alarm!: How to Conquer the Anxiety Disorders.* Cape Town, South Africa, University of Stellenbosch, 2000. Used with permission.

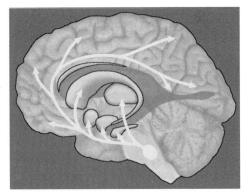

FIGURE 17–2. Serotonergic circuits project to key regions involved in the mediation of anxiety disorders: prefrontal cortex, orbitofrontal cortex, anterior cingulate, amygdala, hippocampus, basal ganglia, thalamus.

For a color version of this figure, please see the color insert at the back of this book.

Source. Reprinted from Stein DJ: *False Alarm!: How to Conquer the Anxiety Disorders.* Cape Town, South Africa, University of Stellenbosch, 2000. Used with permission.

attempt across the anxiety disorders to suppress subcortically mediated anxiety or which may arguably reflect more specific GAD symptoms of excessive worrying and planning (Figure 17–1).

Neurochemical Studies

Serotonergic mediation of GAD is supported by several findings. First, reduced cerebrospinal fluid levels of serotonin and reduced platelet paroxetine binding have been observed in this disorder. Second, administration of the pharmacological probe *m*-chlorophenylpiperazine (m-CPP), a serotonergic agonist, results in increased anxiety and hostility. Third, serotonergic compounds (e.g., buspirone, selective serotonin reuptake inhibitors [SSRIs]) appear effective in the pharmacotherapy of GAD. Serotonergic neurons branch widely throughout the brain, affecting each of the main regions postulated to mediate anxiety symptoms (Figure 17–2); it might be hypothesized that SSRI treatment results in a normalization of limbic, paralimbic, and frontal hyperactivity in GAD.

Animal work has long demonstrated the involvement of the locus coeruleus–norepinephrine–sympathetic nervous system in fear and arousal. Administration of dynamic adrenergic probes has indicated reduced adrenergic receptor sensitivity in GAD, perhaps an adaptation to high circulating catecholamines. The locus coeruleus system projects to the amygdala and to other structures involved in anxiety responses, so that noradrenergic involvement is not inconsistent with the neuroanatomic model outlined earlier.

Involvement of the γ-aminobutyric acid (GABA)/benzodiazepine receptor complex in GAD is supported by several studies, including the responsiveness of this disorder to benzodiazepine treatment. Thus, anxious subjects and GAD patients have reduced benzodiazepine binding capacity, with normalization of findings after benzodiazepine treatment. GABA is the brain's predominant inhibitory neurotransmitter, and GABAergic pathways are widely distributed; nevertheless, the distribution of GABA/benzodiazepine receptors is particularly dense in limbic and paralimbic areas.

Neuroanatomic Studies

Neuroimaging research on GAD is at a relatively preliminary stage. Nevertheless, findings are arguably consistent with involvement of limbic, paralimbic, and prefrontal regions. Work with positron emission tomography (PET) found that GAD patients had increased relative metabolic rates in the right posterior temporal lobe, right precentral frontal gyrus, and left inferior area 17 in the occipital lobe but reduced absolute basal ganglia metabolic rates. Furthermore, benzodiazepine treatment resulted in decreases in absolute metabolic rates for limbic system and cortical surface.

Imaging studies that have pooled or compared findings across different anxiety disorders may also shed light on the underlying neuroanatomy of anxiety symptoms that are not disorder specific. An analysis of pooled PET symptom provocation data from patients with OCD, PTSD, and specific phobia, for example, reported activation of paralimbic structures, right inferior frontal cortex, bilateral lenticulate nuclei, and bilateral brain stem foci. This finding would arguably provide indirect support for a role for the paralimbic system, which serves as a conduit from sensory, motor, and association cortex to the limbic system itself, as well as for inferior frontal regions, in GAD.

Preliminary imaging data on receptor binding in GAD are also available. In a study of female GAD patients, for example, left temporal pole benzodiazepine receptor binding was significantly reduced. This work provides persuasive support for a role for temporolimbic regions, and the GABA/benzodiazepine

receptor complex, in mediating GAD symptoms.

Obsessive-Compulsive Disorder

The characteristic obsessions and compulsions of OCD have a strikingly similar form and content across different patients, raising the question of a specific neuropsychiatric basis for this condition. OCD has a lifetime prevalence of 2%–3% in most countries in which data are available, again supporting a biomedical model. Also remarkable is the recent finding that OCD is the tenth most disabling of all medical conditions worldwide.

There is growing realization of the importance of various CSTC loops in a range of behavior disorders (Cummings 1993); ventral cognitive circuits, involving anterior and lateral orbitofrontal cortex, ventromedial caudate, and dorsomedial nuclei of the thalamus appear to play a role in response inhibition, particularly in relation to certain kinds of cognitive affective cues, and appear most relevant to OCD (Figure 17–3). This kind of model of OCD was first suggested by early findings of an association between neurological lesions of the striatum and OCD (see the section at the beginning of this chapter, "Neurological Disorders With Anxiety Symptoms") and has been supported by a range of subsequent additional studies.

Similar CSTC circuits also have been hypothesized to be involved in various putative OCD spectrum disorders (such as Tourette's disorder). An early "striatal topography" model of OCD spectrum disorders suggested that, whereas the ventral cognitive system mediated OCD symptoms, the sensorimotor cortex and putamen would instead be involved in Tourette's disorder and perhaps trichotillomania (Rauch and Baxter 1998). The data have not, however, fully supported such a model, and it is possible rather that particular striatal projection fields or cell

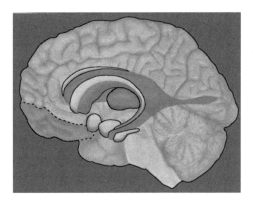

FIGURE 17–3. Neuroanatomic model of obsessive-compulsive disorder.

Note the increased activity in the ventromedial cortico-striatal-thalamic-cortical circuit.

For a color version of this figure, please see the color insert at the back of this book.

Source. Reprinted from Stein DJ: *False Alarm!: How to Conquer the Anxiety Disorders.* Cape Town, South Africa, University of Stellenbosch, 2000. Used with permission.

types are involved in specific kinds of symptoms.

Neurochemical Studies

Interest in the neurochemical substrate of OCD received significant impetus from the early finding that the disorder responded to clomipramine, a serotonin reuptake inhibitor. Subsequent studies confirmed that clomipramine is more robust than desipramine, a noradrenergic reuptake inhibitor, in OCD. Furthermore, each of the SSRIs studied to date has been effective for the treatment of OCD (D.J. Stein et al. 1995). During effective treatment with a serotonin reuptake inhibitor, cerebrospinal fluid 5-hydroxyindoleacetic acid decreases (Thoren et al. 1980), and exacerbation of obsessive-compulsive symptoms by m-CPP is no longer seen after treatment with an SSRI (Zohar et al. 1988).

The serotonergic system innervates not only the basal ganglia but also the orbitofrontal cortex. Serotonergic abnor-

malities in OCD may be region specific. Of particular interest is recent animal work showing that downregulation of serotonin terminal autoreceptors in orbitofrontal cortex occurs only after relatively long periods and with relatively high doses of medication and does not occur after electroconvulsive therapy. This provides an elegant parallel with clinical findings that OCD pharmacotherapy differs from that used for depression.

Nevertheless, it is notable that only about 50%–60% of OCD patients respond to serotonin reuptake inhibitors and that not all patients show abnormal responses to m-CPP, suggesting that other neurochemical systems also are important. Of particular interest, administration of dopamine agonists results in stereotypic behavior in animals and in tics in humans, and conversely, dopamine blockers are effective for the treatment of tics. Furthermore, it turns out that OCD patients with comorbid tics are less likely to respond to serotonin reuptake inhibitors but more likely to respond to augmentation of serotonin reuptake inhibitors with classical neuroleptics.

Given the dopaminergic innervation of the striatum and the interaction between the serotonin and the dopaminergic systems, these findings are consistent with the CSTC model. Indeed, infusion of dopamine into the caudate results in stereotyped orofacial behaviors, whereas infusion of dopamine blockers into the same areas reduces amphetamine-induced stereotypy. Dopaminergic striatal circuits are presumably likely to be particularly important in OCD patients with tics and in patients with OCD spectrum disorders, such as Tourette's disorder, that are characterized by involuntary movements.

Other neurochemical systems, including glutamate and GABA, also play an important role in CSTC circuits.

Neuroanatomic Studies

A range of evidence indicates that cortico-striatal circuits are important in mediating stereotypic behavior. Isolation of primates during development, for example, results in basal ganglia cytoarchitectural abnormalities and stereotypic behavior. MacLean (1978) noted that lesions of the striatum resulted in stereotypic behavior and suggested that this was a repository for fixed action patterns or inherited motor sequences (e.g., grooming, nest-building). Indeed, the animal literature on stereotypies and disorders of grooming parallels not only the phenomenology of OCD but also its psychopharmacology.

There is, however, a growing appreciation of the role of the striatum in cognition and learning. In particular, striatal function has increasingly been associated with the development, maintenance, and selection of motoric and cognitive procedural strategies. Different terms given to allude to this group of functions include *habit system*, *response set*, and *procedural mobilization*. Basal ganglia may play a particularly important role in the implicit learning of procedural strategies and their subsequent automatic execution. Certainly, neurological soft sign abnormalities and neuropsychological dysfunction in patients with OCD are consistent with dysfunction in CSTC circuits.

Structural imaging studies also are consistent with a role for CSTC circuits in OCD. An early study found reduced caudate volume in OCD patients, but not all subsequent research has replicated this finding. The finding that patients with PANDAS have increased basal ganglia volume may partly explain this inconsistency; in some OCD patients, basal ganglia volume initially may be increased, with subsequent reduction over time. Structural studies also have shown neuronal abnormalities or volume loss in orbitofrontal cortex, cingulate, amygdala, and thalamus in OCD. Also, putamen volume may be reduced in certain putative OCD spectrum disorders such as Tourette's disorder and trichotillomania.

Functional imaging studies, however, provide some of the most persuasive evidence of the role of CSTC circuits in OCD. OCD patients at rest, and especially when exposed to feared stimuli, have increased activity in the orbitofrontal cortex, anterior cingulate, and basal ganglia (Rauch and Baxter 1998). A range of functional abnormalities has also been found in Tourette's disorder; one study, for example, found increased metabolism in the orbitofrontal cortex and putamen that correlated with complex behavioral and cognitive features.

Functional imaging findings may have particular explanatory power when they also integrate cognitive neuroscience constructs and findings. During brain imaging of an implicit sequence learning task, control subjects without OCD showed striatal activation, but patients with OCD instead appeared to recruit medial temporal regions. These latter regions are typically involved in conscious cognitive-affective processing. Control subjects can process procedural strategies outside of awareness, but in OCD, intrusion of these into consciousness occurs.

An additional important set of findings that relate to the CSTC hypothesis of OCD emerges from work on neurosurgical treatments for OCD. Several different procedures have been used, but the general effect of these interventions is to interrupt CSTC circuits.

The "standard" neuroanatomic model of OCD may, however, be insufficiently complex to account for all cases. There is, for example, a literature on temporal lobe involvement in OCD. Certainly, although OCD is in many ways a homogeneous entity, further research is necessary to delineate different neurobiological mechanisms in subtypes of the disorder.

Several studies have successfully integrated neurochemical and neuroimaging data. An early study reported that m-CPP exacerbation of OCD symptoms was associated with increased frontal regional cerebral blood flow (rCBF). A later single photon emission computed tomography (SPECT) study that used the 5-HT$_{1D}$ probe sumatriptan also confirmed correlations between symptom changes and prefrontal rCBF, supporting a role for the terminal autoreceptor in OCD. In OCD, there is now preliminary evidence of altered serotonin synthesis in frontostriatal circuitry. In contrast, in Tourette's disorder, striatal dopamine transport densities were increased, and in monozygotic twins with Tourette's disorder, increased caudate dopamine D$_2$ receptor binding was associated with increased tic severity. Finally, a seminal publication reported that patients with OCD treated with either serotonin reuptake inhibitors or behavior therapy had normalization of activity in CSTC circuits (Baxter et al. 1992); effective interventions appear to work via a final common pathway of specific brain structures.

Nevertheless, several important questions remain unresolved about the CSTC model of OCD. It is unclear, for example, how presumptive lesions to the CSTC circuit occur. Despite the documentation of cases of PANDAS, the extent to which autoimmune processes contribute to OCD in general is not known. Also, there may be differential pathogenic mechanisms across different OCD spectrum disorders; for example, Tourette's disorder has been associated with autoantibodies against putamen but not caudate or globus pallidus. Finally, genetic variability may play some role; for example, some studies have found differences in dopamine system polymorphisms in OCD patients with and without tics.

Panic Disorder

Panic disorder is a highly prevalent disorder, with rates fairly similar across different social and cultural settings. It is now well recognized that panic disorder may be associated with significant morbidity (mood, anxiety, and substance use disorders) as well as with severe impairments in occupational and social functioning.

Over the past decade or two, models of panic disorder have become increasingly sophisticated (Gorman et al. 1989, 2000). Current neuroanatomic models of panic (Figure 17–4) emphasize 1) afferents from viscerosensory pathways to thalamus to lateral nucleus of the amygdala, as well as from thalamus to cortical association areas to the lateral nucleus of the amygdala; 2) the extended amygdala, which is thought to play a central role in conditioned fear and anxiety; 3) the hippocampus, which is thought crucial for conditioning to the context of the fear (and so perhaps for phobic avoidance); and 4) efferent tracts from the amygdala to the hypothalamus and brain stem structures, which mediate many of the symptoms of panic. Thus, efferents of the central nucleus of the amygdala include the lateral nucleus (autonomic arousal and sympathetic discharge) and paraventricular nucleus (increased adrenocorticoid release) of the hypothalamus, and the locus coeruleus (increased norepinephrine release), parabrachial nucleus (increased respiratory rate), and periaqueductal gray (defensive behaviors and postural freezing) in the brain stem.

Neurochemical Studies

Early animal studies found that the locus coeruleus plays a key role in fear and anxiety. The locus coeruleus contains the highest concentration of noradrenergic-producing neurons in the brain. Viscerosensory input reaches the locus coeruleus via the nucleus tractus solitarius and the

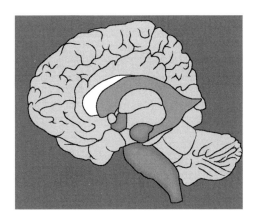

FIGURE 17–4. Neuroanatomic model of panic disorder.

Note the activation of the amygdala, which has efferents to hypothalamus and brain stem sites.

For a color version of this figure, please see the color insert at the back of this book.

Source. Reprinted from Stein DJ: *False Alarm!: How to Conquer the Anxiety Disorders.* Cape Town, South Africa, University of Stellenbosch, 2000. Used with permission.

medullary nucleus paragigantocellularis, and the locus coeruleus sends efferents to a range of important structures, including the amygdala, hypothalamus, and brain stem periaqueductal gray.

Several clinical studies of panic disorder provide support for the role of the locus coeruleus; administration of yohimbine, for example, resulted in greater increases in 3-methoxy-4-hydroxyphenylglycol (MHPG) in panic disorder patients than in control subjects without panic disorder. However, not all studies have replicated such findings, suggesting that additional neurochemical factors are important in the mediation of panic attacks.

Certainly, increasing evidence indicates that the serotonergic system plays a crucial role in panic disorder. A range of studies provides evidence for this; for example, several studies have found that m-CPP administration leads to an acute exacerbation of panic symptoms in panic disorder

patients. Particularly compelling, however, is growing evidence of the effectiveness of the SSRIs in panic disorder, with some indications that they may in fact be more effective than earlier classes of agents.

The serotonergic system interacts at several points with neuroanatomic structures thought important in panic disorder. Thus, modulation of the serotonin system has the potential to influence the major regions of the panic disorder circuit, resulting in decreased noradrenergic activity, diminished release of corticotropin-releasing factor, and modification of defense/escape behaviors.

Peripheral benzodiazepine receptor binding is decreased in panic disorder, and benzodiazepines are effective in treating this condition. In animal models, direct administration of a benzodiazepine agonist into the amygdala produces anxiolytic effects, which are weakened by pretreatment with a benzodiazepine receptor antagonist (Coplan and Lydiard 1998).

A consideration of the various afferents to the locus coeruleus and amygdala is relevant to considering the extensive literature on panicogenic stimuli. It has been argued that respiratory panicogens (e.g., carbon dioxide, lactate), baroceptor stimulation (β-agonists), and circulating peptides (cholecystokinin) promote panic via a limbic viscororeceptor pathway. In contrast, panic attacks that are conditioned by visuospatial, auditory, or cognitive cues may be mediated by pathways from cortical association areas to the amygdala (Coplan and Lydiard 1998). Ultimately, it may be possible to determine particular genetic loci that are involved in contextual fear conditioning, allowing for an integration of the neurochemical, genetic, and environmental data on panic disorder.

Neuroanatomic Studies

Preliminary evidence from brain imaging shows the importance of the amygdala and paralimbic structures in panic disorder. Preliminary studies in nonanxious control subjects reported activation of amygdala and periamygdaloid cortical areas during conditioned fear acquisition and extinction. Furthermore, an early magnetic resonance imaging study reported focal abnormalities in the temporal lobe, particularly on the right side, in patients with panic disorder. Finally, PET scanning during anxious anticipation in control subjects and lactate-induced panic attacks in panic disorder patients both identified increased activity in paralimbic regions (temporal poles).

An early study suggested that only panic patients susceptible to lactate-induced panic had abnormal asymmetry of a parahippocampal region at rest. Subsequent functional imaging studies have confirmed dysfunctions of hippocampus or parahippocampal regions in panic disorder, although the precise abnormalities documented have not always been consistent. Hypocapnia-induced vasoconstriction has made the results of certain imaging studies in panic disorder difficult to interpret.

Additional abnormalities have been documented in some imaging studies of panic disorder. Although it has been hypothesized that cognitive-behavioral treatments exert effects in panic disorder by behavioral desensitization of hippocampal-mediated contextual conditioning, or by cognitive techniques that strengthen medial prefrontal cortex inhibition of amygdala (Gorman et al. 2000; LeDoux 1998), the relevant empirical studies have not yet been undertaken.

Advances in brain imaging methods have, however, begun to tackle the integration of neuroanatomic and neurochemical data. Some groups, for example, have reported decreased benzodiazepine binding in left temporal regions; right orbitofrontal cortex and right insula; and frontal, temporal, and occipital cortex. However, not all studies have been consistent.

Posttraumatic Stress Disorder

PTSD begins, by definition, in the aftermath of exposure to a trauma. Three sets of subsequent symptoms characterize PTSD: reexperiencing phenomena, avoidant and numbing symptoms, and hyperarousal. It should be emphasized that the prevalence of exposure to trauma is significantly higher than the prevalence of PTSD, indicating that most trauma does not lead to this disorder.

Indeed, an important development in the PTSD literature is a growing emphasis that this is not a "normal" reaction to an abnormal event. Rather, PTSD is increasingly viewed as a serious disorder that is associated with significant morbidity and mediated by neurobiological and psychological dysfunctions.

Features of current neuroanatomic models of PTSD (Figure 17–5) include the following: 1) amygdalothalamic pathways are involved in the rapid, automatic (implicit) processing of incoming information; 2) the amygdala, which sends afferents to other regions involved in the anxiety response (hypothalamus, brain stem nuclei) is hyperactivated; 3) the hippocampus is involved in (explicitly) remembering the context of traumatic memories; and 4) activity is decreased in certain frontal-cortical areas, such as Broca's area, consistent with the decreased verbalization during the processing of trauma and with the inability to override automatic amygdala processing.

Neurochemical Studies

A range of neurochemical findings in PTSD are consistent with sensitization of various neurotransmitter systems (Charney et al. 1993). In particular, there is evidence of hyperactive noradrenergic function and dopaminergic sensitization.

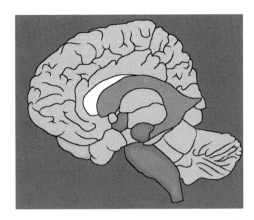

FIGURE 17–5. Neuroanatomic model of posttraumatic stress disorder.

Note the increased activity in the amygdala and its efferents (Rauch et al. 1996), decreased activity in Broca's area (Shin et al. 1997), and decreased volume of the hippocampus (Bremner et al. 1997; M.B. Stein et al. 1997).

For a color version of this figure, please see the color insert at the back of this book.

Source. Reprinted from Stein DJ: *False Alarm!: How to Conquer the Anxiety Disorders.* Cape Town, South Africa, University of Stellenbosch, 2000. Used with permission.

Such sensitization is also consistent with the role of environmental traumas in PTSD; it turns out that dopamine agonists and environmental traumas act as cross-sensitizers of each other. Evidence indicates that the amygdala and related limbic regions may play a particularly important role in the final common pathway of such hyperactivation.

Also, growing evidence suggests the importance of the serotonin system in mediating PTSD symptoms. Clinical studies of abnormal paroxetine binding and exacerbations of symptoms in response to administration of m-CPP are certainly consistent with a role for serotonin in PTSD. Furthermore, evidence is increasing for the efficacy of serotonin reuptake inhibitors in PTSD, with preliminary indications that these agents may be more effective than other classes of medication. These agents may act on amygdala

circuits, helping to inhibit efferents to structures such as hypothalamus and brain stem nuclei, which mediate fear.

A third set of neurochemical findings in PTSD has focused on the hypothalamic-pituitary-adrenal system. PTSD is characterized by decreased plasma levels of cortisol, as well as increased glucocorticoid receptor responsiveness, suggesting that negative feedback inhibition may play an important role in the pathogenesis of the disorder. Such findings differ from those found in other anxiety disorders and in depression. Notably, cortisol-releasing factor receptors are also prominent in the amygdala, particularly in the central nucleus.

One important implication of the hypothalamic-pituitary-adrenal findings is the possibility that dysfunction in this system results in neuronal damage, particularly to the hippocampus. Animal studies have documented hippocampal damage after exposure to either glucocorticoids or naturalistic psychosocial stressors. Parallel neurotoxicity in human PTSD could account for some of the cognitive impairments that are characteristic of this disorder.

Neuroanatomic Studies

A range of structural imaging studies are in fact consistent with the possibility of hippocampal dysfunction occurring in PTSD. In an early magnetic resonance imaging study, combat veterans with PTSD had smaller right hippocampal volumes than did healthy control subjects, and in PTSD patients, hippocampal volume reduction correlated with deficits in short-term verbal memory. A different group of investigators reported consistent findings; both right and left hippocampal volumes were significantly reduced in combat veterans with PTSD compared with both combat control subjects and healthy subjects. Furthermore, hippocampal volume was directly correlated with combat exposure.

A similar set of findings has been reported in adult patients with PTSD secondary to childhood abuse. PTSD patients have increased neurological soft signs and neurodevelopmental abnormalities, and it is theoretically possible that diminished hippocampal size is a risk factor for the development of psychiatric complications following trauma exposure rather than a consequence of trauma. Nevertheless, these preliminary findings are consistent in pointing to a role for the hippocampus in PTSD.

Functional imaging studies have provided additional information to help build a neuroanatomic model of PTSD. First, several studies in control subjects without PTSD have provided evidence for subcortical processing of masked emotional stimuli by the amygdala. Furthermore, in an early study, PTSD patients exposed to audiotaped traumatic and neutral scripts during PET had increases in normalized blood flow in right-sided limbic, paralimbic, and visual areas and decreases in blood flow in left inferior frontal and middle temporal cortex (Rauch et al. 1996). The authors concluded that emotions associated with the PTSD symptomatic state were mediated by the limbic and paralimbic systems within the right hemisphere, with activation of visual cortex perhaps corresponding to visual reexperiencing. It has been suggested that decreased activity in Broca's area during exposure to trauma in PTSD is consistent with patients' inability to verbally process traumatic memories (Rauch et al. 1998).

Once again, modern techniques have recently allowed for the integration of neurochemical and neuroanatomic data. PET was undertaken in combat veterans with PTSD and healthy control subjects after administration of yohimbine. Yohimbine resulted in a significant increase in anxiety in the patients with PTSD, and this group of subjects also had a decrease in several areas, including prefrontal, temporal, parietal, and orbitofrontal cortex. This is perhaps consistent with previous literature suggesting that during intense anxiety states, rCBF decreases.

Social Phobia (Social Anxiety Disorder)

Social phobia (social anxiety disorder) is characterized by a fear of social situations in which the individual may be exposed to the scrutiny of others. These fears may be divided into those that concern social interaction situations (e.g., dating, meetings) and performance fears (e.g., of talking, eating, or writing in public). These fears result in avoidance of social situations or endurance of these situations with considerable distress. Growing evidence indicates that social phobia is a chronic disorder, with substantial comorbidity (particularly of mood and substance use disorders) and significant morbidity.

Detailed neuroanatomic models of social phobia remain to be delineated. Nevertheless, it may be hypothesized again that temporolimbic circuitry is important in mediating the fear responses that characterize this disorder. Furthermore, serotonin and dopamine neurocircuitry, presumably involving prefrontal and basal ganglia regions, also may play a crucial role (Figure 17–6).

Neurochemical Studies

A range of evidence supports the role of serotonergic circuits in social phobia. A pharmacological probe study was performed with agents that affect the serotonergic (fenfluramine), dopaminergic (levodopa), and noradrenergic (clonidine) systems; the only positive finding was an augmented cortisol response to fenfluramine administration in patients with social phobia. The authors concluded that

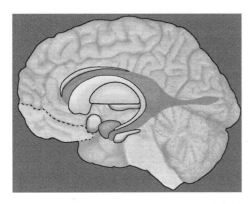

FIGURE 17–6. Neuroanatomic model of social phobia.

Note the increased temporolimbic activity, decreased basal ganglia dopaminergic activity, and perhaps some increased prefrontal activity.

For a color version of this figure, please see the color insert at the back of this book.

Source. Reprinted from Stein DJ: *False Alarm!: How to Conquer the Anxiety Disorders.* Cape Town, South Africa, University of Stellenbosch, 2000. Used with permission.

patients with social phobia may have selective supersensitivity of serotonergic systems.

Also, a range of evidence indicates involvement of the dopaminergic system in social phobia. Timid mice have decreased cerebrospinal fluid dopamine levels, and introverted depressed patients also may have decreased cerebrospinal fluid dopamine levels (Nutt et al. 1998). Social status in monkeys may be reflected in differences in dopamine D_2 striatal density. More persuasively, social phobia may be associated with Parkinson's disease or may appear after the administration of neuroleptics (M.B. Stein 1998).

Evidence that the hypothalamic-pituitary-adrenal axis may be dysfunctional in social phobia is inconsistent to date. Social phobia patients, however, have normal levels of urinary and plasma cortisol and normal dexamethasone suppression test results, although some evidence shows an association between social phobia and hypothalamic growth hormone dysfunction.

Neuroanatomic Studies

Some evidence suggests that patients with social phobia have selective activation of the amygdala when exposed to potentially fear-relevant stimuli (Nutt et al. 1998). Furthermore, after treatment with an SSRI, patients with social phobia had significantly reduced activity in the anterior and lateral part of the left temporal cortex; the left cingulum; and the anterior, lateral, and posterior part of the left midfrontal cortex.

Furthermore, some imaging studies suggest that the striatum also may play a role in social phobia. Indeed, a recent study of the density of dopamine reuptake sites found that striatal dopamine reuptake site densities were markedly lower in patients than in nonphobic control subjects. Moreover, striatal D_2 receptor binding was lower in social phobia patients than in control subjects (Schneier et al. 2000). These findings support the hypothesis that social phobia may be associated with a dysfunction of the striatal dopaminergic system.

Conclusions

Several lessons emerge from a review of the neuropsychiatry of anxiety disorders. First, the anxiety disorders are common and disabling disorders not only in general clinical settings but also in patients with neurological illnesses such as Alzheimer's disease, stroke, and traumatic brain injury. Although the link between depression and neuropsychiatric disorders is increasingly recognized, the importance of anxiety disorders in this context has perhaps been relatively overlooked, paralleling the underdiagnosis and undertreatment of anxiety disorders in primary care settings. The anxiety disorders deserve to be carefully diagnosed and rigorously treated.

Second, both animal and clinical studies increasingly indicate that the amygdala and paralimbic structures play an important role in conditioned fear and in anxiety disorders. Amygdala lesions are classically associated with decreased fear responses, and conversely, hyperactivation of the limbic system is characteristic of several different anxiety disorders. Paralimbic regions, such as the anterior cingulate, appear to play a key role at the interface of cognition and emotion. The apparent centrality of such systems to different anxiety disorders may account in part for their high comorbidity. Additional features of limbic involvement may, however, be specific to particular disorders (e.g., hippocampal shrinkage in PTSD or parahippocampal asymmetry in panic disorder). Serotonin reuptake inhibitors are increasingly viewed as first-line treatments for anxiety disorders, and innervation of amygdala and paralimbic structures by serotonergic neurons may be crucial in explaining their efficacy.

Finally, CSTC pathways also may be important in anxiety disorders, particularly in OCD and certain putative OCD spectrum disorders, such as Tourette's disorder. There is growing consolidation of imaging, immunologic, genetic, and treatment data around this model. It is particularly remarkable that CSTC pathways can be normalized by pharmacotherapy, by psychotherapy, and by neurosurgery. In some ways, it can be argued that although OCD was once viewed as the key to a psychodynamic understanding of the mind, OCD and some OCD spectrum disorders such as Tourette's disorder are now the neuropsychiatric disorders par excellence. Certainly, such disorders provide a key paradigm and challenge for those who are interested in integrating "brain" and "mind" approaches to psychiatric disorders.

References

American Psychiatric Association: Diagnostic and Statistical Manual of Mental Disorders, 3rd Edition. Washington, DC, American Psychiatric Association, 1980

Baxter LR, Schwartz JM, Bergman KS: Caudate glucose metabolic rate changes with both drug and behavior therapy for OCD. Arch Gen Psychiatry 49:681–689, 1992

Bremner JD, Randall P, Vermetten E, et al: Magnetic resonance imaging-based measurement of hippocampal volume in posttraumatic stress disorder related to childhood physical and sexual abuse—a preliminary report. Biol Psychiatry 41:23–32, 1997

Charney DS, Deutch AY, Krystal JH, et al: Psychobiologic mechanisms of posttraumatic stress disorder. Arch Gen Psychiatry 50:295–305, 1993

Coplan JD, Lydiard RB: Brain circuits in panic disorder. Biol Psychiatry 44:1264–1276, 1998

Cummings JL: Frontal-subcortical circuits and human behavior. Arch Neurol 50:873–880, 1993

Cummings JL, Cunningham K: Obsessive-compulsive disorder in Huntington's disease. Biol Psychiatry 31:263–270, 1992

Dupont RL, Rice DP, Miller LS, et al: Economic costs of anxiety disorders. Anxiety 2:167–172, 1996

Gorman JM, Liebowitz MR, Fyer AJ, et al: A neuroanatomical hypothesis for panic disorder [see comments]. Am J Psychiatry 146:148–161, 1989

Gorman JM, Kent JM, Sullivan GM, et al: Neuroanatomical hypothesis of panic disorder, revised. Am J Psychiatry 157:493–505, 2000

Kessler RC, McGonagle KA, Zhao S, et al: Lifetime and 12-month prevalence of DSM-III-R psychiatric disorders in the United States: results from the National Comorbidity Survey. Arch Gen Psychiatry 51:8–19, 1994

Klüver H, Bucy PC: Preliminary analysis of functions of the temporal lobes in monkeys. AMA Archives of Neurology and Psychiatry 42:979–1000, 1939

Lauterbach EC, Cummings JL, Duffy J, et al: Neuropsychiatric correlates and treatment of lenticulostriatal diseases: a review of literature and overview of research opportunities in Huntington's, Wilson's, and Fahr's diseases. J Neuropsychiatry Clin Neurosci 10:249–266, 1998

LeDoux J: Fear and the brain: where have we been, and where are we going? Biol Psychiatry 44:1229–1238, 1998

MacLean PD: Effects of lesions of globus pallidus on species-typical display behavior of squirrel monkeys. Brain Res 149:175–196, 1978

Nutt DJ, Bell CJ, Malizia AL: Brain mechanisms of social anxiety disorder. J Clin Psychiatry 59 (suppl 17):4–11, 1998

Rauch SL, Baxter LR: Neuroimaging in obsessive-compulsive and related disorders, in Obsessive-Compulsive Disorders: Practical Management, 3rd Edition. Edited by Jenike MA, Baer L, Minichiello WE. St. Louis, MO, Mosby, 1998, pp 289–316

Rauch SL, van der Kolk BA, Fisler RE, et al: A symptom provocation study of posttraumatic stress disorder using positron emission tomography and script-driven imagery. Arch Gen Psychiatry 53:380–387, 1996

Rauch SL, Shin LM, Whalen PJ, et al: Neuroimaging and the neuroanatomy of posttraumatic stress disorder. CNS Spectr 3:31–41, 1998

Schneier FR, Liebowitz MR, Abi-Dargham A, et al: Low dopamine D(2) receptor binding potential in social phobia. Am J Psychiatry 157(3):457–459, 2000

Shin LM, Kosslyn SM, McNally RJ, et al: Visual imagery and perception in posttraumatic stress disorder: a positron emission tomographic investigation. Arch Gen Psychiatry 54:233–241, 1997

Stein DJ: False Alarm!: How to Conquer the Anxiety Disorders. Cape Town, South Africa, University of Stellenbosch, 2000

Stein DJ, Spadaccini E, Hollander E: Meta-analysis of pharmacotherapy trials for obsessive compulsive disorder. Int Clin Psychopharmacol 10:11–18, 1995

Stein MB: Neurobiological perspectives on social phobia: from affiliation to zoology. Biol Psychiatry 44:1277–1285, 1998

Stein MB, Koverola C, Hanna C, et al: Hippocampal volume in women victimized by childhood sexual abuse. Psychol Med 27:951–959, 1997

Swedo SE, Rapoport JL, Cheslow DL, et al: High prevalence of obsessive-compulsive symptoms in patients with Sydenham's chorea. Am J Psychiatry 146:246–249, 1989

Swedo SE, Leonard HL, Garvey M: Pediatric autoimmune neuropsychiatric disorders associated with streptococcal infections: clinical description of the first 50 cases. Am J Psychiatry 155:264–271, 1998

Thoren P, Asberg M, Bertilsson L: Clomipramine treatment of obsessive-compulsive disorder, II: biochemical aspects. Arch Gen Psychiatry 37:1289–1294, 1980

Wise MG, Rundell JR: Anxiety and neurological disorders. Semin Clin Neuropsychiatry 4:98–102, 1999

Zohar J, Insel TR, Zohar-Kadouch RC: Serotonergic responsivity in obsessive-compulsive disorder: effects of chronic clomipramine treatment. Arch Gen Psychiatry 45:167–172, 1988

Neuropsychiatric Disorders of Childhood and Adolescence

Martin H. Teicher, M.D., Ph.D.

Susan L. Andersen, Ph.D.

Carryl P. Navalta, Ph.D.

Ann Polcari, Ph.D., R.N.

Dennis Kim, M.D.

In this chapter, we emphasize brain-based psychiatric disorders that invariably emerge during childhood and adolescence. Virtually all neuropsychiatric disorders can appear in pediatric patients; however, certain disorders such as attention-deficit/hyperactivity disorder (ADHD), mental retardation, and Tourette's syndrome (TS) must present before adulthood for diagnosis. These disorders are the focus of this chapter.

Brain Development

The human brain is an enormously complex organ consisting, at the simplest level, of billions of neurons and trillions of synaptic interconnections. Genetic information from 60% of our 100,000 genes provides the basic architecture, but the final form and function is sculpted by experience. Such an intrinsically complex process is inherently vulnerable to numerous errors, which set the stage for the emergence of childhood and adolescent neuropsychiatric disorders.

The brain develops through a series of overlapping stages, which are illustrated in Figure 18–1. The first stage is mitosis, in which neural progenitor cells multiply and divide in the neural tube in the area destined to become the ventricular surface. Eventually the germinal cells undergo their final mitotic division to form immature nerve cells that can no longer reproduce. These neuroblasts are laid down inside out, with larger cells generally

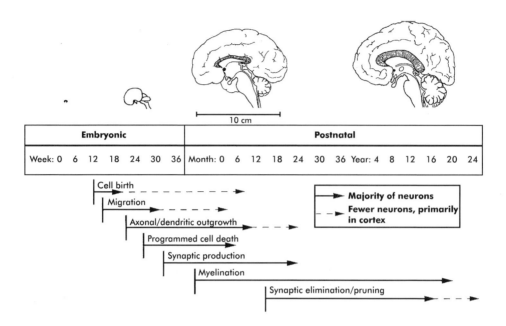

FIGURE 18–1.   Major overlapping stages of human brain development and approximate temporal sequence.

appearing at an earlier stage than smaller cells. During this period the brain produces two to three times the full adult complement of neurons. Although neurogenesis ceases in most brain regions at birth, stem cells continue to generate neurons within the subventricular zone and hippocampal dentate gyrus throughout life (Gage 2000).

The second stage involves the migration of neurons to their final destination. This is a complex process in which immature neurons follow chemical, spatial, and mechanical gradients to reach their destination and establish connections with appropriate targets (Landis 1983; Purves 1980). Learning disorders and some forms of mental retardation can arise from abnormal migration. Once neurons reach their final destination at about the sixteenth fetal week, they branch in an attempt to establish appropriate connections (Sidman and Rakic 1973). In a striking turn of events, more than 50% of these neurons are eliminated before birth in a

process known as *cell death* or *apoptosis* (Landmesser 1980). Cell survival depends on the level of activity the neuron receives and the presence of trophic factors that stabilize its growth (Cowan et al. 1984).

Synaptic development is also characterized by distinct waves of overproduction and elimination. Synaptic density in the human brain increases dramatically during the early postnatal period. Formation of synapses in the cerebellum peaks during the first 2–4 months, whereas synaptic density of the cortex continues to increase throughout early childhood (Huttenlocher 1979). From birth to age 5, the brain triples in mass from 350 g to a near-adult weight of 1.2 kg. Part of this increase is a result of the marked arborization and enhanced connection of neurons. Much of the gain stems from the vigorous myelination of fiber tracts.

During the transition from childhood to adulthood, a second dramatic elimination phase occurs in which synaptic contacts and neurotransmitter receptors overproduced during childhood are pruned back to final adult configuration. Between ages 7 and 15 years, synaptic density in the frontal cortex decreases by approximately 40% (Huttenlocher 1979). Similar changes occur in the density of dopamine (Seeman et al. 1987) (Figure 18–2), glutamate (Barks et al. 1988), and neurotensin (Mailleux et al. 1990) receptors. Overly extensive or insufficient pruning has been associated with some forms of mental retardation (Huttenlocher 1979) and has been hypothesized to play a key role in the emergence of schizophrenia (Feinberg 1982–1983; Keshaven et al. 1994). Teicher and Andersen (Andersen et al. 2000; Teicher et al. 1995) found that dopamine receptors prune very rapidly after the onset of puberty in the nigrostriatal system of rats, prune in early adulthood in the prefrontal cortex, but do not prune in the limbic connections to the nucleus accumbens. Synaptic pruning may represent an important developmental stage in which high synaptic density, facilitating acquisition of new knowledge and skills at considerable metabolic cost, is partially traded for a lower density, facilitating rapid analysis and performance through established patterns (Teicher et al. 1995). In concert with this transition, there is a reduction in synaptic plasticity, attenuating capacity to recover from injury. Synaptic pruning may also be responsible for the plateau in the growth of intellectual capacity (*mental age*) that occurs at about 16 years (Walker 1994).

Development of Lateralization and Hemispheric Asymmetry

The human brain is anatomically, neurochemically, and functionally asymmetric. Lateralization is largely established before age 5 years (Krashen 1973) and emerges through a multistage process that begins in utero (Chi et al. 1972; Molfese et al.

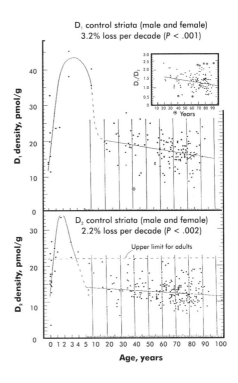

FIGURE 18–2. Overproduction and pruning of dopamine D_1 and D_2 receptors in human corpus striatum during childhood and adolescence.

Source. Seeman P, Bzowej N, Guan H, et al.: "Human Brain Receptors in Children and Aging Adults." *Synapse* 1:399–404, 1987. Copyright © 1987 Wiley-Liss, Inc. Reprinted by permission of Wiley-Liss, Inc., a subsidiary of John Wiley & Sons, Inc.

1975; Wada et al. 1975). Delayed myelination of the corpus callosum enables the two hemispheres to develop relatively independently. During the first few months, the right hemisphere develops more rapidly than the left, with more advanced dendritic outgrowth in Broca's area and motor cortex (Galaburda 1984; Simonds and Scheibel 1989). However, by age 5–6 months, dendritic growth in the left hemisphere surpasses that in the right and continues at a rapid pace for the next 2 years. Between ages 3 and 6 years, the right hemisphere accelerates in its development and helps provide the prosodic components of language that flower between ages 5 and 6 years. The left hemisphere, however, remains more differentiated. Early experience can exert marked effect on lateralization in laboratory animals (Bulman-Fleming et al. 1992; Camp et al. 1984; Denenberg and Yutzey 1985). This may also be true for humans and may be an important factor in the genesis of psychiatric disorders (Teicher et al. 1994, 1996a).

Disorders of Excessive Motor Activity, Movement, Impulse, and Thought

One of the most prevalent and treatable clusters of childhood neuropsychiatric disorders includes ADHD, TS, and obsessive-compulsive disorder (OCD). These conditions often co-occur or run in families (Knell and Comings 1993; Pauls 1991; Pauls and Leckman 1986). They likely occur as a consequence of different but interrelated defects in corticolimbic-basal ganglia circuits (Lou et al. 1990; Luxenberg et al. 1988; Peterson et al. 1993; Singer et al. 1993; Zametkin et al. 1990). TS and ADHD are discussed together to emphasize their commonality. OCD is discussed elsewhere in this book.

Attention-Deficit/ Hyperactivity Disorder

ADHD was first identified as a medical disorder after the 1917 pandemic of von Economo's encephalitis. It is one of the most common neuropsychiatric disorders of childhood, estimated to affect 3%–9% of school-age children (J.C. Anderson et al. 1987; Bird et al. 1988; Szatmari et al. 1989). This is a serious disorder that persists beyond childhood in about 40% of affected individuals (Klein and Mannuzza 1991). It is associated with a dramatically increased incidence of antisocial personal-

ity, drug abuse, delinquency, and criminality (Gittelman et al. 1985; Klein and Mannuzza 1991; Mannuzza et al. 1989; Satterfield et al. 1982; G. Weiss et al. 1985).

Characteristic Features

ADHD is characterized by a triad of symptoms involving age-inappropriate problems with attention, impulse control, and hyperactivity (Barkley 1990; Tryon 1993). Currently, DSM-IV (American Psychiatric Association 1994) divides the symptom triad into two factors: inattention and hyperactivity-impulsivity. To meet criteria for the disorder, children need to have, during the previous 6 months, at least six symptoms of inattention or six symptoms of hyperactivity-impulsivity. If they meet criteria for both inattention and hyperactivity-impulsivity, they are diagnosed with ADHD combined type, which is the most prevalent form. Otherwise, they are diagnosed as either ADHD predominantly inattentive type or ADHD predominantly hyperactive-impulsive type. In addition to meeting symptom criteria, accurate diagnosis requires that some of these symptoms emerge before age 7 years and be of sufficient severity to cause impairment. Symptoms must also be present in at least two different settings, must produce significant impairment in social or school endeavors, and not be better accounted for by another mental disorder or occur exclusively during the course of a pervasive developmental disorder or psychotic disorder.

Although many sources state that ADHD is predominantly a disorder of males, substantial disparity exists in reported gender ratios (J.C. Anderson et al. 1987; Bird et al. 1988; Safer and Krager 1988). McGee et al. (1987) argued that gender differences were purely an artifact of the higher overall baseline rate of behavioral disturbance in boys. The Ontario Child Health Study (Szatmari et al. 1989) provides an interesting epidemiological perspective. According to parents' reports, boys had only a slightly greater prevalence of inattention, impulsivity, and hyperactivity. Even more striking was the observation that adolescent girls report that they had the same prevalence of symptoms as adolescent boys. Only teachers found these symptoms to be significantly more prevalent in boys. In short, it is conceivable that gender differences may be relatively minor.

Studies using objective tests have documented the presence of hyperactivity (see Teicher 1995 for review) and have verified that this is not merely a subjective problem (Henker and Whalen 1989). Using a precise infrared motion analysis system to track body movement patterns during a computerized attention task, Teicher et al. (1996b) found that children with ADHD spent 66% less time immobile than normal, moved their head 3.4 times as far, and covered a 3.8 times greater area. Hyperactivity is most apparent when children with ADHD are required to sit still, and it is also present while they are asleep (Porrino et al. 1983). However, they are no more active than normal when allowed to play (Porrino et al. 1983). Hence, their motor problem appears to stem from a diminished ability to inhibit activity to low levels (Teicher 1995). Deficient inhibition may also explain symptoms of inattention and impulsivity. Inattention usually manifests as failure to sustain interest in tasks that are boring or challenging and in distraction by irrelevant stimuli. These difficulties may arise from failure to inhibit initiation of competing actions. Impulsivity in ADHD largely manifests as impatience and social intrusion, which can be explained by a failure to inhibit immature behaviors through social learning.

ADHD commonly occurs in conjunction with several other psychiatric disorders. Conduct disorder occurs in 40%–70% of subjects with ADHD. This is a serious behavioral problem in which patients violate major societal rules and fail to respect individual rights. Conduct disorder appears to arise specifically in children who show signs of excessive aggressiveness (August et al. 1983). Learning disorders are also prevalent in children with ADHD (Semrud-Clikeman et al. 1992), as are mood disorders. Children abused early in life who develop symptoms of posttraumatic stress disorder (PTSD) also frequently meet criteria for ADHD. McLeer et al. (1994) found that 23% of children with PTSD met criteria for ADHD. More recently, Glod and Teicher (1996) found that 38% of hospitalized abused children with PTSD met criteria for ADHD and that on average the entire group of children with PTSD were more active than normal children or abused children without PTSD. It is, however, unclear whether this is true ADHD or a look-alike state (phenocopy). There is also a high incidence of ADHD among boys with TS (Comings and Comings 1987). Generalized resistance to thyroid hormone has also been associated with a high incidence of ADHD (P. Hauser et al. 1993), but it is a rare disorder almost never found in children diagnosed with ADHD (R.E. Weiss et al. 1993). ADHD-like symptoms may also emerge as an indicator of genetic risk in children with a family history of schizophrenia (Marcus et al. 1985).

Clinical Course

Mothers often indicate that children with ADHD were extremely active in utero and that they started running and climbing as soon as they learned to walk. However, it is hard to diagnose ADHD before age 4 or 5, and most cases remain undiagnosed until school. Using older criteria it has been estimated that remission occurs in 30% by adolescence and in 50%–70% by adulthood (Barkley 1990; Gittelman et al. 1985). In persisting cases it is often stated that the hyperactivity abates but problems with inattention continue. Objective measures of activity in adults with ADHD indicate that many continue to have difficulty inhibiting activity to low levels (Teicher 1995).

Etiology and Pathophysiology

ADHD should be regarded as a syndrome in which the clinical phenotype can arise from multiple etiologies, probably through a number of different pathways. Worldwide, the leading cause of ADHD may be severe early malnutrition during the first year of life (Galler et al. 1983). In the United States, low birth weight, fetal alcohol exposure, and prenatal or postnatal lead exposure can be more common etiological factors. Genetic factors also play a major role. ADHD runs in families, particularly in the male relatives of ADHD children (Pauls 1991). Girls with ADHD have a stronger family history than do boys, suggesting even greater genetic loading but lower penetrance. Twin studies indicate that heritability may be as high as 0.91 (Levy et al. 1997).

Efforts to identify a selective neurochemical imbalance in blood, urine, or cerebrospinal fluid (CSF) have been disappointing. Zametkin and Rapoport (1987) concluded that no reliable differences were found between control subjects without ADHD and boys with ADHD on measures of dopamine or norepinephrine metabolites. However, molecular studies of polymorphism of dopamine transporter and receptor genes have produced some exciting initial findings. Cook et al. (1995) first suggested that there was a highly significant associa-

tion between polymorphism of the dopamine transporter (reuptake) gene locus (DAT1) and ADHD, and this observation has been replicated in other studies (Comings et al. 1996; Daly et al. 1999; Gill et al. 1997; Waldman et al. 1998; but see Palmer et al. 1999). Complete deletion (knockout) of the dopamine transporter gene produces incessant hyperactivity in mice (Giros et al. 1996). Winsberg and Comings (1999) found that homozygosity of the 10-repeat allele was associated with nonresponse to methylphenidate (reviewed by Swanson et al. 2000).

Other molecular studies have failed to find an association with the DAT1 gene, but have found an association with the dopamine D_4 receptor gene (e.g., LaHoste et al. 1996). The D_4 receptor has been associated with novelty seeking (Benjamin et al. 1996; Ebstein et al. 1996), and individuals with high levels of this trait are impulsive, excitable, and quick-tempered, as are patients with ADHD. The D_4 receptor is an interesting candidate gene in that it is preferentially located in frontal and prefrontal cortical regions in the brain (Sunahara et al. 1993) that are involved in executive control and regulation of attention. This gene has a 48–base pair variable repeat in the third cytoplasmic loop that is associated with functional differences in response to dopamine (Asghari et al. 1995). In particular, the 7-repeat allelic variant that has been linked to ADHD is hyporesponsive to dopamine. LaHoste et al. (1996) found that 49% of the subjects with ADHD had at least one 7-repeat allele in comparison with only 21% of ethnically matched case control subjects. These researchers replicated this observation in a refined sample that met both DSM-IV and ICD-10 (World Health Organization 1992) diagnostic criteria for ADHD and confirmed the significance of the genetic association using more stringent haplotype relative risk analysis (Swanson et al. 1998). This association has been replicated in some studies (Barr et al. 2000, Comings et al. 1999b, Faraone et al. 1999; Tahir et al. 2000), but not others (Castellanos et al. 1998, Eisenberg et al. 2000).

Comings et al. (2000) viewed ADHD as a complex disorder that emerged from the interaction of multiple genes. They examined the relationship between 20 genes for dopamine, serotonin, and noradrenergic metabolism and quantitative score for ADHD in 336 unrelated subjects. Multivariate linear regression indicated that three dopamine genes, three serotonin genes, and six adrenergic genes contributed 2.3%, 3%, and 6.9%, respectively, to the variance. Altogether, 12 genes contributed 11.6% to the total variance, which, though highly significant, also means that the amassed genetic knowledge of ADHD is still vastly incomplete. The Comings et al. (1999a, 2000) research also suggests that noradrenergic genes may contribute substantially to ADHD, particularly to patients with both ADHD and learning disabilities.

Imaging studies have helped to delineate and define a network of brain regions involved in ADHD. Morphometric magnetic resonance imaging (MRI) studies have identified abnormalities in the size or symmetry of the frontal cortex, caudate nucleus, corpus callosum, and cerebellar vermis. Castellanos et al. (1996) performed volumetric analysis of the cerebrum, caudate nucleus, putamen, globus pallidus, amygdala, hippocampus, temporal lobe, cerebellum, and prefrontal cortex in 57 boys with ADHD and 55 control subjects. Children with ADHD had a 4.7% smaller cerebral volume, a significant loss of normal right-greater-than-left caudate asymmetry, smaller right globus pallidus, smaller right anterior frontal region, smaller cerebellum, and reversal of

normal lateral ventricular asymmetry. For boys without ADHD, caudate volume decreased substantially with age, whereas in boys with ADHD, caudate volume showed no age-related change. Semrud-Clikeman et al. (2000) found that reversed caudate asymmetry was associated with poorer performance on measures of inhibition. Casey et al. (1997) found that impaired performance on three tests of response inhibition was associated with abnormalities in the prefrontal cortex, caudate, and globus pallidus, but not in the putamen. Results suggested a role of the right prefrontal cortex in suppressing responses to salient but otherwise irrelevant events, whereas the basal ganglia appeared to be involved in executing these behavioral responses (Casey et al. 1997).

Early studies also found that the anterior portion of the corpus callosum, which relays information between the left and right frontal cortex, was decreased in size in boys with ADHD (Giedd et al. 1994; Hynd et al. 1991). A significant inverse correlation was found between size of the anterior corpus callosum and indices of impulsivity/hyperactivity on the Conners' Rating Scale (Giedd et al. 1994). Other reports have documented a decrease in size of the posterior corpus callosum, which may be related to certain aspects of attention (Hynd et al. 1991; Semrud-Clikeman et al. 1994). However, Castellanos et al. (1996), in the most comprehensive study with the largest sample sizes, failed to find a difference in any region of the corpus callosum. Overmeyer et al. (2000) also found no differences in the corpus callosum between a subgroup of children with a refined subtype of ADHD and control subjects without ADHD who had siblings with ADHD.

Animal and human studies have expanded our understanding of cerebellar processes and indicated that the cerebellum plays a role in executive function normally attributed to the prefrontal cortex (Thach et al. 1992). Mostofsky et al. (1998) measured the cerebellar vermis in 12 males with ADHD and 23 male control subjects matched for age and IQ. The researchers found a significant reduction in the size of the inferior posterior lobe (lobules VIII–X). Berquin et al. (1998) also reported a significant reduction in the size of the inferior posterior lobe in 46 right-handed boys with ADHD versus 47 matched control subjects without ADHD. These findings suggest that a cerebello-striatal-prefrontal circuit dysfunction may underlie the motor control, inhibition, and executive function deficits encountered in ADHD.

Functional imaging studies have confirmed and expanded the anatomical studies. First, a number of studies documented basal state differences in metabolism and regional blood flow in the prefrontal cortex and striatum (caudate nucleus and putamen). Lou et al. (1990) found that 11 of 11 children with ADHD had hypoperfusion of the frontal lobes, and 7 of 11 had hypoperfusion of the striatum. Stimulant drugs increased blood flow in the striatum and decreased blood flow in primary sensory and motor cortex. Using positron emission tomography (PET), Zametkin et al. (1990) found that adults with a history of childhood ADHD had an overall 8% reduction in cerebral glucose metabolism, with a significant reduction in 30 of 60 cortical regions. The largest decreases were in the premotor and superior prefrontal cortex. Ernst et al. (1994) found a reduction in global cerebral blood flow in adolescent girls with ADHD compared with that in female control subjects without ADHD. However, a comparable effect was not observed in adolescent boys. Sieg et al. (1995) used [123I]-iodoamphetamine (IMP) single photon emission computed

tomography (SPECT) to assess regional distribution of blood flow and metabolism in 10 children or adolescents with ADHD and 6 control subjects without ADHD. ADHD patients had a greater cortical asymmetry characterized by diminished left frontal and left parietal activity.

More recently, Teicher et al. (2000b) developed a novel functional magnetic resonance imaging (fMRI) procedure called T_2 relaxometry that provides a noninvasive indirect assessment of steady-state regional cerebral blood volume. Using this technique, we compared 11 boys with ADHD with 6 control subjects without ADHD. We found significant elevations of T_2 relaxation time (T_2RT) in the putamen, suggestive of diminished blood flow and neuronal activity. A robust relationship was found between T_2RT in the putamen and objective measures of hyperactivity and attention using infrared motion analysis. Additional correlates with hyperactivity and attention emerged in left dorsolateral prefrontal cortex (Teicher et al. 1996b) and cerebellar vermis (C.M. Anderson et al. 1999). Chronic treatment with methylphenidate altered T_2RT in each region, though the direction and magnitude of the effect was strongly dependent on the basal level of hyperactivity (Teicher et al. 2000b). In those children with ADHD who were objectively hyperactive, methylphenidate reduced T_2RT in putamen and increased T_2RT in the cerebellar vermis. T_2RT changed in the opposite manner in ADHD children who had a more normal capacity to sit still. Similarly, methylphenidate markedly reduced seated activity in the objectively hyperactive children but either increased or exerted no effect on activity of nonhyperactive children with ADHD.

Functional imaging studies have also revealed corticostriatal defects during performance of cognitive tasks, particularly those that measure aspects of inhibitory control or working memory. Schweitzer et al. (2000) found, using [^{15}O]H$_2$O PET, that a working memory task enhanced regional cerebral blood flow in the prefrontal and temporal cortex of six men without ADHD. The same task produced more diffuse and predominantly occipital activation in six men with ADHD. These findings suggested that adults with ADHD used compensatory mental and neural strategies, particularly internalized speech, to guide behavior. Similar results emerged in a blood oxygen level–dependent (BOLD) fMRI study of eight adults with ADHD and eight adults without ADHD during performance of the Counting Stroop. Both groups showed an interference effect, and a prominent activation of the cognitive division of their anterior cingulate was demonstrated in control subjects but not in patients with ADHD (Bush et al. 1999). Rubia et al. (1999) found hypofunction of the right mesial prefrontal cortex during motor inhibition and motor timing tasks and hypofunction of the right inferior prefrontal cortex and left caudate during motor inhibition using BOLD fMRI. Vaidya et al. (1998) found that ADHD children had greater BOLD fMRI activation in frontal cortex on one attention task and reduced striatal activation on another. Methylphenidate increased frontal activation to an equal extent in both groups. However, it increased striatal activation in children with ADHD but reduced striatal activation in control subjects.

Most recently, imaging studies have been used to measure neurochemistry. Dougherty et al. (1999) assessed dopamine transporter density in six adults with ADHD and found a 70% increase in age-corrected transporter density relative to control subjects without ADHD. Similarly, Krause et al. (2000) assessed binding to the dopamine transporter using Tc-99m tropane dopamine transporter (TRO-DAT)–1 SPECT. Ten previously untreated adults with ADHD had a highly significant increase in specific binding of the ligand to the transporter. Specific binding to the transporter was markedly reduced after 4 weeks of treatment with methylphenidate. Ernst et al. (1998, 1999b) assessed 3,4-dihydroxyphenylalanine (DOPA) decarboxylase activity (a measure of dopamine innervation) with [^{18}F]DOPA PET. They found that DOPA decarboxylase activity was reduced by approximately 50% in the prefrontal cortex (Ernst et al. 1998) of adults with ADHD and suggested that a prefrontal dopamine dysfunction mediated ADHD symptoms. They also found a significantly higher accumulation of DOPA in the midbrain of 10 children with ADHD. This region contains the substantia nigra and ventral tegmental area, and higher DOPA accumulation is consistent with a secondary increase in dopamine turnover in this region.

Animal studies indicate that many forms of early brain injury produce hyperactivity. Of particular interest is the neonatal dopamine depletion model (B.A. Shaywitz et al. 1976a, 1976b), which is based on the von Economo's encephalitis paradox (i.e., that affected adults become parkinsonian, whereas affected children develop hyperactivity). Chemical ablation of dopamine nerve fibers produces a profound parkinsonian state in adult rats (Stricker and Zigmond 1976) but causes neonates to become hyperactive (B.A. Shaywitz et al. 1976b). These hyperactive rats perform poorly on a range of learning tasks, and stimulant drugs partially ameliorate these deficits (B.A. Shaywitz et al. 1976a). The hyperactivity often abates after puberty (B.A. Shaywitz et al. 1976b) unless the depletion is extremely profound (F.E. Miller et al. 1981). Curiously, the rats' hyperactivity is situationally specific (Teicher et al. 1981), and the degree and time course of the impairments are influenced by the rats' early experience (Pearson et al. 1980). Heffner et al. (1983) found that the critical feature of this model was depletion of dopamine within the frontal cortex. Early postnatal depletions of dopamine produced a concomitant increase in D_4 receptor binding in rats (Zhang et al. 2000). Shaywitz et al. (Raskin et al. 1983; B.A. Shaywitz et al. 1984) also found that relatively selective neonatal norepinephrine depletions produced impaired learning performance without hyperactivity. Thus, neonatal norepinephrine depletion may provide a model for the inattentive form of ADHD.

Pathophysiological Models of ADHD

A detailed pathophysiological model of ADHD needs to incorporate several factors. First, ADHD has a discrete time course. Symptoms emerge early in childhood (generally before age 7) and often abate or wane by adulthood. Second, many more boys than girls are diagnosed and treated for ADHD. However, ADHD symptoms are less likely to abate with age in girls. Third, pharmacological studies demonstrate that the most highly effective drugs for ADHD target either dopamine or norepinephrine. Fourth, imaging studies provide converging evidence for a disturbance in corticostriatal loops. Fifth, reverse asymmetries are found in brain structure and function in patients with ADHD. Malone et al. (1994) have argued that an imbalance exists between a left hemisphere (or anterior) attention system that provides focused sustained attention on a task (Jutai 1984) and a right (or posterior) attention system that regulates overall arousal and rapidly shifts attention to peripheral stimuli for processing novel information (Goldberg and Costa 1981; Heilman and Van Den Abell 1980).

Finally, emerging evidence suggests that the cerebellar vermis is affected in ADHD and may play a pivotal role in symptomatology.

We believe that the waxing and waning of symptoms with age, gender differences in prevalence, and greater persistence of ADHD symptoms in girls are all a consequence of the normal process of synaptic overproduction and pruning (Andersen and Teicher 2000). As illustrated in Figure 18–2, a marked overproduction of dopamine receptors in the striatum during childhood is pruned by adulthood. Furthermore, we have shown that this process occurs in male rats but is hardly apparent in female rats (Andersen et al. 1997). Gender differences in overproduction of dopamine receptors and other neural elements may account for the apparent shrinkage that occurs in the caudate nucleus of boys without ADHD but not girls with age (Castellanos et al. 1996). Our hypothesis is that at least one class of overexpressed receptors is a permissive factor in the clinical manifestation of ADHD. Overexpression in boys leads to greater clinical prevalence during the period of overproduction, but may explain why fewer girls develop ADHD because this permissive factor is not expressed. Greater abatement of symptoms in boys occurs with pruning; however, girls with ADHD who remain symptomatic do so because the permissive factor is not pruned. By adulthood, striatal D_2 density becomes equal (Teicher et al. 1995), and gender differences in prevalence largely disappear (Biederman et al. 1994). Further, it appears that the caudate nucleus does not shrink with age in boys who meet diagnostic criteria for ADHD (Castellanos et al. 1996). We would hypothesize that it shrinks in boys with ADHD who are no longer symptomatic. Andersen et al. (2000) also found that pruning of dopamine receptors in the prefrontal cortex occurs later in adulthood than pruning in the striatum. This may help explain why symptoms of motor hyperactivity remit or diminish at an earlier age than attentional symptoms.

It is possible that the permissive factor may be a member of the dopamine D_2 receptor family (D_2, D_3, or D_4). D_2 family receptor density is a permissive factor in the expression of TS. Wolf et al. (1996) has shown that differences in Tourette's symptomatology between identical twins is completely explained by their differences in striatal D_2 receptor binding. However, this is an open question in ADHD because other neural elements are also overproduced and pruned in the striatum during the same period.

Figure 18–3 provides a schematic that integrates findings regarding drug response, hemispheric asymmetries in attention, and the role of corticostriatal circuits and the cerebellar vermis. As reviewed below, drugs that effectively treat ADHD act on catecholamine systems. Stimulant drugs bind to the dopamine transporter attenuating dopamine reuptake and stimulating dopamine release (Breese et al. 1975; Gatley et al. 1996). This effect is attenuated and checked by the action of released dopamine on autoreceptors that control pulsatile release rates (Grace 1995; Seeman and Madras 1998). Stimulants also affect other monoamine systems and increase serotonin neurotransmission to variable degrees (Hernandez et al. 1987; Kuczenski et al. 1987). Methylphenidate appears to augment noradrenergic neurotransmission in humans, whereas dextroamphetamine decreases noradrenergic tone (Zametkin et al. 1985). This occurs because the primary amphetamine metabolite, p-hydroxyamphetamine, is taken up in noradrenergic neuron, where it is converted into p-hydroxynorephedrine, a false neurotransmitter that displaces some

of the active transmitter (Lewander 1971a, 1971b; Rangno et al. 1973). Hence, treatment with methylphenidate increases levels of the norepinephrine metabolite 3-methoxy-4-hydroxyphenyl glycol (MHPG), whereas amphetamine causes MHPG levels to fall (Zametkin et al. 1985). ADHD symptoms are also attenuated by clonidine, which is an α_2-adrenoreceptor agonist (Hunt 1987; Hunt et al. 1985). Clonidine generally acts on noradrenergic autoreceptors within the locus coeruleus to attenuate noradrenergic neurotransmission. However, clonidine also acts as a partial agonist at postsynaptic α_2 receptors and can preserve or augment transmission through a component of the noradrenergic signal pathway, enhancing prefrontal cortex function (Arnsten et al. 1996). Selective norepinephrine reuptake inhibitors such as desipramine and nortriptyline have been shown to be effective in ADHD when administered in high doses (Popper 1997). Although these agents are highly selective in their action on the norepinephrine transporter, microdialysis studies show that they markedly increase levels of dopamine in the prefrontal cortex (Gresch et al. 1995).

Dopamine and norepinephrine play pivotal roles in our two attentional systems. Dopamine is primarily involved in the left/anterior attention system that is predominantly a motor control system. This system modulates sustained focused attention within the foveal field of vision, facilitates visually guided motor behavior, and suppresses unnecessary movement in order to focus and attend (Malone et al. 1994). In contrast, norepinephrine is primarily involved in the right/posterior attention system that is primarily a sensory alerting system (Aston-Jones and Bloom 1981; Foote et al. 1980). This system modulates rapid phasic shifts in our attention, particularly to events in our

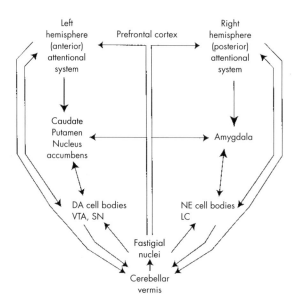

FIGURE 18–3. Simplified neural circuit diagram indicating the interconnections between brain regions and neurotransmitter systems involved in the regulation of activity and attention.

Dysfunction in any component could induce symptoms of ADHD.

DA = dopamine; VTA = ventral tegmental area; SN = substsantia nigra; NE = norepinephrine; LC = locus coeruleus.

peripheral field of vision. The central amygdala, a key component of the fear and anxiety system (LaBar et al. 1998; LeDoux et al. 1988), connects to the locus coeruleus through corticotropin-releasing factor terminals that enhance noradrenergic activity (Van Bockstaele et al. 1998). Hence, the noradrenergically mediated right/posterior attentional system is coupled to fight-or-flight and startle responses.

The primary components of the left/anterior attention system are the cortico-striatal pathways (prefrontal cortex, cingulate cortex, caudate, putamen, globus pallidus, and ventrolateral thalamus) along with dopamine projections from the substantia nigra and ventral tegmental area. Major components of the right/posterior attention system are temporal and parietal cortex, locus coeruleus, amygdala, hippocampus, and thalamus. In general,

patients with ADHD have a deficiency in the left/anterior attention system that leads to impaired focused attention, diminished capacity to suppress motor activity, and increased impulsivity (Malone et al. 1994). Some patients with ADHD may have (or also have) an overactive right/posterior system that can produce high distractibility and rapid intense shifts in attention and affect. It is also possible that some children with ADHD have an underactive right/posterior system, which can lead to left hemisphere–driven hyperfocus coupled with diminished awareness of the environment or external events. This may occur in some inattentive ADHD patients who are "spacey" and hypoactive.

Coordinated interplay and balance between these attentional systems is crucial for safety and success. The cerebellar vermis is in a key position to coordinate balance between these systems. First, the vermis receives multimodal sensory information (Brons et al. 1990; Donaldson and Hawthorne 1979; Huang and Liu 1990) and is intimately involved in the control of eye movements (Suzuki and Keller 1988). The vermis also receives vestibular (Denoth et al. 1979) and proprioceptive (Eccles et al. 1971) information to rapidly guide or adjust body position through its motor pathways. The vermis receives projections from prefrontal cortex (Schmahmann and Pandya 1995) along with noradrenergic and dopaminergic projections from the midbrain (Ariano et al. 1997; Dennett and Hubbard 1988; Melchitzky and Lewis 2000). The vermis outputs through the deep cerebellar fastigial nuclei. These nuclei exert robust effects on global cerebral blood flow and metabolism (Doba and Reis 1972; Goadsby and Lambert 1989). They also modulate the turnover of dopamine and norepinephrine (Dempsey and Richardson 1987). Hence, the vermis is ideally wired to affect cortical arousal and catecholamine neurotransmission in response to input from the prefrontal cortex and multimodal sensory systems. These observations underscore the tight association emerging between cerebellar vermis and prefrontal cortex in normal function and psychiatric disorders (Andreasen et al. 1996; Ciesielski et al. 1997; Diamond 2000; Sweeney et al. 1998).

We suspect that ADHD can arise in a number of possible ways from defects or imbalances in the activity and regulation of these attentional systems. The defect may be located specifically within an attentional system or may be vermal in origin, leading to an impaired capacity to balance and coordinate the systems. A variety of defects can produce similar syndromic manifestations and benefit from one or more drugs that enhance catecholamine neurotransmission. We suspect that, in the near future, use of objective behavioral measures, newer imaging technologies, and molecular studies will identify a number of specific etiologies that comprise the ADHD behavioral syndrome.

Treatment

Comprehensive treatment of ADHD includes both pharmacological and non-pharmacological interventions. Primary medication options include psychostimulants, antidepressants, and antihypertensives. Stimulants, the use of which continues to be clouded by unfounded concerns, remain the mainstay of treatment. In numerous studies, stimulants have been shown to attenuate hyperactivity, improve attention, and diminish impulsivity (Wilens and Biederman 1992). Methylphenidate, in daily doses of 10–60 mg, and dextroamphetamine, given in daily doses of 5–40 mg, are the major agents of choice. Unfortunately, both have a brief duration of action (as short as 3 hours). Effective treatment usually requires multiple daily doses, and children typically receive their first dose in the morning shortly before school and a second dose at lunchtime. Many children also benefit from a smaller dose after school. Older longer-acting preparations of methylphenidate and dextroamphetamine often fail to significantly extend therapeutic duration (G.L. Brown et al. 1980; Pelham et al. 1987, 1990). Adderall, a mixture of amphetamine and dextroamphetamine, has gained popularity as a single-dose preparation. It is a mixture of four amphetamine salts that provide a more gradual onset and longer duration. Pliszka et al. (2000) found that Adderall was at least as effective as regular methylphenidate, and 70% of their sample responded well to Adderall taken as a single dose. Average daily Adderall dose was 25 mg for preadolescents. Concerta has recently been developed as a new delivery system for methylphenidate. Briefly, an osmotic minipump delivers methylphenidate in a manner that produces escalating blood levels throughout the day. The pump is surrounded by a shell of methylphenidate that provides an initial bolus. Studies suggest that once-daily Concerta is as effective as regular methylphenidate delivered in three equal doses throughout the day. Methamphetamine, a much less frequently prescribed stimulant, is available in a sustained release form (Desoxyn Gradumet) that seems to work reasonably well (Wender 1993). Pemoline is another effective stimulant with a longer duration of action and reduced potential for abuse. However, a relatively high (1%–3%) incidence of adverse hepatic effects has markedly restricted its use. High initial doses (37.5–112.5 mg) have been found to produce rapid and sustained beneficial effects (Pelham et al. 1995). An average effective dose of pemoline for a child would be approximately 56 mg (Pelham et al. 1990).

Common side effects of stimulants include anorexia, stomachaches, insomnia, and mood changes (irritability, mood lability, dysphoria). Tics and stereotypic movements occur less commonly (discussion follows). Concerns about diminishing growth and stature from using stimulants are unfounded. If stimulants attenuate final height, the consequence is less than an inch (Popper and Steingard 1995). Spencer et al. (1996) provide data that suggest that ADHD, as a disorder, is associated with delayed growth during early childhood, with compensatory growth by late adolescence. They found that stimulants played no role in the process. Risk for stimulant abuse in the ADHD population appears small. Stimulants exert dysphoric, rather than euphoriant, effects on children (Rapoport et al. 1980), and compliance can be a significant problem. Biederman et al. (1999), in an important

study, found that stimulant treatment of ADHD in childhood actually diminished risk for substance abuse in adulthood. Overall, psychostimulants are effective in the treatment of the core features of ADHD. Consistent and appropriate use can lead to enhanced self-esteem and improved quality of life.

The second major class of medications with demonstrated effectiveness in ADHD is the antidepressants, most notably the selective noradrenergic tricyclics desipramine and nortriptyline (Popper 1997). Studies also indicated that bupropion (Wellbutrin, 0.7 mg/kg/day) can be as effective as methylphenidate in improving attention and reducing conduct problems (Barrickman et al. 1995). Although monoamine oxidase inhibitors are also effective, dietary restrictions preclude their use in pediatric populations. Tricyclic antidepressants have the advantage of sustained effect and can be well suited for children with comorbid mood disorders. Reports of sudden death in prepubertal children receiving desipramine have raised serious concerns about this agent and other tricyclics (Abromowicz 1990; Popper and Zimnitzky 1995; Riddle et al. 1991, 1993). The most common cardiac effects of tricyclics in pediatric patients include sinus tachycardia, intraventricular conduction delay of the right bundle branch block type (QRS > 100 msec), and increased QTc intervals (Biederman et al. 1989; Leonard et al. 1995). As a consequence, maximum desipramine doses should be 5 mg/kg/day, cardiac status and family cardiac history need to be carefully evaluated, and electrocardiogram and plasma levels need to be closely monitored. Although no direct causal relationship has been established between desipramine use and sudden death, cardiovascular toxicity remains a potential risk, and parents need to be informed of this possibility. Selective noradrenergic reuptake inhibitors have been developed that appear to be free of the adverse cardiac affects of tricyclics. Studies suggest that they are effective in ADHD and await U.S. Food and Drug Administration approval. The antidepressant venlafaxine (Effexor) exerts strong effects on both noradrenergic and serotonergic reuptake and should theoretically be beneficial for ADHD with a much more benign cardiac profile than that of tricyclics. However, data are only beginning to emerge about its utility (Olvera et al. 1996; Pleak and Gormly 1995; Wilens et al. 1995). The more selective serotonin reuptake inhibitors (SSRIs), such as fluoxetine, have been reported to be useful in an open trial (Barrickman et al. 1991) and await further testing. The general clinical consensus is that SSRIs provide little effect on core symptoms of ADHD, can be helpful with comorbid mood and anxiety symptoms, but can also worsen symptoms (Popper 1997).

Emerging evidence suggests that the α_2-adrenergic agonists clonidine and guanfacine are potentially effective treatments. Hunt et al. (1985; Hunt 1987) reported in a small sample that clonidine may be comparable in efficacy to methylphenidate in reducing hyperactivity and impulsivity. Oral doses are generally initiated at 0.025–0.05 mg and increased to a maximum of 3–10 µg/kg. Transdermal patches can provide more consistent drug effects and decreased propensity for allergic reactions. Common side effects include sedation, rash, and increased appetite and weight gain, whereas less common reactions include headaches, rebound insomnia, cardiovascular effects, and mood lability. Rebound hypertension can occur upon abrupt cessation. In an open trial, guanfacine has also been reported to be efficacious in children with ADHD (Hunt et al. 1995) and those with comorbid TS (Chappell et al. 1995).

Guanfacine may produce less sedation and hypotension. Common initial doses are 0.25–0.5 mg, which can be titrated to up to 4 mg/day (Hunt et al. 1995).

Selection of a particular pharmacological agent depends on clinical presentation, comorbidity, duration of effect, and abuse potential by other family members. We find it useful to fully inform family members about potential risks and benefits of treatment and to have them decide which option they prefer. Effectiveness should be based on reports from the child, parents, and teachers. Standardized rating scales have been well validated and are often indispensable. Dosage adjustments are needed to optimize treatment and to compensate for growth and development. Some children and families tolerate reemergence of symptoms with medication discontinuation during weekends and summers. Most children require long-term treatment continuing into adolescence and possibly adulthood.

Despite the benefits of pharmacotherapy, additional treatment and support is often required. Environmental manipulation, such as reducing stimuli and distractions, may help modulate symptoms, and education tailored to the student's learning style may be necessary to improve academic performance. A variety of behavioral management programs have been created for parents (Barkley 1987; Robin and Foster 1989). Barkley et al. (1992) compared three different programs and found that they were all helpful, although clinically significant change was evident in only 5%–30% of subjects (Barkley et al. 1992). In a detailed and elaborate study, the Multimodal Treatment Group evaluated the effects of behavioral therapy versus medication management. Altogether, 579 children with ADHD combined type, ages 7 to 9.9 years, were assigned to 14 months of medication management (titration followed by monthly visits); intensive behavioral treatment (parent, school, and child components); the two combined; or standard community care. Children in the combined treatment and medication management groups showed significantly greater improvement than those given intensive behavioral treatment or community care. No significant differences were seen on any measure between combined treatment and medication management. Combined treatment may have advantages in more complex cases. Medication management was superior to community treatment, in part, because average methylphenidate dose was twice as high in the study, suggesting that subjects in the community did not receive an optimal dose. Methylphenidate was usually administered three times a day in the study versus twice daily in the community. No studies support the effectiveness of psychotherapy alone, sugar withdrawal, or restriction of salicylates or food dyes, although omitting food dyes may be helpful in a small minority. Electroencephalograph biofeedback has been touted as an alternative to medications that can exert sustained beneficial effects (J.F. Lubar et al. 1995; J.O. Lubar and Lubar 1984; Nash 2000). Despite the availability of instruments and practitioners providing this service, controlled efficacy studies are absent.

Tourette's Syndrome and Other Tic Disorders

TS is an intriguing neuropsychiatric disorder, presumably arising from deep within the basal ganglia, that illustrates the prominent associations between hyperactivity, impulsivity, tics, obsessions, and compulsions. Tics are stereotyped, brief, repetitive, purposeless, nonrhythmic motor and vocal responses. Although temporarily suppressible, tics are not under full voluntary control, and the individual often experiences increasing internal tension that is only relieved when the tic is released.

Clinically, tic disorders are divided into four categories: transient tic disorder, chronic tic disorder, TS, and tic disorder not otherwise specified. Transient tic disorder is diagnosed when an individual experiences either single or multiple motor and/or vocal tics many times a day on a near daily basis for at least 4 consecutive weeks, but for no more than 12 months (American Psychiatric Association 1994). The tics must be distressing or cause significant impairment. Onset must occur before 18 years, and tics may not be due to the direct effect of a drug or a more generalized neurological disorder such as Huntington's disease or postviral encephalitis. Transient tic disorder can be a single episode or can reoccur after a period of remission. Chronic tic disorder is diagnosed when an individual has motor tics or vocal tics (but not both) for more than a year with no more than a 3-month consecutive hiatus. Onset must be before 18 years, and the same exclusionary criteria apply as in transient tic disorder. TS is diagnosed when an individual meets criteria for a chronic tic disorder involving the presence of both motor and vocal tics. Tic disorder not otherwise specified is used for cases that fail to fall into one of these three primary categories.

Characteristic Features

Tics can be simple or complex. Simple motor tics include jerking movements, shrugging, and eye blinking. Simple vocal tics include grunting, sniffing, and throat clearing. More complex motor tics involve grimacing, banging, or temper tantrums, whereas complex vocal tics include echolalia and coprolalia. Tics wax and wane over time, and the primary muscle groups affected gradually change as well.

TS is a chronic condition in which both motor and vocal tics are observable. The tics are often presaged by premonitory sensory urges that build in tension until the tic is released (Leckman et al. 1993). Many patients feel more troubled by the pre-tic tension than by the tics themselves (Leckman et al. 1993), and some patients can successfully control their tics in public and unleash them when they are alone. Tics are markedly attenuated by sleep (Fish et al. 1991; Hashimoto et al. 1981). TS waxes and wanes over time and can vary enormously in severity from mild and undiagnosed to disabling. Anxiety and stress can increase symptoms.

The modal age at onset is 6–7 years but can range from 2 to 17 years (Leckman et al. 1995b). Tic symptoms are generally most severe during the period preceding puberty (average 10 ± 2.4 years of age) and gradually improve thereafter, except in the most severe cases (Leckman et al. 1998). For this reason, it is important to note that tic severity during childhood is not a predictor of tic severity at 18 years of age (Leckman et al. 1998).

In half of patients, symptoms start as a single tic involving eyes, face, or head and progress in a rostrocaudal manner. Before the first appearance of tics, 25%–50% of TS patients have a history of hyperactivity, inattention, and impulsivity consistent with ADHD (Comings and Comings 1987). Phonic and vocal tics generally emerge at about 11 years of age, often starting with a single syllable and then progressing to longer exclamations. Coprolalia occurs in about 60% of patients and emerges in early adolescence. Complex motor tics may be purposeless or camouflaged by a sequence of intentional actions and can be self-destructive or violent. In a pilot study, Budman et al. (1998) concluded that rage attacks are not related to tic severity, but rather reflect an underlying pathophysiology with other comorbid conditions.

Obsessive-compulsive symptoms appear in 60% of cases (Leckman et al. 1995b), and OCD is observed in 7%–10%. Obsessive-compulsive symptoms usually emerge 5–10 years after the first appearance of simple tics (Bruun 1988). Tic-related OCD may differ from the classic OCD with an earlier age of onset; more prominent symptoms of ritualized touching, tapping, and rubbing; less satisfactory response to SSRIs; and an enhanced response to neuroleptic augmentation (Leckman et al. 1995b).

TS is not an uncommon condition of childhood and is believed to affect between one and six boys per thousand. The disorder is three- to fourfold more prevalent in boys than in girls. As TS often wanes after puberty, prevalence rates drop by about an order of magnitude (Leckman et al. 1995b).

Etiology and Pathophysiology

Tic disorders have a substantial genetic basis, but additional factors play a key role. A large study of affected sib-pair families found that first-degree relatives had a tenfold increased risk (Tourette Syndrome Association International Consortium for Genetics 1999). Tics are present in about two-thirds of relatives of TS patients, and linkage studies suggest that TS is transmitted in a Mendelian fashion. Monozygotic twins have about a 53% concordance rate versus an 8% concordance rate for dizygotic twins (Leckman et al. 1995b). However, the relevant environmental risk factors have yet to be identified. Possible candidate genes on chromosome 4q (a recessive gene) and on 8p (a dominant gene) show linkage to TS. Mathematical models suggest that TS and OCD may be transmitted by a single autosomal dominant gene with variable penetrance (Curtis et al. 1992; Eapen et al. 1993; Pauls and Leckman 1986). Gender differences can be explained by a substantially higher penetrance in males than fcmales (Eapen et al. 1993). Although the TS gene is transmitted equally well by mothers and fathers, differences in clinical presentation can occur. Lichter et al. (1995) reported that maternal transmission was characterized by greater motor tic complexity and more frequent noninterfering rituals, whereas paternal transmission was associated with increased vocal tic frequency, earlier onset of vocal tics relative to motor tics, and more prominent ADHD behaviors. Approximately 10% of individuals with TS have a nonfamilial version, which in all other ways is similar to the familial form.

Epigenetic factors play a role in the expression of TS. Examination of monozygotic twins discordant for TS indicates that the affected twin had a lower birth weight, suggesting involvement of perinatal factors. Other potential factors include exposure to high levels of gonadal androgens and stress hormones during early central nervous system (CNS) development or recurrent stress, anabolic steroids, cocaine, or other stimulants during postnatal development (Leckman and Scahill 1990; Leckman et al. 1990). Emerging evidence suggests that Group A, β-hemolytic streptococcal infection can result in some forms of TS and OCD (Swedo 1994). Sydenham's chorea is a well-known neurological manifestation of rheumatic fever. Studies suggest that antibodies produced in response to streptococcal infection target neurons within the basal ganglia, causing inflammation resulting in chorea, muscle weakness, and fatigue. This autoimmune mechanism has been proposed as an etiology for some cases of TS, and the acronym PANDAS (pediatric autoimmune neuropsychiatric disorders associated with streptococcal infection) encompasses this diagnostic classification. Antineuronal antibodies have been isolated from sera of TS patients (Singer et al. 1998), and an 83-kDa protein (β-lymphocyte antigen D8/17) has been identified with a high frequency in TS patients (Murphy et al. 1997; Singer et al. 1998). Injection of sera from TS patients into the striatum of rats produced stereotypies and episodic utterances (Hallett et al. 2000). In a preliminary study, plasmapheresis to remove circulating antibodies produced both short- and long-term clinical improvement in tics and OCD symptoms (Perlmutter et al. 1999). However, Singer et al. (1999) found that the association with streptococcal antibodies was true only for a limited subgroup. Hence, TS patients differed from control subjects in median, but not mean, antibody titers. No phenotypic differences were seen between TS patients with high and low titers (Singer et al. 1999).

Although the definite pathophysiology of TS is not known, consensus has been reached that the basal ganglia and related thalamocortical circuitry is involved. Evidence derives from several sources, including the ameliorative effects of thalamic lesions and surgical disconnection of the prefrontal cortex (Leckman et al. 1991b). MRI studies have revealed abnormalities in lateralization of basal ganglia structures, corpus callosum morphology, and insular and frontocortical paramagnetic properties (Peterson et al. 1993, 1994; Riddle et al. 1992; Singer et al. 1993). When monozygotic twins discordant for degree of TS severity were compared, Hyde et al. (1995) found that the more severely affected twin had a smaller right anterior caudate and smaller left lateral ventricle. Girls with TS alone had smaller lateral ventricles than did girls with TS and ADHD or than did control subjects (Zimmerman et al. 2000).

Functional imaging studies confirm the presence of altered striatal metabolism but also reveal more widespread involvement affecting frontal, cingulate, and insular cortex. George et al. (1992) found that TS subjects had significantly elevated right frontal cortex activity. Braun et al. (1993) found that regional glucose utilization was decreased in left hemispheric regions of the paralimbic and ventral prefrontal cortices (particularly orbitofrontal, inferior insular, and parahippocampal regions) and in subcortical regions including the nucleus accumbens and ventromedial caudate. Concomitant bilateral increases in regional glucose utilization in the supplementary motor, lateral premotor, and Rolandic cortices was also observed. In a more definitive study, Peterson et al. (1998) found that TS patients endeavoring to suppress their tics had increased neuronal activity in the right midfrontal cortex, bilateral superior and temporal gyrus, and right anterior cingulate and decreased neuronal activity in the ventral globus pallidus, putamen, midthalamus, right posterior cingulate, and left sensory motor cortex. When TS patients could freely express their tics, neuronal activity increased in the head of the caudate, primarily on the right side (Peterson et al. 1998).

A variety of neurotransmitter abnormalities have been postulated to explain the pathophysiology of TS. A leading hypothesis describes an abnormality in striatal dopamine function, stemming from either greater presynaptic innervation or release or excessive postsynaptic receptor sensitivity (Leckman et al. 1995b). Compelling support comes indirectly from pharmacological studies that show that drugs that either antagonize dopamine D_2 family receptors (haloperidol, pimozide) or diminish dopamine synthesis suppress tics, whereas agents that increase dopamine activity (e.g., L-dopa, cocaine) increase tics (Leckman et al. 1995b). Actual measures of dopaminergic function have produced mixed results. CSF and tissue levels of the dopamine

metabolite homovanillic acid (HVA) are reduced in TS (Leckman et al. 1995a). Reduced levels of HVA can arise from diminished dopamine turnover, which could result from postsynaptic supersensitivity. However, autopsy studies (Singer et al. 1991) and preliminary PET and SPECT studies (George et al. 1994; Turjanski et al. 1994) have not found an elevation in dopamine D_1 or D_2 receptor density indicative of supersensitivity. Linkage studies have excluded dopamine D_1 and D_2 family receptors and the enzymes dopamine β-hydroxylase, tyrosinase, and tyrosine hydroxylase from being closely linked with TS (Brett et al. 1995a; Gelernter et al. 1990, 1993). Thus, a mutation in a dopamine receptor gene or biosynthetic enzyme does not appear to be responsible for the genetic transmission of TS. Singer et al. (1991) found that TS patients at autopsy had a 37% greater density of dopamine transporter (reuptake) sites in caudate than did control subjects and 50% greater density in putamen. Malison et al. (1995) confirmed this finding with SPECT. Increased transporter density may explain the diminished HVA findings, as released dopamine recaptured by transport is predominantly converted into dihydroxyphenylacetic acid rather than HVA (Keller et al. 1973). TS patients also have greater accumulation of fluorodopa in the left caudate (a 25% increase) and right midbrain (53% increase) that do control subjects, suggesting an increase in DOPA decarboxylase enzyme activity (Ernst et al. 1999a). These findings are consistent with a greater degree of dopamine terminal innervation. Wolf et al. (1996) observed in monozygotic twins discordant for Tourette's severity that the more affected twin had a greater density of dopamine D_2 receptors in the caudate but not the putamen. Furthermore, within each twin pair a precise match was found between the degree of differences in D_2 binding in the head of the caudate and the degree of difference in severity. Thus, it appears that dopamine receptor density may be a modifying factor that explains the high degree of phenotypic variation in this disorder.

Noradrenergic theories about TS have also emerged based on the efficacy of clonidine, an α_2-agonist, which is believed to directly diminish firing rates of noradrenergic neurons and to indirectly modulate the activity of dopamine neurons (Leckman et al. 1995a; Scahill et al. 2000). Adults with TS had elevated levels of CSF norepinephrine (Leckman et al. 1995a), a blunted growth hormone response to clonidine (Muller et al. 1994), and abnormally high secretion of urinary norepinephrine in response to stress (Chappell et al. 1994). However, studies of the norepinephrine metabolite MHPG have been inconclusive (Leckman et al. 1995a).

Preliminary postmortem brain studies have shown that 5-hydroxytryptamine (5-HT) and its major metabolite 5-hydroxyindoleacetic acid (5-HIAA) may be globally decreased in the basal ganglia and other brain regions (G.M. Anderson et al. 1992). CSF studies have sometimes reported diminished levels of 5-HIAA (Leckman et al. 1995a, 1995b), and blood levels of 5-HT and tryptophan are also reduced (Comings 1990). Despite the well-known association between OCD and 5-HT, SSRIs have little efficacy against tics (Kurlan et al. 1993). Genetic studies exclude variation in the 5-HT_{1A} and 5-HT_7 receptor genes and the tryptophan oxygenase gene from the etiology of TS (Brett et al. 1995b; Gelernter et al. 1995).

Cholinergic interneurons play a critical role in modulating and balancing the effects of dopamine in the extrapyramidal system. Nicotine potentiates the thera-

peutic effects of neuroleptics (McConville et al. 1991), and muscarinic receptor binding is reduced in TS lymphocytes (Rabey et al. 1992). Clinical trials of choline, lecithin, and deanol have not been particularly efficacious (Leckman et al. 1995a). Treatment with a nicotine patch, which is believed to inactivate nicotinic receptors during chronic exposure, and mecamylamine, a nicotinic antagonist, has been effective in ameliorating TS symptoms (Sanberg et al. 1997, 1998).

Leckman et al. (1991b) postulated that TS arises from a failure to habituate one or more components of the corticostriatal-thalamocortical circuit (Figure 18–3). Oral facial tics may arise from insufficient habituation or excess excitation in circuits located within the ventromedian areas of the caudate and putamen that receive topographic projections from the orofacial regions of the primary motor and premotor cortex. It is also noteworthy that the amygdala projects to widespread areas of the nucleus accumbens and ventral portions of the caudate and putamen. Electrical stimulation of the amygdala produces motor and vocal responses resembling tics (Jadresic 1992). Based on the age at onset and proclivity for these conditions to attenuate or remit during puberty, we propose that they emerge during the period of synaptic overproduction and hyperinnervation that takes place during childhood (Figure 18–1). Receptor overproduction may alter the balance between excitation and inhibition in circumscribed regions that control specific motor programs. Waning of symptoms after puberty may be related to the pruning of overproduced receptors and dopamine terminals.

Treatment

TS is a complicated and multifaceted condition in which there is enormous variability between patients. In some patients,

ADHD is the major problem and tic symptoms may be relatively mild. For these individuals the risk of exacerbating tics with stimulant treatment may be a significant concern, but treatment can often be accomplished safely. Other patients are beset by tics that are disfiguring and result in social ostracism or unemployment. Still other patients have serious problems with premonitory sensory urges, obsession, and compulsions, but in public have no discernible tics.

In general, neuroleptic drugs are effective in attenuating or suppressing tics in 60%–80% of patients (Popper and Steingard 1995). Traditionally, haloperidol (0.5–5 mg/day) and pimozide (1–3 mg/day) have been the drugs of choice (see Teicher and Glod 1990 for review of neuroleptic use in childhood). Both are high-potency dopamine D_2 receptor antagonists and are relatively nonsedating. Neuroleptic drugs will also attenuate symptoms of hyperactivity and impulsivity that emerge from comorbid ADHD. However, neuroleptics fail to facilitate attention and can cause substantial cognitive blunting. Pimozide may produce less cognitive blunting than haloperidol and can even have a beneficial cognitive effect in children with comorbid ADHD (Sallee et al. 1994). Pimozide is usually reserved for cases in which haloperidol has not proven entirely satisfactory, because pimozide can produce cardiac arrhythmias and requires more extensive monitoring. Case studies suggest that risperidone can also effectively attenuate tics (Lombroso et al. 1995). This is a significant development because risperidone may be associated with a lower incidence of extrapyramidal side effects than are conventional neuroleptics. Localized injections of botulinum toxin into the site of the most problematic tics has been highly effective. This treatment also attenuated premonitory sensations in 21 of 25 patients tested (Kwak et al. 2000).

The most serious side effect of neuroleptic treatment is the emergence of neuroleptic malignant syndrome, a potentially lethal state of muscle tension, hyperpyrexia, and autonomic nervous system lability. Reviews indicate that children are vulnerable to the emergence of neuroleptic malignant syndrome; however, there appear to be no reported cases in children treated with neuroleptics for TS (Steingard et al. 1992). An unusual but significant side effect of neuroleptic treatment is the development of phobic anxiety, which can result in school avoidance and social phobias (Linet 1985; Mikkelsen et al. 1981).

Clonidine is often prescribed as an alternative that may be useful in approximately 50% of cases (Leckman et al. 1991a). It attenuates hyperactivity and impulsivity and may be valuable in children with comorbid ADHD and behavioral problems (Steingard et al. 1993). Clonidine, however, is sedating and can blunt cognitive performance. In a double-blind placebo-controlled study, Singer et al. (1995) found that clonidine was less efficacious than desipramine for children with combined ADHD and TS. Efficacy of clonidine may increase over the course of 2–3 months, and dosage needs to be slowly titrated; blood pressure requires frequent monitoring, even after attaining stable dose. Guanfacine has been discussed as an alternative α_2-adrenoreceptor agonist. It produces less sedation and hypotension but it remains to be determined if it is as efficacious.

Studies have produced a marked revision in our understanding of the use of stimulants to treat ADHD in children with TS. Initially, tics were viewed as a serious contraindication, as stimulants can worsen tics or bring tics forth in an otherwise asymptomatic individual (Denckla et al. 1976). However, studies by Sverd et al. (1989) and Gadow et al. (1992) have shown that children with stable TS can respond to stimulants without worsening of tics. As a general guideline, stimulants should not be used in a child in whom stimulants have previously brought forth or worsened tics. Stimulants can be cautiously administered to patients with stable TS. Patients should be carefully monitored for tic frequency or impairment, and in the absence of symptom exacerbation, treatment can continue and be adjusted for optimal efficacy. Evidence indicates that noradrenergic tricyclic antidepressants such as desipramine and nortriptyline are beneficial in patients with comorbid ADHD and chronic tic disorders (Spencer et al. 1993a, 1993c). Desipramine was more effective than clonidine in controlling comorbid symptoms of ADHD and exerted greater effects on tic symptoms, although neither drug in this study was very effective against tics (Singer et al. 1995). In contrast, bupropion, which affects both dopamine and norepinephrine, is more prone to exacerbate tics (Spencer et al. 1993b). Case reports have suggested that lithium can also attenuate tics (Erickson et al. 1977; Kerbeshian and Burd 1988).

TS with associated OCD can be relatively refractory to treatment with SSRIs and may require augmentation with a neuroleptic (McDougle et al. 1994). Although TS is clearly a brain-based disorder, it can be exacerbated by stress and anxiety and can be a severely stigmatizing illness with grievous psychosocial consequences. Psychotherapy can be useful to help reduce anxiety that can exacerbate symptoms, and it can promote the development of interpersonal comfort and social skills that may be crucial for successful employment and personal relationships (Popper and Steingard 1995).

Mental Retardation

An enormous number of genetic, biochemical, and environmental factors can adversely affect brain development, leading to low general intelligence and limited adaptive capacity. Mental retardation is diagnosed when an individual presents, before 18 years of age, with an intelligence score of approximately 70 or below and concurrent deficits in adaptive functioning (American Psychiatric Association 2000). Mental retardation is a common syndrome, with an estimated prevalence of 1%–3% of the adult population. Clinically, mental retardation is divided by severity.

The most prevalent form is mild mental retardation, in which intelligence scores range from 50 to 70. Nearly 90% of the mentally retarded fall within this range. These individuals can learn many skills and generally achieve the equivalent of a sixth-grade education. They can live in the community, manage a job, and, with effort or assistance, handle financial matters, although they require support from families and communities to maintain this level of integration. Mild mental retardation is a heterogeneous set of disorders that sometimes arise from chromosomal abnormalities, environmental effects, or complex multifactorial polygenic inheritance (Thapar et al. 1994).

The next most prevalent cluster is moderate mental retardation, in which intelligence scores range from a low of 35–40 to a high of 50–55. Approximately 7% of the mentally retarded fall within this range. These individuals can often learn to manage some aspects of daily living, such as making small change. They usually live in supervised residences and attain the equivalent of a second-grade education. They communicate at the level of a preschool or early grade school child.

About 3% of the mentally retarded fall into the severe range, with intelligence scores ranging from 20–25 up to 35–40. These individuals typically learn few adaptive skills and live in highly structured and closely supervised settings. They have an increased prevalence of neurological complications such as seizures and spasticity, and often there is a discernible etiology, such as Down syndrome or fragile X syndrome.

Only about 1% of the mentally retarded fall within the profound range, with IQ scores below 20–25. These individuals typically die within their 20s and have a host of severe neurological and medical problems. They need to live in highly structured and supervised settings, and are completely dependent on others. Self-injurious behavior can occur in half of these patients.

Instead of attempting to distill the generic features of hundreds of different disorders associated with mental retardation, it seems more reasonable to review some of the major known disorders that present with mental retardation.

Down Syndrome

Down syndrome is the most common chromosomal abnormality that produces mental retardation. The incidence varies greatly with maternal age. In all newborns, the incidence is 1 per 1,000. However, if the mother is 45 years of age or older, the incidence approaches 1 in 50. Down syndrome may be lethal, resulting in fetal death or stillbirth. Clinical presentation varies considerably. Characteristic features include microcephaly with large anterior fontanel, depressed nasal bridge, bilateral epicanthic folds, upward slanting (mongoloid) palpebral fissure, low-set and misformed ears with hypoplastic tragus and narrow auditory meatus, and lingual protrusion with small mouth (Gold 1992). Other observable features include short stature, hands with a single transverse (simian) crease, brachyclinodactyly of the fifth finger, and wide separation between the large and second toe (Gold 1992). Neurologically, developmental delays and intellectual deficits are significant. Motor milestones are delayed as a result of generalized hypotonia, and expressive and receptive language is usually delayed and impaired. Hearing is also frequently affected as a result of middle ear disease or sensorineural hearing loss (Gold 1992). Seizures occur in less than 10% of cases, but can emerge at any age. Quadriplegia can result at any time from cervical subluxation of the atlantoaxial process. Life expectancy is approximately 50 years, with about 40% developing Alzheimer's disease by this point (Holland et al. 1998). Factors that influence longevity include coexisting congenital heart disease and gastrointestinal anomalies (Gold 1992). Leukemia occurs with increased frequency, and neural changes characteristic of Alzheimer's disease begins to emerge in all who survive beyond 30 years. Behaviorally, patients with Down syndrome tend to have greater relative social skills and less psychopathology than patients with other forms of mental retardation (State et al. 1997).

Etiology and Pathophysiology

Down syndrome is a prototypic chromosomal disorder involving extra replication of all or part of chromosome 21. The classic cause is nondisjunction during meiosis leading to trisomy 21, which is a noninherited genetic anomaly. The syndrome can also arise from inheritance of a translocation of part of chromosome 21 (most often to chromosomes 14 or 22) from asymptomatic mothers. It appears that extra replication of a 3,000-kilobase fragment of DNA in the 21q22 region is sufficient to produce many of the features of Down syndrome, including mental retardation (Park et al. 1987). Down syndrome arising from either nondisjunction or translocation can be diagnosed prenatally through chorionic villi sampling or amniocentesis. Patients with Down syndrome undergo progressive neuropathological changes leading to formation of neurofibrillary tangles and neuritic plaques at a relatively young adult age (Wisniewski et al. 1985). They also have other Alzheimer's-like neurochemical abnormalities, including a major loss of acetylcholine neurons in the nucleus basalis, somatostatin neurons in the cerebral cortex, and reduced levels of norepinephrine and 5-HT (Godridge et al. 1987). Chromosome 21 contains the precursor gene for β-amyloid, which is the protein that accumulates in neuritic plaques. Additional biochemical abnormalities include elevated levels of CuZn, superoxide dismutase, and protein S100β (Huret et al. 1987; Lejeune 1990).

Fragile X Syndrome

Fragile X is the most common known inherited cause of mental retardation, with an estimated prevalence rate of 1 in 1,250 males and 1 in 2,000 females (Thapar et al. 1994). Fragile X accounts for approximately 7% of moderate and 4% of mild mental retardation in males and 2.5% of moderate and 3% of mild retardation in females (Thapar et al. 1994). The name derives from the observation that the X chromosome shows a "fragile" site, specifically a bent or broken appearing segment, when grown in the appropriate culture medium. The phenotypic presentation of this disorder is varied and more prominent in males. Infants present with relative macrocrania and facial edema, whereas older children and adults have a long face and a prominent chin. Large, floppy, seashell-shaped ears are characteristic at any age. Males entering adolescence have characteristic macroorchidism

(enlarged testes) and a normal-size penis (Gold 1992). Affected individuals have an increased rate of psychiatric difficulties with abnormal speech and language, impaired social relations, and ADHD (Turk 1992). Many affected individuals show autistic features such as gaze avoidance, hand flapping, tactile defensiveness, and perseveration (Hagerman and Sobesky 1989), though social withdrawal and reduced attachment to caregivers are not characteristic (State et al. 1997). Seventy percent of female carriers are not mentally retarded, but they have an increased prevalence of schizotypal features, depression, and below-average intelligence (Freund et al. 1992), and their level of symptomatology correlates with the degree of cytogenetically evident fragility (Chudley et al. 1983; Thapar et al. 1994).

Etiology and Pathophysiology

Fragile X has an unusual and important mode of inheritance that also appears in myotonic dystrophy and Huntington's chorea. In all of these disorders the severity of the syndrome increases in successive generations. Other features of fragile X include the observation that phenotypically and cytogenetically normal males (normal transmitting males) can transmit the defect to apparently normal females who can then produce affected male offspring. These clinical observations have now been explained at the molecular level and stem from a process known as *anticipation*. The gene directly responsible for fragile X syndrome, *FMR1*, is located on the X chromosome at Xq27.3 (Verkerk et al. 1991). The 5′ untranslated region of the *FMR1* gene contains a polymorphic CGG trinucleotide repeat (6–60 repeats in normal subjects), which can be amplified to hundreds or thousands of repeats producing the disorder (Verkerk et al. 1991). Fragile X usually results from expansion of the CGG repeats leading to hypermethylation of the CpG island adjacent to *FMR1*, loss of transcription of the *FMR1* gene, and lack of FMR1 protein (Siomi et al. 1995). *FMR1* messenger RNA (mRNA) and protein are expressed in many tissues, but particularly high levels are found in brain and testes (Siomi et al. 1995). The role of FMR1 protein is incompletely understood but is known to serve as an RNA-binding protein (Siomi et al. 1995). Fragile X carriers, including normal transmitting males, have this elongated sequence of repeats, which increase in size, particularly when transmitted by females. If the permutation is transmitted by a normal transmitting male, the sequence is not elongated in the offspring (Thapar et al. 1994).

Prader-Willi Syndrome and Angelman's Syndrome

Prader-Willi syndrome and Angelman's syndrome are two distinct genetic forms of mental retardation that usually arise from de novo deletion of a segment of chromosome 15. Prader-Willi syndrome is characterized by obesity associated with hyperphagia, hypogenitalism, short stature, small hands and feet, almond-shaped eyes, and strabismus (Thapar et al. 1994). Although about 40% show mental retardation, most affected individuals are of normal or borderline IQ, but some may have associated behavior problems such as temper tantrums, stubbornness, foraging for food (Akefeldt and Gillberg 1999; Thapar et al. 1994), and OCD symptomatology (State et al. 1999). The estimated incidence is approximately 1 in 25,000. Most cases are sporadic with a recurrence risk of less than 1 in 1,000 (Thapar et al. 1994). Angelman's syndrome is characterized by severe mental retardation; stiff, jerky movements; ataxia; seizures; and unprovoked laughter. The estimated incidence is approximately 1 in 20,000, and most cases are sporadic (Thapar et al. 1994).

Etiology and Pathophysiology

Prader-Willi and Angelman's syndromes illustrate an important genetic principle, known as *genomic imprinting*. The majority of individuals with both disorders have remarkably similar deletions of a segment of chromosome 15, particularly surrounding 15q12 (Thapar et al. 1994). It has now been discovered that the difference between Prader-Willi and Angelman's syndromes stems from the gender of the parent from whom the defective chromosome 15 is inherited. Prader-Willi syndrome emerges most frequently from the 15q12 deletion of paternal origin. It can also occur in uniparental disomy where both chromosomes 15 are inherited from the mother (Nicholls et al. 1989) and is usually milder (Cassidy et al. 1997; Dykens et al. 1999; Roof et al. 2000). In contrast, Angelman's syndrome most often emerges from deletion in maternally derived chromosome 15 (15q11–13) or from uniparental disomy when both chromosomes 15 are inherited from the father (Malcolm et al. 1991; Thapar et al. 1994).

Neurochemical studies have found elevated levels of oxytocin (Martin et al. 1998), dopamine, and serotonin (Akefeldt et al. 1998) in the CSF of Prader-Willi patients. Administration of growth hormone has been reported to be helpful for somatic features of this disorder (Lindgren and Ritzen 1999; Ritzen et al. 1999); however, this treatment may not improve the behavioral symptoms (Akefeldt and Gillberg 1999).

Autism and Pervasive Developmental Disorders

Autism is a rare but serious neuropsychiatric syndrome affecting 4–5 children per

10,000 births (Fombonne et al. 1997). Boys are affected three- to fourfold more often than girls (Wing and Gould 1979). Kanner (1943) introduced the term *early infantile autism* to describe a group of 11 such children. DSM-IV-TR (American Psychiatric Association 2000) distinguishes autistic disorder from other pervasive developmental disorders, including Rett's disorder, childhood disintegrative disorder, Asperger's disorder, and pervasive developmental disorder not otherwise specified. These disorders share a common set of severe disturbances in social recognition and interaction, impaired communication, and a restricted stereotypic behavioral repertoire and range of interests.

Characteristic Features

Children with autism often seem indifferent to others. Their lack of interest may be manifested by minimal eye contact, delayed or absent facial signals, and impaired imitation of appropriate social behaviors. Autistic children have few if any friends; they may not engage in comfort seeking when distressed and often exhibit a preference for solitary play. Extreme cases find all physical contact aversive. Children with autism are frequently nonverbal when first diagnosed. If speech is present, it is often highly deviant and of limited communicative function. Autistic children also have deficient nonverbal communication skills.

Stereotypies are common in autism and can involve the flicking, twirling, or spinning of objects, or hand flapping, whirling, and posturing. Autistic children are often fascinated by spinning tops and other devices. Many autistic children resist change in their environment by ordering and arranging objects in precise ways to ensure sameness.

Mental retardation is present in 75%–80% of children with autism and appears to be stable over time (Freeman et al. 1985, 1991). Children with autism may be underresponsive or overresponsive to sensory stimuli (Ornitz 1974; Ornitz and Ritvo 1968). Abnormal mood states can also be present and are often characterized by temper tantrums, aggression, self-injury, or unexplainable giggling. Deviant motility, such as toe walking, can also be observed. Research suggests that the social problems of autistic children may stem, in part, from the inability to establish joint attention, such as pointing or showing objects (Baron-Cohen 1989). Autistic children may also lack the ability to infer another person's state of mind, an inability that may be a core feature of the disorder (Leslie and Frith 1988; Perner et al. 1989; Rutter and Bailey 1993).

Etiology and Pathophysiology

Autism appears to stem from both genetic and nongenetic factors that affect brain development (Cirianello and Cirianello 1995). The concordance rate in monozygotic twins is 60%, but no concordance has been found between dizygotic twins (Bailey et al. 1995). Cognitive and social abnormalities are nearly ubiquitous in monozygotic twins of affected probands. Dizygotic twins and siblings have a significant but much lower incidence of cognitive disturbance (August et al. 1981; Bailey et al. 1995). Although many etiological factors have been proposed, no single cause has been elucidated. Minshew (1991) argued that less than 5% of individuals with autism have an identifiable etiology. Potential causal factors include tuberous sclerosis, cytomegalovirus, encephalitis, meningitis, and fragile X. Immune abnormalities have also been proposed (Warren et al. 1995). Conservative sources estimate that fragile X may be present in 7% of males and 4% of females with autism (Bolton and Rutter 1990). A number of recent reports has documented deletions and duplications of chromosome 15, especially in the 15q11–13 region (Cook 2001); however, no candidate genes have been identified (Tanguay 2000).

Neuroanatomic studies have suggested that autism arises from premature cessation of development in the cerebellum, cerebrum, and limbic system. Postmortem studies have identified regions of cellular loss unaccompanied by gliosis. These findings suggest that the lesion occurred in fetal life or was the result of misdirected development (Bauman 1991). Courchesne et al. (1991) reported a 25% reduction in the size of cerebellar vermal lobes VI and VII in 14 of 18 subjects with autism. Differences in vermal size, however, correlated with low IQ rather than autism per se (Holttum et al. 1992; Levitt et al. 1999). Damage to the cerebellum may manifest as damage to the frontal lobes and affect attention, memory, and language (Riva and Giorgi 2000). Some theories suggest that autism results from coordinated developmental anomalies affecting the posterior-superior vermis and frontal, temporal, and parietal lobes. Kemper and Bauman (1993) observed progressive developmental changes in neurons in the cerebellum, inferior olive, and diagonal band of Broca. Kemper and Bauman theorized that deficient Purkinje cell production resulted in a failure to form appropriate corticocerebellar synaptic connections and that these circuits regressed with age. This process may also explain the high density of small neurons observed in the hippocampus and amygdala (Bauman and Kemper 1985). Bailey et al. (1998) found abnormal neuronal migration patterns in the brain stem and cerebellum, and reduced numbers of Purkinje cells in adult cases. A striking inverse correlation was found between Purkinje cell number and cortical thickness. Carper and Courchesne (2000) also

found a significant inverse correlation between the size of vermal lobules VI–VII and volume of frontal gray matter in patients with autism, but not in control subjects. Deficient development of corticocerebellar connections may have impaired the normal process of cortical development and attenuated the pruning process. Lack of pruning is consistent with the elevated rates of glucose metabolism (Horwitz et al. 1988) and adenosine triphosphate utilization observed in the frontal and parietal lobes of patients with autism. Gyral malformations have also been found in the cortex, including pachygyria, polymicrogyria, heterotopia, and schizencephaly (Piven et al. 1990).

The deficits in cognitive functioning characteristic of autism have not been linked to specific anatomical defects. Individuals with autism perform normally on tasks that assess perception, attention, and classification of stimuli and appear to have intact sensory and basic memory functions (Courchesne 1991). However, in children with autism slowed orienting to visual cues correlates with degree of cerebellar hypoplasia (Harris et al. 1999). Abnormalities have been observed in certain evoked potential responses (e.g., auditory P300) that are probably indicative of deficient auditory processing (Novic et al. 1980). A reversal in hemispheric asymmetry and reduced hemispheric communication have been proposed (Ornitz and Ritvo 1968) and supported by a variety of studies (Belmonte et al. 1995; Egaas et al. 1995; Hardan et al. 2000; Hashimoto et al. 1988; Horwitz et al. 1988).

Social deficits in autism have been examined with fMRI using facial perception tests. Patients with autism had attenuated responses in mesolimbic and temporal lobe cortical regions and in left amygdala and left cerebellum during facial processing (Critchley et al. 2000). Schultz and colleagues (2000) found that individuals with autism relied on feature-based strategies for facial recognition and had greater activation in the inferior temporal gyri.

Neurochemically, the most noted observation has been a significant increase in whole-blood 5-HT levels in 30% of autistic individuals (Young et al. 1985). High levels of 5-HT have also been found in most first-degree relatives (Piven et al. 1991). McBride et al. (2000) found that whole-blood 5-HT levels vary by race and pubertal status. They found, after correcting for race, a significant elevation in whole-blood 5-HT levels in about 25% of prepubertal but not postpubertal children with autism. Chugani and colleagues (1997, 1999) found decreased 5-HT synthesis and uptake in frontal cortex and thalamus, especially in boys. Mixed findings have emerged regarding a possible linkage of the 5-HT transporter gene and autism (Cook et al. 1997; Klauck et al. 1997). Elevated levels of endogenous opioids have also been noted in patients with autism. This observation emerged from the apparently high pain threshold of autistic individuals with self-abusive behaviors. Research suggests that levels of β-endorphin and endorphin fraction II may be elevated in the CSF (Ross et al. 1987).

Treatment

Pharmacotherapy for autism has had mixed results. However, many autistic children have appropriate target symptoms that warrant a therapeutic trial (Campbell et al. 1996). Fenfluramine, which stimulates 5-HT release, has been used in numerous trials. Although initial reports were promising (e.g., Ritvo et al. 1983, 1986), later studies have been disappointing (e.g., Leventhal et al. 1993). There may, however, have been a sub-

group that responds favorably. Fenfluramine has been withdrawn as a result of emergence of adverse effects on the heart. Opiate antagonists such as naltrexone have been used to enhance cognitive processing (Lensing et al. 1995) and reduce self-injury and hyperactivity (Campbell et al. 1993; Gillberg 1995), with equivocal results. Neuroleptics, particularly haloperidol, have been extensively evaluated in double-blind, placebo-controlled protocols (Campbell et al. 1996). Haloperidol reduces symptoms of anger, uncooperativeness, and hyperactivity, and also exerts some effects on core features of autistic behavior and deviant speech (Campbell et al. 1996). Clomipramine has also been found to be effective in controlled studies in attenuating stereotypies, compulsions, ritualized behaviors, and aggression (Campbell et al. 1996). The few published reports indicate that SSRIs are modestly effective in decreasing hyperactivity, restlessness, agitation, obsessive thoughts, and preoccupations (McDougle et al. 1998; Posey et al. 1999). Although anecdotal reports indicated that secretin, a gastrointestinal hormone, had therapeutic benefits, initial controlled studies have been negative (Chez et al. 2000; Sandler et al. 1999).

Long-term interventions focus on community-based special educational programs and subsequent residential services for those who cannot be cared for at home. An initial study by Lovaas (1987) and a follow-up study (McEachin et al. 1993) suggest that as many as half of preschool-age children with autism can attain normal educational and intellectual function with extremely intensive early behavioral treatment. However, long-term care continues to be the norm for children with autism over the course of their lifetime (Nordin and Gillberg 1998).

Rett's Disorder

Rett's disorder is an X-linked dominant progressive degenerative disorder found exclusively in females, as it is lethal in males. Development often appears to be normal until about 18 months of age, followed by the emergence of autistic symptoms, often leading to a diagnosis of autism. Development of distinctive hand stereotypies (i.e., twisting or wringing), deceleration in normal head growth leading to microcephaly, and progressive neurological deterioration help establish the correct diagnosis. Children develop gait ataxia between 1 and 4 years of age and may lose ambulation completely as they mature.

Monozygotic twins show complete concordance, whereas dizygotic twins are not concordant (Lotspeich 1995). Progressive clinical deterioration is mirrored by progressive cortical atrophy and neuronal loss (Zoghbi et al. 1985). There is a marked attenuation in levels of the noradrenergic metabolite MHPG and the dopamine metabolite HVA in the CSF (Zoghbi et al. 1985). Children with Rett's disorder show some of the motor problems observed in Parkinson's disease and suffer from reduced dopaminergic activity in the basal ganglia, substantia nigra, and cortex (Rett 1966, 1977; Wenk et al. 1991). Mutations in a gene called *MeCP2* is responsible for about one-third of cases (Amir et al. 1999).

Imaging and postmortem studies indicate that children with Rett's disorder have curtailed development, characterized by reduced cerebral volume (Jellinger et al. 1988; Reiss et al. 1993), cortical dysplasia with limited gliosis, decreased cell size, increased packing density (Bauman et al. 1995), global reductions in gray- and white-matter volumes (Subramaniam et al. 1997), and greater loss of gray matter versus white matter (Reiss et al. 1993), particularly in the prefrontal, posterior-frontal, and anterior-temporal regions (Subramaniam et al. 1997). Abnormalities in amino acid receptors have been demonstrated in basal ganglia (Blue et al. 1999a) and superior frontal gyrus (Blue et al. 1999b). *N*-methyl-D-aspartate (NMDA) receptor density in the superior frontal gyrus changes dramatically with age. NMDA receptor density is higher in brains of younger patients with Rett's disorder than it is in the brains of control subjects, and it is lower in the brains of older patients with Rett's disorder than it is in the brains of control subjects (Blue et al. 1999b). Dendritic arborization is reduced in many cortical regions (Armstrong et al. 1998).

PET scans demonstrate reduced frontal blood flow, and reveal an immature blood flow and metabolism pattern comparable to that observed in early infancy (Nielsen et al. 1990). Magnetic resonance spectroscopy (MRS) imaging reveals a significant reduction of *N*-acetyl aspartate concentration and increased choline concentration in frontal, parietal, insular, and hippocampal regions. These findings are consistent with reduced neuronal arborization and gliosis in these regions (Horska et al. 2000).

Asperger's Disorder

Asperger's disorder is characterized by social dysfunction, pedantic speech, and idiosyncratic interests. Children with Asperger's disorder are distinguished from autistic children by better social function, normal intelligence, undelayed language development, and greater clumsiness. Although Asperger's disorder is, at present, nosologically distinct from autism, many argue that the disorder is merely a milder form of autism and should be categorized as such (Miller and Ozonoff 2000).

Specific Disorders of Learning

Learning disorders are specific delineated deficits in the acquisition and performance of reading, writing, or arithmetic skills in the presence of normal intelligence and aptitude. These disorders often come to attention in grammar school and are estimated to affect up to 10% of school-age children, though many cases go undiagnosed. Learning disorders frequently persist into adulthood (American Academy of Child and Adolescent Psychiatry 1998; American Psychiatric Association 1994). Learning disorders are thought to be a consequence of neurocortical impairment, yet their expression is affected by parental support, educational resources, and the individual's personality, initiative, and motivation. Although learning disorders can be comorbid with many other psychiatric conditions, it is important to distinguish learning disorders from mental retardation, sensory impairments, and other psychiatric or neurological conditions that can affect attention, motivation, and behavior.

The evaluation of a learning disorder consists of intelligence tests, specific achievement tests, and a description of the child's classroom behavior. Because learning disabilities often entitle children to special services, most states have adopted specific guidelines for their diagnosis based on standardized tests (Frankenberger and Fronzaglio 1991). Typically, the learning-disabled child demonstrates a significant discrepancy between nonverbal (performance) IQ and verbal IQ, with a history of delayed or impaired speech, language, or reading skills (American Academy of Child and Adolescent Psychiatry 1998; Tallal et al. 1991). Overlooked or left untreated, learning disorders can lead to underachievement in a number of domains, along with diminished self-esteem, disinterest in school, truancy, and conduct and substance abuse disorders (Benasich et al. 1993; Karacostas and Fisher 1993; Naylor et al. 1994; Rowe and Rowe 1992). Approximately 40% of children with learning disorders eventually drop out of school (Popper and Steingard 1995). Current data suggest that, although reading disorders can worsen preexisting aggressive behavior, evidence is insufficient to presume that reading disability causes aggression (Cornwall and Bawden 1992).

Characteristic Features

At present, three identifiable learning disorders are recognized: reading disorder, mathematics disorder, and disorders of written expression. *Reading disorder* is characterized by slow acquisition of reading skills despite normal intelligence, education, motivation, and emotional control. Prominent characteristics include letter and word reversals, word omissions and distortions, spelling errors, and substitution of words (American Psychiatric Association 1994). Left-right orientation, sound and phoneme discrimination, rapid visual and auditory sensory processing, and perceptual-motor skills are also impaired. Approximately 4% of school-age children are affected by reading disorder, and boys are affected three to four times more frequently than girls (C. Lewis et al. 1994).

Mathematics disorder is characterized by difficulty with counting, mathematical reasoning, calculations, and object conceptualization (American Psychiatric Association 1994). Impairment in spatial skills and in right-left, up-down, and east-west differentiation is evident. Children with mathematics disorder often have difficulty copying shapes, memorizing numbers, and sequencing tasks. Mathematics disorder affects about 1% of the school-age population, whereas 2% of children are affected by both arithmetic and reading difficulties (C. Lewis et al. 1994). Boys and girls appear to be equally affected (C. Lewis et al. 1994).

Compared with reading and mathematics disorders, the *disorders of written expression* are not well characterized, and prevalence rates are unknown. Children have impairments in spelling, grammar, punctuation, sentence and paragraph formation, and organizational structure. Characteristic features include slow ability to write or produce writing assignments, illegibility, letter reversals, word-finding and syntax errors, and punctuation and spelling problems (American Psychiatric Association 1994).

Etiology and Pathophysiology

Learning disorders have both a genetic and environmental basis. Environmental factors include prenatal ethanol exposure, perinatal complications, postnatal lead exposure, diminished parental and environmental stimulation, and head trauma (Ewing-Cobbs et al. 1998; Pennington and Smith 1983). Evidence also suggests that there are heritable forms of learning disorders (Cardon et al. 1994, 1995; Pennington and Smith 1983). However, critical questions about the nature of learning disorders color any discussion of etiology and pathophysiology. One major view is that learning disorders are relatively discrete neuropsychiatric syndromes affecting a specific set of higher cognitive functions without affecting general intelligence. The contrasting view is that learning disorders are not discrete neurological syndromes and that they merely represent the tail end of a normal distribution of aptitudes and abilities (B.A. Shaywitz et al. 1995; S.E. Shaywitz et al. 1992). Evidence supporting the latter view derives mostly from the realm of psychological testing, in which an important study

showed that reading ability scores were normally distributed without an expected bimodal hump in the lower range, indicative of a second population with lower mean value (S.E. Shaywitz et al. 1992; but see Rutter and Yule 1975). This argues that there is not a discrete population of patients with reading disorders and that such individuals are merely the lower range of a normal population. This does not preclude the possibility that a small subset of patients may have discrete neurological disorders affecting reading ability, but that any such subset would be relatively small and would not account for the preponderance of patients with reading disability (S.E. Shaywitz et al. 1992).

In contrast to this view, burgeoning literature suggests that some children with learning disorders have identifiable neurological abnormalities and that some learning disorders follow simple genetic models. Numerous studies have shown that learning disorders are highly heritable. Concordance for dyslexia may be as high as 91% in monozygotic twin pairs versus 31% for dizygotic twins (Pennington and Smith 1983). Reading, mathematical, and spelling ability are all inherited traits with heritability indices of 0.78 (Gillis et al. 1992), 0.51 (Gillis et al. 1992), and 0.53 (Stevenson et al. 1987), respectively. Cardon et al. (1994, 1995) identified a quantitative trait locus on chromosome 6 (region 6p21.3) for reading disability in two carefully selected, independent groups of sibling pairs. This region is found in the human leukocyte antigen encoding region, supporting the suspected association between autoimmune disorders and dyslexia (Geschwind and Behan 1982; Schacter and Galaburda 1986).

Patterns of family inheritance have also helped to unravel the association between learning disorders and ADHD. Conservative estimates suggest that 8% of children with ADHD have a learning disorder, but actual estimates range from 0% to 92% (Semrud-Clikeman et al. 1992). Most studies show that ADHD and learning disorders are transmitted independently (Faraone et al. 1993; Gilger et al. 1992) and suggest that comorbidity between ADHD and learning disorder may be a consequence of nonrandom mating between individuals with family histories of ADHD and learning disability (Faraone et al. 1993).

Autopsy findings in learning disorders include arteriovenous malformations, atypical gyral patterns in parietal lobes, thin corpus callosum in the region connecting the parietal lobes, and premature cessation of neuronal migration to the cortex, revealed by an excess number of neurons in white matter (Drake 1968; Geschwind and Galaburda 1985). Also, Galaburda et al. (1985, 1994) observed anomalies in medial geniculate and the lateral posterior thalamic nuclei. Perhaps the most interesting anomalies involve the cortex, particularly the left perisylvian region.

Visual information from the retina is transmitted to the cerebral cortex by way of the lateral geniculate nucleus (LGN) in the thalamus. In primates, most of the retinal ganglion cells that project to the LGN belong to one of two classes, P and M, whose axons terminate in the parvocellular or magnocellular subdivisions of the LGN, respectively. These cell classes give rise to two channels that have been distinguished anatomically, physiologically, and behaviorally (DeYoe and Van Essen 1988). The magnocellular pathway has fast conduction velocities, large receptive fields, and operates in a transient manner. In contrast, the parvocellular pathway is slow with much finer receptive fields (Fitch et al. 1997; Stein and Walsh 1997). The visual cortex also can be subdivided into two pathways, one specialized for motion processing and the other for color and form information. Responses in the motion pathway in the cortex depend primarily on magnocellular LGN, whereas visual responses in the color/form pathway depend on both P and M input (Ferrera et al. 1992). Based on electrophysiological studies and autopsy analysis of the LGN from five subjects, Livingstone et al. (1991) proposed that dyslexic subjects have a specific defect in the magnocellular pathway. They further suggested that dyslexic subjects perform poorly on auditory and somatosensory tests that require rapid discrimination and proposed an underlying defect in the fast subdivision of multiple cortical sensory systems. Evidence in support of this theory has been mixed. Studies using motion-based tests of the magnocellular pathway have been more supportive than tests using low-contrast stimuli (Demb et al. 1998; Greatrex and Drasdo 1995; Johannes et al. 1996; Kubova et al. 1996; Skottun 2000). Stein and Walsh (1997) emphasized the importance of the magnocellular pathway in guiding visual attention and suggested that dyslexia in some patients may result from impaired temporal processing in phonological, visual, and motor domains. Steinman et al. (1998) and Facoetti et al. (2000) have also reiterated the association between magnocellular defects and impaired visuospatial attention in dyslexia.

Imaging studies reveal evidence for abnormalities in cerebral lateralization, in which normal asymmetries associated with brain specialization for language function have been reduced. The planum temporale is often abnormally symmetrical in children with reading disorders; that is, subjects have an underdeveloped Broca's area relative to the homologous cortical area in the right hemisphere (Dalby et al. 1998; Haslam et al. 1981; Jernigan et al. 1991). Similarly, children with reading disorders have reduced blood flow in the left hemisphere (left temporoparietal cortex) under challenge conditions (Georgiewa et al. 1999; Lou et al. 1990; Rumsey et al. 1992; Simos et al. 2000) and may have reduced size of the left dorsolateral prefrontal cortex (Jernigan et al. 1991). Similarly, the cerebral blood flow pattern in the left angular gyrus of men with developmental dyslexia is not commensurate with blood flow in the extrastriate occipital and temporal lobes during single-word reading, suggesting a disconnection of the left angular gyrus in dyslexia (Horwitz et al. 1998).

Left hemisphere electroencephalographic activity is diminished relative to right-sided activity in children with reading disorders (Ackerman et al. 1998; Mattson et al. 1992), whereas right hemisphere activity is reduced in children with arithmetic disabilities (Mattson et al. 1992). Differences in the size of the perisylvian region may reflect a familial genetic factor (Plante 1991). Reduced lateralization of language centers is consistent with results from dichotic listening tasks (Morton 1994), which suggest either less efficient callosal transfer or right hemispheric processing of information. The size of the corpus callosum does not vary directly with the severity of learning disorders for all subjects. The corpus callosum is thicker in children with familial history of dysphasia/dyslexia, probably indicative of reduced cerebral dominance in this subgroup (Njiokiktjien et al. 1994). In contrast, children who have suffered from perinatal adverse events that could impair cognitive skills have a corpus callosum that is reduced in comparison with that of family members without learning impairment.

Nongenetic environmental factors clearly influence the appearance of learning disabilities. Fall conception significantly increases the risk of developing reading and arithmetic disabilities as well as mental retardation, presumably as a result of increased risk of viral infections during early stages of brain development (Liederman and Flannery 1994). Early exposure to environmental toxins can also manifest as learning disorders (Pihl and Parkes 1977). Prenatal and postnatal exposure to low-level lead is significantly associated with learning deficits in girls but not in boys (Leviton et al. 1993). Alcohol is another powerful factor that can produce learning disabilities in the presence of normal intelligence (Streissguth et al. 1990). Geschwind and Galaburda (1985) proposed that increased fetal testosterone modifies neuronal, immune, and neural crest development. Testosterone can also inhibit neuronal migration by altering the ability of the CNS to identify trophic markers (Schacter and Galaburda 1986). The Geschwind-Behan-Galaburda theory has been used to explain the relative superiority of males over females in spatial skills, the greater preponderance of learning disorders in males, the association between learning disorder and immune disorder, and giftedness of left-handed individuals in other non-language-based skills (Geschwind and Behan 1982; Geschwind and Galaburda 1985). More recent studies have found that this influential theory is only partially supported by empirical evidence and is not consistent with current data on the development of the neural crest (Bryden et al. 1994).

Treatment

No systematic study supports any one educational intervention for the treatment of learning disorders. Primarily, mandated special education, provided in the least restrictive environment, is the major treatment for children with learning disorders. Special education is characterized by an individual educational plan and can include services provided as part of the usual classroom instruction or removal from the classroom part-time to designated "resource rooms." Specialized full-time classrooms, programs, or residential schools are usually reserved for those with severe learning disorders or concomitant psychiatric disorders. Alternative writing formats, skill building, and use of word processors can aid in the treatment of learning disorders, particularly disorders of written expression. Homework assignments for children with learning disabilities should emphasize simple, short tasks; careful monitoring and reinforcement by teachers; and parental involvement (Cooper and Nye 1994). Practical parent-based programs have become available (Jenson et al. 1994). In addition, efforts to increase the child's self-esteem are essential for successful treatment. Treatment should also include parental guidance to adjust expectations and to provide support and encouragement. No evidence supports the efficacy of medications, diet restrictions, or vitamin therapy. Similarly, sensory integration therapy has little empirical support as a beneficial intervention (Hoehn and Baumeister 1994; Humphries et al. 1992; Kaplan et al. 1993).

Two remediative treatments have demonstrated some promise. Possibly through improving binocular stability, monocular occlusion for 6 months while reading and writing improved reading ability in approximately half of dyslexic children whose primary problem involved gaze control (Stein and Fowler 1985). Through intensive exposure and training using acoustically modified speech, Tallal et al. (1996) demonstrated rapid gains in auditory comprehension in children with combined language-learning disorders. Tallal's group designed a computer program that altered recorded speech by prolonging the duration of the speech signal and enhancing fast speech elements in order to facilitate comprehension of speech elements that involve rapid frequency discrimination. Intensive training over a 4-week period with acoustically modified speech resulted in improved ability of children with language-learning impairment. Further studies of the remediative efficacy of these and other treatments are required.

Seizure Disorders

Epilepsy is a recurrent paroxysmal disorder involving excessive neural firing. It is a relatively common disorder with an incidence of 0.5%. Onset most often occurs before adulthood. Epilepsy is estimated to affect 0.15% of preschoolers and 0.5% of school-age children and adolescents. Seizures are more prevalent in boys than in girls, and the incidence is higher in nonwhites (Hauser and Hesdorffer 1990). Seizure disorders can present at birth and can be associated with chromosomal or structural abnormalities or in utero infections. Epilepsy can develop as a consequence of meningitis, encephalitis, head trauma, exposure to environmental toxins such as lead, inborn errors of metabolism, arteriovenous malformations, abnormalities in brain development, and a host of idiopathic causes. Differential diagnosis is crucial. Many children suspected of having epilepsy have pseudoseizures or other paroxysmal nonepileptiform events (Andriola and Ettinger 1999; Rothner 1992). These include mitral valve prolapse, cardiac arrhythmias, sleep disorders (pavor nocturnus, cataplexy, somnambulism), migraine headaches, movement disorders (e.g., TS, paroxysmal choreoathetosis), episodic dyscontrol, and panic disorder.

Classification and Features

Epilepsies are broadly classified by the location of the seizure focus. Primarily, generalized seizures involve the simultaneous emergence of seizure activity in both hemispheres, presumably from a subcortical focus. Partial seizures, in contrast, begin with discharge arising in a focal cortical area, though seizure activity can then spread (Dreifuss 1989). The major forms of generalized seizures are tonic-clonic seizures, absence seizures, myoclonic seizures, and infantile spasms. The major forms of partial seizures include simple seizures, complex partial seizures, and partial seizures secondarily generalized.

Generalized Seizures

Tonic-clonic seizures are also known as *grand mal seizures*. Both hemispheres are simultaneously involved at the outset, producing immediate loss of consciousness, tonic extension, muscular stiffness, and inhibition of respiration. During the clonic phase of the attack, symmetrical jerking of all extremities occurs and is usually accompanied by oral and fecal incontinence (Rothner 1992). Typically tonic-clonic seizures last 2–5 minutes and are followed by somnolence and confusion. Severe headaches and muscle aches are also common in the postictal period.

Absence seizures are also known as *petit mal seizures*. They are characterized by abrupt onset of impaired consciousness that generally lasts for 10–20 seconds. During this period, children typically stare straight ahead and may flutter their eyelids, but there is usually an absence of movement. Posture is maintained and incontinence does not occur. Immediately after the seizure, consciousness is regained without postictal confusion. However, petit mal seizures can occur frequently, up to 20–30 times per day, taking a serious toll on attention, and can be brought on by stress and exercise. Electroencephalography reveals a highly characteristic 3-Hz spike-and-wave pattern

(Rothner 1992). In some children, absence seizures remit during adolescence; in others, they may be replaced by tonic-clonic seizures.

Infantile spasms are relatively uncommon. They occur in association with mental retardation in children from ages 3 months to 1 year. The spasms involve a brief jackknife-like flexion or extension of arms and legs. The spasms occur in clusters, particularly around sleep-wake transitions. They are associated with characteristic hypsarrhythmic electroencephalogram (EEG), with a chaotic mixture of irregular high-voltage spike-and-wave discharge, multifocal sharp waves, and burst suppression. Most children with infantile spasms demonstrate moderate to profound mental retardation and will suffer from lifelong intractable seizures (Pellock 1998; Rothner 1992).

Myoclonic seizures, including atonic, akinetic, and tonic forms, usually emerge during the first 10 years of life and affect 0.1% of children. The combination of mental retardation, myoclonic seizures, and other seizure types is called *Lennox-Gastaut syndrome*. The myoclonic seizures are brief but occur frequently, and they are largely refractory to treatment. Ketogenic diet and corpus callosotomy can be of benefit for some children (Pellock 1998; Rothner 1992).

Juvenile myoclonic epilepsy often emerges in adolescence and is a more benign and treatment-responsive condition. The seizures most frequently occur in the morning and take the form of myoclonic jerks or tonic-clonic convulsions. The EEG reveals characteristic generalized polyspikes. Children who develop this disorder were often healthy and free of neurological disturbance until the onset of the seizures. This condition persists throughout life but usually responds well to treatment with sodium valproate (Pellock 1998; Rothner 1992).

Partial Seizures

Simple partial seizures may be motor or sensory. A simple partial motor seizure consists of recurrent clonic movements of one part of the body without loss of consciousness. Sometimes motor activity can spread ipsilaterally (jacksonian march) or even spread to the contralateral hemisphere, resulting in a secondarily generalized tonic-clonic seizure. Partial sensory seizures consist of paresthesias or pain referred to a single part of the body. They also can spread. In general, partial seizures last 1–2 minutes and are not associated with loss of consciousness unless secondarily generalized (Rothner 1992).

Rolandic epilepsy is a benign, inherited focal epileptic disorder of childhood that is the most common form of focal seizure seen in children less than 15 years old (Rothner 1992). These seizures are characterized by emergence of sharp waves in the central temporal region and may or may not be accompanied by either seizure or neurological deficits. Children often report an aura around the mouth preceding the seizure, which is followed by the jerking of the mouth and face before spreading to the rest of the body. Children retain consciousness and do not have postictal confusion. The seizure lasts between 30 seconds and 3 minutes and usually occurs during sleep. Prognosis for spontaneous remission is excellent, and treatment is rarely required (Rothner 1992).

Complex partial seizures, also known as psychomotor or temporal lobe seizures, are distinguished from other partial seizures by alterations in consciousness. Auras such as unpleasant odors, tastes, or sensations frequently precede the seizure. The seizure may be characterized by staring, altered consciousness, and eye blinking with maintenance of balance. Approximately 80% of patients with complex partial seizures engage in simple, repetitive, and purposeless automatism,

which can include swallowing, kissing, lip smacking, fumbling, scratching, or rubbing movements. Rarely, special sensory phenomenon can occur that can include visual distortions or hallucinations, auditory hallucinations, dreamlike or dissociative states, and abnormal body sensations (Kaufman 1985). The seizures last about 2 minutes and are often followed by confusion, drowsiness, and amnesia for the events. The EEG often shows sharp waves or spikes from the temporal region (Rothner 1992). Complex partial seizure attacks occur far less frequently than absence spells.

Psychiatric Consequences of Epilepsy

Bear and Fedio (1977) proposed that patients with temporal lobe epilepsy had distinctive personality aberrations. Many were hyposexual, humorless, circumstantial, overly metaphysical, hyperreligious, hypergraphic, and interpersonally viscous. It was also proposed that right-sided foci predisposed a patient to anger, sadness, and elation, whereas left-sided foci led to ruminative and intellectual tendencies. More recent studies, however, have cast doubt on these theories (Kaufman 1985; Rodin and Schmalz 1984).

An association exists between childhood epilepsy and behavioral, academic, and cognitive problems (Dunn and Austin 1999; Metz-Lutz et al. 1999). Children with epilepsy demonstrate more behavioral problems and psychiatric dysfunction than those in the general population and have more physical deformities or other chronic illness such as diabetes mellitus or asthma. In addition, several cognitive difficulties have been associated with epilepsy, including academic underachievement and greater academic difficulties than would be expected from IQ test scores (Dunn and Austin 1999). One prospective study (Metz-Lutz et al. 1999) suggests that, in addition to cognitive deficits, children with benign focal epilepsy demonstrate abnormalities in a attention, response organization, and fine motor skills.

Old literature suggests that psychosis can emerge in patients with temporal lobe epilepsy. The seizure disorder most often emerges in childhood (5–10 years of age), whereas the psychosis is generally delayed in onset until about age 30. Left-handed patients with left-sided seizure foci were believed to be the most susceptible to psychosis (Kaufman 1985; Perez and Trimble 1980). Interestingly, we have found that childhood abuse was associated with an increased incidence of left hemisphere electroencephalographic abnormalities (Ito et al. 1993) and abnormal left but not right electroencephalographic coherence, suggesting decreased left cortical differentiation (Teicher et al. 1997). Davies (1979) previously reported that childhood incest was associated with a high incidence of abnormal EEGs and seizure disorder in 36% of survivors. It is plausible that the stress of childhood trauma can affect aspects of brain development, thereby increasing the risk for emergence of seizure. Moreover, this particular etiology can be associated with development of serious psychopathology, including dissociation and perception of internal voices that can be mistaken for psychosis.

An association is well established between epilepsy and high incidence of criminality. Incarcerated men have a fourfold increased incidence of epilepsy compared with the general population (Kaufman 1985). It is likely that both epilepsy and criminality result from common causes such as head trauma and low socioeconomic status. As suggested above, a common association may exist among childhood abuse, electroencephalographic abnormalities, and criminal behavior. In a study of 14 juvenile murderers condemned to death, 12 had a history of brutal physical abuse and 5 had been sodomized by relatives (D.O. Lewis et al. 1988). Electroencephalographic abnormalities and seizure disorders were common in this group (D.O. Lewis et al. 1988). Sexual trauma has often been identified in the life histories of sex offenders (Groth 1979; Seghorn et al. 1987). Thus, early abuse can lead to a vicious cycle of intergenerational transmission and perpetuation associated with neuropsychiatric sequelae.

Finally, there is a prominent association between epilepsy, suicidality, and self-destructive behavior. One of the earliest pioneering studies on the physiological determinants of suicide reported a strong positive association between paroxysmal EEG disturbances and suicidal ideation, attempts, and assaultive-destructive behavior (Struve et al. 1972). It has also been reported that the risk of completed suicide is four to five times greater in individuals with epilepsy than among patients without epilepsy and that this risk may be 25-fold greater in patients with temporal lobe epilepsy (Barraclough 1981; Mathews and Barabas 1981). As many as one-third of all patients with epilepsy have attempted suicide at some point in their life (Delay et al. 1957; Jensen 1975). This risk is far greater for patients with epilepsy than for patients with other medical disorders producing comparable degrees of handicap or disability (Mendez et al. 1986). Mendez et al. (1989) provided data suggesting that this risk can be related to interictal psychopathological changes, particularly the high prevalence of borderline personality disorder. We have found that children with early abuse and abnormal EEGs have a marked increase in self-destructive behavior (Teicher et al. 1996a) and that abused children's ratings of suicidal ideation and interictal seizure symptomatology correlate very strongly (M.H.Teicher et al., unpublished observations, September 1996). Brent et al. (1987) examined 15 children with epilepsy treated with phenobarbital and 24 children with epilepsy treated with carbamazepine. The groups were similar across a wide range of demographic, seizure-related, familial, and environmental factors. Patients treated with phenobarbital had a much higher prevalence of major depression (40% vs. 4%, $P = 0.02$) and a much greater prevalence of suicidal ideation (47% vs. 4%, $P = 0.005$). It is unclear whether phenobarbital produced these psychiatric disturbances or failed to alleviate them. However, the implications for treatment are clear.

Treatment

Tonic-clonic seizures are often responsive to valproic acid, phenytoin, carbamazepine, and phenobarbital. Phenobarbital and its associated congener primidone are associated with hyperactivity, fussiness, lethargy, disturbed sleep, irritability, depression, and cognitive disturbance in children (Rothner 1992). They should not be used as drugs of first choice in the pediatric population. Chronic administration of phenytoin can lead to gingival hyperplasia and hirsutism. Phenytoin causes behavioral problems less frequently than phenobarbital but can impair attention and coordination and produce dizziness, ataxia, and diplopia. Carbamazepine is structurally similar to tricyclic antidepressants but lacks prominent effects on monoamine reuptake. Common side effects include diplopia, dizziness, drowsiness, and transient leukopenia. Carbamazepine can also impair neuropsychological performance but is usually less problematic than phenobarbital or phenytoin (Rothner 1992). Rarely, aplastic anemia and hepatotoxicity can occur. Sodium valproate is often the most tolerated anticonvulsant for children and adolescents. Common side effects include gastrointestinal distress and thinning of the hair. Rare cases of fetal hepatotoxicity have occurred, though these cases are almost entirely limited to infants and young children, and the majority have followed combination chemotherapy with other drugs that induce hepatic microsomal enzymes, which can foster buildup of a toxic valproate metabolite. Pancreatitis is another rare complication. Occasionally drowsiness may arise, which can be related to elevated ammonia levels.

Absence seizures are treated with ethosuximide or valproic acid. Although ethosuximide is useful in the treatment of absence seizures, it has no effect against possible coexisting major motor seizures. Major side effects include nausea, vomiting, and anorexia. Cognitive and behavioral side effects are uncommon.

Infantile spasms and myoclonic seizures of childhood are often treatment refractory. Potentially useful medications include adrenocorticotropic hormone, valproic acid, and benzodiazepines. Juvenile myoclonic epilepsy often responds favorably to valproic acid. Uncomplicated partial seizures are treated with carbamazepine, phenytoin, or phenobarbital. Neurosurgery to remove an underlying lesion may be the treatment of choice depending on the region affected (Wyllie et al. 1989). Complex partial seizures are also treated with carbamazepine, phenytoin, or phenobarbital. Acetazolamide can also have efficacy with seizures that occur premenstrually. Many cases of complex partial seizure fail to fully respond to monotherapy and may require combination treatment.

Newer anticonvulsants include felbamate, gabapentin, and lamotrigine (Ben-Menachem 2000). Felbamate is not a first-line anticonvulsant, and it is used only in those patients who have not responded to more conventional drugs and whose seizures are so severe as to warrant treatment with a drug that has a markedly elevated risk of aplastic anemia and hepatic failure. In children, the main indication is multiple seizures of Lennox-Gastaut syndrome (Schmidt and Bourgeois 2000). Gabapentin and lamotrigine are indicated for adjunctive therapy of partial seizures with and without generalization. This represents a new approach to seizure management. The old rule was to pursue monopharmacy even to extreme doses to avoid polypharmacy, with the belief that multiple anticonvulsants would produce supra-additive toxicity. Controlled trials of gabapentin and lamotrigine indicate that they can potentiate anticonvulsant efficacy with little increase in side effects. The most common side effects of gabapentin include somnolence ataxia, fatigue, and nausea. Lamotrigine is sometimes associated with development of a rash that can presage serious dermatological consequences. Common side effects include dizziness, ataxia, diplopia, blurred vision, and nausea.

Duration of treatment needs to be individualized. After a child has been free of seizures for 2–5 years, it may be possible to discontinue seizure medications. Discontinuation is less likely to succeed if the child has had a persistently abnormal EEG; known structural lesion; mental retardation; focal, complex partial seizures; or multiple seizure types. Medications should be withdrawn slowly, generally one medication at a time (Rothner 1992).

Trauma, Infections, and Stress

The developing brain is highly susceptible to adverse environmental factors. In the final section, we summarize recent research on the neuropsychiatric consequences of traumatic brain injury, congenital human immunodeficiency virus (HIV) infection, and physical and sexual abuse during childhood. These are widespread and largely preventable environmental insults that can produce severe neuropsychiatric sequelae.

Traumatic Brain Injury

The leading cause of disability in children between birth and 19 years of age is injury. Data from the National Pediatric Trauma Registry (1993) indicate that more than 25% of children injured and admitted for hospital care receive a diagnosis of head injury. Traumatic brain injury is generally classified as penetrating or closed. Outcome is most strongly related to the severity of brain injury, although posttraumatic amnesia, length of coma, presence of brain stem injury, seizures, and increased intracranial pressure also affect prognosis (Beers 1992; Lieh-Lai et al. 1992). Intelligence, fine motor skills, sensorimotor function, problem-solving ability, memory, adaptive function, attention, and language processing can all be affected (for a review, see Fletcher and Levin 1988). In addition, the presence of posttraumatic behavioral disorders compounds these problems (Michaud et al. 1993). Aggression, poor anger control, hyperactivity, and deficient social skills are typical behavioral symptoms (Asarnow et al. 1991). The symptoms are exacerbated by premorbid factors, including substance abuse, psychiatric disability, and dysfunctional family relations (Rivara et al. 1993).

The remarkable capacity of the developing brain to adapt to certain congenital anomalies and injuries has led many to believe that children will invariably show greater recovery than adults to traumatic brain injury (Rosner 1974). Others have hypothesized that children can be more vulnerable than adults. The relationship between age of injury and extent of disability is complex. Before puberty a high density of synaptic connections allows for considerable adaptive plasticity, which is most evident in the capacity to develop language after severe left hemisphere injury. However, there are also sensitive and critical periods for establishment of connections and synaptic relations, and if these opportunities are lost, enduring consequences can result. Children with brain injury can also require rehabilitation and special education services as well as neurological and psychiatric treatment.

Max and colleagues (Max and Dunisch 1997; Max et al. 1997a, 1997b, 1997c, 1998a, 1998b, 1998c, 1998d) have published extensively on the psychiatric consequences of head trauma. A retrospective analysis revealed that 5.6% of 1,333 consecutive patients presenting to a child psychiatry outpatient clinic had a definite history of traumatic brain injury and that children with such a history were clinically indistinguishable from children without such a history (Max and Dunisch 1997). In a large prospective study, 50 subjects were evaluated upon hospitalization for traumatic brain injury and reassessed upon follow-up at 3, 6, 12, and 24 months (Max et al. 1997a, 1997b, 1997c). The most consistently significant factors associated with the development of subsequent psychiatric disorders were increased severity of injury, family psychiatric history, and family dysfunction. Posttraumatic psychiatric disorders included organic personality syndrome, major depression, ADHD, oppositional defiant disorder, PTSD, simple phobia, separation anxiety disorder, OCD, adjustment disorder, mania, hypomania, and marijuana dependence. Some psychiatric sequelae were clinically apparent by 3 months after injury.

Further analysis of individual disorders revealed mixed results. The change in ADHD symptomatology after brain injury was directly and proportionally related to the severity of brain injury, suggesting a "dose-response" relationship (Max et al. 1998a). Development of oppositional symptomatology in the first year after injury was strongly associated with psychosocial factors, whereas its persistence in the second year was more significantly related to severity of brain injury (Max et al. 1998b). Sixty-eight percent of subjects experienced at least one PTSD symptom in the first 3 months, decreasing to 12% at 2 years. Only 4% of subjects met criteria for PTSD at any point in the study (Max et al. 1998c). Overall, severe traumatic brain injury is significantly associated with a greater incidence of psychiatric disorders (63%) compared with mild injury (21%) and orthopedic injury (4%) (Max et al. 1998d). Psychosocial intervention and family support may contribute to the care of brain-injured patients throughout the first 2 years after injury (Kinsella et al. 1999; Max et al. 1997c), although their therapeutic efficacy remains to be established.

Neuropsychiatric Features of HIV-1 Infection in Children and Young Adults

Approximately 1.5 million individuals in the United States are infected with HIV-1, and 20%–30% can eventually develop dementia. The incidence in parts of Asia and Africa is substantially higher. In the United States and in Europe, the incidence of childhood HIV infection has reportedly plateaued after a period of growth (Dal Maso et al. 1999). According to data published in 1995 by the Centers for Disease Control and Prevention (CDC), 14,920 HIV-infected infants were born in the United States between 1978 and 1993. In the data collected by the CDC through December 2001, 2,905 children under the age of 13 years were living with HIV-1 infection in the United States, while 2,410 children were living with AIDS (Centers for Disease Control and Prevention 2001). These numbers represent an underestimate, since mandated reporting practices have varied considerably from state to state. HIV-1 has become the most frequent cause of dementia in young people (Janssen et al. 1992). HIV-1 infection also results in encephalopathy that can affect between 30% and 60% of children with acquired immunodeficiency syndrome (AIDS) (Simpson 1999). Infants are more susceptible to encephalopathy compared with children and adults with AIDS (Tardieu et al. 2000). Infants with perinatally acquired AIDS have a 4% risk of developing encephalopathy by 12 months of age, making HIV encephalopathy a common condition in this population (Lobato et al. 1995).

The American Academy of Neurology has defined the clinical features of HIV-1 dementia, or AIDS dementia complex (ADC), as cognitive impairment, motor skill impairment, and behavioral changes (Janssen et al. 1991). ADC presents as a subcortical dementia in which primary language abnormalities and seizures are uncommon (Navia et al. 1986). People with ADC usually have rapid progression of symptoms, with a mean survival time of approximately 6 months (McArthur 1987). Progressive neurological deficits do not occur during the latent phases of HIV-1 infection but rather occur after the onset of severe immunodeficiency (McArthur 1987; McArthur et al. 1989). McArthur et al. (1993) estimated that 20%–30% of all individuals with AIDS will eventually develop dementia, though this may change with new treatments.

HIV-1 infection of the CNS results in neurological abnormalities in 40%–90% of children and can be associated with neurological complications such as stroke, seizure, vasculitis, vasculopathy, or myelopathy (Mintz 1996; Pontrelli et al. 1999). A bimodal distribution appears to exist in children with congenital HIV-1 infection: children who present with HIV-1 symptoms by 4 months of age and children who present with symptoms by 6 years of age (Auger et al. 1988). Three types of clinical presentations are found in children with HIV-1 infection: children with encephalopathy, children with neuropsychological dysfunction, and children without evidence of neuropsychological impairment (Working Group of the American Academy of Neurology AIDS Task Force 1991). Children with encephalopathy have clinical findings that include microcephaly, spastic diparesis or quadriparesis, extrapyramidal signs, and ataxia. Children with encephalopathy can have a clinical course characterized by a progressive subacute loss of previously acquired motor and language milestones. Other children with encephalopathy have neurological plateaus during which they neither acquire nor lose motor or cognitive milestones. In contrast, children with neuropsychological deficits, but without encephalopathy, can exhibit diminished speech production and difficulties with articulation (Epstein et al. 1985; Ultmann et al. 1987). Receptive language skills are typically less affected (Wolters et al. 1995). Cognitive deficits can manifest in older children as attention deficits (Cohen et al. 1991). Interestingly, adults with HIV-1–associated dementia appear to benefit from methylphenidate treatment (Fernandez et al. 1988). No large-scale study has established whether children show similar benefits. Another important neuropsychological consequence of HIV-1 is impaired social interactions (Ultmann et al. 1987). Children often become withdrawn and apathetic.

Those with progressive encephalopathy can have features similar to autism, including flat affect, mutism, and minimal interest in their environment. The association of AIDS with poverty, poor social support, and limited resources compounds the problem (Starace et al. 1998; Zierler et al. 2000).

In contrast to those in adults, the neurological abnormalities seen in children are largely a result of a primary HIV-1 encephalopathy. In one series, only 5% of children had opportunistic infections of their CNS. The pathological hallmarks of HIV-1 encephalopathy include HIV-1–infected macrophages and multinucleated giant cells, astrogliosis, microglial activation, and myelin pallor. Neuronal loss takes place in discrete areas of the retina, neocortex, and subcortical brain (Scarmato et al. 1996); loss of synaptic density and vacuolation of dendritic spines also occurs (Everall et al. 1991; Ketzler et al. 1990; Sharer 1992; Sharer et al. 1986; Tenhula et al. 1992; Wiley et al. 1986).

This disease complex is most striking in infected children (Sharer 1992). A direct relationship between the stage of HIV-1 infection, neuroimaging abnormalities, and neurobehavioral measures in HIV-infected children has been reported (Brouwers et al. 1995). MRS reveals reduced *N*-acetyl aspartate/creatine ratios in childhood AIDS encephalopathy and includes the basal ganglia (Lu et al. 1996; Pavlakis et al. 1995, 1998; Salvan et al. 1998). HIV-1 RNA has been found to be elevated in the CSF independently of plasma RNA levels in AIDS subjects with cognitive impairment (Brew et al. 1997; Ellis et al. 1997). Neurons do not appear to be productively affected by HIV-1 (Epstein and Gendelman 1993; Sharer et al. 1996), even though substantial loss of large neurons occurs through apoptosis (Fischer et al. 1999; Gelbard et al. 1995). Preclinical studies demonstrate that infected brain macrophages and microglia produce HIV-1 gene products and soluble neurotoxins (Epstein and Gendelman 1993) and that apoptotic neurons cluster in close proximity to these HIV-1–infected cells (Gelbard et al. 1995). These findings suggest that neurological dysfunction can result from the production of HIV-1–associated neurotoxins by macrophages or microglia that activate pathways for neuronal apoptosis (Dewhurst et al. 1996; Epstein and Gelbard 1999; Gelbard and Epstein 1995; James et al. 1999).

The cascade of events leading from HIV-1–infected macrophages and microglia to neuronal apoptosis and neurological dysfunction remains unclear. Recent studies suggest the involvement of the HIV-1 regulatory protein Tat as a neurotoxic activator of apoptosis (Bonwetsch et al. 1999; Maggirwar et al. 1999; New et al. 1997, 1998). Alternatively, HIV-1 gene products such as *Tat* can induced secretion of human tumor necrosis factor-α and other inflammatory products (New et al. 1998) that cause apoptosis (Perry et al. 1998; Talley et al. 1995). Numerous additional theories have also been proposed. Human herpesvirus 6 has become a focus of attention. Previously, human herpesvirus 6 was considered to be a benign commensal organism. It has now been found to be neuroinvasive, associated with progressive multifocal leukoencephalopathy and multiple sclerosis and is potentially involved in the pathogenesis of HIV encephalopathy (Blumberg et al. 2000; Saito et al. 1995). Novel treatment strategies may emerge from the elucidation of the mechanism of HIV-1 apoptosis (Gelbard et al. 1997).

Therapeutic advances have extended the survival of HIV-infected children past 5 years of age for more than 65% of cases (L. K. Brown et al. 2000). Prevention of vertical transmission has the most potential in reducing the neuropsychiatric sequelae of HIV, given the greater vulnerability of the developing brain before birth. Antiretroviral treatment of HIV-infected women during pregnancy and labor may decrease vertical transmission by 50% (Giaquinto et al. 1998). Zidovudine has been the most thoroughly investigated antiretroviral therapy for children with HIV encephalopathy (Bakashi et al. 1997; Brady et al. 1996; Sei et al. 1996). Administration of zidovudine has been associated with improved neuropsychological functioning (Simpson 1999) and reductions in the typically elevated levels of HIV-1 RNA in CSF (Sei et al. 1996). Also, antiretroviral therapies have been associated with reversal of reduced *N*-acetyl aspartate/creatine ratios on MRS, suggesting some recovery in neuronal arborization (Pavlakis et al. 1998). Ritonavir has also produced neurodevelopmental recovery (Tepper et al. 1998). The addition of zalcitabine to zidovudine in stable pediatric patients can be helpful (Bakashi et al. 1997).

Neuropsychiatric Consequences of Childhood Abuse

Physical or sexual traumatization during childhood can contribute to the development of a spectrum of psychiatric disorders. Early traumatization can be a risk factor in dissociative identity disorder (Wilbur 1984), refractory psychosis (Beck and van der Kolk 1987), borderline personality disorder (Herman et al. 1989; Stone 1981), somatoform disorder (Krystal 1978), and panic disorder (Faravelli et al. 1985). Childhood physical abuse can also sensitize patients to the development of PTSD (Bremner et al. 1993). Animal studies clearly suggest that early deprivation or stress can result in neurobiological abnormalities (Hofer 1975; Hubel 1978;

Teicher 1989). However, little evidence for this has been shown in humans (van der Kolk and Greenberg 1987). Green et al. (1981; Green 1983) found that many abused children had evidence of neurological damage and nonspecific electroencephalographic abnormalities, even in the absence of apparent or reported head injury. Childhood incest has been associated with reports of abnormal electroencephalographic activity. Davies (1979) found in a sample of 22 patients involved as a child or as the younger member of an incestuous relationship that 77% had abnormal EEGs, and 36% had clinical seizures. Davies suggested that these children were more at risk for being sexually abused by family members because of their neurological handicap. Teicher and colleagues (Ito et al. 1993, 1998; Schiffer et al. 1995; Teicher 1989; Teicher et al. 1993, 1994, 1997) hypothesized that early traumatic experience, in the form of childhood abuse, could affect the development of the cerebral cortex and limbic system. Using a scale to evaluate the frequency of symptoms suggestive of temporal lobe epilepsy, they found prominent effects of early abuse (Teicher et al. 1993). Physical abuse was associated with a 38% increase, sexual abuse with a 49% increase, and combined abuse with a 113% increase in symptom scores. Physical or sexual abuse alone were associated with elevated scores only if the abuse occurred before age 18. A blind chart review examined the association between abuse history and neurological abnormalities in 115 consecutive patients admitted to a child and adolescent psychiatric inpatient unit (Ito et al. 1993). Abused children had a greater incidence of electrophysiological abnormalities compared with that in nonabused patients (54.4% versus 26.9%). Interestingly, abused and nonabused patients differed only in the prevalence of left hemisphere abnormalities. Neuropsychological testing also indicated that left hemisphere deficits were 6.7-fold more prevalent than right hemisphere deficits in the abused group, whereas this ratio was threefold less in nonabused patients.

Schiffer et al. (1995) used probe auditory–evoked potentials as an indirect measure of auditory cortex activity. They compared 10 unmedicated adults, with no currently active psychopathology, who grew up in psychologically abusive families, to 10 control subjects from nonabusive families. Probe-evoked potentials were measured while subjects focused on a neutral work-related memory or a distressing childhood memory. Compared to control subjects, adults from psychologically abusive families had highly lateralized evoked potential patterns. During the neutral memory task, evoked potentials were strongly suppressed over the left cortex in the abused group (indicative of enhanced left cortex cognitive activity), and this pattern switched to right cortical suppression during recall of the distressing memory. Control subjects showed no significant degree of laterality or switch between these two tasks, even though they had equally strong emotional reactions. These findings suggest that the two hemispheres may function more autonomously in patients with childhood abuse.

To more precisely evaluate the effects of abuse on electroencephalographic asymmetry and cortical development, a quantitative electroencephalographic study was conducted (Ito et al. 1998; Teicher et al. 1997). Fifteen child and adolescent inpatients with a history of documented intense abuse were recruited, as were 15 control subjects. Artifact-free awake EEGs were analyzed to compare the power of paired right and left hemisphere leads in the alpha frequency band and to calculate global hemispheric and regional electroencephalographic coherence. (Coherence is a measure of cortical interconnectivity and displays a prominent developmental sequence that parallels cortical maturation.) Abused children had higher overall levels of left hemisphere coherence and a reversed hemispheric asymmetry. Further, left hemisphere coherence decayed more slowly across electrode distance in abused children. These findings strongly suggest that increased left hemisphere coherence in abused patients is a consequence of deficient left-cortical differentiation and development.

Evidence for left hemisphere disturbance was also found in MRI studies. Stein et al. (1997) and Bremner et al. (1997) found evidence for reduced left hippocampal volume in adults with a history of childhood abuse and current symptoms of PTSD. Bremner et al. (1997) compared MRI scans of 17 adults with physical or sexual abuse and PTSD with scans of 17 matched subjects with no abuse history or PTSD. The left hippocampus was 12% smaller in the abused group than that in the nonabused adults. Stein et al. (1997) measured hippocampal volume in 21 women with childhood sexual abuse. Fifteen patients had current PTSD and 15 had dissociative disorder. There was a significant reduction in left hippocampal size, which also correlated inversely with dissociative symptoms.

Because childhood abuse appeared to be associated with altered left hemisphere development and diminished right/left hippocampal development, we examined the corpus callosum as the major fiber tract connecting the hemispheres. MRI scans were obtained from 51 child psychiatric patients and 97 carefully screened control subjects from the National Institute of Mental Health. We found that there was a major reduction in the middle portions of the corpus callosum in hospitalized boys with a history of abuse or neglect. No differences emerged between psychiatrically healthy control subjects and hospitalized boys with psychiatric illness but no history of maltreatment (Teicher et al. 1997). Stepwise regression analysis showed that childhood neglect was the determining factor for corpus callosum shrinkage in boys (Teicher et al. 2000a). The corpus callosum of girls was less affected, and in these subjects sexual abuse appeared to be the major decisive factor. De Billis (1999) has also measured the corpus callosum in children with a history of abuse and PTSD. They also found that the midportion of the corpus callosum was markedly diminished in size, and they found that boys were more affected than girls. Sanchez et al. (1998) also reported that differential rearing experiences affected the development of the corpus callosum and cognitive function of male rhesus monkeys, emphasizing the importance of the environment.

More recently we used fMRI with T_2 relaxometry as an indirect measure of blood flow into the cerebellar vermis. The vermis is an interesting target for stress-mediated effects because it has a protracted ontogeny and high density of glucocorticoid receptors. Previous work by Harlow on the effects of isolation rearing in primates showed that the adverse effects were partially ameliorated by rocking and swinging, which provides robust sensory stimulation of the vermis. We found that T_2 relaxation time was strongly affected by degree of irritability on the limbic system checklist in both adults with a history of abuse and in control subjects without an abuse history. However, control subjects had lower adjusted T_2 relaxation time measures, suggesting hypoperfusion of the vermis in abused subjects (C.M. Anderson et al. 1999).

It should be noted that these studies are correlational and do not prove causation. They are, however, consistent with animal studies that indicate that early experience and stress affect brain development, including laterality and neurotransmitter levels (Denenberg and Yutzey 1985; Plotsky and Meaney 1993). These studies do suggest that early experience can be a powerful chisel that shapes the developing brain in enduring ways and can be associated with the emergence of neuropsychiatric consequences (Teicher 2000).

Conclusions

As noted at the outset of this chapter, brain development is a plastic process programmed by genes and sculpted by experience. Anomalous experience can exert persisting deleterious effects. In contrast, research in autism (Lovaas 1987; McEachin et al. 1993) and in communicative disorders (Merzenich et al. 1996) suggests that early directed interventions can have the capacity to correct developmental disabilities. Increased understanding of the processes regulating brain development may eventually lead to new strategies that not only treat but also prevent these disorders.

References

Abromowicz M (ed): Sudden death in children treated with a tricyclic antidepressant. Med Lett Drugs Ther 32(819):53, 1990

Ackerman PT, McPherson WB, Oglesby DM, et al: EEG power spectra of adolescent poor readers. J Learn Disabil 31:83–90, 1998

Akefeldt A, Gillberg C: Behavior and personality characteristics of children and young adults with Prader-Willi syndrome: a controlled study. J Am Acad Child Adolesc Psychiatry 38:761–769, 1999

Akefeldt A, Ekman R, Gillberg C, et al: Cerebrospinal fluid monoamines in Prader-Willi syndrome. Biol Psychiatry 44 (12):1321–1328, 1998

American Academy of Child and Adolescent Psychiatry: Practice parameters for the assessment and treatment of children and adolescents with language and learning disorders. J Am Acad Child Adolesc Psychiatry 37 (10 suppl):46S–62S, 1998

American Psychiatric Association: Diagnostic and Statistical Manual of Mental Disorders, 4th Edition. Washington, DC, American Psychiatric Association, 1994

American Psychiatric Association: Diagnostic and Statistical Manual of Mental Disorders, 4th Edition, Text Revision. Washington, DC, American Psychiatric Association, 2000

Amir RE, Van den Veyver IB, Wan M, et al: Rett syndrome is caused by mutations in X-linked MECP2, encoding methyl-CpG-binding protein 2. Nat Genet 23:185–189, 1999

Andersen SL, Teicher MH: Sex differences in dopamine receptors and their relevance to ADHD. Neurosci Biobehav Rev 24:137–141, 2000

Andersen SL, Rutstein M, Benzo J, et al: Sex differences in brain development: dopamine receptor overproduction and elimination. Neuroreport 8:1495–1498, 1997

Andersen SL, Thomphson AP, Rutstein M, et al: Dopamine receptor pruning in prefrontal cortex during the periadolescent period in rats. Synapse 37:167–169, 2000

Anderson CM, Polcari AM, McGreenery CE, et al: Childhood abuse: Limbic System Checklist–33 and cerebellar vermis blood flow (NR384), in 1999 New Research Program and Abstracts, American Psychiatric Association 152nd Annual Meeting, Washington, DC, May 15–20, 1999. Washington, DC, American Psychiatric Association, 1999, p 171

Anderson GM, Pollak ES, Chatterjee D, et al: Postmortem analyses of brain monoamine and amino acids in Tourette's syndrome: a preliminary study of subcortical regions. Arch Gen Psychiatry 49:584–586, 1992

Anderson JC, Williams S, McGee R, et al: DSM-III disorders in preadolescent children: prevalence in a large sample from the general population. Arch Gen Psychiatry 44:69–76, 1987

Andreasen NC, O'Leary DS, Cizadlo T, et al: Schizophrenia and cognitive dysmetria: a positron-emission tomography study of dysfunctional prefrontal-thalamic-cerebellar circuitry. Proc Natl Acad Sci U S A 93:9985–9990, 1996

Andriola MR, Ettinger AB: Pseudoseizures and other nonepileptic paroxysmal disorders in children and adolescents. Neurology 53 (5 suppl 2):S89–95, 1999

Ariano MA, Wang J, Noblett KL, et al: Cellular distribution of the rat D4 dopamine receptor protein in the CNS using anti-receptor antisera. Brain Res 752:26–34, 1997

Armstrong DD, Dunn K, Antalffy B: Decreased dendritic branching in frontal, motor and limbic cortex in Rett syndrome compared with trisomy 21. J Neuropathol Exp Neurol 57:1013–1017, 1998

Arnsten AFT, Steere JC, Hunt RD: The contribution of noradrenergic mechanisms to prefrontal cortex cognitive function: potential significance for attention-deficit hyperactivity disorder. Arch Gen Psychiatry 53:448–455, 1996

Asarnow RF, Saltz P, Light R, et al: Behavioral problems and adaptive functioning in children with mild and severe closed head injury. J Pediatr Psychol 16:543–555, 1991

Asghari V, Sanyal S, Vuchwaldt S, et al: Modulation of intracellular cyclic AMP levels by different human D4 receptor variants. J Neurochem 65:1157–1165, 1995

Aston-Jones G, Bloom FE: Norepinephrine-containing locus coeruleus neurons in behaving rats exhibit pronounced responses to non-noxious environmental stimuli. J Neurosci 1:887–900, 1981

Auger I, Thomas P, De Gruttola V, et al: Incubation periods for paediatric AIDS patients. Nature 336:575–577, 1988

August GJ, Stewart MA, Tsai L: The incidence of cognitive disabilities in the siblings of autistic children. Br J Psychiatry 138:416–422, 1981

August GJ, Stewart MA, Holmes CS: A four-year follow-up of hyperactive boys with and without conduct disorder. Br J Psychiatry 143:192–198, 1983

Bailey A, Le Couteur A, Gottesman I, et al: Autism as a strongly genetic disorder: evidence from a British twin study. Psychol Med 25:63–77, 1995

Bailey A, Luthert P, Dean A, et al: A clinico-pathological study of autism. Brain 121:889–905, 1998

Bakashi SS, Britto P, Capparelli E, et al: Evaluation of pharmacokinetics, safety, tolerance, and activity of combination of zalcitabine and zidovudine in stable, zidovudine-treated pediatric patients with human immunodeficiency virus infection. J Infect Dis 175:1039–1050, 1997

Barkley RA: Defiant Children: A Clinician's Manual for Parent Training. New York, Guilford, 1987

Barkley RA: A critique of current diagnostic criteria for attention deficit hyperactivity disorder: clinical and research implications. J Dev Behav Pediatr 11:343–352, 1990

Barkley RA, Guevremont DC, Anastopoulos AD, et al: A comparison of three family therapy programs for treating family conflicts in adolescents with attention-deficit hyperactivity disorder. J Consult Clin Psychol 60:450–462, 1992

Barks JD, Silverstein FS, Sims K, et al: Glutamate recognition sites in human fetal brain. Neurosci Lett 84:131–136, 1988

Baron-Cohen S: Perceptual role-taking and protodeclarative pointing in autism. British Journal of Developmental Psychology 7:113–127, 1989

Barr CL, Wigg KG, Bloom S, et al: Further evidence from haplotype analysis for linkage of the dopamine D4 receptor gene and attention-deficit hyperactivity disorder. Am J Med Genet 96:262–267, 2000

Barraclough B: Suicide and epilepsy, in Epilepsy and Psychiatry. Edited by Reynolds E, Trimble MR. New York, Churchill Livingstone, 1981, pp 72–76

Barrickman L, Noyes R, Kuperman S, et al: Treatment of ADHD with fluoxetine: a preliminary trial. J Am Acad Child Adolesc Psychiatry 30:762–767, 1991

Barrickman LL, Perry PJ, Allen AJ, et al: Bupropion versus methylphenidate in the treatment of attention-deficit hyperactivity disorder. J Am Acad Child Adolesc Psychiatry 34:649–657, 1995

Bauman ML: Microscopic neuroanatomic abnormalities in autism. Pediatrics 87:791–795, 1991

Bauman ML, Kemper TL: Histoanatomic observations of the brain in early infantile autism. Neurology 35:866–874, 1985

Bauman ML, Kemper TL, Arin DM: Pervasive neuroanatomic abnormalities of the brain in three cases of Rett's syndrome. Neurology 45:1581–1586, 1995

Bear DM, Fedio P: Quantitative analysis of interictal behavior in temporal lobe epilepsy. Arch Neurol 34:454–467, 1977

Beck JC, van der Kolk B: Reports of childhood incest and current behavior of chronically hospitalized psychotic women. Am J Psychiatry 144:1474–1476, 1987

Beers SR: Cognitive effects of mild head injury in children and adolescents. Neuropsychol Rev 3:281–320, 1992

Belmonte M, Egaas B, Townsend J, et al: NMR intensity of corpus callosum differs with age but not with diagnosis of autism. Neuroreport 6:1253–1256, 1995

Benasich AA, Curtiss S, Tallal P: Language, learning, and behavioral disturbances in childhood: a longitudinal perspective. J Am Acad Child Adolesc Psychiatry 32:585–594, 1993

Benjamin J, Li L, Patterson C, et al: Population and familial association between the D4 dopamine receptor gene and measures of novelty seeking. Nat Genet 12:81–84, 1996

Ben-Menachem E: New antiepileptic drugs and non-pharmacological treatments. Curr Opin Neurol 13:165–170, 2000

Berquin PC, Giedd JN, Jacobsen LK, et al: Cerebellum in attention-deficit hyperactivity disorder: a morphometric MRI study. Neurology 50:1098–1093, 1998

Biederman J, Baldessarini RJ, Wright V, et al: A double-blind placebo-controlled study of desipramine in the treatment of ADD, II: serum drugs levels and cardiovascular findings. J Am Acad Child Adolesc Psychiatry 28:903–911, 1989

Biederman J, Faraone SV, Spencer T, et al: Gender differences in a sample of adults with attention deficit hyperactivity disorder. Psychiatry Res 53:13–29, 1994

Biederman J, Wilens T, Mick E, et al: Pharmacotherapy of attention-deficit/hyperactivity disorder reduces risk for substance use disorder (electronic article). Pediatrics 104(2): e20, 1999

Bird HR, Canino G, Rubio-Stipec M, et al: Estimates of the prevalence of childhood maladjustment in a community survey in Puerto Rico. Arch Gen Psychiatry 45:1120–1126, 1988

Blue ME, Naidu S, Johnston MV: Altered development of glutamate and GABA receptors in the basal ganglia of girls with Rett syndrome. Exp Neurol 156:345–352, 1999a

Blue ME, Naidu S, Johnston MV: Development of amino acid receptors in frontal cortex from girls with Rett syndrome. Ann Neurol 45:541–545, 1999b

Blumberg BM, Mock DJ, Powers JM, et al: The HHV6 paradox: ubiquitous commensal or insidious pathogen? A two-step in situ PCR approach. J Clin Virol 16:159–178, 2000

Bolton P, Rutter M: Genetic influences in autism. Int Rev Psychiatry 2:67–80, 1990

Bonwetsch R, Croul S, Richardson MW, et al: Role of HIV-1 Tat and CC chemokine MIP-1alpha in the pathogenesis of HIV associated central nervous system disorders. J Neurovirol 5:685–694, 1999

Brady MT, McGrath N, Brouwers P, et al: Randomized study of the tolerance and efficacy of high- versus low-dose zidovudine in human immunodeficiency virus-infected children with mild to moderate symptoms (AIDS Clinical Trials Group 128). Pediatric AIDS Clinical Trials Group. J Infect Dis 173(5):1097–1106, 1996

Braun AR, Stoetter B, Randolph C, et al: The functional neuroanatomy of Tourette's syndrome: an FDG-PET study, I: regional changes in cerebral glucose metabolism differentiating patients and controls. Neuropsychopharmacology 9:277–291, 1993

Breese GR, Cooper BR, Hollister AS: Involvement of brain monoamines in the stimulant and paradoxical inhibitory effects of methylphenidate. Psychopharmacologia 44(1):5–10, 1975

Bremner JD, Southwick SM, Johnson DR, et al: Childhood physical abuse and combat-related posttraumatic stress disorder in Vietnam veterans. Am J Psychiatry 150:235–239, 1993

Bremner JD, Randall P, Vermetten E, et al: Magnetic resonance imaging–based measurement of hippocampal volume in posttraumatic stress disorder related to childhood physical and sexual abuse—a preliminary report. Biol Psychiatry 41:23–32, 1997

Brent DA, Crumrine PK, Varma RR, et al: Phenobarbital treatment and major depressive disorder in children with epilepsy. Pediatrics 80:909–917, 1987

Brett PM, Curtis D, Robertson MM, et al: The genetic susceptibility to Gilles de la Tourette syndrome in a large multiple affected British kindred: linkage analysis excludes a role for the genes coding for dopamine D1, D2, D3, D4, D5 receptors, dopamine beta hydroxylase, tyrosinase, and tyrosine hydroxylase. Biol Psychiatry 37:533–540, 1995a

Brett PM, Curtis D, Robertson MM, et al: Exclusion of the 5-HTIA serotonin neuroreceptor and tryptophan oxygenase genes in a large British kindred multiply affected with Tourette's syndrome, chronic motor tics, and obsessive-compulsive behavior. Am J Psychiatry 152:437–440, 1995b

Brew BJ, Pemberton L, Cunningham P, et al: Levels of human immunodeficiency virus type 1 RNA in cerebrospinal fluid correlate with AIDS dementia stage. J Infect Dis 175(4): 963–966, 1997

Brons J, Robertson LT, Tong G: Somatosensory climbing fiber responses in the caudal posterior vermis of the cat cerebellum. Brain Res 519:243–248, 1990

Brouwers P, Tudor-Williams G, DeCarli C, et al: Relation between stage of disease and neurobehavioral measures in children with symptomatic HIV disease. AIDS 9:713–720, 1995

Brown GL, Ebert MH, Mikkelsen EJ, et al: Behavior and motor activity response in hyperactive children and plasma amphetamine levels following a sustained release preparation. J Am Acad Child Adolesc Psychiatry 19:225–239, 1980

Brown LK, Lourie KJ, Pao M: Children and adolescents living with HIV and AIDS: a review. J Child Psychol Psychiatry 41:81–96, 2000

Bruun RD: Subtle and underrecognized side effects of neuroleptic treatment in children with Tourette's disorder. Am J Psychiatry 145:621–624, 1988

Bryden MP, McManus IC, Bulman-Fleming MB: Evaluating the empirical support for the Geschwind-Behan-Galaburda model of cerebral lateralization. Brain Cogn 26:103–167, 1994

Budman CL, Bruun RD, Parks KS, et al: Rage attacks in children and adolescents with Tourette's disorder: a pilot study. J Clin Psychiatry 59:576–580, 1998

Bulman-Fleming B, Wainwright PE, Collins RL: The effects of early experience on callosal development and functional lateralization in pigmented BALB/c mice. Behav Brain Res 50:31–42, 1992

Bush G, Frazier JA, Rauch SL, et al: Anterior cingulate cortex dysfunction in attention deficit/hyperactivity disorder revealed by fMRI and the Counting Stroop. Biol Psychiatry 45:1542–1552, 1999

Camp DM, Robinson TE, Becker JB: Sex differences in the effects of early experience on the development of behavioral and brain asymmetries in rats. Physiol Behav 33:433–439, 1984

Campbell M, Anderson LT, Small AM, et al: Naltrexone in autistic children: behavioral symptoms and attentional learning. J Am Acad Child Adolesc Psychiatry 32:1283–1291, 1993

Campbell M, Schopler E, Cueva JE, et al: Treatment of autistic disorder. J Am Acad Child Adolesc Psychiatry 35:134–143, 1996

Cardon LR, Smith SD, Fulker DW, et al: Quantitative trait locus for reading disability on chromosome 6. Science 266:276–279, 1994

Cardon LR, Smith SD, Fulker DW, et al: Quantitative trait locus for reading disability: correction (letter). Science 268:1553, 1995

Carper RA, Courchesne E: Inverse correlation between frontal lobe and cerebellum sizes in children with autism. Brain 123 (pt 4):836–844, 2000

Casey BJ, Castellanos FX, Giedd JN, et al: Implication of right frontostriatal circuitry in response inhibition and attention-deficit/hyperactivity disorder. J Am Acad Child Adolesc Psychiatry 36:374–383, 1997

Cassidy SB, Forsythe M, Heeger S, et al: Comparison of phenotype between patients with Prader-Willi syndrome due to deletion 15q and uniparental disomy 15. Am J Med Genet 68:433–440, 1997

Castellanos FX, Giedd JN, Marsh WL, et al: Quantitative brain magnetic resonance imaging in attention-deficit hyperactivity disorder. Arch Gen Psychiatry 53:607–616, 1996

Castellanos FX, Lau E, Tayebi N, et al: Lack of an association between a dopamine-4 receptor polymorphism and attention-deficit/hyperactivity disorder: genetic and brain morphometric analyses. Mol Psychiatry 3:431–434, 1998

Centers for Disease Control and Prevention: HIV/AIDS Surveillance Report 13(2):7, 2001

Chappell P, Riddle M, Anderson G, et al: Enhanced stress responsivity of Tourette syndrome patients undergoing lumbar puncture. Biol Psychiatry 36:35–43, 1994

Chappell PB, Riddle MA, Scahill L, et al: Guanfacine treatment of comorbid attention-deficit hyperactivity disorder and Tourette's syndrome: preliminary clinical experience. J Am Acad Child Adolesc Psychiatry 34:1140–1146, 1995

Chez MG, Buchanan CP, Bagan BT, et al: Secretin and autism: a two-part investigation. J Autism Dev Disord 30:87–94, 2000

Chi J, Dooling E, Giles F: Left-right asymmetries of the temporal speech areas of the human fetus. Arch Neurol 34:346–348, 1972

Chudley AE, Knoll J, Gerrard JW, et al: Fragile (X) X-linked mental retardation, I: relationship between age and intelligence and the frequency of expression of fragile (X) (q28). Am J Med Genet 14:699–712, 1983

Chugani DC, Muzik O, Rothermel R, et al: Altered serotonin synthesis in the dentatothalamocortical pathway in autistic boys. Ann Neurol 42:666–669, 1997

Chugani DC, Muzik O, Behen M, et al: Developmental changes in brain serotonin synthesis capacity in autistic and nonautistic children. Ann Neurol 45:287–295, 1999

Ciesielski KT, Harris RJ, Hart BL, et al: Cerebellar hypoplasia and frontal lobe cognitive deficits in disorders of early childhood. Neuropsychologia 35:643–655, 1997

Cirianello RD, Cirianello SD: The neurobiology of infantile autism. Annu Rev Neurosci 18:1010–1028, 1995

Cohen SE, Mundy T, Karassik B, et al: Neuropsychological functioning in human immunodeficiency virus type 1 seropositive children infected through neonatal blood transfusion. Pediatrics 88:58–68, 1991

Comings DE: Blood serotonin and tryptophan in Tourette syndrome. Am J Med Genet 36:418–430, 1990

Comings DE, Comings BG: A controlled study of Tourette syndrome; I: attention-deficit disorder, learning disorders, and school problems. Am J Hum Genet 41:701–741, 1987

Comings DE, Wu H, Ring RH, et al: Polygenetic inheritance of Tourette syndrome, stuttering, ADHD, conduct disorder and oppositional defiant disorder: the additive and subtractive effect of the three dopamine genes—DRD2, DBH and DAT1. Am J Med Genet 67:264–288, 1996

Comings DE, Gade-Andavolu R, Gonzalez N, et al: Additive effect of three noradrenergic genes (ADRA2a, ADRA2C, DBH) on attention-deficit hyperactivity disorder and learning disabilities in Tourette syndrome subjects. Clin Genet 55:160–172, 1999a

Comings DE, Gonzalez N, Wu S, et al: Studies of the 48 bp repeat polymorphism of the DRD4 gene in impulsive, compulsive, addictive behaviors: Tourette syndrome, ADHD, pathological gambling, and substance abuse. Am J Med Genet 88:358–368, 1999b

Comings DE, Gade-Andavolu R, Gonzalez N, et al: Comparison of the role of dopamine, serotonin, and noradrenaline genes in ADHD, ODD and conduct disorder: multivariate regression analysis of 20 genes. Clin Genet 57:178–196, 2000

Cook EH Jr: Genetics of autism. Child Adolesc Psychiatr Clin N Am 10(2):333–359, 2001

Cook EH Jr, Stein MA, Krasowski MD, et al: Association of attention-deficit disorder and the dopamine transporter gene. Am J Hum Genet 56:993–998, 1995

Cook EH Jr, Courchesne R, Lord C, et al: Evidence of linkage between the serotonin transporter and autistic disorder. Mol Psychiatry 2:247–250, 1997

Cooper H, Nye B: Homework for students with learning disabilities: the implications of research for policy and practice. J Learn Disabil 27:470–479, 1994

Cornwall A, Bawden HN: Reading disabilities and aggression: a critical review. J Learn Disabil 25:281–288, 1992

Courchesne E: Neuroanatomic imaging in autism. Pediatrics 87:781–790, 1991

Cowan WM, Fawcett JW, O'Leary DDM, et al: Regressive events in neurogenesis. Science 225:1258–1265, 1984

Critchley HD, Daly EM, Bullmore ET, et al: The functional neuroanatomy of social behaviour: changes in cerebral blood flow when people with autistic disorder process facial expressions. Brain 123:2203–2212, 2000

Curtis D, Robertson MM, Gurling HM: Autosomal dominant gene transmission in a large kindred with Gilles de la Tourette syndrome. Br J Psychiatry 160:845–849, 1992

Dalby MA, Elbro C, Stodkilde-Jorgensen H: Temporal lobe asymmetry and dyslexia: an in vivo study using MRI. Brain Lang 62:51–69, 1998

Dal Maso L, Parazzini F, Lo Re A, et al: Paediatric AIDS incidence in Europe and the USA, 1985–96. J Epidemiol Biostat 4:75–81, 1999

Daly G, Hawi Z, Fitzgerald M, et al: Mapping susceptibility loci in attention deficit hyperactivity disorder: preferential transmission of parental alleles at DAT1, DBH and DRD5 to affected children. Mol Psychiatry 4:192–196, 1999

Davies RK: Incest: some neuropsychiatric findings. Int J Psychiatry Med 9:117–121, 1979

De Bellis MD, Keshavan MS, Clark DB, et al: A.E. Bennett Research Award. Developmental traumatology, part II: brain development. Biol Psychiatry 45(10):1271–1284, 1999

Delay J, Deniker P, Barande R: Le suicide des epileptique. Encephale 46:401–436, 1957

Demb JB, Boynton GM, Best M, et al: Psychophysical evidence for a magnocellular pathway deficit in dyslexia. Vision Res 38:1555–1559, 1998

Dempsey CW, Richardson DE: Paleocerebellar stimulation induces in vivo release of endogenously synthesized [3H]dopamine and [3H]norepinephrine from rat caudal dorsomedial nucleus accumbens. Neuroscience 21:565–571, 1987

Denckla MB, Bemporad JR, MacKay MC: Tics following methylphenidate administration: a report of 20 cases. JAMA 235:1349–1351, 1976

Denenberg VH, Yutzey DA: Hemispheric laterality, behavioral asymmetry, and the effects of early experience in rats, in Cerebral Lateralization in Nonhuman Species. Edited by Glick SD. Orlando, FL, Academic Press, 1985, pp 109–133

Dennett ER, Hubbard JI: Noradrenaline excites neurons in the guinea pig cerebellar vermis in vitro. Brain Res Bull 21:245–249, 1988

Denoth F, Magherini PC, Pompeiano O, et al: Responses of Purkinje cells of the cerebellar vermis to neck and macular vestibular inputs. Pflugers Arch 381:87–98, 1979

Dewhurst S, Gelbard HA, Fine SM: Neuropathogenesis of AIDS. Mol Med Today 2:16–23, 1996

DeYoe EA, Van Essen DC: Concurrent processing streams in monkey visual cortex. Trends Neurosci 11(5):219–226, 1988

Diamond A: Close interrelation of motor development and cognitive development and of the cerebellum and prefrontal cortex. Child Dev 71:44–56, 2000

Doba N, Reis DJ: Changes in regional blood flow and cardiodynamics evoked by electrical stimulation of the fastigial nucleus in the cat and their similarity to orthostatic reflexes. J Physiol (Lond) 227:729–747, 1972

Donaldson IM, Hawthorne ME: Coding of visual information by units in the cat cerebellar vermis. Exp Brain Res 34:27–48, 1979

Dougherty DD, Bonab AA, Spencer TJ, et al: Dopamine transporter density in patients with attention deficit hyperactivity disorder (letter). Lancet 354:2132–2133, 1999

Drake W: Clinical and pathological findings in a child with a developmental learning disability. J Learn Disabil 1:468–475, 1968

Dreifuss FE: Classification of epileptic seizures and the epilepsies. Pediatr Clin North Am 36:265–279, 1989

Dunn DW, Austin JK: Behavioral issues in pediatric epilepsy. Neurology 53:S96–100, 1999

Dykens EM, Cassidy SB, King BH: Maladaptive behavior differences in Prader-Willi syndrome due to paternal deletion versus maternal uniparental disomy. Am J Ment Retard 104:67–77, 1999

Eapen V, Puls D, Robertson MM: Evidence for autosomal dominant transmission in Tourette's syndrome. United Kingdom cohort study. Br J Psychiatry 162:593–596, 1993

Ebstein RP, Novick O, Umansky R, et al: Dopamine D4 (D4DR) exon III polymorphism associated with the human personality trait of novelty seeking. Nat Genet 12:78–80, 1996

Eccles JC, Sabah NH, Schmidt RF, et al: Cerebellar Purkyne cell responses to cutaneous mechanoreceptors. Brain Res 30:419–424, 1971

Egaas B, Courchesne C, Saitoh O: Reduced size of corpus callosum in autism. Arch Neurol 52:794–801, 1995

Eisenberg J, Zohar A, Mei-Tal G, et al: A haplotype relative risk study of the dopamine D4 receptor (DRD4) exon III repeat polymorphism and attention deficit hyperactivity disorder (ADHD). Am J Med Genet 96:258–261, 2000

Ellis RJ, Hsia K, Spector SA, et al; Cerebrospinal fluid human immunodeficiency virus type 1 RNA levels are elevated in neurocognitively impaired individuals with acquired immunodeficiency syndrome. HIV Neurobehavioral Research Center Group. Ann Neurol 42(5):679–688, 1997

Epstein LG, Gelbard HA: HIV-1–induced neuronal injury in the developing brain. J Leukoc Biol 65:453–457, 1999

Epstein LG, Gendelman HE: Human immunodeficiency virus type I infection of the nervous system: pathogenetic mechanisms. Ann Neurol 33:429–436, 1993

Epstein LG, Sharer LR, Joshi VV, et al: Progressive encephalopathy in children with acquired immune deficiency syndrome. Ann Neurol 17:488–496, 1985

Erickson HM Jr, Goggin JE, Messiha FS: Comparison of lithium and haloperidol therapy in Gilles de la Tourette syndrome. Adv Exp Med Biol 90:197–205, 1977

Ernst M, Liebenauer LL, King C, et al: Reduced brain metabolism in hyperactive girls. J Am Acad Child Adolesc Psychiatry 33:858–868, 1994

Ernst M, Zametkin AJ, Matochik JA, et al: DOPA decarboxylase activity in attention deficit hyperactivity disorder adults. A [fluorine-18]fluorodopa positron emission tomographic study. J Neurosci 18:5901–5907, 1998

Ernst M, Zametkin AJ, Jons PH, et al: High presynaptic dopaminergic activity in children with Tourette's disorder. J Am Acad Child Adolesc Psychiatry 38:86–94, 1999a

Ernst M, Zametkin AJ, Matochik JA, et al: High midbrain [18F]DOPA accumulation in children with attention deficit hyperactivity disorder. Am J Psychiatry 156:1209–1215, 1999b

Everall IP, Luthbert PJ, Lantos PL: Neuronal loss in the frontal cortex in HIV infection. Lancet 337:1119–1121, 1991

Ewing-Cobbs L, Fletcher JM, Levin HS, et al: Academic achievement and academic placement following traumatic brain injury in children and adolescents: a two-year longitudinal study. J Clin Exp Neuropsychol 20:769–781, 1998

Facoetti A, Paganoni P, Lorusso ML: The spatial distribution of visual attention in developmental dyslexia. Exp Brain Res 132:531–538, 2000

Faraone SV, Biederman J, Lehman BK, et al: Evidence for the independent familial transmission of attention deficit hyperactivity disorder and learning disabilities: results from a family genetic study. Am J Psychiatry 150:891–895, 1993

Faraone SV, Biederman J, Weiffenbach B, et al: Dopamine D4 gene 7-repeat allele and attention deficit hyperactivity disorder. Am J Psychiatry 156:768–770, 1999

Faravelli C, Webb T, Ambonetti A: Prevalence of traumatic early life events in 31 agoraphobic patients with panic attacks. Am J Psychiatry 142:1493–1494, 1985

Feinberg I: Schizophrenia: caused by a fault in programmed synaptic elimination during adolescence? J Psychiatr Res 17:319–334, 1982–1983

Fernandez F, Adams F, Levy JK, et al: Cognitive impairment due to AIDS-related complex and its response to psychostimulants. Psychosomatics 29:38–46, 1988

Ferrera VP, Nealey TA, Maunsell JH: Mixed parvocellular and magnocellular geniculate signals in visual area V4. Nature 358:756–761, 1992

Fischer CP, Jorgen G, Gundersen H, et al: Preferential loss of large neocortical neurons during HIV infection: a study of the size distribution of neocortical neurons in the human brain. Brain Res 828:119–126, 1999

Fish DR, Sawyers D, Allen PJ: The effect of sleep on the dyskinetic movements of Parkinson's disease, Gilles de la Tourette syndrome, Huntington's disease and torsion dystonia. Arch Neurol 48:210–214, 1991

Fitch RH, Miller S, Tallal P: Neurobiology of speech perception. Annu Rev Neurosci 20:331–353, 1997

Fletcher JM, Levin HS: Neurobehavioral effects of brain injury in children, in Handbook of Pediatric Psychology. Edited by Routh DK. New York, Guilford, 1988, pp 258–296

Fombonne E, Du MC, Cans C, et al: Autism and associated medical disorders in a French epidemiological survey. J Am Acad Child Adolesc Psychiatry 36:1561–1569, 1997

Foote S, Aston-Jones G, Bloom FE: Impulse activity of locus coeruleus neurons in awake rats and squirrel monkeys is a function of sensory stimulation and arousal. Proc Natl Acad Sci U S A 77:3033–3037, 1980

Frankenberger W, Fronzaglio K: A review of states' criteria and procedures for identifying children with learning disabilities. J Learn Disabil 24:495–500, 1991

Freeman BJ, Ritvo ER, Needleman R, et al: The stability of cognitive and linguistic parameters in autism: a 5 year study. J Am Acad Child Psychiatry 24:290–311, 1985

Freeman BJ, Rahbar B, Ritvo ER, et al: The stability of cognitive and behavioral parameters in autism: a twelve-year prospective study. J Am Acad Child Adolesc Psychiatry 30:479–482, 1991

Freund LS, Reiss AL, Hagerman R, et al: Chromosome fragility and psychopathology in obligate female carriers of the fragile X chromosome. Arch Gen Psychiatry 49:54–60, 1992

Gadow KD, Nolan EE, Sverd J: Methylphenidate in hyperactive boys with comorbid tic disorder; II: short-term behavioral effects in school settings. J Am Acad Child Adolesc Psychiatry 31:462–471, 1992

Gage FH: Mammalian neural stem cells. Science 287:1433–1438, 2000

Galaburda AM: Anatomical asymmetries, in Cerebral Dominance: The Biological Foundations. Edited by Geschwind N, Galaburda AM. Cambridge, MA, Harvard University Press, 1984, pp 11–25

Galaburda AM, Sherman GF, Rosen GD, et al: Developmental dyslexia: four consecutive patients with cortical anomalies. Ann Neurol 18:222–233, 1985

Galaburda AM, Menard MT, Rosen GD: Evidence for aberrant auditory anatomy in developmental dyslexia. Proc Natl Acad Sci U S A 91:8010–8013, 1994

Galler JR, Ramsey F, Solimano G, et al: The influence of early malnutrition on subsequent behavioral development; II: classroom behavior. J Am Acad Child Psychiatry 22:16–22, 1983

Gatley SJ, Pan D, Chen R, et al: Affinities of methylphenidate derivatives for dopamine, norepinephrine and serotonin transporters. Life Sci 58:231–239, 1996

Gelbard HA, Epstein LG: HIV-1 encephalopathy in children. Curr Opin Pediatr 7:655–662, 1995

Gelbard HA, James H, Sharer L, et al: Apoptotic neurons in brains of pediatric patients with HIV-1 encephalitis and progressive encephalopathy. Neuropathol Appl Neurobiol 21:208–217, 1995

Gelbard HA, Boustany RM, Schor NF: Apoptosis in development and disease of the nervous system, II: apoptosis in childhood neurologic disease. Pediatr Neurol 16:93–97, 1997

Gelernter J, Pakstis AJ, Pauls DL, et al: Gilles de la Tourette syndrome is not linked to D2-dopamine receptor. Arch Gen Psychiatry 47:1073–1077, 1990

Gelernter J, Kennedy JL, Grandy DK, et al: Exclusion of close linkage of Tourette's syndrome to D1 dopamine receptor. Am J Psychiatry 150:449–453, 1993

Gelernter J, Rao PA, Pauls DL, et al: Assignment of the 5HT7 receptor gene (HTR7) to chromosome 10q and exclusion of genetic linkage with Tourette syndrome. Genomics 26:207–209, 1995

George MS, Trimble MR, Costa DC, et al: Elevated frontal cerebral blood flow in Gilles de la Tourette syndrome: a 99Tcm-HMPAO SPECT study. Psychiatry Res 45:143–151, 1992

George MS, Robertson MM, Costa DC, et al: Dopamine receptor availability in Tourette's syndrome. Psychiatry Res 55:193–203, 1994

Georgiewa P, Rzanny R, Hopf JM, et al: fMRI during word processing in dyslexic and normal reading children. Neuroreport 10:3459–3465, 1999

Geschwind N, Behan P: Left-handedness: association with immune disease, migraine, and developmental learning disorder. Proc Natl Acad Sci U S A 79:5097–5100, 1982

Geschwind N, Galaburda AM: Cerebral Lateralization. Cambridge, MA, MIT Press, 1985

Giaquinto C, Ruga E, Giacomet V, et al: HIV: mother to child transmission, current knowledge and on-going studies. Int J Gynaecol Obstet 63 (suppl 1):S161–165, 1998

Giedd JN, Castellanos FX, Casey BJ, et al: Quantitative morphology of the corpus callosum in attention deficit hyperactivity disorder. Am J Psychiatry 151:665–669, 1994

Gilger JW, Pennington BF, DeFries JC: A twin study of the etiology of comorbidity: attention-deficit hyperactivity disorder and dyslexia. J Am Acad Child Adolesc Psychiatry 31:343–348, 1992

Gill M, Daly G, Heron S, et al: Confirmation of association between attention deficit disorder and a dopamine transporter polymorphism. Mol Psychiatry 2:311–313, 1997

Gillberg C: Endogenous opioids and opiate antagonists in autism: brief review of empirical findings and implications for clinicians. Dev Med Child Neurol 37:239–245, 1995

Gillis JJ, DeFries JC, Fulker DW: Confirmatory factor analysis of reading and mathematics performance: a twin study. Acta Genet Med Gemellol (Roma) 41:287–300, 1992

Giros M, Jaber M, Jones SR, et al: Hyperlocomotion and indifference to cocaine and amphetamine in mice lacking the dopamine transporter. Nature 379:606–612, 1996

Gittelman R, Mannuzza S, Shenker R, et al: Hyperactive boys almost grown up; I: psychiatric status. Arch Gen Psychiatry 42:937–947, 1985

Glod CA, Teicher MH: Relationship between early abuse, posttraumatic stress disorder, and activity levels in prepubertal children. J Am Acad Child Adolesc Psychiatry 35:1384–1393, 1996

Goadsby PJ, Lambert GA: Electrical stimulation of the fastigial nucleus increases total cerebral blood flow in the monkey. Neurosci Lett 107:141–144, 1989

Godridge H, Reynolds GP, Czudek C, et al: Alzheimer-like neurotransmitter deficits in adult Down's syndrome. J Neurol Neurosurg Psychiatry 50:775–778, 1987

Gold AP: Evaluation and diagnosis by inspection, in Child and Adolescent Neurology for Psychiatrists. Edited by Kaufman DM, Solomon GE, Pfeffer CR. Baltimore, MD, Williams & Wilkins, 1992, pp 1–12

Goldberg E, Costa LD: Hemisphere differences in the acquisition and use of descriptive systems. Brain Lang 14(1):144–173, 1981

Grace AA: The tonic/phasic model of dopamine system regulation: its relevance for understanding how stimulant abuse can alter basal ganglia function. Drug Alcohol Depend 37(2):111–129, 1995

Greatrex JC, Drasdo N: The magnocellular deficit hypothesis in dyslexia: a review of reported evidence. Ophthalmic Physiol Opt 15:501–506, 1995

Green AH: Dimensions of psychological trauma in abused children. J Am Acad Child Psychiatry 22:231–237, 1983

Green A, Voeller K, Gaines R, et al: Neurological impairment in maltreated children. Child Abuse Negl 5:129–134, 1981

Gresch PJ, Sved AF, Zigmond MJ, et al: Local influence of endogenous norepinephrine on extracellular dopamine in rat medial prefrontal cortex. J Neurochem 65:111–116, 1995

Groth AN: Sexual trauma in the life histories of sex offenders. Victimology 4:6–10, 1979

Hagerman RJ, Sobesky WE: Psychopathology in fragile X syndrome. Am J Orthopsychiatry 59:142–152, 1989

Hallett JJ, Harling-Berg CJ, Knopf PM, et al: Anti-striatal antibodies in Tourette syndrome cause neuronal dysfunction. J Neuroimmunol 111(1-2):195–202, 2000

Hardan AY, Minshew NJ, Keshavan MS: Corpus callosum size in autism. Neurology 55:1033–1036, 2000

Harris NS, Courchesne E, Townsend J, et al: Neuroanatomic contributions to slowed orienting of attention in children with autism. Brain Res Cogn Brain Res 8:61–71, 1999

Hashimoto T, Endo S, Fukuda K, et al: Increased body movements during sleep in Gilles de la Tourette syndrome. Brain Dev 3:31–35, 1981

Hashimoto T, Tayama M, Mori K, et al: Magnetic resonance imaging in autism: preliminary report. Neuropediatrics 20:142–146, 1988

Haslam RH, Dalby JT, Johns RD, et al: Cerebral asymmetry in developmental dyslexia. Arch Neurol 38:679–682, 1981

Hauser P, Zametkin AJ, Martinez P, et al: Attention deficit–hyperactivity disorder in people with generalized resistance to thyroid hormone. N Engl J Med 328:997–1001, 1993

Hauser WA, Hesdorffer DC (eds): Facts About Epilepsy. New York, Demos Publications, 1990

Heffner TG, Heller A, Miller FE, et al: Locomotor hyperactivity in neonatal rats following electrolytic lesions of mesocortical dopamine neurons. Brain Res 285:29–37, 1983

Heilman K, Van Den Abell T: Right hemisphere dominance for attention: the mechanism underlying hemispheric asymmetry of inattention. Neurology 30:327–330, 1980

Henker B, Whalen CK: Hyperactivity and attention deficits. Am Psychol 44:216–223, 1989

Herman JL, Perry JC, van der Kolk BA: Childhood trauma in borderline personality disorder. Am J Psychiatry 146:490–495, 1989

Hernandez L, Lee F, Hoebel BG: Simultaneous microdialysis and amphetamine infusion in the nucleus accumbens and striatum of freely moving rats: increase in extracellular dopamine and serotonin. Brain Res Bull 19:623–628, 1987

Hoehn TP, Baumeister AA: A critique of the application of sensory integration therapy to children with learning disabilities. J Learn Disabil 27:338–350, 1994

Hofer MA: Studies on how early maternal deprivation produces behavioral change in young rats. Psychosom Med 37:245–264, 1975

Holland AJ, Hon J, Huppert FA, et al: Population-based study of the prevalence and presentation of dementia in adults with Down's syndrome. Br J Psychiatry 172:493–498, 1998

Holttum JR, Minshew NJ, Sanders RS, et al: Magnetic resonance imaging of the posterior fossa in autism. Biol Psychiatry 32:1091–1101, 1992

Horska A, Naidu S, Hershovits EH, et al: Quantitative ^{1}H MR spectroscopic imaging in early Rett syndrome. Neurology 54:715–722, 2000

Horwitz B, Rumsey J, Grady C, et al: The cerebral metabolic landscape in autism: intercorrelations of regional glucose utilization. Ann Neurol 22:749–755, 1988

Horwitz B, Rumsey JM, Donohue BC: Functional connectivity of the angular gyrus in normal reading and dyslexia. Proc Natl Acad Sci U S A 95:8939–8944, 1998

Huang C, Liu G: Organization of the auditory area in the posterior cerebellar vermis of the cat. Exp Brain Res 81:377–383, 1990

Hubel DH: Effects of deprivation on the visual cortex of cat and monkey. Harvey Lect 72:1–51, 1978

Humphries T, Wright M, Snider L, et al: A comparison of the effectiveness of sensory integrative therapy and perceptual-motor training in treating children with learning disabilities. J Dev Behav Pediatr 13:31–40, 1992

Hunt RD: Treatment effects of oral and transdermal clonidine in relation to methylphenidate: an open pilot study in ADHD. Psychopharmacol Bull 23: 111–114, 1987

Hunt RD, Minderaa RB, Cohen DJ: Clonidine benefits children with attention deficit disorder and hyperactivity: report of a double-blind placebo-crossover therapeutic trial. J Am Acad Child Adolesc Psychiatry 24:617–629, 1985

Hunt RD, Arnsten AFT, Asbell MD: An open trial of guanfacine in the treatment of attention-deficit hyperactivity disorder. J Am Acad Child Adolesc Psychiatry 34:50–54, 1995

Huret JL, Delabar JM, Marlhens F, et al: Down syndrome with duplication of a region of chromosome 21 containing the CuZn superoxide dismutase gene without detectable karyotypic abnormality. Hum Genet 75:251–257, 1987

Huttenlocher PR: Synaptic density in human frontal cortex—developmental changes and effects of aging. Brain Res 163:195–205, 1979

Hyde TM, Stacey ME, Coppola R: Cerebral morphometric abnormalities in Tourette's syndrome: a quantitative MRI study of monozygotic twins. Neurology 45:1176–1182, 1995

Hynd GW, Semrud-Clikeman M, Lorys AR, et al: Corpus callosum morphology in attention deficit hyperactivity disorder: morphometric analysis of MRI. J Learn Disabil 24:141–146, 1991

Ito Y, Teicher MH, Glod CA, et al: Increased prevalence of electrophysiological abnormalities in children with psychological, physical, and sexual abuse. J Neuropsychiatry Clin Neurosci 5:401–408, 1993

Ito Y, Teicher MH, Glod CA, et al: Preliminary evidence for aberrant cortical development in abused children: a quantitative EEG study. J Neuropsychiatry Clin Neurosci 10:298–307, 1998

Jadresic D: The role of the amygdaloid complex in Gilles de la Tourette's syndrome. Br J Psychiatry 16:532–534, 1992

James HJ, Sharer LR, Zhang Q, et al: Expression of caspase-3 in brains from paediatric patients with HIV-1 encephalitis. Neuropathol Appl Neurobiol 25:380–386, 1999

Janssen RS, Cornblath DR, Epstein LG, et al: Nomenclature and research case definitions for neurological manifestations of human immunodeficiency virus type-1 (HIV-1) infection: report of a working group of the American Academy of Neurology AIDS Task Force. Neurology 41:778–785, 1991

Janssen RS, Nwanyanwu OC, Selik RM, et al: Epidemiology of human immunodeficiency virus encephalopathy in the United States. Neurology 42:1472–1476, 1992

Jellinger K, Armstrong D, Zoghbi HY, et al: Neuropathology of Rett syndrome. Acta Neuropathol (Berl) 76:142–158, 1988

Jensen I: Temporal lobe epilepsy: late morality in patients treated with unilateral temporal lobe resections. Acta Neurol Scand 52:374–380, 1975

Jenson WR, Sheridan SM, Olympia D, et al: Homework and students with learning disabilities and behavior disorders: a practical, parent-based approach. J Learn Disabil 27:538–548, 1994

Jernigan TL, Hesselink JR, Sowell E, et al: Cerebral structure on magnetic resonance imaging in language- and learning-impaired children. Arch Neurol 48:539–545, 1991

Johannes S, Kussmaul CL, Munte TF, et al: Developmental dyslexia: passive visual stimulation provides no evidence for a magnocellular processing defect. Neuropsychologia 34:1123–1127, 1996

Jutai JW: Cerebral asymmetry and the psychophysiology of attention. Int J Psychophysiol 1:219–225, 1984

Kanner L: Autistic disturbances of affective contact. Nervous Child 2:217–250, 1943

Kaplan BJ, Polatajko HJ, Wilson BN, et al: Reexamination of sensory integration treatment: a combination of two efficacy studies. J Learn Disabil 26: 342–347, 1993

Karacostas DD, Fisher GL: Chemical dependency in students with and without learning disabilities. J Learn Disabil 26:491–495, 1993

Kaufman DM: Clinical Neurology for Psychiatrists, 2nd Edition. Orlando, FL, Grune & Stratton, 1985, pp 172–197

Keller HH, Bartholini G, Pletscher A: Spontaneous and drug-induced changes of cerebral dopamine turnover during postnatal development of rats. Brain Res 64:371–378, 1973

Kemper TL, Bauman ML: The contribution of neuropathologic studies to the understanding of autism. Neurol Clin 11:175–187, 1993

Kerbeshian J, Burd L: Differential responsiveness to lithium in patients with Tourette disorder. Neurosci Biobehav Rev 12:247–250, 1988

Keshaven M, Anderson S, Pettegrew JW: Is schizophrenia due to excessive synaptic pruning in the prefrontal cortex? The Feinberg hypothesis revisited. J Psychiatr Res 28:239–264, 1994

Ketzler S, Weis S, Haug H, et al: Loss of neurons in the frontal cortex in AIDS brains. Acta Neuropathol (Berl) 80:92–94, 1990

Kinsella G, Ong B, Murtagh D, et al: The role of the family for behavioral outcome in children and adolescents following traumatic brain injury. J Consult Clin Psychol 67:116–123, 1999

Klauck SM, Poustka F, Benner A, et al: Serotonin transporter (5-HTT) gene variants associated with autism? Hum Mol Genet 6:2233–2238, 1997

Klein RG, Mannuzza S: Long-term outcome of hyperactive children: a review. J Am Acad Child Adolesc Psychiatry 30:383–387, 1991

Knell ER, Comings DE: Tourette's syndrome and attention-deficit hyperactivity disorder: evidence for a genetic relationship. J Clin Psychiatry 54:331–337, 1993

Krashen S: Lateralization, language learning, and the critical period: some new evidence. Language Learning 23:63–74, 1973

Krause KH, Dresel SH, Krause J, et al: Increased striatal dopamine transporter in adult patients with attention deficit hyperactivity disorder: effects of methylphenidate as measured by single photon emission computed tomography. Neurosci Lett 285:107–110, 2000

Krystal H: Trauma and affects. Psychoanal Study Child 33:81–116, 1978

Kubova Z, Kuba M, Peregrin J, et al: Visual evoked potential evidence for magnocellular system deficit in dyslexia. Physiol Res 45:87–89, 1996

Kuczenski R, Segal DS, Leith NJ, et al: Effects of amphetamine, methylphenidate, and apomorphine on regional brain serotonin and 5-hydroxyindole acetic acid. Psychopharmacology (Berl) 93(3):329–335, 1987

Kurlan R, Corno PG, Deeley C, et al: A pilot controlled study of fluoxetine for obsessive-compulsive symptoms in children with Tourette's syndrome. Clin Neuropharmacol 16:167–172, 1993

Kwak CH, Hanna PA, Jankovic J: Botulinum toxin in the treatment of tics. Arch Neurol 57:1190–1193, 2000

LaBar KS, Gatenby JC, Gore JC, et al: Human amygdala activation during conditioned fear acquisition and extinction: a mixed-trial fMRI study. Neuron 20:937–945, 1998

LaHoste GJ, Swanson JM, Wigal SB, et al: Dopamine D4 receptor gene polymorphism is associated with attention deficit hyperactivity disorder. Mol Psychiatry 1:121–124, 1996

Landis SC: Neuronal growth cones. Annu Rev Physiol 45:567–580, 1983

Landmesser LT: The generation of neuromuscular specificity. Annu Rev Neurosci 3:279–302, 1980

Leckman JF, Scahill L: Possible exacerbation of tics by androgenic steroids (letter). N Engl J Med 322:1674, 1990

Leckman JF, Dolnansky ES, Hardin MT, et al: Perinatal factors in the expression of Tourette's syndrome: an exploratory study. J Am Acad Child Adolesc Psychiatry 29:220–226, 1990

Leckman JF, Hardin MT, Riddle MA, et al: Clonidine treatment of Gilles de la Tourette's syndrome. Arch Gen Psychiatry 48:324–328, 1991a

Leckman JF, Knorr AM, Rasmussen AM, et al: Basal ganglia research and Tourette's syndrome (letter). Trends Neurosci 14:94, 1991b

Leckman JF, Walker DE, Cohen DJ: Premonitory urges in Tourette's syndrome. Am J Psychiatry 150:98–102, 1993

Leckman JF, Goodman WK, Anderson GM, et al: Cerebrospinal fluid biogenic amines in obsessive compulsive disorder, Tourette's syndrome, and healthy controls. Neuropsychopharmacology 12:73–86, 1995a

Leckman JF, Pauls DL, Cohen DJ: Tic disorders, in Psychopharmacology: The Fourth Generation of Progress. Edited by Bloom FE, Kupfer DJ. New York, Raven, 1995b, pp 1665–1674

Leckman JF, Zhang H, Vitale A, et al: Course of tic severity in Tourette syndrome: the first two decades. Pediatrics 102:14–19, 1998

LeDoux JE, Iwata J, Cicchetti P, et al: Different projections of the central amygdaloid nucleus mediate autonomic and behavioral correlates of conditioned fear. J Neurosci 8:2517–2529, 1988

Lejeune J: Pathogenesis of mental deficiency in trisomy 21. Am J Med Genet Suppl 7:20–30, 1990

Lensing P, Schimke H, Klimesch W, et al: Clinical case report: opiate antagonist and event-related desynchronization in 2 autistic boys. Neuropsychobiology 31:16–23, 1995

Leonard HL, Meyer MC, Swedo SE, et al: Electrocardiographic changes during desipramine and clomipramine treatment in children and adolescents. J Am Acad Child Adolesc Psychiatry 34:1460–1468, 1995

Leslie AM, Frith U: Autistic children's understanding of seeing, knowing and believing. British Journal of Developmental Psychology 6:315–324, 1988

Leventhal BL, Cook EH Jr, Morford M, et al: Clinical and neurochemical effects of fenfluramine in children with autism. J Neuropsychiatry Clin Neurosci 5:307–315, 1993

Leviton A, Bellinger D, Allred EN, et al: Pre- and postnatal low-level lead exposure and children's dysfunction in school. Environ Res 60:30–43, 1993

Levitt JG, Blanton R, Capetillo-Cunliffe L, et al: Cerebellar vermis lobules VIII-X in autism. Prog Neuropsychopharmacol Biol Psychiatry 23:625–633, 1999

Levy F, Hay DA, McStephen M, et al: Attention-deficit hyperactivity disorder: a category or a continuum? genetic analysis of a large-scale twin study. J Am Acad Child Adolesc Psychiatry 36:737–744, 1997

Lewander T: Displacement of brain and heart noradrenaline by p-hydroxynorephedrine after administration of p-hydroxyamphetamine. Acta Pharmacol Toxicol (Copenh) 29:20–32, 1971a

Lewander T: On the presence of p-hydroxynorephedrine in the rat brain and heart in relation to changes in catecholamine levels after administration of amphetamine. Acta Pharmacol Toxicol (Copenh) 29: 3–8, 1971b

Lewis C, Hitch GJ, Walker P: The prevalence of specific arithmetic difficulties and specific reading difficulties in 9- to 10-year-old boys and girls. J Child Psychol Psychiatry 35:283–292, 1994

Lewis DO, Pincus JH, Bard B, et al: Neuropsychiatric, psychoeducational, and family characteristics of 14 juveniles condemned to death in the United States. Am J Psychiatry 145:584–589, 1988

Lichter DG, Jackson LA, Schachter M: Clinical evidence for genomic imprinting in Tourette's syndrome. Neurology 45:924–928, 1995

Liederman J, Flannery KA: Fall conception increases the risk of neurodevelopmental disorder in offspring. J Clin Exp Neuropsychol 16:754–768, 1994

Lieh-Lai MW, Theodorou AA, Sarnaik AP, et al: Limitations of the Glasgow Coma Scale in predicting outcome in children with traumatic brain injury. J Pediatr 120: 195–199, 1992

Lindgren AC, Ritzen EM: Five years of growth hormone treatment in children with Prader-Willi syndrome. Acta Paediatr Suppl 88:109–111, 1999

Linet LS: Tourette syndrome, pimozide, and school phobia: the neuroleptic separation anxiety syndrome. Am J Psychiatry 142:613–615, 1985

Livingstone MS, Rosen GD, Drislane FW, et al: Physiological and anatomical evidence for a magnocellular defect in developmental dyslexia. Proc Natl Acad Sci U S A 88: 7943–7947, 1991

Lobato MN, Caldwell MB, Ng P, et al: Encephalopathy in children with perinatally acquired human immunodeficiency virus infection. Pediatric Spectrum of Disease Clinical Consortium. J Pediatr 126(5 pt 1):710–715, 1995

Lombroso PJ, Scahill L, King RA, et al: Risperidone treatment of children and adolescents with chronic tic disorders: a preliminary report. J Am Acad Child Adolesc Psychiatry 34:1147–1152, 1995

Lotspeich LJ: Autism and pervasive developmental disorders, in Psychopharmacology: The Fourth Generation of Progress. Edited by Bloom FE, Kupfer DJ. New York, Raven, 1995, pp 1653–1663

Lou HC, Henriksen L, Bruhn P, et al: Striatal dysfunction in attention deficit and hyperkinetic disorder. Arch Neurol 46:48–52, 1990

Lovaas OI: Behavioral treatment and normal educational and intellectual functioning in young autistic children. J Consult Clin Psychol 55:3–9, 1987

Lu D, Pavlakis SG, Frank Y, et al: Proton MR spectroscopy of the basal ganglia in healthy children and children with AIDS. Radiology 199:423–428, 1996

Lubar JO, Lubar JF: Electroencephalographic biofeedback of SMR and beta for treatment of attention deficit disorders in a clinical setting. Biofeedback Self Regul 9:1–23, 1984

Lubar JF, Swartwood MO, Swartwood JN, et al: Evaluation of the effectiveness of EEG neurofeedback training for ADHD in a clinical setting as measured by changes in T.O.V.A. scores, behavioral ratings, and WISC-R performance. Biofeedback Self Regul 20:83–99, 1995

Luxenberg JS, Swedo SE, Flament MF, et al: Neuroanatomical abnormalities in obsessive-compulsive disorder detected with quantitative X-ray computed tomography. Am J Psychiatry 145:1089–1093, 1988

Maggirwar SB, Tong N, Ramirez S, et al: HIV-1 Tat-mediated activation of glycogen synthase kinase-3beta contributes to Tat-mediated neurotoxicity. J Neurochem 73: 578–586, 1999

Mailleux P, Pelaprat D, Vanderhaeghen JJ: Transient neurotensin high-affinity binding sites in the human inferior olive during development. Brain Res 508:345–348, 1990

Malcolm S, Clayton-Smith J, Nichols M, et al: Uniparental disomy in Angelman's syndrome. Lancet 337:694–697, 1991

Malison RT, McDougle CJ, van Dyck CH, et al: [123]beta-CIT SPECT imaging of striatal dopamine transporter binding in Tourette's disorder. Am J Psychiatry 152: 1359–1361, 1995

Malone MA, Kershner JR, Swanson JM: Hemispheric processing and methylphenidate effects in attention-deficit hyperactivity disorder. J Child Neurol 9:181–189, 1994

Mannuzza S, Klein RG, Konig PH, et al: Hyperactive boys almost grown up, IV: criminality and its relationship to psychiatric status. Arch Gen Psychiatry 46:1073–1079, 1989

Marcus J, Hans SL, Mednick SA, et al: Neurological dysfunctioning in offspring of schizophrenics in Israel and Denmark: a replication analysis. Arch Gen Psychiatry 42:753–761, 1985

Martin A, State M, Anderson GM, et al: Cerebrospinal fluid levels of oxytocin in Prader-Willi syndrome: a preliminary report. Biol Psychiatry 44:1349–1352, 1998

Mathews WS, Barabas G: Suicide and epilepsy: a review of the literature. Psychosomatics 22:515–524, 1981

Mattson AJ, Sheer DE, Fletcher JM: Electrophysiological evidence of lateralized disturbances in children with learning disabilities. J Clin Exp Neuropsychol 14:707–716, 1992

Max JE, Dunisch DL: Traumatic brain injury in a child psychiatry outpatient clinic: a controlled study. J Am Acad Child Adolesc Psychiatry 35:404–411, 1997

Max JE, Lindgren SD, Robin DA, et al: Traumatic brain injury in children and adolescents: psychiatric disorders in the second three months. J Nerv Ment Dis 185:394–401, 1997a

Max JE, Robin DA, Lindgren SD, et al: Traumatic brain injury in children and adolescents: psychiatric disorders at two years. J Am Acad Child Adolesc Psychiatry 36:1278–1285, 1997b

Max JE, Smith WL, Sato Y, et al: Traumatic brain injury in children and adolescents: psychiatric disorders in the first three months. J Am Acad Child Adolesc Psychiatry 36:94–102, 1997c

Max JE, Arndt S, Castillo CS, et al: Attention-deficit hyperactivity symptomatology after traumatic brain injury: a prospective study. J Am Acad Child Adolesc Psychiatry 37: 841–847, 1998a

Max JE, Castillo CS, Bokura H, et al: Oppositional defiant disorder symptomatology after traumatic brain injury: a prospective study. J Nerv Ment Dis 186:325–332, 1998b

Max JE, Castillo CS, Robin DA, et al: Posttraumatic stress symptomatology after childhood traumatic brain injury. J Nerv Ment Dis 186(10):589–596, 1998c

Max JE, Koele SL, Smith WL, et al: Psychiatric disorders in children and adolescents after severe traumatic brain injury: a controlled study. J Am Acad Child Adolesc Psychiatry 37:832–840, 1998d

McArthur JC: Neurologic manifestations of AIDS. Medicine (Baltimore) 66:407–437, 1987

McArthur JC, Cohen BA, Selnes OA, et al: Low prevalence of neurological and neuropsychological abnormalities in otherwise healthy HIV-1–infected individuals: results from the multicenter AIDS Cohort Study. Ann Neurol 26:601–611, 1989

McArthur JC, Hoover DR, Bacellar H, et al: Dementia in AIDS patients: incidence and risk factors. Neurology 43:2245–2252, 1993

McBride PA, Anderson GM, Hertzig ME, et al: Effects of diagnosis, race, and puberty on platelet serotonin levels in autism and mental retardation. J Am Acad Child Adolesc Psychiatry 37:767–776, 2000

McConville BJ, Fogelson MH, Norman AB, et al: Nicotine potentiation of haloperidol in reducing tic frequency in Tourette's disorder. Am J Psychiatry 148:793–794, 1991

McDougle CJ, Goddman WK, Price LH: Dopamine antagonists in tic-related and psychotic spectrum obsessive compulsive disorder. J Clin Psychiatry 55 (suppl):24–31, 1994

McDougle CJ, Brodkin ES, Naylor ST, et al: Sertraline in adults with pervasive developmental disorders: a prospective open-label investigation. J Clin Psychopharmacol 18:62–66, 1998

McEachin JJ, Smith T, Lovaas OI: Long-term outcome for children with autism who received early intensive behavioral treatment. Am J Ment Retard 97:359–372, 1993

McGee R, Williams S, Silva OA: A comparison of girls and boys with teacher-identified problems of attention. J Am Acad Child Adolesc Psychiatry 26:711–717, 1987

McLeer SV, Callaghan M, Henry D, et al: Psychiatric disorders in sexually abused children. J Am Acad Child Adolesc Psychiatry 33:313–319, 1994

Melchitzky DS, Lewis DA: Tyrosine hydroxylase- and dopamine transporter–immunoreactive axons in the primate cerebellum. Evidence for a lobular- and laminar-specific dopamine innervation. Neuropsychopharmacology 22: 466–472, 2000

Mendez MF, Cummings JL, Benson DF: Depression in epilepsy: significance and phenomenology. Arch Neurol 43:766–770, 1986

Mendez MF, Lanska DJ, Manon-Espaillat R, et al: Causative factors for suicide attempts by overdose in epileptics. Arch Neurol 46:1065–1068, 1989

Merzenich MM, Jenkins WM, Johnston P, et al: Temporal processing deficits of language-learning impaired children ameliorated by training. Science 271:77–81, 1996

Metz-Lutz MN, Kleitz C, de Saint Martin A, et al: Cognitive development in benign focal epilepsies of childhood. Dev Neurosci 21:182–190, 1999

Michaud LJ, Rivara FP, Jafle KM, et al: Traumatic brain injury as a risk factor for behavioral disorders in children. Arch Phys Med Rehabil 74:368–375, 1993

Mikkelsen EJ, Detlor J, Cohen DJ: School avoidance and social phobia triggered by haloperidol in patients with Tourette's disorder. Am J Psychiatry 138:1572–1576, 1981

Miller FE, Heffner TG, Kotake C, et al: Magnitude and duration of hyperactivity following neonatal 6-hydroxydopamine is related to the extent of brain dopamine depletion. Brain Res 229:123–132, 1981

Miller JN, Ozonoff S: The external validity of Asperger disorder: lack of evidence from the domain of neuropsychology. J Abnorm Psychol 109:227–238, 2000

Minshew NJ: Indices of neural function in autism: clinical and biologic implications. Pediatrics 87:774–780, 1991

Mintz M: Neurological and developmental problems in pediatric HIV infection. J Nutr 126 (10 suppl):2663S–2673S, 1996

Molfese DL, Freeman RB Jr, Palermo DS: The ontogeny of brain lateralization for speech and nonspeech stimuli. Brain Lang 2:356–368, 1975

Morton LL: Interhemispheric balance patterns detected by selective phonemic dichotic laterality measures in four clinical subtypes or reading disabled children. J Clin Exp Neuropsychol 16:556–567, 1994

Mostofsky SH, Mazzocco MM, Aakalu G, et al: Decreased cerebellar posterior vermis size in fragile X syndrome: correlation with neurocognitive performance. Neurology 50: 121–130, 1998

Muller N, Putz A, Klages U, et al: Blunted growth hormone response to clonidine in Gilles de la Tourette syndrome. Psychoneuroendocrinology 19:335–341, 1994

Murphy TK, Goodman WK, Fudge MW, et al: B lymphocyte antigen D8/17: a peripheral marker for childhood-onset obsessive compulsive disorder and Tourette's syndrome? Am J Psychiatry 153:402–407, 1997

Nash JK: Treatment of attention deficit hyperactivity disorder with neurotherapy. Clin Electroencephalogr 31(1):30–37, 2000

National Pediatric Trauma Registry: Facts From the National Pediatric Trauma Registry—Fact Sheet 1. Boston, MA, Research and Training Center in Rehabilitation and Childhood Trauma, 1993

Navia BA, Jordan BD, Price RW: The AIDS dementia complex, I: clinical features. Ann Neurol 19:517–524, 1986

Naylor MW, Staskowski M, Kenney MC, et al: Language disorders and learning disabilities in school-refusing adolescents. J Am Acad Child Adolesc Psychiatry 33:1331–1337, 1994

New DR, Ma M, Epstein LG, et al: Human immunodeficiency virus type 1 Tat protein induces death by apoptosis in primary human neuron cultures. J Neurobiol 3:168–173, 1997

New DR, Maggirwar SB, Epstein LG, et al: HIV-1 Tat induced neuronal death via tumor necrosis factor–alpha and activation of non-N-methyl-D-aspartate receptors by the NFkappaB-independent mechanism. J Biol Chem 273:17852–17858, 1998

Nicholls RD, Knoll JH, Butler MG, et al: Genetic imprinting suggested by maternal heterodisomy in nondeletion Prader-Willi syndrome. Nature 342:281–285, 1989

Nielsen J, Friberg L, Lou H, et al: Immature patterns of brain activity in Rett syndrome. Arch Neurol 47:982–986, 1990

Njiokiktjien C, de Sonneville L, Vaal J: Callosal size in children with learning disabilities. Behav Brain Res 64:213–218, 1994

Nordin V, Gillberg C: The long-term course of autistic disorders: update on follow-up studies. Acta Psychiatr Scand 97:99–108, 1998

Novic B, Vaugham HG Jr, Kurtzberg D, et al: An electrophysiologic indication of auditory processing defects in autism. Psychiatry Res 3:107–114, 1980

Olvera RL, Pliszka SR, Luh J, et al: An open trial of venlafaxine in the treatment of attention-deficit/hyperactivity disorder in children and adolescents. J Child Adolesc Psychopharmacol 6(4):241–250, 1996

Ornitz EM: The modulation of sensory input and motor output in autistic children. J Autism Child Schizophr 4:197–215, 1974

Ornitz EM, Ritvo ER: Perceptual inconstancy in early infantile autism. Arch Gen Psychiatry 18:76–98, 1968

Overmeyer S, Simmons A, Santosh J, et al: Corpus callosum may be similar in children with ADHD and siblings of children with ADHD. Dev Med Child Neurol 42:8–13, 2000

Palmer CG, Bailey JN, Ramsey C, et al: No evidence of linkage or linkage disequilibrium between DAT1 and attention deficit hyperactivity disorder in a large sample. Psychiatr Genet 9(3):157–160, 1999

Park JP, Wurster-Hill DH, Andrews PA, et al: Free proximal trisomy 21 without the Down's syndrome. Clin Genet 32:342–348, 1987

Pauls DL: Genetic factors in the expression of attention-deficit hyperactivity disorder. J Child Adolesc Psychopharmacol 1:353–360, 1991

Pauls DL, Leckman JF: The inheritance of Gilles de la Tourette's syndrome and associated behaviors. N Engl J Med 315:993–997, 1986

Pavlakis SG, Lu D, Frank Y, et al: Magnetic resonance spectroscopy in childhood AIDS encephalopathy. Pediatr Neurol 12:277–282, 1995

Pavlakis SG, Lu D, Frank Y, et al: Brain lactate and N-acetylaspartate in pediatric AIDS encephalopathy. AJNR Am J Neuroradiol 19:383–385, 1998

Pearson DE, Teicher MH, Shaywitz BA, et al: Environmental influences on body weight and behavior in developing rats after neonatal 6-hydroxydopamine. Science 209:715–717, 1980

Pelham WE, Sturges J, Hoza J, et al: Sustained release and standard methylphenidate effects on cognitive and social behavior in children with attention deficit disorder. Pediatrics 80:491–501, 1987

Pelham WE, Greenslade KE, Vodde-Hamilton MA, et al: Relative efficacy of long-acting CNS stimulants on children with attention deficit–hyperactivity disorder: a comparison of standard methylphenidate, sustained-release methylphenidate, sustained-release dextroamphetamine, and pemoline. Pediatrics 86:226–237, 1990

Pelham WE, Swanson JM, Furman MB, et al: Pemoline effects on children with ADHD: a time-response by dose-response analysis on classroom measures. J Am Acad Child Adolesc Psychiatry 34:1504–1513, 1995

Pellock JM: Treatment of seizures and epilepsy in children and adolescents. Neurology 51:S8–14, 1998

Pennington BF, Smith SD: Genetic influences on learning disabilities and speech and language disorders. Child Dev 54:369–387, 1983

Perez MM, Trimble MR: Epileptic psychosis-diagnostic comparison with process schizophrenia. Br J Psychiatry 137:245–249, 1980

Perlmutter SJ, Leitman SF, Garvey MA, et al: Therapeutic plasma exchange and intravenous immunoglobulin for obsessive-compulsive disorder and tic disorders in childhood. Lancet 354:1153–1158, 1999

Perner J, Frith U, Leslie AM, et al: Exploration of the autistic child's theory of mind: Knowledge, belief, and communication. Child Dev 60:689–700, 1989

Perry SW, Hamilton JA, Tjoelker LW, et al: Platelet-activating factor receptor activation. An initiator step in HIV-1 neuropathogenesis. J Biol Chem 273:17660–17664, 1998

Peterson BS, Riddle MA, Cohen DJ, et al: Reduced basal ganglia volumes in Tourette's syndrome using 3-dimensional reconstruction techniques from magnetic resonance images. Neurology 43:941–949, 1993

Peterson BS, Gore JC, Riddle MA, et al: Abnormal magnetic resonance imaging T2 relaxation time asymmetries in Tourette's syndrome. Psychiatry Res 55:205–221, 1994

Peterson BS, Skudlarski P, Anderson AW, et al: A functional magnetic resonance imaging study of tic suppression in Tourette syndrome. Arch Gen Psychiatry 55:326–333, 1998

Pihl RO, Parkes M: Hair element content in learning disabled children. Science 198:204–206, 1977

Piven J, Berthier ML, Starkstein SE, et al: Magnetic resonance imaging evidence for a defect of cerebral cortical development in autism. Am J Psychiatry 147:731–739, 1990

Piven J, Tsai G, Nehme E, et al: Platelet serotonin, a possible marker for familial autism. J Autism Dev Disord 21:51–59, 1991

Plante E: MRI findings in the parents and siblings of specifically language-impaired boys. Brain Lang 41:67–80, 1991

Pleak RR, Gormly LJ: Effects of venlafaxine treatment for ADHD in a child (letter). Am J Psychiatry 152:1099, 1995

Pliszka SR, Browne RG, Olvera RL, et al: A double-blind, placebo-controlled study of Adderall and methylphenidate in the treatment of attention-deficit/hyperactivity disorder. J Am Acad Child Adolesc Psychiatry 39(5):619–626, 2000

Plotsky PM, Meaney JM: Early postnatal experience alters hypothalamic corticotropin-releasing factor (CRF) mRNA, median eminence CRF content and stress-induced release in rats. Brain Res Mol Brain Res 18:195–200, 1993

Pontrelli L, Pavlakis S, Krilov LR: Neurobehavioral manifestations and sequelae of HIV and other infections. Child Adolesc Psychiatr Clin N Am 8:869–878, 1999

Popper CW: Antidepressants in the treatment of attention-deficit/hyperactivity disorder. J Clin Psychiatry 58 (suppl 14):14–29; discussion 30-31, 1997

Popper CW, Steingard RJ: Disorders usually first diagnosed in infancy, childhood, or adolescence, in American Psychiatric Press Textbook of Psychiatry, 2nd Edition. Edited by Hales RE, Yudofsky SC, Talbott JA. Washington, DC, American Psychiatric Press, 1995, pp 729–832

Popper CW, Zimnitzky B: Sudden death putatively related to desipramine treatment in youth: a fifth case and a review of speculative mechanisms. J Child Adolesc Psychopharmacol 5:283–300, 1995

Porrino LJ, Rapoport JL, Behar D: A naturalistic assessment of the motor activity of hyperactive boys, I: comparison with normal controls. Arch Gen Psychiatry 40:681–687, 1983

Posey DJ, Litwiller M, Koburn A, et al: Paroxetine in autism. J Am Acad Child Adolesc Psychiatry 38:111–112, 1999

Purves D: Neural Activity and the Growth of the Brain. Cambridge, England, Cambridge University Press, 1980

Rabey JM, Lewis A, Graff E, et al: Decreased (3H) quinuclidinyl benzilate binding to lymphocytes in Gilles de la Tourette syndrome. Biol Psychiatry 31:889–895, 1992

Rangno RE, Kaufmann JS, Cavanaugh JH, et al: Effects of a false neurotransmitter, p-hydroxynorephedrine, on the function of adrenergic neurons in hypertensive patients. J Clin Invest 52:952–960, 1973

Rapoport JL, Buchsbaum MS, Weingartner H, et al: Dextroamphetamine. Its cognitive and behavioral effects in normal and hyperactive boys and normal men. Arch Gen Psychiatry 37:933–943, 1980

Raskin LA, Shaywitz BA, Anderson GM, et al: Differential effects of selective dopamine, norepinephrine or catecholamine depletion on activity and learning in the developing rat. Pharmacol Biochem Behav 19:743–749, 1983

Reiss AL, Faruque F, Naidu S, et al: Neuroanatomy of Rett syndrome: a volumetric imaging study. Ann Neurol 34:227–234, 1993

Rett A: Uber Ein Zerebral-Atrophisches Syndrom Bei Hyperammonamie. Vienna, Austria, Bruder Hollinek, 1966, pp 1–68

Rett A: Soziale Praventivmassnahmen bei entwicklungsgestorten Kindern. Ther Umsch 34:49–51, 1977

Riddle MA, Nelson JC, Kleinman CS, et al: Case study: sudden death in children receiving Norpramin: a review of three reported cases and commentary. J Am Acad Child Adolesc Psychiatry 30:104–108, 1991

Riddle MA, Rasmussen AM, Woods SW, et al: SPECT imaging of cerebral blood flow in Tourette syndrome, in Tourette Syndrome: Genetics, Neurobiology, and Treatment, Advances in Neurology, Vol 58. Edited by Chase TN, Friedhoff AJ, Cohen DJ. New York, Raven, 1992, pp 207–211

Riddle MA, Geller B, Ryan ND: Case study: another sudden death in a child treated with desipramine. J Am Acad Child Adolesc Psychiatry 32:792–797, 1993

Ritvo ER, Freeman BJ, Geller E, et al: Effects of fenfluramine on 14 outpatients with the syndrome of autism. J Am Acad Child Psychiatry 22:549–558, 1983

Ritvo ER, Freeman BJ, Yuwiler A, et al: Fenfluramine treatment of autism: UCLA collaborative study of 81 patients at nine medical centers. Psychopharmacol Bull 22:133–140, 1986

Ritzen EM, Lindgren AC, Hagenas L, et al: Growth hormone treatment of patients with Prader-Willi syndrome. J Pediatr Endocrinol Metab 12 (suppl 1):345–349, 1999

Riva D, Giorgi C: The cerebellum contributes to higher functions during development: evidence from a series of children surgically treated for posterior fossa tumours. Brain 123 (pt 5):1051–1061, 2000

Rivara JB, Jaffe KM, Fay GC, et al: Family functioning and injury severity as predictors of child functioning one year following traumatic brain injury. Arch Phys Med Rehabil 74:1047–1055, 1993

Robin AL, Foster S: Negotiating Parent-Adolescent Conflict. New York, Guilford, 1989

Rodin E, Schmalz S: The Bear-Fedio personality inventory and temporal lobe epilepsy. Neurology 34:591–596, 1984

Roof E, Stone W, MacLean W, et al: Intellectual characteristics of Prader-Willi syndrome: comparison of genetic subtypes. J Intellect Disabil Res 44:25–30, 2000

Rosner BS: Recovery of function and localization of function in historical perspective, in Plasticity and Recovery of Function in the Central Nervous System. Edited by Stein DG, Rosen JJ, Butters N. New York, Academic Press, 1974, pp 1–29

Ross DL, Klykylo WM, Hitzemann R: Reduction of elevated CSF beta-endorphin by fenfluramine in infantile autism. Am J Psychiatry 3:83–86, 1987

Rothner AD: Epilepsy, in Child and Adolescent Neurology for Psychiatrists. Edited by Kaufman DM, Solomon GE, Pfeffer CR. Baltimore, MD, Williams & Wilkins, 1992, pp 96–113

Rowe KJ, Rowe KS: The relationship between inattentiveness in the classroom and reading achievement. J Am Acad Child Adolesc Psychiatry 31:357–368, 1992

Rubia K, Overmeyer S, Taylor E, et al: Hypofrontality in attention deficit hyperactivity disorder during higher-order motor control: a study with functional MRI. Am J Psychiatry 156:891–896, 1999

Rumsey JM, Andreason P, Zametkin AJ, et al: Failure to activate the left temporoparietal cortex in dyslexia: an oxygen 15 positron emission tomographic study. Arch Neurol 49:527–534, 1992

Rutter M, Bailey A: Thinking and relationships: mind and brain (some reflections on theory of mind and autism), in Understanding Other Minds: Perspectives From Autism. Edited by Baron-Cohen S, Tager-Flusberg H, Cohen D. New York, Oxford University Press, 1993, pp 481–504

Rutter M, Yule W: The concept of specific reading retardation. J Child Psychol Psychiatry 16:181–197, 1975

Safer DJ, Krager JM: A survey of medication treatment for hyperactive/inattentive students. JAMA 260:2256–2258, 1988

Saito Y, Sharer LR, Dewhurst S, et al: Cellular localization of human herpes virus–6 in the brains of children with AIDS encephalopathy. J Neurovirol 1:30–39, 1995

Sallee FR, Sethuraman G, Rock CM: Effects of pimozide on cognition in children with Tourette syndrome: interaction with comorbid attention deficit hyperactivity disorder. Acta Psychiatr Scand 90:4–9, 1994

Salvan AM, Lamoureux S, Michel G, et al: Localized proton magnetic resonance spectroscopy of the brain in children infected with human immunodeficiency virus with and without encephalopathy. Pediatr Res 44:755–762, 1998

Sanberg PR, Silver AA, Shytle RD, et al: Nicotine for the treatment of Tourette's syndrome. Pharmacol Ther 74:21–25, 1997

Sanberg PR, Shytle RD, Silver AA: Treatment of Tourette's syndrome with mecamylamine. Lancet 352:705–706, 1998

Sanchez MM, Hearn EF, Do D, et al: Differential rearing affects corpus callosum size and cognitive function of rhesus monkeys. Brain Res 812:38–49, 1998

Sandler AD, Sutton KA, DeWeese J, et al: Lack of benefit of a single dose of synthetic human secretin in the treatment of autism and pervasive developmental disorder. N Engl J Med 341:1801–1806, 1999

Satterfield JH, Hoppe CM, Schell AM: A prospective study of delinquency in 110 adolescent boys with attention deficit disorder and 88 normal adolescent boys. Am J Psychiatry 139:795–798, 1982

Scahill L, Chappell PB, King RA, et al: Pharmacologic treatment of tic disorders. Child Adolesc Psychiatr Clin N Am 9(1):99–117, 2000

Scarmato V, Frank Y, Rozenstein A, et al: Central brain atrophy in childhood AIDS encephalopathy. AIDS 10:1227–1231, 1996

Schacter SC, Galaburda AM: Development and biological associations of cerebral dominance: review and possible mechanisms. J Am Acad Child Psychiatry 25:7411–7450, 1986

Schiffer F, Teicher MH, Papanicolaou AC: Evoked potential evidence for right brain activity during recall of traumatic memories. J Neuropsychiatry Clin Neurosci 7:169–175, 1995

Schmahmann JD, Pandya DN: Prefrontal cortex projections to the basilar pons in rhesus monkey: implications for the cerebellar contribution to higher function. Neurosci Lett 199:175–178, 1995

Schmidt D, Bourgeois B: A risk-benefit assessment of therapies for Lennox-Gastaut syndrome. Drug Saf 22:467–477, 2000

Schultz RT, Gauthier I, Klin A, et al: Abnormal ventral temporal cortical activity during face discrimination among individuals with autism and Asperger syndrome. Arch Gen Psychiatry 57:331–340, 2000

Schweitzer JB, Faber TL, Grafton ST, et al: Alterations in the functional anatomy of working memory in adult attention deficit hyperactivity disorder. Am J Psychiatry 157:278–280, 2000

Seeman P, Madras BK: Anti-hyperactivity medication: methylphenidate and amphetamine (comments). Mol Psychiatry 3:386–396, 1998

Seeman P, Bzowej N, Guan II, et al: Human brain receptors in children and aging adults. Synapse 1:399–404, 1987

Seghorn TK, Boucher RJ, Prentky RA: Childhood sexual abuse in the lives of sexually aggressive offenders. J Am Acad Child Adolesc Psychiatry 26:262–267, 1987

Sei S, Stewart SK, Farley M, et al: Evaluation of human immunodeficiency virus (HIV) type 1 RNA levels in cerebrospinal fluid and viral resistance to zidovudine in children with HIV-encephalopathy. J Infect Dis 174(6):1200–1206, 1996

Semrud-Clikeman M, Biederman J, Sprich-Buckminster S, et al: Comorbidity between ADHD and learning disability: a review and report in a clinically referred sample. J Am Acad Child Adolesc Psychiatry 31:439–448, 1992

Semrud-Clikeman M, Filipek PA, Biederman J, et al: Attention-deficit hyperactivity disorder: magnetic resonance imaging morphometric analysis of the corpus callosum. J Am Acad Child Adolesc Psychiatry 33:875–881, 1994

Semrud-Clikeman M, Steingard RJ, Filipek P, et al: Using MRI to examine brain-behavior relationships in males with attention deficit disorder with hyperactivity. J Am Acad Child Adolesc Psychiatry 39:477–484, 2000

Sharer LR: Pathology of HIV-1 infection of the central nervous system. A review. J Neuropathol Exp Neurol 51:3–11, 1992

Sharer LR, Epstein LG, Cho E-S, et al: Pathologic features of AIDS encephalopathy in children: Evidence for LAV/HTLV-III infection of brain. Hum Pathol 17:271–284, 1986

Sharer LR, Saito Y, Da Cunha A, et al: In situ amplification and detection of HIV-1 DNA in fixed pediatric AIDS brain tissue. Hum Pathol 27:614–617, 1996

Shaywitz BA, Klopper JH, Yager RD, et al: Paradoxical response to amphetamine in developing rats treated with 6-hydroxy-dopamine. Nature 261:153–155, 1976a

Shaywitz BA, Yager RD, Klopper JH: Selective brain dopamine depletion in developing rats: an experimental model of minimal brain dysfunction. Science 191:305–308, 1976b

Shaywitz BA, Teicher MH, Cohen DJ, et al: Dopaminergic but not noradrenergic mediation of hyperactivity and performance deficits in the developing rat pup. Psychopharmacology (Berl) 82:73–77, 1984

Shaywitz BA, Fletcher JM, Shaywitz SE: Defining and classifying learning disabilities and attention-deficit/hyperactivity disorder. J Child Neurol 10 (suppl):S50–S57, 1995

Shaywitz SE, Escobar MD, Shaywitz BA, et al: Evidence that dyslexia may represent the lower tail of a normal distribution of reading ability. N Engl J Med 326:145–150, 1992

Sidman RL, Rakic P: Neuronal migration with special reference to developing human brain: a review. Brain Res 62:1–35, 1973

Sieg KG, Gaffney GR, Preston DF, et al: SPECT brain imaging abnormalities in attention deficit hyperactivity disorder. Clin Nucl Med 20:55–60, 1995

Simonds RJ, Scheibel AB: The postnatal development of the motor speech area: a preliminary study. Brain Lang 37:42–58, 1989

Simos PG, Breier JI, Fletcher JM, et al: Brain activation profiles in dyslexic children during non-word reading: a magnetic source imaging study. Neurosci Lett 290:61–65, 2000

Simpson DM: Human immunodeficiency virus–associated dementia: review of pathogenesis, prophylaxis, and treatment studies of zidovudine therapy. Clin Infect Dis 29:19–34, 1999

Singer HS, Hahn IH, Moran TH: Tourette's syndrome: abnormal dopamine uptake sites in postmortem striatum from patients with Tourette's syndrome. Ann Neurol 30:558–562, 1991

Singer HS, Reiss AL, Brown JE, et al: Volumetric MRI changes in the basal ganglia of children with Tourette's syndrome. Neurology 43:950–956, 1993

Singer HS, Brown J, Quaskey S, et al: The treatment of attention-deficit hyperactivity disorder in Tourette's syndrome: a double-blind placebo-controlled study with clonidine and desipramine. Pediatrics 95:74–81, 1995

Singer HS, Giuliano JD, Hansen BH, et al: Antibodies against human putamen in children with Tourette syndrome. Neurology 50:1618–1624, 1998

Singer HS, Guulian JD, Hansen BH, et al: Antibodies against a neuron-like (HTB-10 neuroblastoma) cell in children with Tourette syndrome. Biol Psychiatry 15:775–780, 1999

Siomi MC, Siomi H, Sauer WH, et al: FXR1, an autosomal homolog of the fragile X mental retardation gene. EMBO J 14:2401–2408, 1995

Skottun BC: The magnocellular deficit theory of dyslexia: the evidence from contrast sensitivity. Vision Res 40:111–127, 2000

Spencer T, Biederman J, Kerman K, et al: Desipramine treatment of children with attention-deficit hyperactivity disorder and tic disorder or Tourette's syndrome. J Am Acad Child Adolesc Psychiatry 32:354–360, 1993a

Spencer T, Biederman J, Steingard R, et al: Bupropion exacerbates tics in children with attention-deficit hyperactivity disorder and Tourette's syndrome. J Am Acad Child Adolesc Psychiatry 32:211–214, 1993b

Spencer T, Biederman J, Wilens T, et al: Nortriptyline treatment of children with attention-deficit hyperactivity disorder and tic disorder or Tourette's syndrome. J Am Acad Child Adolesc Psychiatry 32:205–210, 1993c

Spencer TJ, Biederman J, Harding M, et al: Growth deficits in ADHD children revisited: evidence for disorder-associated growth delays? J Am Acad Child Adolesc Psychiatry 35(11):1460–1469, 1996

Starace F, Dijkgraaf M, Houweling H, et al: HIV-associated dementia: clinical, epidemiological and resource utilization issues. AIDS Care 10 (suppl 2):S113–S121, 1998

State MW, King BH, Dykens E: Mental retardation: a review of the past 10 years. Part II. J Am Acad Child Adolesc Psychiatry 36(12):1664–1671, 1997

State MW, Dykens EM, Rosner B, et al: Obsessive-compulsive symptoms in Prader-Willi and "Prader-Willi–like" patients. J Am Acad Child Adolesc Psychiatry 38:329–334, 1999

Stein J, Fowler S: Effect of monocular occlusion on visuomotor perception and reading in dyslexic children. Lancet 2:69–73, 1985

Stein J, Walsh V: To see but not to read: the magnocellular theory of dyslexia. Trends Neurosci 20:147–152, 1997

Stein MB, Koverola C, Hanna C, et al: Hippocampal volume in women victimized by childhood sexual abuse. Psychol Med 27:951–959, 1997

Steingard R, Khan A, Gonzalez A, et al: Neuroleptic malignant syndrome: review of experience with children and adolescents. J Child Adolesc Psychopharmacol 2:183–198, 1992

Steingard R, Biederman J, Spencer T, et al: Comparison of clonidine response in the treatment of attention-deficit hyperactivity disorder with and without comorbid tic disorders. J Am Acad Child Adolesc Psychiatry 32:350–353, 1993

Steinman SB, Steinman BA, Garzia RP: Vision and attention, II: is visual attention a mechanism through which a deficient magnocellular pathway might cause reading disability? Optom Vis Sci 75:674–681, 1998

Stevenson J, Graham P, Fredman G, et al: A twin study of genetic influences on reading and spelling ability and disability. J Child Psychol Psychiatry 28:229–247, 1987

Stone MH: Borderline syndromes: a consideration of subtypes and an overview, directions for research. Psychiatr Clin North Am 4:3–13, 1981

Streissguth AP, Barr HM, Sampson PD: Moderate prenatal alcohol exposure: effects on child IQ and learning problems at age 7-1/2 years. Alcohol Clin Exp Res 14:662–669, 1990

Stricker EM, Zigmond MJ: Recovery of function following damage to central catecholamine-containing neurons: a neurochemical model for the lateral hypothalamic syndrome, in Progress in Psychobiology, Physiology, and Psychology, Vol 6. New York, Academic Press, 1976, pp 121–188

Struve FA, Klein DF, Saraf KR: Electroencephalographic correlates of suicide ideation and attempts. Arch Gen Psychiatry 27:363–365, 1972

Subramaniam B, Naidu S, Reiss AL: Neuroanatomy in Rett syndrome: cerebral cortex and posterior fossa. Neurology 48:399–407, 1997

Sunahara RK, Seeman P, Van Tol HH, et al: Dopamine receptors and antipsychotic drug response. Br J Psychiatry Suppl (22):31–38, 1993

Suzuki DA, Keller EL: The role of the posterior vermis of monkey cerebellum in smooth-pursuit eye movement control, II: target velocity-related Purkinje cell activity. J Neurophysiol 59:19–40, 1988

Sverd J, Gadow KD, Paolicelli LM: Methylphenidate treatment of attention-deficit hyperactivity disorder in boys with Tourette's syndrome. J Am Acad Child Adolesc Psychiatry 28:574–579, 1989

Swanson JM, Sunohara GA, Kennedy JL, et al: Association of the dopamine receptor D4 (DRD4) gene with a refined phenotype of attention deficit hyperactivity disorder (ADHD): a family based approach. Mol Psychiatry 3:38–41, 1998

Swanson J, Oosterlaan J, Murias M, et al: Attention deficit/hyperactivity disorder children with a 7-repeat allele of the dopamine receptor D4 gene have extreme behavior but normal performance on critical neuropsychological tests of attention. Proc Natl Acad Sci U S A 97(9):4754–4759, 2000

Swedo SE: Sydenham's chorea: a model for childhood autoimmune neuropsychiatric disorders. JAMA 272:1788–1791, 1994

Sweeney JA, Strojwas MH, Mann JJ, et al: Prefrontal and cerebellar abnormalities in major depression: evidence from oculomotor studies. Biol Psychiatry 43:584–594, 1998

Szatmari P, Offord DR, Boyle MH: Ontario Child Health Study: prevalence of attention deficit disorder with hyperactivity. J Child Psychol Psychiatry 30:219–230, 1989

Tahir E, Yazgan Y, Cirakoglu B, et al: Association and linkage of DRD4 and DRD5 with attention deficit hyperactivity disorder (ADHD) in a sample of Turkish children. Mol Psychiatry 5:396–404, 2000

Tallal P, Townsend J, Curtiss S, et al: Phenotypic profiles of language-impaired children based on genetic/family history. Brain Lang 41:81–95, 1991

Tallal P, Miller SL, Bedi G, et al: Language comprehension in language-learning impaired children improved with acoustically modified speech. Science 271:81–84, 1996

Talley A, Dewhurst S, Perry S, et al: Tumor necrosis factor alpha induces apoptosis in human neuronal cells: protection by the antioxidant N-acetylcysteine and the genes bcl-2 and crmA. Mol Cell Biol 15:2359–2366, 1995

Tanguay PE: Pervasive developmental disorders: a 10-year review. J Am Acad Child Adolesc Psychiatry 39:1079–1095, 2000

Tardieu M, Le Chenadec J, Persoz A, et al: HIV-1–related encephalopathy in infants compared with children and adults. French Pediatric HIV Infection Study and the SEROCO Group. Neurology 54:1089–1095, 2000

Teicher MH: Psychological factors in neurological development, in Neurobiological Development, Vol 12. Edited by Evrard P, Minkowski A. New York, Nestle Nutrition Workshop Series, Raven, 1989, pp 243–258

Teicher MH: Actigraphy and motion analysis: new tools for psychiatry. Harv Rev Psychiatry 3:18–35, 1995

Teicher MH: Wounds that time won't heal: the neurobiology of child abuse. Cerebrum 2:50–67, 2000

Teicher MH, Glod CA: Neuroleptic drugs: indications and guidelines for their rational use in children and adolescents. J Child Adolesc Psychopharmacol 1:33–56, 1990

Teicher MH, Shaywitz BA, Kootz HL, et al: Differential effects of maternal and sibling presence on the hyperactivity of 6-hydroxydopamine treated developing rats. J Comp Physiol Psychol 95:134–135, 1981

Teicher MH, Glod CA, Surrey J, et al: Early childhood abuse and limbic system ratings in adult psychiatric outpatients. J Neuropsychiatry Clin Neurosci 5:301–306, 1993

Teicher MH, Ito Y, Glod CA, et al: Early abuse, limbic system dysfunction, and borderline personality disorder, in Biological and Neurobehavioral Studies of Borderline Personality Disorder. Edited by Silk K. Washington, DC, American Psychiatric Press, 1994, pp 177–207

Teicher MH, Andersen SL, Hostetter JC Jr: Evidence for dopamine receptor pruning between adolescence and adulthood in striatum but not nucleus accumbens. Brain Res Dev Brain Res 89:167–172, 1995

Teicher MH, Ito Y, Glod CA, et al: Neurophysiological mechanisms of stress response in children, in Severe Stress and Mental Disturbance in Children. Edited by Pfeffer C. Washington, DC, American Psychiatric Press, 1996a, pp 59–84

Teicher MH, Ito Y, Glod CA, et al: Objective measurement of hyperactivity and attentional problems in ADHD. J Am Acad Child Adolesc Psychiatry 35:334–342, 1996b

Teicher MH, Ito Y, Glod CA, et al: Preliminary evidence for abnormal cortical development in physically and sexually abused children using EEG coherence and MRI. Ann N Y Acad Sci 821:160–175, 1997

Teicher MH, Andersen SL, Dumont NL, et al: Childhood neglect attenuates development of the corpus callosum. Abstr Soc Neurosci 26:549, 2000a

Teicher MH, Anderson CM, Polcari A, et al: Functional deficits in basal ganglia of children with attention-deficit/hyperactivity disorder shown with functional magnetic imaging relaxometry. Nat Med 6:470–473, 2000b

Tenhula WN, Xu SZ, Madigan MC, et al: Morphometric comparisons of optic nerve axon loss in acquired immunodeficiency syndrome. Am J Ophthalmol 15:14–20, 1992

Tepper BJ, Farley JJ, Rothman MI, et al: Neurodevelopmental/neuroradiologic recovery of a child infected with HIV after treatment with combination antiretroviral therapy using the HIV-specific protease inhibitor ritonavir (case report). Pediatrics 101:E7, 1998

Thach WT, Goodkin HP, Keating JG: The cerebellum and the adaptive coordination of movement. Annu Rev Neurosci 15:403–442, 1992

Thapar A, Gottesman, Owen MJ, et al: The genetics of mental retardation. Br J Psychiatry 164:747–758, 1994

Tourette Syndrome Association International Consortium for Genetics: A complete genome screen in sib pairs affected by Gilles de la Tourette syndrome. Am J Hum Genet 65:1428–1436, 1999

Tryon WW: The role of motor excess and instrumented activity measurement in attention deficit hyperactivity disorder. Behav Modif 17:371–406, 1993

Turjanski N, Sawle GV, Playford ED, et al: PET studies of the presynaptic and postsynaptic dopaminergic system in Tourette's syndrome. J Neurol Neurosurg Psychiatry 57:688–692, 1994

Turk J: The fragile-X syndrome: on the way to a behavioural phenotype. Br J Psychiatry 160:24–35, 1992

Ultmann MH, Belman AL, Ruff HA, et al: Developmental abnormalities in children with acquired immune deficiency syndrome (AIDS): a follow up study. Int J Neurosci 32:661–667, 1987

Vaidya CJ, Austin G, Kirkorian G, et al: Selective effects of methylphenidate in attention deficit hyperactivity disorder: a functional magnetic resonance study. Proc Natl Acad Sci U S A 95:14494–14499, 1998

Van Bockstaele EJ, Colago EE, Valentino RJ: Amygdaloid corticotropin-releasing factor targets locus coeruleus dendrites: substrate for the co-ordination of emotional and cognitive limbs of the stress response. J Neuroendocrinol 10:743–757, 1998

van der Kolk B, Greenberg MS: The psychobiology of the trauma response: hyperarousal, constriction, and addiction to traumatic reexposure, in Psychological Trauma. Edited by van der Kolk B. Washington, DC, American Psychiatric Press, 1987, pp 63–87

Verkerk AJ, Pieretti M, Sutcliffe JS, et al: Identification of a gene (FMR1) containing a CGG repeat coincident with a breakage point cluster region exhibiting length variation in fragile X syndrome. Cell 65:905–914, 1991

Wada JA, Clarke R, Hamm A: Cerebral hemispheric asymmetry in humans. Arch Neurol 32:239–246, 1975

Waldman ID, Rowe A, Abramowitz S, et al: Association and linkage of the dopamine transporter gene and attention deficit hyperactivity disorder in children: heterogeneity owing to diagnostic subtype and severity. Am J Hum Genet 63:1767–1776, 1998

Walker EF: Developmentally moderated expressions of the neuropathology underlying schizophrenia. Schizophr Bull 20:453–480, 1994

Warren RP, Yonk J, Burger RW, et al: DR-positive T cells in autism: association with decreased plasma levels of the complement C4B protein. Neuropsychobiology 31:53–57, 1995

Weiss G, Milroy T, Perlman T: Psychiatric status of hyperactives as adults: a controlled prospective 15-year follow-up of 63 hyperactive children. J Am Acad Child Psychiatry 24:211–220, 1985

Weiss RE, Stein MA, Trommer B, et al: Attention-deficit hyperactivity disorder and thyroid function. J Pediatr 123:539–545, 1993

Wender PH: Methamphetamine in child psychiatry. J Child Adolesc Psychopharmacol 3:iv–vi, 1993

Wenk GL, Naidu S, Casanova MG, et al: Altered neurochemicals markers in Rett's syndrome. Neurology 41:1753–1756, 1991

Wilbur CB: Multiple personality and child abuse. An overview. Psychiatr Clin North Am 7:3–7, 1984

Wilens TE, Biederman J: The stimulants. Psychiatr Clin North Am 41:191–222, 1992

Wilens TE, Biederman J, Spencer TJ: Venlafaxine for adult ADHD (letter). Am J Psychiatry 152:1099–1100, 1995

Wiley CA, Schrier RD, Nelson JA, et al: Cellular localization of human immunodeficiency virus infection within the brains of acquired immune deficiency syndrome patients. Proc Natl Acad Sci U S A 83: 7089–7093, 1986

Wing L, Gould J: Severe impairments of social interaction and associated abnormalities in children: epidemiology and classification. J Autism Child Schizophr 9:11–29, 1979

Winsberg B, Comings DE: Association of the dopamine transporter gene (DAT1) with poor methylphenidate response. J Am Acad Child Adolesc Psychiatry 38:1474–1477, 1999

Wisniewski KE, Wisniewski HM, Wen GY: Occurrence of neuropathological changes and dementia of Alzheimer's disease in Down's syndrome. Ann Neurol 17:278–282, 1985

Wolf SS, Jones DW, Knable MB, et al: Tourette's syndrome: prediction of phenotypic variation in monozygotic twins by caudate nucleus D2 receptor binding. Science 273:1225–1227, 1996

Wolters PL, Brouwers P, Moss HA, et al: Differential receptive and expressive language functioning of children with symptomatic HIV disease and relation to CT scan brain abnormalities. Pediatrics 95: 112–119, 1995

Working Group of the American Academy of Neurology AIDS Task Force: Nomenclature and research case definitions for neurologic manifestations of human immunodeficiency virus type 1 infection. Neurology 41:778–785, 1991

World Health Organization: International Statistical Classification of Diseases and Related Health Problems, 10th Revision. Geneva, Switzerland, World Health Organization, 1992

Wyllie E, Rothner AD, Luders H: Partial seizures in children: clinical features, medical treatment, and surgical considerations. Pediatr Clin North Am 36:343–364, 1989

Young JG, Leven LI, Newcorn JH, et al: Genetic and neurobiological approaches to the pathophysiology of autism and the pervasive developmental disorders, in Psychopharmacology: The Third Generation of Progress. Edited by Meltzer HY. New York, Raven, 1985, pp 825–836

Zametkin AJ, Rapoport JL: Neurobiology of attention deficit disorder with hyperactivity: where have we come in 50 years? J Am Acad Child Adolesc Psychiatry 26:676–686, 1987

Zametkin AJ, Karoum F, Linnoila M, et al: Stimulants, urinary catecholamines, and indoleamines in hyperactivity. A comparison of methylphenidate and dextroamphetamine. Arch Gen Psychiatry 42:251–255, 1985

Zametkin AJ, Nordahl TE, Gross M, et al: Cerebral glucose metabolism in adults with hyperactivity of childhood onset. N Engl J Med 323:1361–1366, 1990

Zhang K, Tarazi FT, Baldessarini RJ: Regulation of dopamine D1- and D2-like receptors in transient hyperactivity following neonatal 6-hydroxydopamine lesions. Abstr Soc Neurosci 26:841, 2000

Zierler S, Krieger N, Tang Y, et al: Economic deprivation and AIDS incidence in Massachusetts. Am J Public Health 90:1064–1073, 2000

Zimmerman AM, Abrams MT, Giuliano JD, et al: Subcortical volumes in girls with Tourette syndrome: support for a gender effect. Neurology 54:2224–2229, 2000

Zoghbi HY, Percy AK, Glaze DG, et al: Reduction of biogenic amine levels in the Rett syndrome. N Engl J Med 313:921–941, 1985

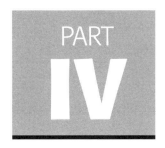

PART

IV

Neuropsychiatric Treatments

Psychopharmacologic Treatments for Patients With Neuropsychiatric Disorders

Peter P. Roy-Byrne, M.D.

Mahendra Upadhyaya, M.D.

Modern neuropsychiatry is concerned with the understanding and treatment of cognitive, emotional, and behavioral syndromes in patients with known neurologic illness or central nervous system (CNS) dysfunction. Although some syndromes (e.g., major depression) in patients with neurologic disease (e.g., cerebrovascular accident [CVA], head trauma) are clinically similar to those seen in well patients experiencing the syndrome de novo, treatment response may be quite different. Furthermore, the neuropsychiatric sequelae of a number of neurologic disorders frequently seem an amalgam of several syndromes and often do not fit neatly into DSM-IV (American Psychiatric Association 1994) syndromal definitions. Does the combative, irritable, agitated, brain-injured patient have dysphoric mania, agitated depression, or posttraumatic stress disorder (PTSD)? Does the apathetic, withdrawn, poststroke patient really have major depression? Although DSM-IV may be a useful starting point, departing from it is a frequent necessity.

Despite likely dissimilarities in the clinical presentation and treatment response of neuropsychiatric and psychiatric syndromes, the treatment of patients with neuropsychiatric illness has largely been modeled on known treatments of whatever syndrome (e.g., depression, psychosis) seems to be present. Unfortunately, the paucity of double-blind, placebo-controlled treatment studies in neuropsychiatric patients and the scarcity of even large case series make treatment at this point more art than science.

For this reason, this chapter does not duplicate material commonly found in numerous textbooks of psychopharmacology and psychiatric treatment. The neuropsychiatrist needs information on the psychopharmacologic treatment of neuropsychiatric patients and their syndromes rather than drug treatment of psychiatric illness in general. The chapter is not organized by medication but rather by syndrome so that the interested physician and trainee can more easily locate information relevant to a specific patient with a specific array of cognitive, emotional, and behavioral abnormalities. Side effects, drug interactions, and pharmacokinetic considerations are included only as they are pertinent to the neuropsychiatric context.

This chapter focuses on five major syndromes commonly seen by the treating neuropsychiatrist: depression, including apathetic, "deficit" states; psychosis; states of agitation, including anxiety and mania; aggression, impulsivity, and behavioral dyscontrol; and cognitive disturbance (amnesia, dementia). A common organization is employed throughout the chapter. Each syndrome is defined in enough detail to appreciate how it borders on and overlaps with the others. Following this, studies, case series, and isolated case reports are reviewed. Issues of dosage, treatment duration, and response course are considered. Finally, side effects, pharmacokinetic considerations, and drug interactions are highlighted.

Approach to the Neuropsychiatric Patient

The psychiatrist who is asked to assess a neuropsychiatric patient for pharmacologic treatment must first become familiar with the nature and course of the underlying neurologic illness because apparently distinct neurologic and psychiatric symptoms often arise from similar mechanisms intrinsic to the neurologic disorder (e.g., psychosis in CNS neoplasms). Conversely, similar symptoms can be caused

by distinct neurologic and psychiatric disorders as well as by the side effects of both neurologic and psychotropic medications (e.g., both Parkinson's bradykinesia and phenytoin-induced lethargy may be mistaken for signs of depression).

Many patients have no prior experience with the mental health system and may feel surprised and even threatened that a psychiatrist has been called. The fear of further loss of control in a situation that already feels out of control may be quite profound. Usually, however, once the patient's psychological and behavioral symptoms are explained as those that are frequently encountered as part of the symptom complex of the neurologic disorder—and can potentially be treated—the patient will be placed at ease and relieved. Presenting the pharmacologic intervention as a way to assist recovery during a period of intense stress and adaptation will help the patient feel more hopeful and maintain an internal locus of control. Realistic expectations, including the possibility of incomplete remission of symptoms, must be conveyed from the outset so that the patient who is already frustrated with an often slow and arduous rehabilitation process does not become even more hopeless if some symptoms persist.

The next step in evaluating a neurologic patient's appropriateness for psychotropic medication involves obtaining a careful history of premorbid psychiatric problems, personality traits, and coping styles. Multiple informants often will minimize informational bias (Strauss et al. 1997). The psychiatric symptoms may have predated the onset of neurologic symptoms and will provide clues regarding diagnosis and subsequent treatment. Because CNS, particularly frontal lobe, insults frequently amplify underlying character traits (Prigatano 1992), it may be unrealistic to attempt to completely attenuate specific behaviors and traits that appear to be a direct result of the neurologic insult. Optimal treatment must take into account whether the psychiatric symptoms preexisted the neurologic disorder, arose as a neurologically or psychologically mediated result of the neurologic insult, or surfaced as a reaction to the resulting disability and loss. Certain premorbid traits, such as IQ, may have implications for course of illness (Palsson et al. 1999).

Documentation of symptoms will help in tracking what is often slow improvement that appears subjectively inapparent to the patient and caregivers but may be real improvement in functioning. Although it may be impractical to completely document all symptoms, specific target symptoms and functional goals should be measured and documented in as great detail as possible. Caregivers, significant others, and, in certain cases, patients can be asked to use simple, anchored 0–10 scales to rate the severity of symptoms and functional impairment over time. Figure 19–1 depicts one simple example of such a scale, which allows the clinician to fill in items tailored to the particular patient's symptoms and problems.

A basic tenet of treating psychiatric symptoms in patients with neurologic disorders is to treat as many signs and symptoms with as few medications as possible. Therefore, a patient with a severe head injury who may be having complex partial seizures and is exhibiting labile affect and impulsivity should be considered for treatment with carbamazepine or valproate, which may treat both the patient's seizure disorder and his or her affective and behavioral symptoms, rather than combining phenytoin and lithium. Potential "neuroprotective" effects of psychotropic medications should be considered in stroke or head-injury patients (Alexopoulos et al. 1997),

as should the rare possibility that the effects of medications could worsen the underlying illness.

Detailed knowledge of the patient's stage in rehabilitation as well as the patient's current social, occupational, and interpersonal status is required to tailor the pharmacologic regimen to specific practical needs and limitations. For example, starting a potentially sedating medication at a time when a rigorous physical therapy regimen is being initiated or during a long-awaited reentry into the workplace would be ill-advised.

Before administering psychotropic medications, pertinent laboratory tests must be obtained. Because of the patient's susceptibility to medication side effects, the clinician should start at a lower dose of medication and titrate more slowly, although the patient may ultimately require the same dose of medication as the nonneurologic patient (i.e., "Start low and go slow, but go"). Side effects should be well documented, using standardized measures, whenever possible.

Treatment of symptoms secondary to the primary neurologic disorder, such as pain and sleep disturbance, may decrease psychiatric symptoms sufficiently to allow avoidance of further psychopharmacotherapy. Similarly, appropriately treating a psychiatric symptom early in its presentation before it can exacerbate the neurologic disorder may significantly improve the patient's overall functioning.

Once medication has been initiated, all available tools to subjectively follow pharmacokinetics and pharmacologic efficacy must be considered. For example, medication blood levels, physiologic response (such as vital signs), laboratory monitoring (such as electroencephalography), and neuropsychological testing can all be helpful. Figure 19–2 sums up many of the points in this section.

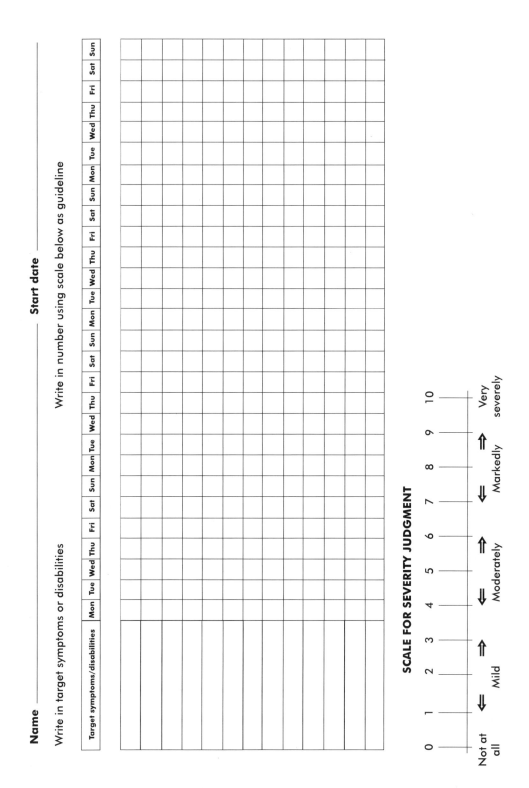

FIGURE 19–1.   Rating scale for the assessment of medication efficacy.

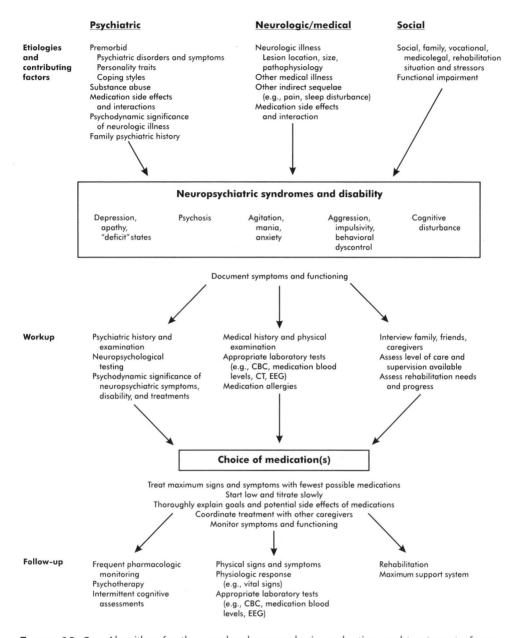

FIGURE 19–2.   Algorithm for the psychopharmacologic evaluation and treatment of neuropsychiatric patients.

CBC = complete blood cell count; CT = computed tomography; EEG = electroencephalogram.

Depression, Apathy, and "Deficit" States

Major depression and dysthymia are among the most common psychiatric disorders. Although decades of clinical observation and research have clearly delineated retarded and agitated subtypes of depression, few consistent clinical or biological differences between the two have emerged (Goodwin and Jamison 1990), and even the clinical maxim of avoiding the use of "activating" antidepressants in anxious depressed individuals has been disproved (Tollefson et al. 1994). In contrast, this distinction is more important in the assessment and treatment of neuropsychiatric patients. In these patients, the overlap of agitated states with behavioral dyscontrol, delirium, and occasionally psychosis, along with the greater prevalence of states of apathy—in which cognitive and behavioral slowing occur in the absence of mood disturbance (Levy et al. 1998)—argues for separate consideration of retarded depression, in conjunction with apathetic and other deficit-like states. However, admixtures of subjective anxiety, nervousness, and worry, without significant (i.e., clinically predominant) agitation, is also considered in this section.

Treatment

In contrast to the plethora of double-blind, placebo-controlled trials of various antidepressants in major depression, there are relatively few such studies in depressed patients with neurologic illness.

Placebo-controlled studies have examined the efficacy of nortriptyline (Lipsey et al. 1984), trazodone (Reding et al. 1986), and citalopram (G. Andersen et al. 1994) in depressed CVA patients; of imipramine (Strang 1965), nortriptyline (J. Andersen et al. 1980), desipramine (Laitinen 1969), and bupropion (Goetz et al. 1984) in depressed Parkinson's disease patients; of desipramine in depressed multiple sclerosis patients (Schiffer and Wineman 1990); of imipramine (Reifler et al. 1989), clomipramine (Petracca et al. 1996), moclobemide (M. Roth et al. 1996), maprotiline (Fuchs et al.1993), citalopram (Nyth et al. 1992), and sertraline (Magai et al. 2000) in depressed Alzheimer's disease patients; of desipramine in depressed traumatic brain injury (TBI) patients (Wroblewski et al. 1996); and of fluoxetine in depressed

patients with Huntington's disease (Como et al. 1997). Although studies have documented selective serotonin reuptake inhibitor (SSRI) (Elliott et al. 1998; Zisook et al. 1998) and imipramine (Elliott et al. 1998; Rabkin et al. 1994) efficacy in depressed patients with human immunodeficiency virus (HIV) disease, most patients in these studies were not in the late stages of HIV illness and likely had major depression relatively little affected by CNS viral involvement. Several studies of the monoamine oxidase B (MAO-B) inhibitor selegiline in Parkinson's disease patients measured effects on depression as a secondary phenomenon (Klaassen et al. 1995).

All but four of the studies cited above report a greater efficacy of the active drug compared with placebo in the course of trial durations between 4 and 8 weeks. Type of illness (Huntington's disease; Como et al. 1997) and patient (advanced Alzheimer's disease; Magai et al. 2000) may have affected response in these negative studies. The group of Parkinson's disease studies reported response rates somewhat lower (i.e., 60%) than in non–medically ill depressed patients. Many studies have purposely employed lower (e.g., trazodone 200 mg [Reding et al. 1986]) doses, as would be used in elderly patients, and earlier studies using normal doses of tricyclics have sometimes shown a high frequency of side effects (e.g., 18% rate of delirium in CVA patients [Lipsey et al. 1984]) and an inability to reach therapeutic blood levels in multiple sclerosis due to side effects [Schiffer and Wineman 1990]).

A provocative 12-week comparison study (Robinson et al. 2000) showed that nortriptyline was superior to fluoxetine in depressed CVA patients, although a similar comparison of amitriptyline and fluoxetine in depressed patients with Alzheimer's disease (Taragano et al.

1997) showed equal efficacy, and a study of nondepressed CVA patients with hemiplegia showed that fluoxetine was superior to both maprotiline and placebo in facilitating rehabilitation therapy, supporting a distinct functional effect in the absence of depression (Dam et al. 1996). This finding, effects of SSRIs on "emotional incontinence" (i.e., pathologic crying in the absence of depression) (Nahas et al. 1998; Seliger et al. 1992), and the broader spectrum of action of SSRIs in general probably make them advantageous in many situations, despite the findings of Robinson et al. (2000).

Uncontrolled reports of antidepressant treatment are mixed, with two early reports showing little effect of amitriptyline and phenelzine in moderately injured TBI patients (Dinan and Mobayed 1992; Saran 1985), whereas a more recent trial in mild TBI patients showed good effect with sertraline (Fann et al. 2000).

Except for the possibility that anticholinergic activity could be a theoretical advantage in Parkinson's disease, the sedation, postural hypotension, modest hypertensive, and seizure threshold lowering effects of tricyclic antidepressants (TCAs) limit their usefulness in most neuropsychiatric patients. In one study of 68 brain-injured patients (Wroblewski et al. 1990), 20% of them developed seizures, largely due to TCAs they were taking. In HIV disease patients, imipramine was much less tolerable than paroxetine (Elliott et al. 1998), and in multiple sclerosis patients TCAs produced twice the side-effect rate of SSRIs (Scott et al. 1996). With the substantial experience with SSRIs during the last decade, there is good reason to believe their lower side-effect profile and once-daily dosing would make them preferable agents in neurologically compromised depressed patients. Among isolated reports noting CNS side effects with SSRIs, extrapyramidal side effects (EPS) are most common (Leo 1996), although large case series suggest these effects are not typical for more obviously vulnerable patients with either Parkinson's disease (Caley and Friedman 1992) or multiple sclerosis (Flax et al. 1991).

There would seem to be little reason to use nonselective monoamine oxidase inhibitors (MAOIs). Selegiline, a selective MAO-B inhibitor, would seem to be a good choice for Parkinson's disease patients because it has primary effects on the underlying illness. However, the lower doses used to treat Parkinson's disease symptoms have not usually been effective in studies of primary major depression, which usually requires higher doses that also inhibit MAO-A. Finally, bupropion was found to be effective in fewer than half of Parkinson's disease patients in one study (Goetz et al. 1984). Although its potential to lower seizure threshold is a particular liability in a neurologically ill population, the dose dependence of this side effect may make lower doses more acceptable.

Although strategies using dopaminergic agents have been particularly recommended for states of apathy often seen in Parkinson's disease patients, sometimes without accompanying depression (Marin et al. 1995), Parkinson's disease patients do not experience euphoria in response to methylphenidate, possibly reflecting degeneration of dopaminergic neurons with decreased dopamine availability (Cantello et al. 1989). However, more direct-acting agonists such as bromocriptine and amantadine have been found to be effective in these groups of patients (Jouvent et al. 1983) as well as in individual patients with TBI-associated apathy (Van Reekum et al. 1995). Stimulants such as methylphenidate have been extremely effective in Alzheimer's dementia and vascular dementia (Galynker et al.

1997) and in CVA patients (Grade et al. 1998); can work within 2 days (Masand et al. 1991); and promote improved participation in rehabilitation and enhanced functioning (Crisostomo et al. 1988). One retrospective case series documented efficacy in depressed CVA patients comparable to that of nortriptyline, with a more rapid onset of effect and a similar side-effect profile (Lazarus et al. 1994). A tendency for stimulants to reduce seizure frequency (Wroblewski et al. 1992) or to enhance neuronal recovery (Feeney et al. 1982) in brain injury patients may be other advantages. Methylphenidate has also been effective in improving impairments in psychomotor speech and arousal in three apathetic patients with brain tumors (Weitzner et al. 1995). A documented effect of pemoline compared with placebo on fatigue in 50% of multiple sclerosis patients is noteworthy (Weinshenker et al. 1992), although the drug was not very well tolerated because of anorexia, irritability, and insomnia. Patients with HIV-related apathetic depression have done particularly well with methylphenidate in case reports (White et al. 1992). However, other reports have claimed that dopaminergic agents, while improving affect and cognitive function, may be less effective on core symptoms of apathy such as lack of initiative (Salloway 1994), and they could provoke psychosis in Parkinson's disease and other vulnerable patients.

Finally, electroconvulsive therapy (ECT) is an effective treatment in Parkinson's disease patients that also transiently improves core motor symptoms (Kellner et al. 1994). Five of six patients with Huntington's disease also improved with ECT, although one patient developed delirium and another developed a worsening of the movement disorder (Ranen et al. 1994). ECT has been used to treat depression in

a patient with frontal craniotomy and residual meningioma (Starkstein and Migliorelli 1993). Reports of a high rate of ECT-induced delirium in Parkinson's disease patients, alone (Oh et al. 1992) and in comparison with CVA patients (Fiegel 1992), have been interpreted as being due to denervation supersensitivity of dopamine receptors, and reduction of dopaminergic drugs before ECT has been advised (Rudorfer et al. 1992). In general, patients with more severe depression often accompanied by psychosis may be the best candidates for ECT. States of catatonia are extreme examples of deficit states and are known to be most strongly related to affective illness rather than psychosis. Although ECT is certainly effective in these conditions as well, parenteral benzodiazepines are also highly effective (Gaind et al. 1994) and can result in reversal of the catatonic state, usually within hours to days.

In summary, SSRIs may be the treatment of choice in neuropsychiatrically ill patients with depression, especially if there is more anxiety or at least a relative absence of apathy. The question of whether tricyclics really are superior to SSRIs in CVA patients requires further study. SSRIs with relatively shorter half-lives (paroxetine, fluvoxamine) or absence of inhibition of select microsomal enzyme systems (citalopram, sertraline, paroxetine, fluvoxamine) may be advantageous in some cases. Because of the potentially activating properties of the SSRIs, they should be started at about half the usual starting dose and titrated up to standard antidepressant doses in the first 1–3 weeks. Brain-injured patients may also be at an increased risk for sedation with the SSRIs (Cassidy 1989). Venlafaxine at lower doses is less likely to cause hypertension but also acts more like a pure SSRI, with noradrenergic properties requiring higher (≥225 mg) doses. Nefazodone, a serotonin type 2 (5-HT$_2$) receptor blocker with mild reuptake blocking effects, may also have a place in treating patients with anxiety (Balon 1998) or HIV depression (Elliott et al. 1999). Mirtazapine's effect in increasing appetite could be advantageous in HIV (Elliott and Roy-Byrne 2000) or Alzheimer's (Raji and Brady 2001) patients with wasting, although sedative side effects may limit its use in some patients. More apathetic states could be treated with dopaminergic strategies, including bupropion, bromocriptine, amantadine, and stimulants. TCAs, if used, should probably be limited to desipramine (lowest anticholinergic effects) and nortriptyline (lowest hypotensive effects, low anticholinergic effects, and good blood level data for interpretation). If an MAOI is to be used, tranylcypromine should probably be avoided because of occasional spontaneous hypertensive crises, even when an MAOI diet is followed (Keck et al. 1989). Table 19–1 lists characteristic antidepressants recommended in this section, dose ranges, side effects, and relevant drug interactions.

Psychosis

Psychotic states (hallucinations, delusions, and formal thought disorder) principally occur in schizophrenia and less commonly in mania and depression. Psychosis occurs less frequently overall in neurologic patients than does depression, agitation, or cognitive impairment and often may be associated with and a result of cognitive impairment, as in the paranoid delusions of Alzheimer's disease patients. When it occurs, psychosis can have a serious impact on patient care, causing noncompliance with needed medical interventions, behavior that may lead to self-harm or injury, and caregiver with-

drawal from the patient. In these circumstances, rapid and definitive treatment of psychosis is always indicated whether it occurs in isolation or, more commonly, in combination with states of agitation, cognitive impairment, and occasionally aggression.

Treatment

Neuroleptic (antipsychotic) medications remain the mainstay in pharmacologic treatment of psychosis. There is little evidence that other agents sometimes used as effective adjuncts to neuroleptics (e.g., anticonvulsants, benzodiazepines) have primary antipsychotic effects of their own. The recent introduction of the atypical neuroleptics risperidone, olanzapine, and quetiapine offers for the first time both a chance of expanded efficacy and diminished side effects. These advantages are even more prominent in neuropsychiatric patients, who are more prone to neurologic side effects.

Typical neuroleptics have been most often studied in the mixed psychosis and agitation of dementia patients. Although an early placebo-controlled study showing superiority of both haloperidol (mean dose, 4.6 mg) and loxapine (mean dose, 22 mg) (Petrie et al. 1982) reported that only one-third of patients showed significant improvement, a more recent study (Devanand et al. 1998) showed a response rate of 55%–60% with 2–3 mg haloperidol, superior to the 30% rate with 0.5 mg and consistent with the surprisingly high correlations obtained between blood levels of haloperidol and change on the psychosis factor of the Brief Psychiatric Rating Scale (BPRS) in the earlier study by the same researchers (Devanand et al. 1992). In contrast, correlations between blood level and hostility/agitation were much lower. Unfortunately, studies still suggest that patients with dementia are overtreated with neuroleptics, with 20 of

TABLE 19–1. Antidepressants

Drug	Starting daily dose (mg)	Target daily dose (mg)	Neuropsychiatric side effects	Neuropsychiatric drug interactions	Comments
Tricyclic antidepressants (TCAs)					
Nortriptyline	10	30–100	Dizziness, fatigue, drowsiness, tremor, nervousness, confusion (esp. w/nortriptyline), insomnia (esp. w/desipramine), headache, seizures, anticholinergic effects Other: orthostatic hypotension, ECG alterations, cardiac conduction delay, tachycardia, sexual dysfunction, weight gain	↑ Blood level w/SSRIs, methylphenidate, neuroleptics, valproate, opioids ↓ Blood level w/CBZ, phenytoin, barbiturates ↑ Blood level of neuroleptics, CBZ, opioids ↓ Blood level of levodopa Additive anticholinergic effects w/neuroleptics, antiparkinsonians, antihistamines	Low, but present, anticholinergic and hypotensive potential Blood level monitoring available Antiarrhythmic properties Analgesic effects, including for neuropathic pain
Desipramine	25	75–200			
Selective serotonin reuptake inhibitors (SSRIs)					
Fluoxetine	5	10–80	Drowsiness (esp. w/paroxetine, fluvoxamine), nervousness (esp. w/fluoxetine), fatigue (esp. w/paroxetine), insomnia, tremor, dizziness, headache, confusion, paresthesia Other: nausea, sexual dysfunction, weight loss	Sedation w/antihistamines, chloral hydrate Lethargy, impaired consciousness w/metoprolol, propranolol Excitation and hallucinations w/narcotics EPS w/neuroleptics Neurotoxicity w/lithium Serotonergic effects w/lithium, buspirone, sumatriptan Serotonin syndrome w/other serotonergic drugs (e.g., MAOIs, opioids)	*Fluoxetine:* May have "therapeutic window" May require up to 8 weeks to reach steady state Most inhibition of hepatic cytochrome P450 2D6 enzymes of the SSRIs; also inhibits 2C and $3A_4$ Potential use in cataplexy Antimyoclonic adjunct w/oxitriptan *Sertraline:* ↑ Plasma level w/food Most likely to cause diarrhea
Sertraline	25	50–200			
Paroxetine	10	20–60			
Fluvoxamine	25	50–300			
Citalopram	10	20–60			

TABLE 19–1. Antidepressants (*continued*)

Drug	Starting daily dose (mg)	Target daily dose (mg)	Neuropsychiatric side effects	Neuropsychiatric drug interactions	Comments
Selective serotonin reuptake inhibitors (SSRIs) (*continued*)				Contraindicated w/MAOIs ↑ Blood level w/valproate ↓ Blood level w/CBZ ↑ Blood level of TCAs, neuroleptics, BZDs, CBZ, valproate, phenytoin, propranolol (esp. w/fluoxetine, paroxetine)	Least inhibition of cytochrome P450 2D6 but does inhibit 2C and 3A$_4$ *Paroxetine:* More sedating, less stimulating, and shorter half-life than sertraline and fluoxetine; withdrawal syndrome more likely Inhibition of cytochrome P450 2D6 but not 2C and 3A$_4$; can inhibit trazodone metabolism; withdrawal syndrome more likely *Fluvoxamine:* Twice-daily administration Most sedating and shortest half-life of SSRIs; withdrawal syndrome most likely Least bound to plasma proteins and no inhibition of hepatic cytochrome P450 2D6 enzymes; does inhibit 1A2, 2C, and 3A$_4$ enzymes Least ejaculatory delay of SSRIs *Citalopram:* Minimal to no cytochrome inhibition Most purely serotonergic in vitro

TABLE 19–1.   Antidepressants (continued)

Drug	Starting daily dose (mg)	Target daily dose (mg)	Neuropsychiatric side effects	Neuropsychiatric drug interactions	Comments
Atypical antidepressants					
Bupropion	75–100	200–450	Nervousness, tremor, dizziness, insomnia, headache, confusion, paresthesia, drowsiness, seizures	Contraindicated w/MAOIs Caution w/levodopa ↑ Blood level w/CBZ	↑ Risk of seizures, esp. w/doses >450 mg/day, >150 mg/dose Contraindicated in seizure disorders, bulimia, anorexia nervosa Fewer drug interactions than SSRIs
Trazodone	50–100	150–400	Drowsiness, dizziness, confusion, fatigue, nervousness, incoordination, headache, tremor, paresthesia Other: hypotension, priapism	Additive CNS depressant effects w/ other CNS depressants Serotonin syndrome w/other serotonergic drugs ↑ Blood level w/paroxetine, phenytoin ↑ Blood level of phenytoin Inhibits antihypertensive effects of clonidine	Risk of hypotension Occasionally enhances sex drive Two to three divided doses May be useful in drug-induced dyskinesia Priapism very rare but serious
Venlafaxine	18.75–50.0	75–225	Drowsiness, nervousness, dizziness, anorexia, insomnia, fatigue, tremor, headache, confusion, paresthesia Other: sexual dysfunction, hypertension	Contraindicated w/MAOIs	Risk of hypertension, esp. w/doses >200 mg No known cytochrome P450 effects

TABLE 19–1.   Antidepressants (continued)

Drug	Starting daily dose (mg)	Target daily dose (mg)	Neuropsychiatric side effects	Neuropsychiatric drug interactions	Comments
Atypical antidepressants (continued)					
Nefazodone	50–100	200–500	Dizziness, drowsiness, confusion, fatigue, headache, insomnia, paresthesia, tremor	Potential interaction w/MAOIs; ↑ Blood levels of triazolam, alprazolam; Potential ↑ of nefazodone and other drugs that are highly protein bound	Risk of hypotension; Two divided doses; Potent inhibitor of P450 $3A_4$
Mirtazapine	15	30–45	Sedation (less with higher doses), weight gain, agranulocytosis (very rare)	Contraindicated w/MAOIs	No in vitro cytochrome enzyme inhibition; Minimal controlled data in conditions other than depression
Psychostimulants					
Methylphenidate	5–30	10–90	Nervousness, insomnia, dizziness, headache, dyskinesia, drowsiness, confusion, delusions, rebound depression, hallucinations, Tourette's, tics; Other: anorexia, palpitations, blood pressure and pulse changes, cardiac arrhythmia, weight loss	Hypertension w/MAOIs; ↑ Blood levels of TCAs, phenytoin, phenobarbital, primidone; Antagonistic effect by neuroleptics, phenobarbital	Contraindicated in marked anxiety, tension, agitation; Fast onset of action; Give early in day, divided doses (methylphenidate three times daily, dextroamphetamine twice daily); Dependence rare in medically ill; May precipitate or worsen Tourette's or dyskinesia
Dextroamphetamine	2.5–20	5–60			

Note.   BZDs = benzodiazepines; CBZ = carbamazepine; CNS = central nervous system; ECG = electrocardiogram; EPS = extrapyramidal symptoms; MAOIs = monoamine oxidase inhibitors; OCD = obsessive-compulsive disorder; SSRIs = selective serotonin reuptake inhibitors; TCAs = tricyclic antidepressants.

22 nursing-home patients able to successfully discontinue these drugs in a recent study (Bridges-Parlet et al. 1997).

Despite a long history of use of typical neuroleptics in epilepsy-related psychosis, the treatment of psychosis in epilepsy has not been subjected to controlled study, and even uncontrolled reports are scarce. The often-cited phenomenon of forced normalization (i.e., worsening psychosis with better seizure control) is actually quite rare. More likely, chronic interictal psychosis should be treated with neuroleptics, with careful attention to effects on seizure frequency. In one report (Onuma et al. 1991), 11 of 21 patients (52%) showed aggravation of symptoms with decrease or discontinuation of neuroleptics. This suggests that patients should be carefully monitored to determine if ongoing neuroleptics are truly required.

Much of the recent literature on atypical neuroleptics has focused on Parkinson's disease patients, who, because of their unique sensitivity to EPS, provide the most sensitive test for neuroleptic side effects. The only medication with confirmed antipsychotic benefit without worsening Parkinson's disease is clozapine, based on a recent double-blind, placebo-controlled trial (Parkinson Study Group 1999) with a mean dose of 25 mg. This is consistent with a review (Musser and Akil 1996) citing 16 reports in 167 patients documenting antipsychotic efficacy, often with several days' onset and usually at very low doses. Long-term treatment (1–2 years) continued to be effective in many patients. In many patients, doses of levodopa can be increased without motor or psychotic decompensation. Experts recommend starting with very low doses (e.g., 6.25 mg), because sedation is a major problem.

Clozapine significantly lowers the seizure threshold and produces electroencephalographic abnormalities in most non–neurologically ill patients at some time during treatment (Malow et al. 1994; Welch et al. 1994). In schizophrenic patients, seizures are dose dependent (Haller and Binder 1990), and both slow titration and lower ceiling doses (below 600 mg) may reduce the likelihood of seizures. In the neuropsychiatric population, doses far lower than these are likely to provoke seizures. Both seizures and myoclonus due to clozapine may respond to valproate (Meltzer and Ranjan 1994). Reports in neuropsychiatric groups suggest that preexisting electroencephalographic abnormalities predict liability to develop delirium (Duffy and Kant 1996).

Although risperidone, olanzapine, and quetiapine have all been shown to produce minimal EPS in schizophrenic patients, the emerging data in Parkinson's disease patients suggest that, although they are a vast improvement over typical neuroleptics, clozapine is probably superior to them (Gimenez-Roldan et al. 2001), and they may still produce EPS to varying degrees. Hence, in Parkinson's disease, reports show that olanzapine and risperidone can either worsen (Ford et al. 1994; Graham et al. 1998) or have no effect on (Aarsland et al. 1999; Wolters et al. 1996; Workman et al. 1997) underlying Parkinson's disease. The less widely used drug quetiapine has mostly been reported to work without worsening underlying disease (Dewey and O'Suilleabhain 2000; Fernandez et al. 1999; Parsa and Bastani 1998; Targum and Abbott 2000), consistent with a recent study suggesting that it produces fewer EPS in a heterogeneous group of psychotic elderly patients compared with risperidone (Yeung et al. 1999). However, switching patients from olanzapine to quetiapine is only variably successful (Fernandez et al. 1999), and in one report quetiapine was only useful for visual hallucinations and had poor efficacy against delusions. Nonetheless, one recent review suggests that quetiapine probably produces less worsening of motor features of Parkinson's disease than does olanzapine, which may cause fewer EPS compared with risperidone (Friedman and Factor 2000), although its limited use and distribution compared with the others may compromise this interpretation. This review also emphasized more fine-tuning of antiparkinsonian medications, with lowering doses of both anticholinergics and dopaminergics before initiation of neuroleptics. Although many patients may be unable to switch from clozapine to olanzapine (J.H. Friedman et al. 1998) or quetiapine (Fernandez et al. 1999), the side-effect burden of clozapine suggests that other agents may be preferable first-line medications in Parkinson's disease.

There is a growing number of recent reports on the efficacy of atypical neuroleptics in dementia-related psychoses. A 12-week double-blind, placebo-controlled study in 625 patients with severe dementia and significant psychosis tested three daily doses of risperidone and found 1 and 2 mg, but not 0.5 mg, to be effective. Only the 1-mg dose gave a frequency of EPS not different from placebo (Katz et al. 1999). In open studies in dementia using mean doses closer to 2 mg, the rate of EPS was 32% (Irizarry et al. 1999) and 50% (Herrmann et al. 1998), supporting a narrow dose window for this drug. A 6-week double-blind, placebo-controlled study of 206 nursing home patients with Alzheimer's disease showed antipsychotic effects with 5 mg and 10 mg, but not 20 mg, of olanzapine (Street et al. 2000). Reports in the more severe Lewy body dementia suggest marked side effects of confusion with clozapine (Burke et al. 1998) and intolerance in 3 of 8 patients with olanzapine (Walker et al. 1999), although other reports (Allen et al. 1995 with risperidone; Chacko et al. 1993 with

clozapine) indicate efficacy with good tolerability.

Results are mixed in other patient groups. Singh et al. (1997) reported substantial efficacy without EPS for risperidone in 20 of 21 psychotic HIV patients, and Lera and Zirulnik (1999) reported good efficacy for clozapine in psychotic HIV patients who experienced EPS with typical neuroleptics, although other reports indicate both EPS with risperidone and akathisia with olanzapine (Meyer et al. 1998). Use of atypicals in movement disorders such as Huntington's disease indicate benefits on chorea as well as psychosis only when higher doses of 6 mg of risperidone are used (Dallocchio et al. 1999; Parsa et al. 1997); studies also show problems with Huntington's disease patients tolerating the high doses of clozapine needed to be effective, with marked disability in most of these patients with doses of 150 mg (van Vugt et al. 1997). Risperidone has been effective in 5 of 6 patients with TBI without EPS (Duffy and Kant 1996) and, in other reports, was superior to conventional neuroleptics in improving TBI psychosis, sleep and daytime alertness (Schreiber et al. 1998), and psychosis following ischemic brain damage (Zimnitzky et al. 1996). Finally, risperidone has been effective for psychosis associated with neurosarcoidosis (Popli 1997). Doses between 3 and 6 mg were used in these studies.

In summary, neuroleptic medications appear to be the mainstay treatments for psychosis although they still have side effects in some patients. Clozapine is least likely to have motor side effects, although seizure threshold–lowering effects are more problematic in neurologically compromised patients. It may be preferred in unusually EPS-sensitive patients with Parkinson's disease, Huntington's disease, and other conditions with basal ganglia involvement. The use of very low doses may mitigate this effect. In most neurologic disorders, patients will show exaggerated sensitivity to motor side effects, making atypical neuroleptics the treatment of choice. Studies of discontinuation of neuroleptics have also shown that long-term treatment in Alzheimer's disease patients is often unnecessary (Risse et al. 1987). Table 19–2 lists characteristic antipsychotics recommended in this section, dose ranges, side effects, and relevant drug interactions.

Agitated States, Including Anxiety and Mania

Syndromes of agitation span the entire spectrum of psychiatric illness, occurring in mood, anxiety, psychotic, dementing, and impulse dyscontrol disorders. In the absence of frank psychosis, dementia, or delirium, the differential diagnosis of prominent agitation is still extremely difficult, as states of agitated depression, mixed bipolar affective state/dysphoric mania, and severe panic anxiety merge with frequently ambiguous boundaries. This section highlights this symptom complex, principally as it presents in states of anxiety, mania, and severe agitated depression. We use this syndrome to discuss two major classes of drugs: the anxiolytics (e.g., benzodiazepines and azapirones) and the thymoleptics (e.g., lithium, valproic acid, and carbamazepine). Effects of antidepressants and neuroleptics on agitation are also highlighted.

Treatment

Despite the high prevalence of agitated states in various neuropsychiatric conditions, there are far fewer double-blind, placebo-controlled studies than for depressed states. Although virtually every psychotropic agent has been, and will continue to be, used for agitation, there is emerging evidence that the anticonvulsants may have particular utility in managing secondary mania, withdrawal-related anxiety states, panic anxiety associated with electroencephalographic abnormalities, and the agitation seen in some dementias. However, there is still only scattered scientific validation of the following treatment suggestions.

In the management of manic states, anticonvulsants have been recommended for some time in cases in which "neurologic" factors, including substance abuse, have been present (Pope et al. 1988). Scattered reports have suggested efficacy for carbamazepine in elderly neurologic manic patients intolerant to lithium (McFarland et al. 1990); in mentally retarded manic patients (Glue 1989); in patients with HIV-related mania resistant to lithium (Halman et al. 1993); in TBI patients with agitation (Azouvi et al. 1999); and in patients with Alzheimer's-related agitation resistant to neuroleptics (Gleason and Schneider 1990; Lemke 1995). Valproate has reportedly been effective in mentally retarded manic patients (Sovner 1989); in agitated patients with dementia (8 of 10, Lott et al. 1995; 7 of 15, Narayan and Nelson 1997; 6 of 13, Porsteinsson et al. 1997; but see also only 1 of 15, Herrmann 1998); and in agitated patients with brain injury (Horne and Lindley 1995). Blood levels have varied widely (14–107 µg/mL), although all reports showed some responders at levels below 50 µg/mL. These uncontrolled reports have now been validated for both drugs in placebo-controlled trials. For carbamazepine, a placebo-controlled trial in 51 patients showed such superior efficacy (71% vs. 21% response; mean level, 5.3 µg/mL) that the trial was prematurely terminated (Tariot et al. 1998b). More recently, Porsteinsson et al. (2001) documented effi-

TABLE 19–2.   Antipsychotics

Drug	Starting daily dose (mg)	Target daily dose (mg)	Neuropsychiatric side effects	Neuropsychiatric drug interactions	Comments
Haloperidol	1–5	2–20	Parkinsonism, dystonia, akathisia, perioral (rabbit) tremor, anticholinergic effects, sedation, confusion, impaired psychomotor performance, TD, NMS, orthostatic hypotension, ejaculatory inhibition, priapism, dysphagia, urinary incontinence, temperature dysregulation, sudden death	Additive CNS depressant effects w/other CNS depressants	*Haloperidol:* Most EPS potential, esp. w/low calcium, akathisia w/low iron
Perphenazine	4–16	8–40		Additive anticholinergic effects w/ other anticholinergic drugs	Intravenous route provides rapid onset of action w/ potentially lower risk of EPS
Thioridazine	10–200	100–800		↑ EPS w/SSRIs, lithium, buspirone	Available in decanoate form
				Neurotoxicity w/lithium	Useful in Huntington's, Tourette's
				↑ Blood level w/TCAs, SSRIs, MAOIs, alprazolam, buspirone, β-adrenergic blockers	*Thioridazine:* Most anticholinergic, sedating, and risk for hypotension at doses >800 mg
			Other: slowed cardiac conduction (esp. w/thioridazine), photosensitivity, hyperthermia, hyperprolactinemia, weight gain	↓ Blood level w/lithium, CBZ, phenytoin, phenobarbital, antiparkinsonians	Has been used for symptomatic management of agitation, anxiety, depressed mood, sleep disturbances, and fears in geriatric patients
				↓ Blood level of TCAs, valproate, phenytoin, β-adrenergic blockers	
Risperidone	1–2	2–10	Insomnia, agitation, EPS, headache, anxiety, dizziness, sommolence, aggressive reaction, NMS, risk of TD not yet determined	May antagonize effects of levodopa and dopamine agonists	Maximum efficacy for most patients at 4–6 mg/day
				↑ Blood level w/clozapine, inhibitors of cytochrome P450 2D6	Less EPS potential than haloperidol at doses <8 mg/ day
				↓ Blood level w/CBZ	Two divided doses

TABLE 19–2. Antipsychotics (continued)

Drug	Starting daily dose (mg)	Target daily dose (mg)	Neuropsychiatric side effects	Neuropsychiatric drug interactions	Comments
Clozapine	15–50	200–600	Drowsiness, dizziness, headache, tremor, syncope, insomnia, restlessness, hypokinesia/ akinesia, agitation, seizures, rigidity, akathisia, confusion, fatigue, hyperkinesia, weakness, lethargy, ataxia, slurred speech, depression, abnormal movements, anxiety, EPS, NMS, obsessive-compulsive symptoms Other: salivation, agranulocytosis	Additive CNS depressant effects w/other CNS depressants Occasional collapse (hypotension, respiratory depression, loss of consciousness) w/BZDs ↑ Risk of bone marrow suppression w/CBZ, possibly lithium ↑ Risk of NMS w/other antipsychotics, lithium, CBZ ↓ Blood level w/CBZ, phenytoin	Monitor WBC weekly More effective for negative schizophrenic symptoms, lower risk of EPS, TD, NMS, and higher risk of lowering seizure threshold (dose related) than standard neuroleptics May improve motor function in Tourette's, Huntington's, drug-induced persistent dyskinesia, spasmodic torticollis, Parkinson's, essential tremor
Olanzapine	5	10–20	Somnolence, dry mouth, weight gain with increased lipid abnormalities and possible diabetes risk, nausea, dizziness, constipation, headache, transient elevation transaminase	↓ Blood level w/smoking and CBZ ↑ Blood level w/fluoxetine	Once-daily dosing Antimanic effect
Quetiapine	25	300–450	Sedation, moderate weight gain, EPS, dizziness, agitation, postural hypotension, dry mouth, elevated transaminase	—	? Lower EPS risk, no prolactin elevation, twice-daily dosing, less experience than w/other atypicals

Note. BZDs = benzodiazepines; CBZ = carbamazepine; CNS = central nervous system; EPS = extrapyramidal side effects; MAOIs = monoamine oxidase inhibitors; NMS = neuroleptic malignant syndrome; SSRIs = selective serotonin reuptake inhibitors; TCAs = tricyclic antidepressants; TD = tardive dyskinesia; WBC = white blood count.

cacy for valproate, with a much higher rate of "marked improvement" (about 40%) compared with the only carbamazepine study (about 5%) (Tariot et al. 1998a). Both carbamazepine and valproate have been effective in alcohol withdrawal (Myrick et al. 2000; Stuppaeck et al. 1992), and valproate has some efficacy in panic (Roy-Byrne and Cowley 1998). Because of carbamazepine's potential for bone marrow suppression and valproate's potential for hepatotoxicity, complete blood cell count and liver function tests should be monitored. Carbamazepine and valproate blood levels do not necessarily correlate with clinical response but should be used to monitor compliance and drug metabolism. Preliminary evidence of efficacy of gabapentin for agitation is mixed (3 of 4, Roane et al. 2000; but only 2 of 12, Herrmann et al. 2000). Because gabapentin also has anxiolytic properties, nonhepatic clearance, and better tolerance, it could be a safer, easier-to-use alternative in the future.

Lithium is considerably less useful in secondary mania in neuropsychiatric patients. In addition to the previously cited reports in which carbamazepine was preferable, two reports have shown that lithium at low levels lost its previous efficacy and produced severe side effects after head trauma (Hornstein and Seliger 1989) and CVA (Moskowitz and Altshuler 1991). Lithium has also been shown to be inadequate without clozapine augmentation in Parkinson's disease (E. Kim et al. 1994) and to be less effective in mental retardation (Glue 1989). The elderly are well known to be more sensitive to lithium neurotoxicity, which can occur at low-normal lithium levels (Bell et al. 1993) and can persist for some period of time after lithium discontinuation (Saxena and Mallikarjuna 1988). Except for a possibly unique effect on steroid-induced mania and agitation (Falk et

al. 1979), and utility in treating the "on-off" phenomenon of Parkinson's disease (Coffey et al. 1982), lithium would appear not to be a first-line choice for many neuropsychiatric patients. Its proconvulsant effect (Moore 1981; Parmelee and O'Shannick 1988; Sacristan et al. 1991) and ability to cause or aggravate EPS (Lecamwasam et al. 1994) are other shortcomings. In dementia, most reports show that it has minimal effect (Holton and George 1985; Kunik et al. 1994), although it may be useful in certain HIV-related manic syndromes (Halman et al. 1993). Lithium has no known effects in primary anxiety disorders.

Benzodiazepines are potent inhibitors of both primary mania and anxiety. However, in agitated states secondary to neurologic illness, these agents have many drawbacks. They can cause confusion, cognitive impairment, psychomotor slowing, and disinhibition presenting as a paradoxical reaction. Earlier controlled studies in Alzheimer's disease patients showed that superiority over placebo for oxazepam is lost at 8 weeks due to tolerance (Sanders 1965) and that diazepam is worse than thiothixene (Kirven and Montero 1973). One study suggested that oxazepam was inferior to haloperidol and diphenhydramine in elderly institutionalized patients (Coccaro et al. 1990). Another single-case design report (Herz et al. 1992) also suggested that oxazepam was inferior to thiothixene. A double-blind study in hospitalized acquired immunodeficiency syndrome (AIDS) patients with delirium showed that lorazepam was markedly inferior to both haloperidol and chlorpromazine and was associated with such severe, treatment-limiting adverse effects that this arm of the study was prematurely terminated (Breitbart et al. 1996). A drug discontinuation study showed that dementia patients tapered from long-term use of benzodiazepines had improved memory without worsening of anxiety (Salzman et al. 1992). All this is consistent with the fact that less than 10% of benzodiazepine use in the elderly is for dementia (Kirby et al. 1999). Nonetheless, judicious use of these agents, often in combination with other medications such as neuroleptics (which may allow lower doses to be used) and antidepressants (which can reverse activating side effects), can be extremely beneficial. Extremely low doses and careful titration are necessary. Agents with short half-lives and without active metabolites (e.g., lorazepam, oxazepam) are the benzodiazepines of choice.

The nonbenzodiazepine anxiolytic buspirone has shown some efficacy in agitated states associated with dementia (Colenda 1988; Sakauye et al. 1993) and TBI (Levine 1988), especially when no severe motor or cognitive deficits were present (Gualtieri 1991). In Huntington's disease, one study reported improvement in both agitation and choreoathetoid movements with 120 mg/day (Hamner et al. 1996). In developmentally delayed patients, 16 of 22 had a good response to 15–45 mg/day (Buitelaar et al. 1998). Although one study (Cantillon et al. 1996) showed that low-dose buspirone was superior to haloperidol in agitated dementia, the effects were extremely modest.

Neuroleptics are frequently used as a nonspecific treatment to calm agitated patients, even when they are not obviously psychotic, with reasonably good effect (Salzman 1987). The use of the parenteral route, including intravenous injection, is not uncommon (Tesar et al. 1985), especially with medically ill patients in cardiac and intensive care units (Sanders et al. 1991). The neuroleptic pimozide, because of unique effects on reducing intracellular calcium influx, has been found especially helpful in agitated

delirium associated with hypercalcemia (Mark et al. 1993). Breitbart et al. 1996 documented significant improvement in symptoms in hospitalized AIDS patients using either haloperidol or chlorpromazine. However, major EPS, sedation, and hypotension limit the use of neuroleptics, and there are questions about how specific their effect is beyond a generally powerful sedating and motor-inhibiting one. In patients with dementia, several placebo-controlled studies have shown these drugs to be only marginally more effective in the absence of more classic psychotic symptoms (Raskind 1993). Because neurologic patients appear to be at increased risk for developing tardive dyskinesia and akathisia (Rifkin et al. 1975) and because animal studies have implicated typical neuroleptics in being deleterious to cortical recovery (Feeney et al. 1982), the potential utility of atypical neuroleptics for agitation or delirium is of special interest. Unfortunately, only risperidone has been studied, and it was effective at low dose in the controlled study by Katz et al. (1999). However, Herrmann et al. (1998) reported a 58% rate of EPS with similar low doses. Effects on agitation also take longer than effects on psychosis (7 vs. 3 weeks, Lavretsky and Sulzer 1998). Other reports have noted efficacy for both risperidone (Sipahimalani and Masand 1997a, 1997b) and olanzapine (K.S. Kim et al. 2001; Passik and Cooper 1999; Sipahimalani and Masand 1998) in agitated delirium at low doses. Periodic trials of neuroleptic discontinuation in agitated patients with dementia may show these drugs to be unnecessary (Bridges-Parlet et al. 1997).

Antidepressants have also been shown, not surprisingly, to have some efficacy. The SSRI citalopram was effective for anxiety, fear, and panic in 65 Alzheimer's dementia patients but not in 24 patients with vascular dementia (Nyth and Gottfries 1990); fluoxetine reduced anxiety, fear-panic, and irritability (but not depressed mood) in 10 Alzheimer's disease patients (Lebert et al. 1994), although in a small ($N = 15$) study it was no more effective than placebo (Auchus and Bissey-Black 1997). Although SSRIs are known to cause agitation as a side effect in primary depression, they work equally well in patients with agitated and retarded primary depression (Tollefson et al. 1994). Other reports have noted the utility of TCAs in brain injury–related agitation (Mysiw et al. 1988), in states of pathologic emotional lability in stroke (Robinson et al. 1993), and in multiple sclerosis (Schiffer et al. 1985). Fluoxetine has also reportedly been effective for emotional lability in stroke, multiple sclerosis, brain injury, amyotrophic lateral sclerosis, and encephalitis (Iannaccone and Ferini-Strambi 1996; Sloan et al. 1992; W.C. Tsai et al. 1998) and, remarkably, works in 2–6 days. Sertraline is also effective (Burns et al. 1999; Peterson et al. 1995). One crossover study (Lawlor et al. 1994) showed trazodone (150 mg) to be superior to both buspirone (30 mg) and placebo in agitated Alzheimer's disease patients, and a parallel group study showed efficacy equal to that of haloperidol in patients who were not psychotic (Sultzer et al. 1997).

Finally, there is preliminary evidence that calcium channel blockers, such as verapamil, have utility in both primary mania (Dubovsky et al. 1986) and panic disorder (Klein and Uhde 1988). Although no reports exist regarding the use of calcium channel blockers in neuropsychiatric patients with agitation, reports that HIV-related mania may be associated with direct increases in intracellular calcium triggered by the HIV coat protein gp 120 (Dreyer et al. 1990) provide a rationale for their use in these patients. Evidence is also emerging that cholinergic medications, discussed in detail in the final section of this chapter, also have antiagitation effects (Lanctot and Herrmann 2000; Mega et al. 1999; Rösler et al. 1998).

In summary, anticonvulsants are emerging as an extremely useful strategy for agitated neuropsychiatric patients with mania, dementia, or anxiety. When significant dysphoria is present, suggesting an element of depression, antidepressants may be indicated as an adjunct. Low-dose neuroleptics, long a mainstay in the treatment of agitation with dementia, may exacerbate dysphoria and depression in some patients, lower seizure threshold, impair cortical recovery, and have major motor side effects; they should be avoided if psychosis is absent. Newer antipsychotic agents such as risperidone and olanzapine, although imperfect, are likely an improvement, and they usually reduce agitation along with psychosis (see previous section). Of the primary anxiolytics, the azapirones are more effective and have fewer side effects than benzodiazepines. These latter agents should probably be reserved as an adjunct to be used with other agents. Tables 19–3 and 19–4 list characteristic mood stabilizers, anxiolytics, and sedative/hypnotics recommended in this section, with dose ranges, side effects, and relevant drug interactions.

Aggression, Impulsivity, and Behavioral Dyscontrol

Behavioral dyscontrol is often associated with psychotic (Chemerinski et al. 1998), agitated, or manic states; depression (Lyketsos et al. 1999); and cognitive impairment (Paradiso et al. 1996). It also may be part of acute delirium or chronic severe brain dysfunction. Less often, dyscontrol (e.g., aggression, hypersexuality) may emerge from more specific neurologic lesions (Mendez et al. 2000). The severity of symptoms can range from mild irritability to marked physical violence. Aggressive behavior may occur in 10%–40% of brain-injured individuals. As more severely compromised neurologic patients survive due to improved medical care, the neuropsychiatrist will increasingly confront this problem. Although behavioral management remains a core treatment of impulsivity and aggression (Wong et al. 1988), psychopharmacologic interventions have become increasingly important.

Behavioral dyscontrol is extremely varied in nature and includes aggressive acts, paraphilias, compulsions, rituals, self-mutilation, and socially inappropriate behaviors (Collacott et al. 1998). It is important to document the behavioral dysfunction and its potential response to treatment with observer ratings, because self-rating scales can be unreliable. The Overt Aggression Scale (Yudofsky et al. 1986) is one reliable and valid method. The Aberrant Behavior Checklist, measuring irritability, social withdrawal, stereotyping, hyperactivity, and excessive speech in mentally retarded populations, is another (Aman et al. 1985).

Treatment

There are no U.S. Food and Drug Administration (FDA)–approved medications for the treatment of aggression and impulsivity, few standardized classification and assessment tools, and few randomized controlled trials. Treatment often targets the clinical syndromes associated with the maladaptive behavior. Thus, the irritable, depressed patient should first be given an antidepressant; the agitated, paranoid patient should receive a trial of a neuroleptic; and the hyperaroused, angry patient may benefit from an anticonvulsant. However, common side effects of medications used to treat anger and aggression can themselves exacerbate

the symptoms (e.g., akathisia from neuroleptics; benzodiazepine-induced disinhibition; overactivation from antidepressants), and anticholinergic agents can aggravate cognitive deficits, lower seizure threshold, and promote delirium, particularly when combined with other delirium-promoting agents.

β-Adrenergic receptor blockers—such as propranolol, pindolol, and nadolol—have been studied in both open (Alpert et al. 1990; Connor et al. 1997; Greendyke and Kanter 1986; Greendyke et al. 1986; Ratey et al. 1992b) and double-blind, placebo-controlled trials (Allan et al. 1996; Ratey et al. 1992b) and have been found to be effective in reducing anger and aggression in a wide range of neuropsychiatric disorders. However, more recent studies using placebo-control (Allan et al. 1996) and placebo-discontinuation (Silver et al. 1999) designs show only modest changes and low rates (30%) of response, respectively. Investigation is plagued by heterogeneous diagnosis, and it is possible that patients with more clear-cut brain damage, as in developmental disability (Connor et al. 1997), may do better. Many of these patients did not respond to other medications, such as neuroleptics, anxiolytics, anticonvulsants, and lithium. Response may take up to 8 weeks, and both central and peripheral effects may contribute to therapeutic action (Ruedrich 1996). Pindolol is less likely to cause bradycardia, and nadolol and long-acting propranolol allow once-daily dosing, which may be necessary in the noncompliant or cognitively impaired patient. Secondary depression due to β-blockers appears to be a rare occurrence, but these medications are contraindicated in patients with asthma, chronic obstructive pulmonary disease, insulin-dependent diabetes, congestive heart failure, persistent angina, significant peripheral vascular disease, and hyperthyroidism (Yudofsky

TABLE 19–3. Mood stabilizers

Drug	Starting daily dose (mg)	Target daily dose (mg)	Neuropsychiatric side effects	Neuropsychiatric drug interactions	Comments
Lithium	300–900	600–2,400	Lethargy, fatigue, muscle weakness, tremor, headache, confusion, dulled senses, ataxia, dysarthria, aphasia, muscle hyperirritability, hyperactive deep tendon reflexes, hypertonia, choreoathetoid movements, cogwheel rigidity, dizziness, drowsiness, disturbed accommodation, dystonia, seizures, EPS Other: nausea, diarrhea, polyuria, nephrogenic diabetes insipidus, hypothyroidism, hyperparathyroidism, T-wave depression, acne, leukocytosis	EPS and NMS w/neuroleptics Neurotoxicity w/SSRIs, neuroleptics, CBZ, valproate, phenytoin, calcium channel blockers ↑ Blood level w/SSRIs ↑ or ↓ Blood level of neuroleptics	Lowers seizure threshold Predominantly renally excreted Once-daily dosing more tolerable w/less renal toxicity Blood levels correlate w/ therapeutic response Used in Huntington's, cluster headaches, torticollis, Tourette's, SIADH, leukopenia
Carbamazepine	200–600	400–2,000	Dizziness, drowsiness, incoordination, confusion, headache, fatigue, blurred vision, hallucinations, diplopia, oculomotor disturbance, nystagmus, speech disturbance, abnormal involuntary movement, peripheral neuritis, paresthesia, depression, agitation, talkativeness, tinnitus, hyperacusis Other: nausea, bone marrow suppression, hepatotoxicity, SIADH	Additive CNS depressant effects w/ other CNS depressants Contraindicated w/MAOIs Neurotoxicity w/lithium, neuroleptics Bone marrow suppression w/clozapine ↑ Blood level w/SSRIs, verapamil ↓ Blood level w/TCAs, haloperidol, valproate, phenytoin, phenobarbital ↓ Blood level of TCAs, BZDs, neuroleptics, valproate, phenytoin, phenobarbital, methadone, propranolol	Induces own hepatic metabolism (2–5 weeks) Monitor CBC, LFTs, electrolytes Blood level of approx. 4–12 µg/mL Useful in trigeminal neuralgia, neuropathic pain, sedative/hypnotic withdrawal

TABLE 19–3. Mood stabilizers (*continued*)

Drug	Starting daily dose (mg)	Target daily dose (mg)	Neuropsychiatric side effects	Neuropsychiatric drug interactions	Comments
Valproate	250–750	500–3,000	Sedation, tremor, paresthesia, headache, lethargy, dizziness, diplopia, confusion, incoordination, ataxia, dysarthria, psychosis, nystagmus, asterixis, "spots before eyes" Other: nausea, hair loss, thrombocytopenia, impaired platelet aggregation, elevated liver transaminases, hepatotoxicity, pancreatitis	Additive CNS depressant effects w/other CNS depressants ↑ Blood level w/chlorpromazine ↓ Blood level w/SSRIs, CBZ, phenytoin, phenobarbital ↑ Blood level of TCAs, chlorpromazine, CBZ, phenytoin, phenobarbital, primidone, BZDs	Monitor CBC w/platelets, LFTs Blood level of approx. 50–150 μg/mL Useful in neuropathic pain
Neurontin	100–300	600–1,800	Somnolence, fatigue, ataxia, dizziness, GI upset	Exclusively renal clearance, not bound to plasma protein, pharmacodynamic interactions possible but unknown	6-hour half-life, dose dependent ↓ Bioavailability, need three-times-daily schedule w/ larger doses, otherwise twice daily may suffice

Note. BZDs = benzodiazepines; CBC = complete blood count; CBZ = carbamazepine; CNS = central nervous system; EPS = extrapyramidal side effects; GI = gastrointestinal; LFTs = liver function tests; MAOIs = monoamine oxidase inhibitors; NMS = neuroleptic malignant syndrome; SIADH = syndrome of inappropriate antidiuretic hormone; SSRIs = selective serotonin reuptake inhibitors; TCAs = tricyclic antidepressants.

TABLE 19–4. Anxiolytics and sedative/hypnotics

Drug	Starting daily dose (mg)	Target daily dose (mg)	Neuropsychiatric side effects	Neuropsychiatric drug interactions	Comments
Benzodiazepines			Drowsiness, incoordination, confusion, dysarthria, fatigue, agitation, dizziness, akathisia, anterograde amnesia (esp. alprazolam, lorazepam) Other: sexual dysfunction	Augments respiratory depression w/opioids Neurotoxicity and sexual dysfunction w/lithium Additive CNS depressant effects w/other CNS depressants ↑ Blood level w/SSRIs, phenytoin ↓ Blood level w/CBZ ↓ Blood level of levodopa, phenytoin	May develop tolerance to psychotropic and anticonvulsant effects Do not induce own metabolism Addictive potential May cause withdrawal syndrome Alprazolam has antidepressant properties May cause EEG changes May worsen delirium and dementia Useful in treating akathisia *Clonazepam:* May accumulate in bloodstream May have utility in pain syndromes, movement disorders
Alprazolam	0.25–0.50	0.75–6.00			
Lorazepam	0.5–1.0	1.5–12.0			
Clonazepam	0.25–0.5	1–5			

TABLE 19–4. Anxiolytics and sedative/hypnotics (*continued*)

Drug	Starting daily dose (mg)	Target daily dose (mg)	Neuropsychiatric side effects	Neuropsychiatric drug interactions	Comments
Nonbenzodiazepines					
Buspirone	10–15	15–60	Nervousness, headache, confusion, weakness, numbness, drowsiness, paresthesia, incoordination, tremor	EPS w/neuroleptics Hypertension w/MAOIs ↑ ALT w/trazodone ↑ Blood level of BZDs, haloperidol	Has antidepressant effects but may produce dysphoria at higher doses Slow onset of action Nonaddictive Usually does not impair psychomotor performance
Diphenhydramine	25–50	25–200	Drowsiness, dizziness, anticholinergic effects, incoordination, fatigue, confusion, nervousness, tremor, insomnia, euphoria, paresthesia	Additive CNS depressant effects w/ other CNS depressants ↑ Anticholinergic effects w/MAOIs, TCAs	Minimal effects on EEG Anticholinergic effects may decrease EPS but may exacerbate delirium May help with insomnia; tolerance may develop Unpredictable antianxiety properties
Zolpidem	5–10	5–10	Drowsiness, dizziness, lethargy, depression, abnormal dreams, anterograde amnesia, sleep disorder	Additive CNS depressant effects w/ other CNS depressants	Used for short-term treatment of insomnia No significant anxiolytic or anticonvulsant effects Abuse and withdrawal reported

Note.   ALT = alanine aminotransferase; BZDs = benzodiazepines; CBZ = carbamazepine; CNS = central nervous system; EEG = electroencephalogram; EPS = extrapyramidal side effects; MAOIs = monoamine oxidase inhibitors; SSRIs = selective serotonin reuptake inhibitors; TCAs = tricyclic antidepressants.

et al. 1987). Yudofsky et al. (1987) proposed titrating the dose of propranolol as high as 12 mg/kg or up to 800 mg and maintaining maximum tolerable dosages for up to 8 weeks to achieve the desired clinical response, although doses in the range of 160–320 mg/day have been effective.

Parenteral benzodiazepines are often used to manage both acute aggression and behavioral dyscontrol and can be as effective as neuroleptics (Dorevitch et al. 1999). However, they can also produce disinhibition, which worsens agitation and arousal (Yudofsky et al. 1987). Benzodiazepines with rapid onset of action and relatively short half-lives that can be given intramuscularly or intravenously, such as lorazepam, are most useful in the acute situation. Diazepam and chlordiazepoxide are less reliably and rapidly absorbed intramuscularly (Garza-Trevino et al. 1989). Although longer-acting benzodiazepines, such as clonazepam (Feinbar and Alvarez 1986), can be useful in patients with more chronic agitation and aggression, particularly when symptoms of anxiety coexist, their use in treating or preventing more chronic aggression is not supported (Salzman 1988). Impairment of cognitive functioning by benzodiazepines could potentially aggravate aggression by increasing confusion.

Buspirone can reduce anxiety-associated agitation and has a benign side-effect profile. It has been reported to be effective in treating aggression in patients with head injury (Gualtieri 1991), developmental disability (Ratey et al. 1991a; Verhoeven and Tuinier 1996), dementia (Levy 1994; Tiller 1989), and Huntington's disease (Byrne et al. 1994). Although the effect of buspirone on anxiety can reduce agitation, its effect on aggression is probably independent of anxiolysis. Although doses between 30 and 60 mg are usually employed (Verhoe-

ven and Tuinier 1996), lower doses (5–15 mg) have been useful in some reports (Ratey et al. 1991a, 1991b, 1992a).

Serotonergic antidepressants have also been effective in the treatment of aggression and behavioral dyscontrol. In open trials, this includes fluoxetine in depressed (Fava et al. 1983), brain-injured (Sobin et al. 1989), and mentally retarded (King 1991; Markowitz 1992) patients; sertraline in mentally retarded (Hellings et al. 1996), Huntington's disease (Ranen et al. 1996), developmentally disabled (Campbell and Duffy 1995), and intermittent explosive disorder (Feder 1999) patients; paroxetine in mentally retarded patients (although the effect wore off after 1 month) (Davanzo et al. 1998) and in patients with dementia (Swartz et al. 1997); and citalopram in patients with dementia (Pollock et al. 1997). Standard dose ranges were used. Trazodone is also effective in reducing aggression secondary to organic mental disorders and dementia (Greenwald et al. 1986; Mashiko et al. 1996; Pinner and Rich 1988; Simpson and Foster 1986; Zubieta and Alessi 1992). Concomitant use of tryptophan in some of these reports confounds interpretation of efficacy, however. Because of its potential for causing orthostatic hypotension, use of trazodone should be monitored closely, particularly in elderly and motorically compromised patients. Although sedation can be a problem initially, it often goes away in a few days.

Although anticonvulsants are particularly effective in treating mood lability, impulsivity, and aggression in patients with known seizure disorders, lack of electroencephalographic abnormalities does not preclude potential benefit from anticonvulsants (Mattes 1990). Carbamazepine has been effective in managing aggression and irritability in a variety of patients with CNS impairment, including dementia, developmental disorders, schizophrenia, seizures, and TBI (Chatham-Showalter 1996; Evans and Gualtieri 1985; Luchins 1984; Mattes 1990; McAllister 1985; Yatham and McHale 1988). However, a placebo-controlled trial in children with conduct disorder showed no benefit (Cueva et al. 1996). Valproate has also been found to be effective for aggression in patients with mental retardation (Ruedrich et al. 1999), TBI (Wroblewski et al. 1997), dementia (Haas et al. 1997), and personality disorder (Kavoussi and Coccaro 1998) and may be better tolerated than carbamazepine. Blood levels below 50 µg/mL have been effective in some reports (Mazure et al. 1992). A recent review of 17 reports showed a 77% response rate with normal blood level range (Lindenmayer and Kotsaftis 2000). Phenytoin has been effective for impulsive aggression in inmates using placebo crossover (Barratt et al. 1997), whereas lamotrigine (Beran and Gibson 1998) and gabapentin (Tallian et al. 1996) have worsened aggression in epileptic patients.

Lithium was effective in treating aggressive behavior and affective instability in brain-injured patients (Glenn et al. 1989) and in a double-blind, placebo-controlled trial with 42 adult mentally retarded patients (M. Craft et al. 1987). Open trials in aggressive children with mental retardation and patients chronically hospitalized for severe aggression (Bellus et al. 1996) also support its use (Campbell et al. 1995). Although higher plasma levels are more likely to result in clinical improvement, the potential neurotoxic side effects of lithium at lower levels than in psychiatric patients may limit its use in the neurologically compromised patient.

Neuroleptics are effective in treating aggression in neuropsychiatric patients (Rao et al. 1985). They should be reserved, however, for patients who exhibit psychotic symptoms or who require rapid behavioral control, as the extrapyramidal and anticholinergic properties of these medications can further increase agitation (Tune et al. 1992). Akathisia can be confused with worsening aggression, thus prompting a detrimental rise in neuroleptic dosage. Neuroleptics can also, in some cases, impair executive cognitive functioning (Medalia et al. 1988). Despite these risks, a very effective means of rapid tranquilization in the agitated patient is the combination of haloperidol (2–5 mg) with lorazepam (1–2 mg), either orally, intramuscularly, or intravenously. In the chronically aggressive psychotic patient, clozapine at doses of 300–500 mg may be the most effective antipsychotic (Cohen and Underwood 1994; Michals et al. 1993). Risperidone is certainly better tolerated, but placebo-controlled evidence that it is more effective for aggression than typical neuroleptics is conflicting, with two studies (Czobor et al. 1995; De Deyn et al. 1999) showing superior effects to haloperidol in schizophrenia and dementia, whereas another study (Beck et al. 1997) found no difference in a small but select group of forensic schizophrenic subjects. Open studies show good effects in autistic (Horrigan and Barnhill 1997) and mentally retarded (Cohen et al. 1998) patients. However, recent reviews emphasize that atypicals should not be used for acute management (Buckley 1999). No data have been published for quetiapine or olanzapine.

Methylphenidate and dextroamphetamine can be useful in patients with distractibility, impaired attention, impulsivity, and irritability (Mooney and Haas 1993), symptoms also seen in attention-deficit/hyperactivity disorder. These stimulants are generally well tolerated in the neurologic patient (Kaufman et al.

1984), do not appear to lower the seizure threshold at therapeutic doses (Wroblewski et al. 1992), and may even enhance cortical recovery (Feeney et al. 1982). However, they should be used with caution due to their potential to aggravate irritability and delusional thought content.

Although an emerging body of literature on the treatment of the developmentally disabled suggests that opiate antagonists such as naltrexone (up to 2 mg/kg) decrease self-injury behavior by 30%–50% (Buzan et al. 1995), the only double-blind, placebo-controlled study (in autistic, mentally retarded adults) did not show an effect (Willemsen-Swinkels et al. 1995). However, a small crossover study showed good effects of 50-mg doses of naltrexone in females with self-mutilation behavior and bipolar disorder (Sonne et al. 1996), and open studies with the same population showed similar effects (A.S. Roth et al. 1996). A retrospective study showed good response in 50% of 56 children with self-injurious behavior (Casner et al. 1996), and an open report showed effects in patients with impulse control disorders (S.W. Kim 1998). Nonetheless, use of naltrexone for this indication should not at present be routine.

Other medications, such as amantadine, a dopamine agonist, and clonidine, an α-adrenergic agonist, have been used to treat aggression. Gualtieri et al. (1989) used amantadine successfully in doses of 50–400 mg/day in agitated patients recovering from coma. Clonidine at 0.6 mg/day reduced violent outbursts in an autistic adult (Koshes and Rock 1994), but its depressogenic and hypotensive risks may be problematic in the neurologic patient. Although a novel class of 5-HT_{1B} receptor agonists called serenics are prompting excitement (Olivier et al. 1994), they currently are not available in the United States and require more testing. Finally, a recent randomized, placebo-controlled study showed an antiaggressive effect of estrogen in both men and women with dementia that was rapid and sustained (Kyomen et al. 1999).

Because of the heterogeneity of symptoms and pathophysiology in this population, and the ethical issues involved in carrying out placebo-controlled studies in aggressive neuropsychiatric patients, animal studies must continue to be used, and the adoption of single-subject research designs may prove to be the most practical approach in studying this population (Eichelman 1992). Table 19–5 lists characteristic antihypertensives recommended in this section, dose ranges, side effects, and relevant drug interactions.

Cognitive Disturbance

Unlike depression, anxiety, mania, and psychosis, all of which can occur as "primary" disorders independent of gross neurologic disease, cognitive disturbance is almost always a result of etiologically identifiable brain dysfunction and has previously served to largely define disorders known as organic brain syndromes. Moreover, cognitive impairment is often associated with other mood and behavioral features (e.g., agitation and depression predict greater cognitive disturbance in Alzheimer's disease and Parkinson's disease, respectively [Chen et al. 1998; Kuzis et al. 1997]), as well as with functional status and survival time (e.g., in HIV illness [Wilkie et al. 1998]). However, difficulties with concentration, memory, and more complicated executive cognitive functions occur not just as primary components of neurologic disease and CNS dysfunction but also as epiphenomena in the course of major mood disturbance (i.e., pseudodementia) and as a core fea-

TABLE 19–5. Antihypertensives

Drug	Starting daily dose (mg)	Target daily dose (mg)	Neuropsychiatric side effects	Neuropsychiatric drug interactions	Comments
Propranolol	20–80	40–800	Light-headedness, insomnia, lassitude, weakness, fatigue, catatonia, visual disturbance, hallucinations, vivid dreams, confusion, emotional lability, clouded sensorium, impaired psychomotor	Hypotension w/MAOIs ↑ Blood level of both propranolol and chlorpromazine when taken together ↓ Blood level w/CBZ, phenytoin, phenobarbital performance	Discontinue if heart rate <50 bpm, SBP <90 mm Hg Clinical response may take 4–8 weeks Useful for migraine, essential tremor, akathisia, performance anxiety, lithium tremor, aggression, mania, social phobia
Verapamil	80–240	160–480	Confusion, equilibrium disorders, insomnia, muscle cramps, paresthesia, psychosis, akathisia, somnolence, headache, CVA	Hypotension w/MAOIs ↑ Neurotoxicity w/lithium, CBZ ↑ Parkinsonism w/neuroleptics ↓ Blood level w/TCAs, phenobarbital ↑ Blood level of CBZ ↑ or ↓ Blood level of lithium	Useful in mania, migraine, TD, Tourette's, panic disorder
Clonidine	0.05–0.20	0.15–0.80	Nervousness, agitation, mental depression, headache, insomnia, vivid dreams or nightmares, behavioral changes, restlessness, anxiety, hallucinations, delirium, sedation, weakness, fatigue	Additive CNS depressant effects w/other CNS depressants Impaired BP control w/ neuroleptics ↓ Blood level w/TCAs	Useful in opiate withdrawal, Tourette's, and possibly mania, anxiety, akathisia, ADHD, aggression Available in transdermal form

Note. ADHD = attention-deficit/hyperactivity disorder; BP = blood pressure; bpm = beats per minute; CBZ = carbamazepine; CNS = central nervous system; CVA = cerebrovascular accident; MAOIs = monoamine oxidase inhibitors; SBP = systolic blood pressure; TCAs = tricyclic antidepressants; TD = tardive dyskinesia.

ture of schizophrenia (Lancon et al. 2000) and chronic bipolar disorder (Ferrier et al. 1999), as a measurable but more subtle aspect of PTSD and obsessive-compulsive disorder, and secondary to many medications used to treat neurologic and other medical illnesses.

Treatment

The majority of treatment studies continue to focus on Alzheimer's dementia, the most prevalent cause of cognitive impairment in the U.S. population. A growing number of studies have documented the palliative efficacy of reversible cholinesterase inhibitors in these patients. Tacrine hydrochloride, the first FDA-approved agent for this indication, clearly has a beneficial, though small, effect on cognition (0.62 points on Mini-Mental State Exam score) compared with placebo declines of about a point (Qizilbash et al. 1998) over 3 months. The effect may delay the need for nursing home placement (Knopman et al. 1996), although it does not appear to alter the long-term trajectory of the illness. Because of gastrointestinal side effects and liver transaminase elevations, tolerability is poor, with more than 75% of patients in a representative clinic population declining open treatment in one report (Lyketsos et al. 1996).

Donepezil, also now FDA approved and similar to tacrine except for less peripheral activity and the absence of liver transaminase effects, is better tolerated with comparable efficacy for both short-term (24 weeks) and longer-term (5 years) treatment (Greenberg et al. 2000; S.L. Rogers et al. 1998, 2000). Evidence also suggests beneficial psychotropic effects in patients with problematic depression, psychosis, agitation, and disinhibition, although other patients without obvious behavioral problems may experience behavioral worsening (Mega et al.

1999). It may also have efficacy in vascular dementia (Mendez et al. 1999) and for psychotropic-induced memory loss in patients without dementia (Jacobsen and Comas-Díaz 1999).

Other cholinesterase inhibitors, including rivastigmine (Farlow et al. 2000; McKeith et al. 2000; Rösler et al. 1999), galantamine (Wilcock et al. 2000; Wilkinson and Murray 2001), and metrifonate (Cummings et al. 1998), have shown efficacy and tolerability comparable to donepezil. Effect sizes of metrifonate are similar to those of the three marketed agents (improvements of 3–5 points on the Alzheimer's Disease Assessment Scale [ADAS-cog] over 6 months compared with placebo). Demonstration that metrifonate also lowers caregiver burden (Shikiar et al. 2000) provides another more novel measure of beneficial outcome. Extended-release physostigmine also is effective, but, because tolerability is poorer and efficacy perhaps a bit less (Thal et al. 1996; van Dyck et al. 2000), it is unlikely to be used except in patients nonresponsive to other agents.

Although muscarinic agonists have not been practical to employ due to requirements for either frequent intravenous (arecoline) or intracerebroventricular (bethanechol) administration and because of high rates of nausea and other side effects, studies have documented the efficacy of arecoline (Raffaele et al. 1991) and bethanechol (Penn et al. 1988). The results of these studies suggest that newer muscarinic agonists, now under development, may prove to be more practically effective. Nicotine agonists may also prove useful in both Alzheimer's (Potter et al. 1999) and Parkinson's (Newhouse et al. 1997) dementias. Although galantamine has nicotinic effects in addition to its cholinesterase inhibition (Maelicke et al. 2001), no advantage over other marketed inhibitors has been identified.

Selegiline, an MAO-B inhibitor commonly used in Parkinson's disease, was initially shown at an open daily dose of 20 mg to improve cognitive performance of 14 Alzheimer's dementia patients (Schneider et al. 1991). Subsequently, double-blind studies at low 10-mg doses likely to act principally by increasing CNS dopamine showed superiority to placebo (Finali et al. 1991), to phosphatidylserine (Monteverde et al. 1990), and to oxiracetam (Falsaperla et al. 1990) on a variety of cognitive tests. However, as summarized in a negative crossover study (Tariot et al. 1998b), positive effects of this drug on agitation and depression in some patients make it hard to separate mood state–dependent effects on cognition from a primary cognitive effect. The two most recent studies show no effect (Freedman et al. 1998) and a modest effect on delaying functional impairment (Sano et al. 1997). Because the former study was one of the few longer-term evaluations, the utility of the agent requires further study.

A number of naturalistic case control studies have shown that anti-inflammatory drugs may help Alzheimer's dementia patients. In one study, patients taking daily nonsteroidal anti-inflammatory drugs (NSAIDs) or aspirin had shorter duration of illness and better cognitive performance (Rich et al. 1995). In another study, the onset of Alzheimer's dementia in monozygotic twin pairs was inversely proportional to prior use of steroids or adrenocorticotropic hormone (ACTH) (Breitner et al. 1994). Finally, a third naturalistic study (Prince et al. 1998) showed that NSAID use was associated with less cognitive decline, particularly in younger subjects. One placebo-controlled study of 44 patients actually supported an effect for indomethacin (J. Rogers et al. 1993), and NSAIDs are associated with histopathologic evidence of slowed progression of Alzheimer's

dementia (Alafuzoff et al. 2000). However, another study failed to show an effect for diclofenac/misoprostol (Scharf et al. 1999), and a study of prednisone was also negative (Aisen et al. 2000), although the dose was quite low and adverse effects on hippocampal cells could have counteracted anti-inflammatory effects.

Before the approval of tacrine, donepezil, and rivastigmine, the only approved cognitive drugs were ergoloid mesylates (Hydergine). Their cognitive benefits have always been said to be modest at best and hard to distinguish from nonspecific activating properties. A review (Schneider and Olin 1994) confirms this, showing effect sizes of 0.56 for clinical ratings but only 0.27 for neuropsychological measures. A previous study in 80 Alzheimer's dementia patients that failed to show an effect (Thompson et al. 1990) may have been compromised by its 3-mg/day dose, because there is a strong dose-response relationship with this drug, and some authors believe higher doses (e.g., 8 mg) might be better (Schneider and Olin 1994).

Two studies support very modest effects of antioxidants. Le Bars et al. (1997) showed that Ginkgo biloba was superior to placebo by 1.4 ADAS-cog points in a mixed Alzheimer's and vascular dementia group. These results are inferior to those seen with tacrine or donepezil, and the predominance of mild cases makes the generalizability of results unclear. A meta-analysis of studies with this agent (Oken et al. 1998) shows that few reports were well designed with clearly described patient groups, although these few also show similar modest effects. An increase in bleeding risk, especially for patients taking anticoagulants, warrants caution, however. A second study (Sano et al. 1997) showed that 2,000 IU of α-tocopherol slowed functional decline in Alzheimer's disease patients, with a delay of roughly a half year over a 2-year period. However, no cognitive improvements were noted, despite these functional benefits.

Initial studies showing that fewer Alzheimer's and vascular dementia patients take replacement estrogen than do matched control subjects (Mortel and Meyer 1995) and that those who do have better cognitive function than those who do not (Henderson et al. 1994) have been replicated in several other uncontrolled naturalistic designs showing that estrogen use is associated with reduced incidence of Alzheimer's disease (Slooter et al. 1999). These associations were convergent with preclinical studies showing genomic and receptor-mediated effects of estrogen on learning, memory, and neuronal growth and connections (Shaywitz and Shaywitz 2000). Unfortunately, a recent well-designed study (Mulnard et al. 2000) failed to show a beneficial effect of estrogen supplements for mild to moderate elderly (75 years) women with Alzheimer's disease, although beneficial effects in postmenopausal women without dementia (Kampen and Sherwin 1994) suggest that preventive effects might be possible.

Based on the possibility that calcium blockade will slow mechanisms of neuronal death that depend on increased free intracellular calcium in Alzheimer's disease, studies of 90 mg/day nimodipine in these patients have shown some promise. Ban et al. (1990) showed 12 weeks of nimodipine to be more effective than placebo on the Mini-Mental State Exam and the Wechsler Memory Scale. Improvement continued between 60 and 90 days. Tollefson (1990) also showed that the same dose improved recall on the Buschke test, although 180 mg proved worse than placebo. However, one naturalistic study (Maxwell et al. 1999) showed that elderly patients taking calcium channel blockers are more likely to develop dementia. Unique calcium channel effects of nimodipine could explain some of these differences.

A variety of other agents have been either tested briefly or reported on. Stimulants (methylphenidate or dextroamphetamine) have been found in one open trial to improve scores on several neuropsychological tests in HIV disease patients (Angrist et al. 1992) and have been found in a placebo-controlled crossover trial to improve cognition in cognitively impaired HIV disease patients (van Dyck et al. 1997). Opiate antagonists have helped improve TBI-associated memory impairment in one case series (Tennant and Wild 1987). The 5-HT antidepressant fluvoxamine has improved memory impairment in Korsakoff's dementia in two studies (Martin et al. 1989, 1995). Clonidine variably improved memory in Korsakoff's dementia, and this was correlated with increased cingulate gyrus and thalamic blood flow (Moffoot et al. 1994). Both clonidine and another α_2 agonist, guanfacine, improve various aspects of cognition in healthy humans (Jäkälä et al. 1999a, 1999b, 1999c). Phosphatidylserine, a lipid membrane processor, improved several cognitive measures in Alzheimer's dementia patients (Crook et al. 1992). Citicoline, a metabolic intermediate that enhances the formation of neural membranes and promotes acetylcholine biosynthesis, improved verbal memory in older individuals with "inefficient" memories who did not have dementia (Spiers et al. 1996). Milacemide, a prodrug for glycine (Dysken et al. 1992), did not work in Alzheimer's dementia patients despite the plausibility of N-methyl-D-aspartate (NMDA)–glutamate theories of cognition (Ingram et al. 1994) and increased word retrieval in young and old subjects without dementia treated with it (Schwartz et al. 1991). However, cycloserine improved cognition relative to placebo in 17 Alzheimer's disease patients, suggesting that NMDA strategies need to be pursued further (G.E. Tsai et al. 1999). Finally, preliminary studies show a beneficial effect for both insulin and somatostatin acutely administered to Alzheimer's disease patients (S. Craft et al. 1999), whereas peptide T may be associated with improved performance in more cognitively impaired HIV disease patients with relatively preserved immunologic status (Heseltine et al. 1998).

In conclusion, few approved treatments for cognitive impairment, principally in Alzheimer's dementia, are available. Tacrine is perhaps a bit more effective than ergoloid mesylates but with more side-effect morbidity. Donepezil is a much more tolerable alternative, although its efficacy is also only modest. NSAIDs could be employed more readily if there are no medical contraindications. Patients with hypertension might take nimodipine to address both blood pressure and dementia. Selegiline is an option, as are psychostimulants, although activating effects may obscure true cognitive effects. Antioxidants may have some utility, and estrogens deserve further exploration in at-risk patients. Emerging strategies are now emphasizing the use of combinations of agents, especially because effect sizes for all agents are quite modest (Knopman et al. 1998). Studies have already shown effects for both estrogen (Schneider et al. 1997) and selegiline (Schneider et al. 1993) when added to cholinesterase inhibitors. This strategy is consistent with differential effects of these agents on separable cognitive processes (Riekkinen and Riekkinen 1999) and the unique prominence of different individual transmitter abnormalities in different diseases associated with cognitive impairment (J.I. Friedman et al. 1999).

References

Aarsland D, Larsen JP, Lim NG, et al: Olanzapine for psychosis in patients with Parkinson's disease with and without dementia. J Neuropsychiatry Clin Neurosci 11:392–394, 1999

Aisen PS, Davis KL, Berg JD, et al: A randomized controlled trial of prednisone in Alzheimer's disease. Neurology 54:588–593, 2000

Alafuzoff P: Lower counts of astroglia and activated microglia in patients with Alzheimer's disease with regular use of NSAIDs. J Alzheimers Dis 2:37–46, 2000

Alexopoulos GS, Meyers BS, Young RC, et al: "Vascular depression" hypothesis. Arch Gen Psychiatry 54:915–922, 1997

Allan ER, Alpert M, Sison CE, et al: Adjunctive nadolol in the treatment of acutely aggressive schizophrenic patients. J Clin Psychiatry 57:455–459, 1996

Allen RL, Walker Z, D'Ath PJ, et al: Risperidone for psychotic and behavioural symptoms in Lewy body dementia (letter). Lancet 346:185, 1995

Alpert M, Allan ER, Citrome L, et al: A double-blind, placebo-controlled study of adjunctive nadolol in the management of violent psychiatric patients. Psychopharmacol Bull 28:367–371, 1990

Aman MG, Singh NN, Stewart AW, et al: The Aberrant Behavior Checklist: a behavior rating scale for the assessment of treatment effects. Am J Ment Defic 89:485–491, 1985

American Psychiatric Association: Diagnostic and Statistical Manual of Mental Disorders, 4th Edition. Washington, DC, American Psychiatric Association, 1994

Andersen G, Vestergaard K, Lauritzen L: Effective treatment of poststroke depression with the selective serotonin reuptake inhibitor citalopram. Stroke 25:1099–1104, 1994

Andersen J, Aabro E, Gulmann N, et al: Antidepressive treatment in Parkinson's disease: a controlled trial of the effect of nortriptyline in patients with Parkinson's disease treated with L-dopa. Acta Neurol Scand 62:210–219, 1980

Angrist B, d'Hollosy M, Sanfilipo M, et al: Central nervous system stimulants as symptomatic treatments for AIDS-related neuropsychiatric impairment. J Clin Psychopharmacol 12:268–272, 1992

Auchus AP, Bissey-Black C: Pilot study of haloperidol, fluoxetine, and placebo for agitation in Alzheimer's disease. J Neuropsychiatry Clin Neurosci 9:591–593, 1997

Azouvi P, Jokic C, Attal N, et al: Carbamazepine in agitation and aggressive behaviour following severe closed-head injury: results of an open trial. Brain Inj 13:797–804, 1999

Balon R: Nefazodone for mood disorder associated with epilepsy (letter). J Clin Psychiatry 59:690, 1998

Ban TA, Morey L, Aguglia E, et al: Nimodipine in the treatment of old age dementias. Prog Neuropsychopharmacol Biol Psychiatry 14:525–551, 1990

Barratt ES, Stanford MS, Felthous AR, et al: The effects of phenytoin on impulsive and premeditated aggression: a controlled study. J Clin Psychopharmacol 17:341–349, 1997

Beck NC, Greenfield SR, Gotham H, et al: Risperidone in the management of violent, treatment-resistant schizophrenics hospitalized in a maximum security forensic facility. J Am Acad Psychiatry Law 25:461–468, 1997

Bell AJ, Cole A, Eccleston D, et al: Lithium neurotoxicity at normal therapeutic levels. Br J Psychiatry 162:689–692, 1993

Bellus SB, Stewart D, Vergo JG, et al: The use of lithium in the treatment of aggressive behaviours with two brain-injured individuals in a state psychiatric hospital. Brain Inj 10:849–860, 1996

Beran RG, Gibson RJ: Aggressive behaviour in intellectually challenged patients with epilepsy treated with lamotrigine. Epilepsia 39:280–282, 1998

Breitbart W, Marotta R, Platt MM, et al: A double-blind trial of haloperidol, chlorpromazine, and lorazepam in the treatment of delirium in hospitalized AIDS patients. Am J Psychiatry 153:231–237, 1996

Breitner JC, Gau BA, Welsh KA, et al: Inverse association of anti-inflammatory treatments and Alzheimer's disease: initial results of a co-twin control study. Neurology 44:227–232, 1994

Bridges-Parlet S, Knopman D, Steffes S: Withdrawal of neuroleptic medications from institutionalized dementia patients: results of a double-blind, baseline-treatment-controlled pilot study. J Geriatr Psychiatry Neurol 10:119–126, 1997

Buckley PF: The role of typical and atypical antipsychotic medications in the management of agitation and aggression. J Clin Psychiatry 10:52–60, 1999

Buitelaar JK, van der Gaag RJ, van der Hoeven J: Buspirone in the management of anxiety and irritability in children with pervasive developmental disorders: results of an open-label study. J Clin Psychiatry 59:56–59, 1998

Burke WJ, Pfeiffer RF, McComb RD: Neuroleptic sensitivity to clozapine in dementia with Lewy bodies. J Neuropsychiatry Clin Neurosci 10:227–229, 1998

Burns A, Russell E, Stratton-Powell H, et al: Sertraline in stroke-associated lability of mood. Int J Geriatr Psychiatry 14:681–685, 1999

Buzan RD, Thomas M, Dubovsky SL: The use of opiate antagonists for recurrent self-injurious behavior. J Neuropsychiatry Clin Neurosci 7:437–444, 1995

Byrne A, Martin W, Hnatko G: Beneficial effects of buspirone therapy in Huntington's disease (letter). Am J Psychiatry 151:1097, 1994

Caley CF, Friedman JH: Does fluoxetine exacerbate Parkinson's disease? J Clin Psychiatry 53:278–282, 1992

Campbell JJ III, Duffy JD: Sertraline treatment of aggression in a developmentally disabled patient (letter). J Clin Psychiatry 56:123–124, 1995

Campbell M, Kafanteris V, Cueva JE: An update on the use of lithium carbonate in aggressive children and adolescents with conduct disorder. Psychopharmacol Bull 31:93–102, 1995

Cantello R, Aquaggia M, Gilli M, et al: Major depression in Parkinson's disease and the mood response to intravenous methylphenidate: possible role of the hedonic dopamine synapse. J Neurol Neurosurg Psychiatry 52:724–731, 1989

Cantillon M, Brunswick R, Molina D, et al: Buspirone vs haloperidol: a double-blind trial for agitation in a nursing home population with Alzheimer's disease. Am J Geriatr Psychiatry 4:263–267, 1996

Casner JA, Weinheimer B, Gualtieri CT: Naltrexone and self-injurious behavior: a retrospective population study. J Clin Psychopharmacol 16:389–394, 1996

Cassidy JW: Fluoxetine: a new serotonergically active antidepressant. J Head Trauma Rehabil 4:67–69, 1989

Chacko RC, Hurley RA, Jankovic J: Clozapine use in diffuse Lewy body disease. J Neuropsychiatry Clin Neurosci 5:206–208, 1993

Chatham-Showalter PE: Carbamazepine for combativeness in acute traumatic brain injury. J Neuropsychiatry Clin Neurosci 8:96–99, 1996

Chemerinski E, Petracca G, Tesón A, et al: Prevalence and correlates of aggressive behavior in Alzheimer's disease. J Neuropsychiatry Clin Neurosci 10:421–425, 1998

Chen ST, Sultzer DL, Hinkin CH, et al: Executive dysfunction in Alzheimer's disease: association with neuropsychiatric symptoms and functional impairment. J Neuropsychiatry Clin Neurosci 10:426–432, 1998

Coccaro EF, Zemishlany Z, Thorne A: Pharmacologic treatment of noncognitive behavioral disturbance in elderly demented patients. Am J Psychiatry 147:1640–1645, 1990

Coffey CE, Ross DR, Ferren EL, et al: Treatment of the "on-off" phenomenon in parkinsonism with lithium carbonate. Ann Neurol 12:375–379, 1982

Cohen SA, Underwood MT: The use of clozapine in a mentally retarded and aggressive population. J Clin Psychiatry 55:440–444, 1994

Cohen SA, Ihrig K, Lott RS, et al: Risperidone for aggression and self-injurious behavior in adults with mental retardation. J Autism Dev Disord 28:229–233, 1998

Colenda CC: Buspirone in treatment of agitated demented patients (letter). Lancet 1:1169, 1988

Collacott RA, Cooper S-A, Branford D, et al: Epidemiology of self-injurious behaviour in adults with learning disabilities. Br J Psychiatry 173:428–432, 1998

Como PG, Rubin AJ, O'Brien CF, et al: A controlled trial of fluoxetine in nondepressed patients with Huntington's disease. Mov Disord 12:397–401, 1997

Connor DF, Ozbayrak KR, Benjamin S, et al: A pilot study of nadolol for overt aggression in developmentally delayed individuals. J Am Acad Child Adolesc Psychiatry 36:826–834, 1997

Craft M, Ismail A, Krishnamurti D, et al: Lithium in the treatment of aggression in mentally handicapped patients. Br J Psychiatry 150:685–689, 1987

Craft S, Asthana S, Newcomer JW, et al: Enhancement of memory in Alzheimer disease with insulin and somatostatin, but not glucose. Arch Gen Psychiatry 56:1135–1140, 1999

Crisostomo EA, Duncan PW, Propst M, et al: Evidence that amphetamine with physical therapy promotes recovery of motor function in stroke patients. Ann Neurol 23:94–97, 1988

Crook T, Petrie W, Wells C, et al: Effects of phosphatidylserine in Alzheimer's disease. Psychopharmacol Bull 28:61–66, 1992

Cueva JE, Overall JE, Small AM, et al: Carbamazepine in aggressive children with conduct disorder: a double-blind and placebo-controlled study. J Am Acad Child Adolesc Psychiatry 35:480–490, 1996

Cummings JL, Cyrus PA, Bieber F, et al: Metrifonate treatment of the cognitive deficits of Alzheimer's disease. Neurology 50:1214–1221, 1998

Czobor P, Volavka J, Meibach RC: Effect of risperidone on hostility in schizophrenia. J Clin Psychopharmacol 15:243–249, 1995

Dallocchio C, Buffa C, Tinelli C, et al: Effectiveness of risperidone in Huntington chorea patients (letter). J Clin Psychopharmacol 19:101–103, 1999

Dam M, Tonin P, De Boni A, et al: Effects of fluoxetine and maprotiline on functional recovery in poststroke hemiplegic patients undergoing rehabilitation therapy. Stroke 27: 1211–1214, 1996

Davanzo PA, Belin TR, Widawski MH, et al: Paroxetine treatment of aggression and self-injury in persons with mental retardation. Am J Ment Retard 102:427–437, 1998

De Deyn PP, Rabheru K, Rasmussen A, et al: A randomized trial of risperidone, placebo, and haloperidol for behavioral symptoms of dementia (comments). Neurology 53:946–955, 1999

Devanand DP, Cooper T, Sackeim HA, et al: Low dose oral haloperidol and blood levels in Alzheimer's disease: a preliminary study. Psychopharmacol Bull 28:169–173, 1992

Devanand DP, Marder K, Michaels KS, et al: A randomized, placebo-controlled dose-comparison trial of haloperidol for psychosis and disruptive behaviors in Alzheimer's disease. Am J Psychiatry 155: 1512–1520, 1998

Dewey RB Jr, O'Suilleabhain PE: Treatment of drug-induced psychosis with quetiapine and clozapine in Parkinson's disease Neurology 55(11):1753–1754, 2000

Dinan TG, Mobayed M: Treatment resistance of depression after head injury: a preliminary study of amitriptyline response. Acta Psychiatr Scand 85:292–294, 1992

Dorevitch A, Katz N, Zemishlany Z, et al: Intramuscular flunitrazepam versus intramuscular haloperidol in the emergency treatment of aggressive psychotic behavior. Am J Psychiatry 156:142–144, 1999

Dreyer EB, Kaiser PK, Offermann JT, et al: HIV-1 coat protein neurotoxicity prevented by calcium channel antagonists. Science 248:364–367, 1990

Dubovsky SL, Franks RD, Allen S, et al: Calcium antagonists in mania. Psychiatry Res 18:309–320, 1986

Duffy JD, Kant R: Clinical utility of clozapine in 16 patients with neurological disease. J Neuropsychiatry Clin Neurosci 8:92–95, 1996

Dysken MW, Mendels J, Lewitt P, et al: Milacemide: a placebo-controlled study in senile dementia of the Alzheimer type. J Am Geriatr Soc 40:503–506, 1992

Eichelman B: Aggressive behavior: from laboratory to clinic. Arch Gen Psychiatry 49:488–492, 1992

Elliott AJ, Roy-Byrne PP: Mirtazapine for depression in patients with human immunodeficiency virus. J Clin Psychopharmacol 20:265–267, 2000

Elliott AJ, Uldall KK, Bergam K, et al: Randomized, placebo-controlled trial of paroxetine versus imipramine in depressed HIV-positive outpatients. Am J Psychiatry 155: 367–372, 1998

Elliott AJ, Russo J, Bergam K, et al: Antidepressant efficacy in HIV-seropositive outpatients with major depressive disorder: an open trial of nefazodone. J Clin Psychiatry 60:226–231, 1999

Evans RW, Gualtieri CT: Carbamazepine: a neuropsychological and psychiatric profile. Clin Neuropharmacol 8:221–241, 1985

Falk WE, Mahnke MW, Poskanzer DC: Lithium prophylaxis of corticotropin-induced psychosis. JAMA 241:1011–1012, 1979

Falsaperla A, Monici-Preti PA, Oliani C: Selegiline versus oxiracetam in patients with Alzheimer-type dementia. Clin Ther 12: 376–384, 1990

Fann JR, Uomoto JM, Katon WJ: Sertraline in the treatment of major depression following mild traumatic brain injury. J Neuropsychiatry Clin Neurosci 12(2):226–232, 2000

Farlow M, Anand R, Messina J Jr, et al: A 52-week study of the efficacy of rivastigmine in patients with mild to moderately severe Alzheimer's disease. Eur Neurol 44(4): 236–241, 2000

Fava M, Rosenbaum JF, Pava JA: Anger attacks in unipolar depression, I: clinical correlates and response to fluoxetine treatment. Am J Psychiatry 150:1158–1163, 1983

Feder R: Treatment of intermittent explosive disorder with sertraline in 3 patients. J Clin Psychiatry 60:195–196, 1999

Feeney D, Gonzales A, Law W: Amphetamine, haloperidol and experience interact to affect rate of recovery after motor cortex injury. Science 217:855–857, 1982

Feinbar JP, Alvarez WA: Clonazepam treatment of organic brain syndromes in three elderly patients. J Clin Psychiatry 47:525–526, 1986

Fernandez HH, Friedman JH, Jacques C, et al: Quetiapine for the treatment of drug-induced psychosis in Parkinson's disease. Mov Disord 14:484–487, 1999

Ferrier IN, Stanton BR, Kelly TP, et al: Neuropsychological function in euthymic patients with bipolar disorder. Br J Psychiatry 175:246–251, 1999

Fiegel GS: ECT and delirium in Parkinson's disease (letter). Am J Psychiatry 149:1759, 1992

Finali G, Piccirilli M, Oliani C, et al: L-Deprenyl therapy improves verbal memory in amnesic Alzheimer patients. Clin Neuropharmacol 14:523–536, 1991

Flax JW, Gray J, Herbert J: Effect of fluoxetine on patients with multiple sclerosis (letter). Am J Psychiatry 148:1603, 1991

Ford B, Lynch T, Greene P: Risperidone in Parkinson's disease (letter). Lancet 344:681, 1994

Freedman M, Rewilak D, Xerri T, et al: L-Deprenyl in Alzheimer's disease: cognitive and behavioral effects. Neurology 50: 660–668, 1998

Friedman JH, Factor SA: Atypical antipsychotics in the treatment of drug-induced psychosis in Parkinson's disease. Mov Disord 15:201–211, 2000

Friedman JH, Goldstein S, Jacques C: Substituting clozapine for olanzapine in psychiatrically stable Parkinson's disease patients: results of an open label pilot study. Clin Neuropharmacol 21:285–288, 1998

Friedman JI, Adler DN, Davis KL: The role of norepinephrine in the pathophysiology of cognitive disorders: potential applications to the treatment of cognitive dysfunction in schizophrenia and Alzheimer's disease. Biol Psychiatry 46:1243–1252, 1999

Fuchs A, Hehnke U, Erhart C, et al: Video rating analyses of effect of maprotiline in patients with dementia and depression. Pharmacopsychiatry 26:37–41, 1993

Gaind GS, Rosebush PI, Mazurek MF: Lorazepam treatment of acute and chronic catatonia in two mentally retarded brothers. J Clin Psychiatry 55:20–30, 1994

Galynker I, Ieronimo C, Miner C, et al: Methylphenidate treatment of negative symptoms in patients with dementia. J Neuropsychiatry Clin Neurosci 9:231–239, 1997

Garza-Trevino ES, Hollister LE, Overall JE, et al: Efficacy of combinations of intramuscular antipsychotics and sedative-hypnotics for control of psychotic agitation. Am J Psychiatry 146:1598–1601, 1989

Gimenez-Roldan S, Mateo D, Navarro E, et al: Efficacy and safety of clozapine and olanzapine: an open-label study comparing two groups of Parkinson's disease patients with dopaminergic-induced psychosis. Parkinsonism Relat Disord 7(2):121–127, 2001

Gleason RP, Schneider LS: Carbamazepine treatment of agitation in Alzheimer's outpatients refractory to neuroleptics. J Clin Psychiatry 51:115–118, 1990

Glenn MB, Wroblewski B, Parziale J: Lithium carbonate for aggressive behavior or affective instability in ten brain injured patients. Am J Phys Med Rehabil 68:221–226, 1989

Glue P: Rapid cycling affective disorders in the mentally retarded. Biol Psychiatry 26: 250–256, 1989

Goetz GG, Tanner CM, Klawans HL: Bupropion in Parkinson's disease. Neurology 34: 1092–1094, 1984

Goodwin FK, Jamison KR: Manic Depressive Illness. New York, Oxford University Press, 1990

Grade C, Redford B, Chrostowski J, et al: Methylphenidate in early poststroke recovery: a double-blind, placebo-controlled study. Arch Phys Med Rehabil 79:1047–1050, 1998

Graham JM, Sussman JD, Ford KS, et al: Olanzapine in the treatment of hallucinosis in idiopathic Parkinson's disease: a cautionary note. J Neurol Neurosurg Psychiatry 65:774–777, 1998

Greenberg SM, Tennis MK, Brown LB, et al: Donepezil therapy in clinical practice. Arch Neurol 57:94–99, 2000

Greendyke RM, Kanter DR: Therapeutic effects of pindolol on behavioral disturbances associated with organic brain disease. J Clin Psychiatry 47:423–426, 1986

Greendyke RM, Kanter DR, Schuster DB, et al: Propranolol in the treatment of assaultive patients with organic brain disease. J Nerv Ment Dis 174:290–294, 1986

Greenwald BS, Marin DB, Silvermans M: Serotonergic treatment of screaming and banging in dementia. Lancet 2:1464–1465, 1986

Gualtieri CT: Buspirone for the behavior problems of patients with organic brain disorders. J Clin Psychopharmacol 11:280–281, 1991

Gualtieri CT, Chandler M, Coons TB, et al: Amantadine: a new clinical profile for traumatic brain injury. Clin Neuropharmacol 12:258–270, 1989

Haas S, Vincent K, Holt J, et al: Divalproex: a possible treatment alternative for demented, elderly aggressive patients. Ann Clin Psychiatry 9:145–147, 1997

Haller E, Binder RL: Clozapine and seizures. Am J Psychiatry 147:1069–1071, 1990

Halman MH, Worth JL, Sanders KM, et al: Anticonvulsant use in the treatment of manic syndromes in patients with HIV-1 infection. J Neuropsychiatry Clin Neurosci 5: 430–434, 1993

Hamner M, Huber M, Gardner VT: Patient with progressive dementia and choreoathetoid movements treated with buspirone. J Clin Psychopharmacol 16:261–262, 1996

Hellings JA, Kelley LA, Gabrielli WF, et al: Sertraline response in adults with mental retardation and autistic disorder. J Clin Psychiatry 57:333–336, 1996

Henderson VW, Paganini-Hill A, Emanuel CK, et al: Estrogen replacement therapy in older women: comparisons between Alzheimer's disease cases and nondemented control subjects. Arch Neurol 51: 896–900, 1994

Herrmann N: Valproic acid treatment of agitation in dementia. Can J Psychiatry 43:69–72, 1998

Herrmann N, Rivard M-F, Flynn M, et al: Risperidone for the treatment of behavioral disturbances in dementia: a case series. J Neuropsychiatry Clin Neurosci 10:220–223, 1998

Herrmann N, Lanctot K, Myszak M: Effectiveness of gabapentin for the treatment of behavioral disorders in dementia. J Clin Psychopharmacol 20:90–93, 2000

Herz LR, Volicer L, Rheume Y: Pharmacotherapy of agitation in dementia. Am J Psychiatry 149:1757–1758, 1992

Heseltine PNR, Goodkin K, Atkinson JH, et al: Randomized double-blind placebo-controlled trial of peptide T for HIV-associated cognitive impairment. Arch Neurol 55:41–51, 1998

Holton A, George K: The use of lithium in severely demented patients with behavioral disturbance. Br J Psychiatry 146:99–100, 1985

Horne M, Lindley SE: Divalproex sodium in the treatment of aggressive behavior and dysphoria in patients with organic brain syndromes. J Clin Psychiatry 56:430–431, 1995

Hornstein A, Seliger G: Cognitive side effects of lithium in closed head injury. J Neuropsychiatry Clin Neurosci 1:446–447, 1989

Horrigan JP, Barnhill LJ: Risperidone and explosive aggressive autism. J Autism Dev Disord 27:313–323, 1997

Iannaccone S, Ferini-Strambi L: Pharmacologic treatment of emotional lability. Clin Neuropharmacol 19:532–535, 1996

Ingram DK, Spangler EL, Iijima S, et al: New pharmacological strategies for cognitive enhancement using a rat model of age-related memory impairment. Ann N Y Acad Sci 717:16–32, 1994

Irizarry MC, Ghaemi SN, Lee-Cherry ER, et al: Risperidone treatment of behavioral disturbances in outpatients with dementia. J Neuropsychiatry Clin Neurosci 11:336–342, 1999

Jacobsen FM, Comas-Díaz L: Donepezil for psychotropic-induced memory loss. J Clin Psychiatry 60:698–704, 1999

Jäkälä P, Riekkinen M, Sirviö J, et al: Clonidine, but not guanfacine, impairs choice reaction time performance in young healthy volunteers. Neuropsychopharmacology 21:495–502, 1999a

Jäkälä P, Riekkinen M, Sirviö J, et al: Guanfacine, but not clonidine, improves planning and working memory performance in humans. Neuropsychopharmacology 20:460–470, 1999b

Jäkälä P, Sirviö J, Riekkinen M, et al: Guanfacine and clonidine, alpha2-agonists, improve paired associates learning, but not delayed matching to sample, in humans. Neuropsychopharmacology 20:119–130, 1999c

Jouvent R, Absensour P, Bonnet AM, et al: Antiparkinsonian and antidepressant effects of high doses of bromocriptine: an independent comparison. J Affect Disord 5:141–145, 1983

Kampen DL, Sherwin BB: Estrogen use and verbal memory in healthy postmenopausal women. Obstet Gynecol 83:979–983, 1994

Katz IR, Jeste DV, Mintzer JE, et al: Comparison of risperidone and placebo for psychosis and behavioral disturbances associated with dementia: a randomized, double-blind trial. J Clin Psychiatry 60:107–115, 1999

Kaufman M, Cassem N, Murray G, et al: Use of psychostimulants in medically ill patients with neurologic disease and major depression. Can J Psychiatry 29:46–49, 1984

Kavoussi RJ, Coccaro EF: Divalproex sodium for impulsive aggressive behavior in patients with personality disorder. J Clin Psychiatry 59:676–680, 1998

Keck PE Jr, Pope HG Jr, Nierenberg AA: Autoinduction of hypertensive reactions by tranylcypromine? J Clin Psychopharmacol 9:48–51, 1989

Kellner CH, Beale MD, Pritchett JT, et al: Electroconvulsive therapy and Parkinson's disease: the case for further study. Psychopharmacol Bull 30:495–500, 1994

Kim E, Zwil AS, McAllister TW, et al: Treatment of organic bipolar mood disorders in Parkinson's disease. J Neuropsychiatry Clin Neurosci 6:181–184, 1994

Kim KS, Pae CU, Chae JH, et al: An open pilot trial of olanzapine for delirium in the Korean population. Psychiatry Clin Neurosci 55(5):515–519, 2001

Kim SW: Opioid antagonists in the treatment of impulse-control disorders. J Clin Psychiatry 59:159–164, 1998

King BH: Fluoxetine reduced self-injurious behavior in an adolescent with mental retardation. J Child Adolesc Psychopharmacol 1:321–329, 1991

Kirby M, Denihan A, Bruce I, et al: Benzodiazepine use among the elderly in the community. Int J Geriatr Psychiatry 14:280–284, 1999

Kirven LE, Montero EF: Comparison of thioridazine and diazepam in the control of nonpsychotic symptoms associated with senility: double-blind study. J Am Geriatr Soc 21: 546–551, 1973

Klaassen T, Verhey FRJ, Sneijders GHJM, et al: Treatment of depression in Parkinson's disease: a meta-analysis. J Neuropsychiatry Clin Neurosci 7:281–286, 1995

Klein E, Uhde TW: Controlled study of verapamil for treatment of panic disorder. Am J Psychiatry 145:431–434, 1988

Knopman D, Schneider L, Davis K, et al: Long-term tacrine (Cognex) treatment: effects on nursing home placement and mortality. Neurology 47:166–177, 1996

Knopman D, Kahn J, Miles S: Clinical research designs for emerging treatments for Alzheimer disease. Arch Neurol 55:1425–1429, 1998

Koshes RJ, Rock NL: Use of clonidine for behavioral control in an adult patient with autism (letter). Am J Psychiatry 151:11, 1994

Kunik ME, Yudofsky SC, Silver JM, et al: Pharmacologic approach to management of agitation associated with dementia. J Clin Psychiatry 55 (suppl):13–17, 1994

Kuzis G, Sabe L, Tiberti C, et al: Cognitive functions in major depression and Parkinson's disease. Arch Neurol 54:982–986, 1997

Kyomen HH, Satlin A, Hennen J, et al: Estrogen therapy and aggressive behavior in elderly patients with moderate-to-severe dementia: results from a short-term, randomized, double-blind trial. Am J Geriatr Psychiatry 7:339–348, 1999

Laitinen L: Desipramine in treatment of Parkinson's disease. Acta Neurol Scand 45:109–113, 1969

Lancon C, Auquier P, Nayt G, et al: Stability of the five-factor structure of the positive and negative syndrome scale. Schizophr Res 42:231–239, 2000

Lanctot KL, Herrmann N: Donepezil for behavioural disorders associated with Lewy bodies: a case series. Int J Geriatr Psychiatry 15:338–345, 2000

Lavretsky H, Sultzer D: A structured trial of risperidone for the treatment of agitation in dementia. Am J Geriatr Psychiatry 6:127–135, 1998

Lawlor BA, Radcliffe H, Molchan SE, et al: A pilot placebo-controlled study of trazodone and buspirone in Alzheimer's disease. Int J Geriatr Psychiatry 9:55–59, 1994

Lazarus LW, Moberg PJ, Langsley PR, et al: Methylphenidate and nortriptyline in the treatment of poststroke depression: a retrospective comparison. Arch Phys Med Rehabil 75:403–406, 1994

Le Bars PL, Katz MM, Berman N, et al: A placebo-controlled, double-blind, randomized trial of an extract of Ginkgo biloba for dementia. JAMA 278:1327–1332, 1997

Lebert F, Pasquier F, Petit H: Behavioral effects of fluoxetine in dementia of the Alzheimer type. International Journal of the Geriatric Society 9:590–591, 1994

Lecamwasam D, Synek B, Moyles K, et al: Chronic lithium neurotoxicity presenting as Parkinson's disease. Int Clin Psychopharmacol 9:127–129, 1994

Lemke MR: Effect of carbamazepine on agitation in Alzheimer's inpatients refractory to neuroleptics. J Clin Psychiatry 56:354–357, 1995

Leo RJ: Movement disorders associated with the serotonin selective reuptake inhibitors. J Clin Psychiatry 57:449–454, 1996

Lera G, Zirulnik J: Pilot study with clozapine in patients with HIV-associated psychosis and drug-induced parkinsonism. Mov Disord 14:128–131, 1999

Levine AM: Buspirone and agitation in head injury. Brain Inj 2:165–187, 1988

Levy MA: A trial of buspirone for the control of disruptive behaviors in community-dwelling patients with dementia. Int J Geriatr Psychiatry 9:841–848, 1994

Levy ML, Cummings JL, Fairbanks LA, et al: Apathy is not depression. J Neuropsychiatry Clin Neurosci 10:314–319, 1998

Lindenmayer J-P, Kotsaftis A: Use of sodium valproate in violent and aggressive behaviors: a critical review. J Clin Psychiatry 61:123–128, 2000

Lipsey JR, Robinson RG, Pearlson GD, et al: Nortriptyline treatment of post-stroke depression: a double-blind study. Lancet 8372:297–300, 1984

Lott AD, McElroy SL, Keys MA: Valproate in the treatment of behavioral agitation in elderly patients with dementia. J Neuropsychiatry Clin Neurosci 7:314–319, 1995

Luchins DI: Carbamazepine in psychiatric syndromes: clinical and neuropharmacological perspectives. Psychopharmacol Bull 20:269–271, 1984

Lyketsos CG, Corazzini K, Steele CD, et al: Guidelines for the use of tacrine in Alzheimer's disease: clinical application and effectiveness. J Neuropsychiatry Clin Neurosci 8:67–73, 1996

Lyketsos CG, Steele C, Galik E, et al: Physical aggression in dementia patients and its relationship to depression. Am J Psychiatry 156:66–71, 1999

Maelicke A, Samochocki M, Jostock R, et al: Allosteric sensitization of nicotinic receptors by galantamine, a new treatment strategy for Alzheimer's disease. Biol Psychiatry 49(3):279–288, 2001

Magai C, Kennedy G, Cohen CI, et al: A controlled clinical trial of sertraline in the treatment of depression in nursing home patients with late-stage Alzheimer's disease. Am J Geriatr Psychiatry 8:66–74, 2000

Malow BA, Reese KB, Sato S, et al: Spectrum of EEG abnormalities during clozapine treatment. Electroencephalogr Clin Neurophysiol 91:205–211, 1994

Marin RS, Fogel BS, Hawkins J, et al: Apathy: a treatable syndrome. J Neuropsychiatry Clin Neurosci 7:23–30, 1995

Mark BZ, Kunkel EJS, Fabi MB, et al: Pimozide is effective in delirium secondary to hypercalcemia when other neuroleptics fail. Psychosomatics 34:446–449, 1993

Markowitz P: Effect of fluoxetine on self-injurious behavior in the developmentally disabled: a preliminary study. J Clin Pharmacol 12:27–31, 1992

Martin PR, Adinoff B, Eckardt MJ, et al: Effective pharmacotherapy of alcoholic amnestic disorder with fluvoxamine. Arch Gen Psychiatry 46:617–621, 1989

Martin PR, Adinoff B, Lane E, et al: Fluvoxamine treatment of alcoholic amnestic disorder. Eur Neuropsychopharmacol 5:27–33, 1995

Masand P, Murray GB, Pickett P: Psychostimulants in post-stroke depression. J Neuropsychiatry Clin Neurosci 3:23–27, 1991

Mashiko H, Yokoyama H, Matsumoto H, et al: Trazodone for aggression in an adolescent with hydrocephalus. J Neuropsychiatry Clin Neurosci 50:133–136, 1996

Mattes JA: Comparative effectiveness of carbamazepine and propranolol for rage outbursts. J Neuropsychiatry Clin Neurosci 2:159–164, 1990

Maxwell CJ, Hogan DB, Ebly EM: Calcium-channel blockers and cognitive function in elderly people: results from the Canadian Study of Health and Aging. CMAJ 161:501–506, 1999

Mazure CM, Druss BG, Cellar JS: Valproate treatment of older psychotic patients with organic mental syndromes and behavioral dyscontrol. J Am Geriatr Soc 40:914–916, 1992

McAllister TW: Carbamazepine in mixed frontal lobe and psychiatric disorders. J Clin Psychiatry 46:393–394, 1985

McFarland BH, Miller MR, Straumfjord AA: Valproate use in the older manic patients. J Clin Psychiatry 51:479–481, 1990

McKeith I, Del Ser T, Spano P, et al: Efficacy of rivastigmine in dementia with Lewy bodies: a randomised, double-blind, placebo-controlled international study. Lancet 356(9247): 2031–2036, 2000

Medalia A, Gold J, Merriam A: The effects of neuroleptics on neuropsychological test results of schizophrenics. Arch Clin Neuropsychol 3:249–271, 1988

Mega MS, Masterman DM, O'Connor SM, et al: The spectrum of behavioral responses to cholinesterase inhibitor therapy in Alzheimer disease. Arch Neurol 56:1388–1393, 1999

Meltzer HY, Ranjan R: Valproic acid treatment of clozapine induced myoclonus. Am J Psychiatry 151:1246–1247, 1994

Mendez MF, Younesi FL, Perryman KM: Use of donepezil for vascular dementia: preliminary clinical experience. J Neuropsychiatry Clin Neurosci 11:268–270, 1999

Mendez MF, Chow T, Ringman J, et al: Pedophilia and temporal lobe disturbances. J Neuropsychiatry Clin Neurosci 12: 71–76, 2000

Meyer JM, Marsh J, Simpson G: Differential sensitivities to risperidone and olanzapine in a human immunodeficiency virus patient. Biol Psychiatry 44:791–794, 1998

Michals ML, Crismon ML, Roberts S, et al: Clozapine response and adverse effects in nine brain-injured patients. J Clin Psychopharmacol 13:198–203, 1993

Moffoot A, O'Carroll RE, Murray C, et al: Clonidine infusion increases uptake of 99mTc-exametazime in anterior cingulate cortex in Korsakoff's psychosis. Psychol Med 24:53–61, 1994

Monteverde A, Gnemmi P, Rossi F, et al: Selegiline in the treatment of mild to moderate Alzheimer-type dementia. Clin Ther 12:315–322, 1990

Mooney GF, Haas LJ: Effect of methylphenidate on brain-related anger. Arch Phys Med Rehabil 74:153–160, 1993

Moore DP: A case of petit mal epilepsy aggravated by lithium. Am J Psychiatry 138: 690–691, 1981

Mortel KF, Meyer JS: Lack of postmenopausal estrogen replacement therapy and the risk of dementia. J Neuropsychiatry Clin Neurosci 7:334–337, 1995

Moskowitz AS, Altshuler L: Increased sensitivity to lithium-induced neurotoxicity after stroke: a case report. J Clin Psychopharmacol 11:272–273, 1991

Mulnard RA, Cotman CW, Kawas C, et al: Estrogen replacement therapy for treatment of mild to moderate Alzheimer disease: a randomized controlled trial. JAMA 283: 1007–1015, 2000

Musser WS, Akil M: Clozapine as a treatment for psychosis in Parkinson's disease: a review. J Neuropsychiatry Clin Neurosci 8:1–9, 1996

Myrick H, Brady KT, Malcolm R: Divalproex in the treatment of alcohol withdrawal. Am J Drug Alcohol Abuse 26:155–160, 2000

Mysiw WJ, Jackson RD, Corrigan JD: Amitriptyline for post-traumatic agitation. Am J Phys Med Rehabil 67:29–33, 1988

Nahas Z, Arlinghaus KA, Kotrla KJ, et al: Rapid response of emotional incontinence to selective serotonin reuptake inhibitors. J Neuropsychiatry Clin Neurosci 10:453–455, 1998

Narayan M, Nelson JC: Treatment of dementia with behavioral disturbance using divalproex or a combination of divalproex and a neuroleptic. J Clin Psychiatry 58:351–354, 1997

Newhouse PA, Porter A, Corwin J, et al: The potential for nicotinic modulation of cognitive and motor functioning in Parkinson's disease. Paper presented at the 4th Symposium on Neurodegenerative Disorders, Ocho Rios, Jamaica, February 23–28, 1997

Nyth AL, Gottfries CG: The clinical efficacy of citalopram in treatment of emotional disturbances in dementia disorders: a Nordic multicentre study. Br J Psychiatry 157:894–901, 1990

Nyth AL, Gottfries CE, Lyby K, et al: A controlled multicenter clinical study of citalopram and placebo in elderly depressed patients with and without concomitant dementia. Acta Psychiatr Scand 86:138–145, 1992

Oh JJ, Rummans TA, O'Connor MK, et al: Cognitive impairment after ECT in patients with Parkinson's disease and psychiatric illness (letter). Am J Psychiatry 149:271, 1992

Oken BS, Storzbach DM, Kaye JA: The efficacy of Ginkgo biloba on cognitive function in Alzheimer disease. Arch Neurol 55:1409–1415, 1998

Olivier B, Mos J, Raghoebar M, et al. Serenics. Prog Drug Res 42:167–308, 1994

Onuma T, Adachi N, Hisano T, et al: 10-year follow-up study of epilepsy with psychosis. Journal of Neurosurgery and Psychiatry 45:360–361, 1991

Palsson S, Aevarsson O, Skoog I: Depression, cerebral atrophy, cognitive performance and incidence of dementia: population study of 85-year-olds. Br J Psychiatry 174:249–253, 1999

Paradiso S, Robinson RG, Arndt S: Self-reported aggressive behavior in patients with stroke. J Nerv Ment Dis 184:746–753, 1996

Parkinson Study Group: Low-dose clozapine for the treatment of drug-induced psychosis in Parkinson's disease. N Engl J Med 340:757–763, 1999

Parmelee DX, O'Shannick GH: Carbamazepine-lithium toxicity in brain damaged adolescents. Brain Inj 2:305–308, 1988

Parsa MA, Bastani B: Quetiapine (Seroquel) in the treatment of psychosis in patients with Parkinson's disease. J Neuropsychiatry Clin Neurosci 10:216–219, 1998

Parsa MA, Szigethy E, Voci JM, et al: Risperidone in treatment of choreoathetosis of Huntington's disease (letter). J Clin Psychopharmacol 17:134–135, 1997

Passik SD, Cooper M: Complicated delirium in a cancer patient successfully treated with olanzapine. J Pain Symptom Manage 17:219–223, 1999

Penn RD, Martin EM, Wilson RS, et al: Intraventricular bethanechol infusion for Alzheimer's disease: results of double-blind and escalating dose trials. Neurology 39:219–222, 1988

Peterson K, Armstrong S, Moseley J: Pathologic crying responsive to treatment with sertraline (letter). Am J Psychiatry 152:953–954, 1995

Petracca G, Teson A, Chemerinski E, et al: A double-blind placebo-controlled study of clomipramine in depressed patients with Alzheimer's disease. J Neuropsychiatry Clin Neurosci 8:270–275, 1996

Petrie WM, Ban TA, Berney S, et al: Loxapine in psychogeriatrics: a placebo and standard controlled clinical investigation. J Clin Psychopharmacol 2:122–126, 1982

Pinner AE, Rich C: Effects of trazodone on aggressive behavior in seven patients with organic mental disorders. Am J Psychiatry 145:1295–1296, 1988

Pollock BG, Mulsant BH, Sweet R, et al: An open pilot study of citalopram for behavioral disturbances of dementia: plasma levels and real-time observations. Am J Geriatr Psychiatry 5:70–78, 1997

Pope HG, McElroy SL, Satlin A, et al: Head injury, bipolar disorder, and response to valproate. Compr Psychiatry 29:34–38, 1988

Popli AP: Risperidone for the treatment of psychosis associated with neurosarcoidosis (letter). J Clin Psychopharmacol 17:132–133, 1997

Porsteinsson A, Tariot PN, Erb R, et al: An open trial of valproate for agitation in geriatric neuropsychiatric disorders. Am J Geriatr Psychiatry 5:344–351, 1997

Porsteinsson AP, Tariot PN, Erb R, et al: Placebo-controlled study of divalproex sodium for agitation in dementia. Am J Geriatr Psychiatry 9(1):58–66, 2001

Potter A, Corwin J, Lang J, et al: Acute effects of the selective nicotine agonist ABT-418 in Alzheimer's disease. Psychopharmacology (Berl) 142:334–342, 1999

Prigatano G: Personality disturbances associated with traumatic brain injury. J Consult Clin Psychol 60:360–368, 1992

Prince M, Rabe-Hesketh S, Brennan P: Do antiarthritic drugs decrease the risk for cognitive decline? An analysis based on data from the MRC Treatment Trial of Hypertension in Older Adults. Neurology 50:374–379, 1998

Qizilbash N, Whitehead A, Higgins J, et al: Cholinesterase inhibition for Alzheimer disease: a meta-analysis of the tacrine trials. JAMA 280:1777–1782, 1998

Rabkin JG, Rabkin R, Harrison W, et al: Effect of imipramine on mood and enumerative measures of immune status in depressed patients with HIV illness. Am J Psychiatry 151:516–523, 1994

Raffaele KC, Berardi A, Asthana S, et al: Effects of long-term continuous infusion of the muscarinic cholinergic agonist arecoline on verbal memory in dementia of the Alzheimer type. Psychopharmacol Bull 27:315–320, 1991

Raji MA, Brady SR: Mirtazapine for treatment of depression and comorbidities in Alzheimer disease. Ann Pharmacother 35(9): 1024–1027, 2001

Ranen NG, Peyser CE, Folstein SE: ECT as a treatment for depression in Huntington's disease. J Neuropsychiatry Clin Neurosci 6:154–159, 1994

Ranen NG, Lipsey J, Treisman G, et al: Sertraline in the treatment of severe aggressiveness in Huntington's disease. J Neuropsychiatry Clin Neurosci 8:338–339, 1996

Rao N, Jellinek HM, Woolston DC: Agitation in closed head injury: haloperidol effects on rehabilitation outcome. Arch Phys Med Rehabil 66:30–34, 1985

Raskind MA: Geriatric psychopharmacology: management of late-life depression and the noncognitive behavioral disturbances of Alzheimer's disease. Psychopharmacology (Berl) 16:815–827, 1993

Ratey JJ, Sovner R, Parks A, et al: Buspirone treatment of aggression and anxiety in mentally retarded patients: a multiple-baseline, placebo lead in study. J Clin Psychiatry 52:159–162, 1991a

Ratey JJ, Sovner R, Parks A, et al: The use of buspirone in the treatment of aggression and anxiety in mentally retarded patients. J Clin Psychiatry 52:159–162, 1991b

Ratey JJ, Leveroni CL, Miller AC, et al: Low-dose buspirone to treat agitation and maladaptive behavior in brain-injured patients: two case reports. J Clin Psychopharmacol 12:362–364, 1992a

Ratey JJ, Sorgi P, O'Driscoll GA, et al: Nadolol to treat aggression and psychiatric symptomatology in chronic psychiatric inpatients: a double-blind, placebo-controlled study. J Clin Psychiatry 53:41–46, 1992b

Reding MJ, Orto LA, Winter SW, et al: Antidepressant therapy after stroke: a double-blind trial. Arch Neurol 43:763–765, 1986

Reifler BV, Teri L, Raskind M, et al: Double blind trial of imipramine in Alzheimer's disease patients with and without depression. Am J Psychiatry 146:45–49, 1989

Rich JB, Rasmusson DX, Folstein MF, et al: Nonsteroidal anti-inflammatory drugs in Alzheimer's disease. Neurology 45:51–55, 1995

Riekkinen P Jr, Riekkinen M: THA improves word priming and clonidine enhances fluency and working memory in Alzheimer's disease. Neuropsychopharmacology 20: 357–364, 1999

Rifkin A, Quitkin F, Klein D: Akinesia: a poorly recognized drug-induced extrapyramidal behavioral disorder. Arch Gen Psychiatry 32:672–674, 1975

Risse SC, Cubberly Z, Lawpe JH, et al: Acute effects of neuroleptic withdrawal in elderly dementia patients. Journal of Geriatric Drug Therapy 2:65–67, 1987

Roane DM, Feinberg TE, Meckler L, et al: Treatment of dementia-associated agitation with gabapentin. J Neuropsychiatry Clin Neurosci 12:40–43, 2000

Robinson RG, Parikh RM, Lipsey JR, et al: Pathological laughing and crying following stroke: validation of a measurement scale and a double-blind treatment study. Am J Psychiatry 150:290–291, 1993

Robinson RG, Schultz SK, Castillo C, et al: Nortriptyline versus fluoxetine in the treatment of depression and in short-term recovery after stroke: a placebo-controlled, double-blind study. Am J Psychiatry 157:351–359, 2000

Rogers J, Kirby LC, Hempelman SR, et al: Clinical trial of indomethacin in Alzheimer's disease. Neurology 43:1609–1611, 1993

Rogers SL, Farlow MR, Doody RS, et al: A 24-week, double-blind, placebo-controlled trial of donepezil in patients with Alzheimer's disease. Donepezil Study Group. Neurology 50(1):136–145, 1998

Rogers SL, Doody RS, Pratt RD, et al: Long-term efficacy and safety of donepezil in the treatment of Alzheimer's disease: final analysis of a US multicentre open-label study. Eur Neuropsychopharmacol 10(3):195–203, 2000

Rösler M, Retz W, Retz-Junginger P, et al: Effects of two-year treatment with the cholinesterase inhibitor rivastigmine on behavioural symptoms in Alzheimer's disease. Behav Neurol 11(4):211–216, 1998

Rösler M, Anand R, Cicin-Sain A, et al: Efficacy and safety of rivastigmine in patients with Alzheimer's disease: international randomised controlled trial. BMJ 318: 633–640, 1999

Roth AS, Ostroff RB, Hoffman RE: Naltrexone as a treatment for repetitive self-injurious behavior: an open-label trial. J Clin Psychiatry 57:233–237, 1996

Roth M, Mountjoy CQ, Amrein R, et al: Moclobemide in elderly patients with cognitive decline and depression: an international double-blind, placebo-controlled trial. Br J Psychiatry 168:149–157, 1996

Roy-Byrne P, Cowley DS: Clinical approach to treatment-resistant panic disorder, in Panic Disorder and Its Treatment. Edited by Rosenbaum JF, Pollack MH. New York: Marcel Dekker, 1998, pp 207–227

Rudorfer MU, Manji HK, Potter WZ: ECT and delirium in Parkinson's disease. Am J Psychiatry 149:1758–1759, 1992

Ruedrich SL: Beta adrenergic blocking medications for treatment of rage outbursts in mentally retarded persons. Semin Clin Neuropsychiatry 1:115–121, 1996

Ruedrich S, Swales TP, Fossaceca C, et al: Effect of divalproex sodium on aggression and self-injurious behaviour in adults with intellectual disability: a retrospective review. J Intellect Disabil Res 43:105–111, 1999

Sacristan JA, Iglesias C, Arellano F, et al: Absence seizures induced by lithium: possible interaction with fluoxetine. Am J Psychiatry 148:146–147, 1991

Sakauye KM, Camp CJ, Ford PA: Effects of buspirone on agitation associated with dementia. Am J Geriatr Psychiatry 1:82–84, 1993

Salloway SP: Diagnosis and treatment of patients with "frontal lobe" syndromes. J Neuropsychiatry Clin Neurosci 6:388–398, 1994

Salzman C: Treatment of the elderly agitated patient. J Clin Psychiatry 48 (suppl 5): 19–21, 1987

Salzman C: Use of benzodiazepines to control disruptive behavior in inpatients. J Clin Psychiatry 49 (suppl 12):13–15, 1988

Salzman C, Fisher J, Nobel K, et al: Cognitive improvement following benzodiazepine discontinuation in elderly nursing home residents. Int J Geriatr Psychiatry 7:89–93, 1992

Sanders JF: Evaluation of oxazepam and placebo in emotionally disturbed aged patients. Geriatrics 20:739–746, 1965

Sanders KM, Murray GB, Cassem NH: High-dose intravenous haloperidol for agitated delirium in a cardiac patient on intra-aortic balloon pump. J Clin Psychopharmacol 11:146–147, 1991

Sano M, Ernesto C, Thomas RG, et al: A controlled trial of selegiline, alpha-tocopherol, or both as treatment for Alzheimer's disease. N Engl J Med 336:1216–1222, 1997

Saran AS: Depression after minor closed head injury: role of dexamethasone suppression test and antidepressants. J Clin Psychiatry 46:335–338, 1985

Saxena S, Mallikarjuna P: Severe memory impairment with acute overdose lithium toxicity: a case report. Br J Psychiatry 152: 853–854, 1988

Scharf S, Mander A, Ugoni A, et al: A double-blind, placebo-controlled trial of diclofenac/misoprostol in Alzheimer's disease. Neurology 53:197–201, 1999

Schiffer RB, Wineman NM: Antidepressant pharmacotherapy of depression associated with multiple sclerosis. Am J Psychiatry 147:1493–1497, 1990

Schiffer RB, Herndon RM, Rudick RA: Treatment of pathologic laughing and weeping with amitriptyline. N Engl J Med 312: 1480–1482, 1985

Schneider LS, Olin JT: Overview of clinical trials of Hydergine in dementia. Arch Neurol 51:787–798, 1994

Schneider LS, Pollock VE, Zemansky MF, et al: A pilot study of low dose L-deprenyl in Alzheimer's disease. J Geriatr Psychiatry Neurol 4:143–148, 1991

Schneider LS, Olin JT, Pawluczyk S: A double-blind crossover pilot study of L-deprenyl (selegiline) combined with cholinesterase inhibitor in Alzheimer's disease. Am J Psychiatry 150:321–323, 1993

Schneider LS, Farlow MR, Pogoda JM: Potential role for estrogen replacement in the treatment of Alzheimer's dementia. Am J Med 103:46S–50S, 1997

Schreiber S, Klag E, Gross Y, et al: Beneficial effect of risperidone on sleep disturbance and psychosis following traumatic brain injury. Int Clin Psychopharmacol 13:273–275, 1998

Schwartz BL, Hashtroudi S, Herting RL, et al: Glycine prodrug facilitates memory retrieval in humans. Neurology 41: 341–1343, 1991

Scott TF, Allen D, Price TRP, et al: Characterization of major depression symptoms in multiple sclerosis patients. J Neuropsychiatry Clin Neurosci 8:318–323, 1996

Seliger GM, Hornstein A, Flax J, et al: Fluoxetine improves emotional incontinence. Brain Inj 6:267–270, 1992

Shaywitz BA, Shaywitz SE: Estrogen and Alzheimer disease: plausible theory, negative clinical trial. JAMA 283:1055–1056, 2000

Shikiar R, Shakespeare A, Sagnier P-P, et al: The impact of metrifonate therapy on caregivers of patients with Alzheimer's disease: results from the MALT clinical trial. J Am Geriatr Soc 48:268–274, 2000

Silver JM, Yudofsky SC, Slater JA, et al: Propranolol treatment of chronically hospitalized aggressive patients. J Neuropsychiatry Clin Neurosci 11:328–335, 1999

Simpson DM, Foster D: Improvement in organically disturbed behavior with trazodone treatment. J Clin Psychiatry 47: 191–193, 1986

Singh AN, Golledge H, Catalan J: Treatment of HIV-related psychotic disorders with risperidone: a series of 21 cases. J Psychosom Res 42:489–493, 1997

Sipahimalani A, Masand PS: Treatment of delirium with risperidone. International Journal of Geriatric Psychopharmacology 1:24–26, 1997a

Sipahimalani A, Masand PS: Use of risperidone in delirium: case reports. Ann Clin Psychiatry 9:105–107, 1997b

Sipahimalani A, Masand PS: Olanzapine in the treatment of delirium. Psychosomatics 39:422–430, 1998

Sloan RL, Brown KW, Pentland B: Fluoxetine as a treatment for emotional lability after brain injury. Brain Inj 6:315–319, 1992

Slooter AJ, Bronzova J, Witteman JC, et al: Estrogen use and early onset Alzheimer's disease: a population-based study. J Neurol Neurosurg Psychiatry 67:779–781, 1999

Sobin P, Schneider L, McDermott H: Fluoxetine in the treatment of agitated dementia (letter). Am J Psychiatry 146: 1636, 1989

Sonne S, Rubey R, Brady K, et al: Naltrexone treatment of self-injurious thoughts and behaviors. J Nerv Ment Dis 184:192–195, 1996

Sovner R: The use of valproate in the treatment of mentally retarded persons with typical and atypical bipolar disorders. J Clin Psychiatry 50 (suppl):40–43, 1989

Spiers P, Myers D, Hochanadel G, et al: Citicoline improves verbal memory in aging. Arch Neurol 53:441–448, 1996

Starkstein SE, Migliorelli R: ECT in a patient with frontal craniotomy and residual meningioma. J Neuropsychiatry Clin Neurosci 5:428–430, 1993

Strang RR: Imipramine in treatment of parkinsonism: a double-blind placebo study. BMJ 2:33–34, 1965

Strauss ME, Lee MM, DiFilippo JM: Premorbid personality and behavioral symptoms in Alzheimer's disease: some cautions. Arch Neurol 54:257–259, 1997

Street JS, Clark WS, Gannon KS, et al: Olanzapine treatment of psychotic and behavioral symptoms in patients with Alzheimer disease in nursing care facilities: a double-blind, randomized, placebo-controlled trial. The HGEU Study Group. Arch Gen Psychiatry 57(10):968–976, 2000

Stuppaeck CH, Pycha R, Miller C, et al: Carbamazepine versus oxazepam in the treatment of alcohol withdrawal: a double-blind study. Alcohol Alcohol 27:153–158, 1992

Sultzer DL, Gray KF, Gunay I, et al: A double-blind comparison of trazodone and haloperidol for treatment of agitation in patients with dementia. Am J Geriatr Psychiatry 5:60–69, 1997

Swartz JR, Miller BL, Lesser IM, et al: Frontotemporal dementia: treatment response to serotonin selective reuptake inhibitors. J Clin Psychiatry 58:212–216, 1997

Tallian KB, Nahata MC, Lo W, et al: Gabapentin associated with aggressive behavior in pediatric patients with seizures. Epilepsia 37:501–502, 1996

Taragano FE, Lyketsos CG, Mangone CA, et al: A double-blind, randomized, fixed-dose trial of fluoxetine vs amitriptyline in the treatment of major depression complicating Alzheimer's disease. Psychosomatics 38:246–252, 1997

Targum SD, Abbott JL: Efficacy of quetiapine in Parkinson's patients with psychosis. J Clin Psychopharmacol 20:54–60, 2000

Tariot PN, Erb R, Podgorski CA, et al: Efficacy and tolerability of carbamazepine for agitation and aggression in dementia. Am J Psychiatry 155:54–61, 1998a

Tariot PN, Goldstein B, Podgorski CA, et al: Short-term administration of selegiline for mild-to-moderate dementia of the Alzheimer's type. Am J Geriatr Psychiatry 6:145–154, 1998b

Tennant FS, Wild J: Naltrexone treatment for postconcussional syndrome. Am J Psychiatry 144:813–814, 1987

Tesar GE, Murray GB, Cassem NH: Use of high-dose intravenous haloperidol in the treatment of agitated cardiac patients. J Clin Psychopharmacol 5:344–347, 1985

Thal LJ, Schwartz G, Sano M, et al: A multicenter double-blind study of controlled-release physostigmine for the treatment of symptoms secondary to Alzheimer's disease. Neurology 47:1389–1395, 1996

Thompson TL, Filley CM, Mitchell WD, et al: Lack of efficacy of Hydergine in patients with Alzheimer's disease. N Engl J Med 323:445–448, 1990

Tiller JG: Short-term buspirone treatment in disinhibition with dementia (letter). Lancet 1:1169, 1989

Tollefson GD: Short-term effects of the calcium channel blocker nimodipine (Bay-e-9736) in the management of primary degenerative dementia. Biol Psychiatry 27: 1133–1142, 1990

Tollefson GD, Greist JH, Jefferson JW, et al: Is baseline agitation a relative contraindication for a selective serotonin reuptake inhibitor: a comparative trial of fluoxetine versus imipramine. J Clin Psychopharmacol 14:385–391, 1994

Tsai GE, Falk WE, Gunther J, et al: Improved cognition in Alzheimer's disease with short-term D-cycloserine treatment. Am J Psychiatry 156:470–473, 1999

Tsai WC, Lai JS, Wang TG: Treatment of emotionalism with fluoxetine during rehabilitation. Scand J Rehabil Med 30:145–149, 1998

Tune L, Carr S, Hoag E, et al: Anticholinergic effects of drugs commonly prescribed for the elderly: potential means for assessing risk of delirium. Am J Psychiatry 149: 1393–1394, 1992

van Dyck CH, McMahon TJ, Rosen MI, et al: Sustained-release methylphenidate for cognitive impairment in HIV-1–infected drug abusers: a pilot study. J Neuropsychiatry Clin Neurosci 9:29–36, 1997 van Dyck CH, Newhouse P, Falk WE, et al: Extended-release physostigmine in Alzheimer disease: a multicenter, double-blind, 12-week study with dose enrichment. Arch Gen Psychiatry 57:157–164, 2000

Van Reekum R, Bayley M, Garner S, et al: N of 1 study: amantadine for the amotivation syndrome in patient with traumatic brain injury. Brain Inj 9:49–53, 1995

van Vugt JP, Siesling S, Vergeer M, et al: Clozapine versus placebo in Huntington's disease: a double blind randomised comparative study. J Neurol Neurosurg Psychiatry 63:35–39, 1997

Verhoeven WM, Tuinier S: The effect of buspirone on challenging behaviour in mentally retarded patients: an open prospective multiple-case study. J Intellect Disabil Res 40:502–508, 1996

Walker Z, Grace J, Overshot R, et al: Olanzapine in dementia with Lewy bodies: a clinical study. Int J Geriatr Psychiatry 14:459–466, 1999

Weinshenker BG, Penman M, Bass B, et al: A double-blind, randomized, crossover trial of pemoline in fatigue associated with multiple sclerosis. Neurology 42:1468–1471, 1992

Weitzner MA, Meyers CA, Valentine AD: Methylphenidate in the treatment of neurobehavioral slowing associated with cancer and cancer treatment. J Neuropsychiatry Clin Neurosci 7:347–350, 1995

Welch J, Manschreck T, Redmond D: Clozapine-induced seizures and EEG changes. J Neuropsychiatry Clin Neurosci 6:250–256, 1994

White JC, Christensen JF, Singer CM: Methylphenidate as a treatment for depression in acquired immunodeficiency syndrome: an n-of-1 trial. J Clin Psychiatry 53:153–156, 1992

Wilcock GK, Lilienfeld S, Gaens E: Efficacy and safety of galantamine in patients with mild to moderate Alzheimer's disease: multicentre randomised controlled trial. Galantamine International-1 Study Group. BMJ 321(7274):1445–1449, 2000

Wilkie FL, Goodkin K, Eisdorfer C, et al: Mild cognitive impairment and risk of mortality in HIV-1 infection. J Neuropsychiatry Clin Neurosci 10:125–132, 1998

Wilkinson D, Murray J: Galantamine: a randomized, double-blind, dose comparison in patients with Alzheimer's disease. Int J Geriatr Psychiatry 16(9):852–857, 2001

Willemsen-Swinkels S, Buitelaar JK, Nijof GJ, et al: Failure of naltrexone hydrochloride to reduce self-injurious and autistic behavior in mentally retarded. Arch Gen Psychiatry 52:766–773, 1995

Wolters EC, Jansen EN, Tuynman-Qua HG, et al: Olanzapine in the treatment of dopaminomimetic psychosis in patients with Parkinson's disease. Neurology 47:1085–1087, 1996

Wong SE, Woolsey JE, Innocent AJ, et al: Behavioral treatment of violent psychiatric patients. Psychiatr Clin North Am 11:569–580, 1988

Workman RH Jr, Orengo CA, Bakey AA, et al: The use of risperidone for psychosis and agitation in demented patients with Parkinson's disease. J Neuropsychiatry Clin Neurosci 9:594–597, 1997

Wroblewski BA, McColgan K, Smith K, et al: The incidence of seizures during tricyclic antidepressant drug treatment in a brain-injured population. J Clin Psychopharmacol 10:124–125, 1990

Wroblewski BA, Leary JM, Phelan AM, et al: Methylphenidate and seizure frequency in brain injured patients with seizure disorders. J Clin Psychiatry 53:86–89, 1992

Wroblewski BA, Joseph AB, Cornblatt RR: Antidepressant pharmacotherapy and the treatment of depression in patients with severe traumatic brain injury: a controlled, prospective study. J Clin Psychiatry 57:582–587, 1996

Wroblewski BA, Joseph AB, Kupfer J, et al: Effectiveness of valproic acid on destructive and aggressive behaviours in patients with acquired brain injury. Brain Inj 11:37–47, 1997

Yatham LN, McHale PA: Carbamazepine in the treatment of aggression: a case report and a review of the literature. Acta Psychiatr Scand 78:188–190, 1988

Yeung PP, Mintzer JE, Mullen JA, et al: Extrapyramidal symptoms in elderly outpatients treated with either quetiapine or risperidone. Paper presented at Annual Meeting of the American College of Neuropsychopharmacology, Acapulco, Mexico, December 12–16, 1999

Yudofsky SC, Silver JM, Jackson W, et al: The Overt Aggression Scale for the objective rating of verbal and physical aggression. Am J Psychiatry 143:35–39, 1986

Yudofsky SC, Silver JM, Schneider SE: Pharmacologic treatment of aggression. Psychiatr Ann 17:397–407, 1987

Zimnitzky BM, DeMaso DR, Steingard RJ: Use of risperidone in psychotic disorder following ischemic brain damage. J Child Adolesc Psychopharmacol 6:75–78, 1996

Zisook S, Peterkin J, Goggin KJ, et al: Treatment of major depression in HIV-seropositive men. J Clin Psychiatry 59: 217–224, 1998

Zubieta JK, Alessi NE: Acute and chronic administration of trazodone in the treatment of disruptive behavior disorders in children. J Clin Psychopharmacol 12: 346–351, 1992

Cognitive Rehabilitation and Behavior Therapy for Patients With Neuropsychiatric Disorders

Michael D. Franzen, Ph.D.

Mark R. Lovell, Ph.D.

There is increasing evidence and awareness that treatment of central nervous system (CNS) disorders is a viable and productive endeavor. For example, although traumatic brain injury has been typically conceptualized as permanently devastating, some agreement exists that certain treatments can have positive effects (NIH Consensus Statement 1998). The role of the psychiatrist in the diagnosis and treatment of the sequelae of CNS dysfunction has become a crucial one and promises to become even more central with the continued development of sophisticated neuropharmacologic treatments for both the cognitive and the psychosocial components of brain impairment (Gualtieri 1988).

An understanding of nonpharmacologic, behavioral methods of assessment and treatment can greatly enhance the patient's recovery from cognitive deficits as well as provide a useful adjunct treatment for behavioral deficits and excesses that are commonly associated with CNS dysfunction. In this chapter, we review the role of psychologic treatments for the neuropsychologic (cognitive) and behavioral consequences of CNS dysfunction.

In response to the increase in the number of patients requiring treatment for CNS dysfunction, there has been a proliferation of treatment agencies structured to provide rehabilitation services, as well as an accompanying increase in research efforts designed to assess the efficacy of these treatment programs. There has been a particularly intense focus over the last few years on the development of rehabilitation programs designed specifically to treat the neuropsychologic and psychosocial sequelae of neuropsychiatric disorders. Before turning to a discussion of specific treatment modalities that may be useful with neuropsychiatric patients, we briefly review neuroanatomic influences on the recovery process.

Neuroanatomic and Neurophysiologic Determinants of Recovery

Recovery from brain injury or disease can be conceptualized as involving a number of separate but interacting processes. Although a complete discussion of existing research concerning neuroanatomic and neurophysiologic aspects of the recovery process is beyond the scope of this chapter, Gouvier et al. (1986) has provided an early complete review of current theories of recovery from brain injury.

After an acute brain injury, such as a stroke or head injury, some degree of improvement is likely because of a lessening of the temporary or treatable consequences of the injury. Factors such as degree of cerebral edema and extent of increased intracranial pressure are well known to temporarily affect brain function after a closed head injury or stroke (Lezak 1995). Extracellular changes after injury to the cell also have been shown to affect neural functioning. In addition, the regrowth of neural tissue to compensate for an injured area has been shown to occur to some minimal extent in animal studies on both anatomic (Kolata 1983) and physiologic (Wall and Egger 1971) levels. However, with degenerative illnesses, such as Alzheimer's disease and Huntington's disease, the condition actually worsens over time.

The differences in prognosis among various neurologic disorders obviously affect the structure of the rehabilitation

program. The expectations and goals of a rehabilitation program that is structured to improve memory function in patients with head injury are likely to be much different from those of a program for patients with Alzheimer's disease. Similarly, the goals will vary as a function of the severity of memory impairment in patients with closed head injury. A program designed for patients with head injury and consequent moderate memory impairment is likely to focus on teaching alternative strategies for remembering new information. In contrast, a program designed for a patient with Alzheimer's disease would probably focus on improving the patient's functioning with regard to activities of daily living. Previously, the amount of time since the injury also was seen as a determining variable in the design of rehabilitation efforts, with treatment aimed at improving the skill or substituting other cognitive mechanisms used in the early stages of recovery and treatment aimed at compensatory behaviors in the late stages of recovery. However, some intriguing data suggest that at least for stroke, brain reorganization for motor skills may be possible even a decade past the time of the stroke (Liepert et al. 2000).

Cognitive Rehabilitation of Patients With Neuropsychiatric Disorders

The terms *cognitive rehabilitation* and *cognitive retraining* have been variously used to describe treatments designed to maximize recovery of the individual's abilities in the areas of intellectual functioning, visual processing, language, and particularly, memory. It is important to note that the techniques used to improve cognitive functioning after a neurologic event represent an extremely heterogeneous group of procedures that vary widely in their focus according to the nature of the patient's cognitive difficulties, the specific skills and training of the staff members, and the medium through which information is presented (i.e., computer vs. individual therapy vs. group therapy).

Because patients with different neurologic or neuropsychiatric syndromes often have different cognitive deficits, the focus of the treatment is likely to vary greatly. For example, a treatment program designed primarily to treat patients with head injury is likely to focus on the amelioration of attentional and memory deficits, whereas a rehabilitation program designed for stroke patients is likely to focus on a more specific deficit, such as language disorders or other disorders that tend to occur after lateralized brain damage, and to have less emphasis on co-occurring attentional and memory deficits.

Attention to psychiatric problems in patients with neurologic impairment is an increasingly important component of rehabilitation efforts (e.g., Robinson 1997). The use of pharmacologic agents in the treatment of affective and behavior changes following traumatic brain injury has been reported in case studies (Khouzam and Donnelly 1998; Mendez et al. 1999). Carbamazepine has been used in the treatment of behavioral agitation following severe traumatic brain injury (Azouvi et al. 1999).

The systematic research concerning the effectiveness of cognitive and behavioral treatment strategies in this group is still a developing endeavor. Some work has been reported in the area of treating social skills deficits and anger control. Medd and Tate (2000) reported the effects of anger management training in individuals with traumatic brain injury. In addition to psychologically based methods, pharmacologic methods have been used to treat the physical and emotional symptoms (Holzer 1998; McIntosh 1997; Wroblewski et al. 1997). Although amantadine was at first promising, it has not provided robust effects in improving cognitive and behavioral functioning in brain-injured subjects (Schneider et al. 1999). The treatment of frontal lobe injury with dopaminergic agents may beneficially affect other rehabilitation efforts (Kraus and Maki 1997). The use of psychostimulants in facilitating treatment effects has been reported for pediatric subjects with traumatic brain injury (Williams et al. 1998) as well as for adults (Glen 1998).

The results of psychologic treatment methods for the cognitive deficits associated with traumatic brain injury generally show larger effects for skills as measured by standardized tests than as measured by ecologically relevant behaviors (Ho and Bennett 1997). This is a vexing problem because the ultimate goal of the treatment is to provide some socially relevant and valid effect. Future research is needed to investigate the variables that govern generalizability and ecologic validity.

Flesher (1990) presented an intriguing discussion of an approach to using this type of intervention with schizophrenic patients; however, there have been limited reports of applications, an exception being Benedict et al. (1994), who reported on the use of information-processing rehabilitation. Although it may be too early to critically evaluate the efficacy of this approach (Bellak and Mueser 1993), it certainly bears watching. In contrast, the use of behavioral methods for training in social skills in schizophrenic patients is well documented.

Attentional Processes

Disorders of attention are common sequelae of several neurologic disorders, particularly traumatic brain injury. Recognition and treatment of attentional disorders are extremely important because an inability to focus and sustain attention may directly limit the patient's ability to actively participate in the rehabilitation program and may therefore affect progress in other areas of cognitive functioning. Attention is not a unitary process. A number of components of attention have been identified, including alertness and the ability to selectively attend to incoming information, as well as the capacity to focus and maintain attention or vigilance (Posner and Rafal 1987).

Rehabilitation programs designed to improve attention usually attempt to address all of these processes. One such program is the Orientation Remedial module developed by Ben-Yishay and associates (Ben-Yishay and Diller 1981) at New York University. The Orientation Remedial program consists of five separate tasks that are presented by microcomputer and vary in degree of difficulty; they involve training in the following areas:

1. Attending and reacting to environmental signals
2. Timing responses in relation to changing environmental cues
3. Being actively vigilant
4. Estimating time
5. Synchronizing of response with complex rhythms

Progress on these tasks is a prerequisite for further training on higher-level tasks.

Memory

Much emphasis has been placed on the development of treatment approaches to improve memory. In reviewing the empirical literature, Franzen and Haut (1991) divided the strategies into three basic categories: 1) the use of spared skills in the form of mnemonic devices or alternative functional systems, 2) direct retraining with the use of repetitive practice and drills, and 3) the use of behavioral prosthetics or external devices or strategies to improve memory.

Use of Spared Skills

Mnemonic strategies are approaches to memory rehabilitation that are specifically designed to promote the encoding and remembering of a specific type of information, depending on the patient's particular memory impairment, by capitalizing on the spared skills. Currently, several different types of mnemonic strategies may be of use in neuropsychiatric settings. Visual imagery is one of the most well-known and commonly used mnemonic strategies (Glisky and Schacter 1986) and involves the use of visual images to assist in the learning and retention of verbal information. The method of loci involves the association of verbal information to be remembered with locations that are familiar to the patient (e.g., the room in a house or the location on a street). When recall of the information is required, the patient visualizes each room and the item(s) that are to be remembered in each location (Moffat 1984). Initial research suggested that this method may be particularly useful for elderly patients (Robertson-Tchabo et al. 1976).

Peg mnemonics requires the patient to learn a list of peg words and to associate these words with a given visual image, such as "one bun," "two shoes," and so on. After the learned association of the numbers with the visual image, sequential information can be remembered in order by association with the visual image (Gouvier et al. 1986). This strategy showed some early promise in patients with brain injuries (Patten 1972). More recent research, however, suggested that this approach may not be highly effective because patients with brain injuries are unable to generate visual images (Crovitz et al. 1979) and have difficulty maintaining this information over time.

Another type of visual-imagery procedure that has been widely used in clinical settings and has been studied extensively is face-name association. For example, the name "Angela Harper" might be encoded by the patient by visualizing an angel playing a harp. Obviously, the ease with which this method can be used by patients with brain injuries depends on their ability to form internal visual images, as well as the ease with which the name can be transferred into a distinct visual image. Whereas it may be relatively easy to find visual associations for a name such as "Angela Harper," a name such as "Jane Johnson" may be much more difficult to encode in this manner.

Overall, visual-imagery strategies may be useful for specific groups of patients (e.g., those with impairments in verbal memory who need to use nonverbal cues to assist them in recall) and in patients whose impairments are mild enough to allow them to recall the series of steps necessary to spontaneously use these strategies once they return to their natural environments. A series of single-subject experiments reported by Wilson (1987) indicated that the strategy of visual imagery to learn peoples' names may be differentially effective for different individuals, even when the etiology of memory impairment is similar.

The use of verbally based mnemonic strategies also has become quite popular, particularly with patients who have difficulty using visual imagery.

This procedure was originally demonstrated by Gardner (1977) with a globally amnesic patient who was able to recall pertinent personal information by the learning and subsequent singing of the following rhyme:

Henry's my name/Memory's my game/I'm in the V.A. in Jamaica Plain

My bed's on 7D/The year is '73/Every day I make a little gain.

For patients who have difficulty learning and remembering written information, Glasgow et al. (1977) used a structured procedure called *PQRST*. This strategy involves application of the following five steps:

1. **P**review the information.
2. Form **Q**uestions about the information.
3. **R**ead the information.
4. **S**tate the questions.
5. **T**est for retention by answering the questions after the material has been read.

Repetitive Practice

Cognitive rehabilitation strategies that emphasize repetitive practice of the information to be remembered has little experimental evidence. Although it is generally accepted that patients with brain injuries can learn specific pieces of information through repeated exposure, studies designed to show generalization of this training to new settings or tasks have not been encouraging.

Glisky and Schacter (1986) suggested that attempts to remedy memory disorders should be focused on the acquisition of domain-specific knowledge that is likely to be specifically relevant to the patient's ability to function in everyday life. The goal of this treatment is not to improve memory functioning in general but rather to deal with specific problems associated with memory impairment. Initial research has established that even patients with severe brain injuries are indeed capable of acquiring discrete pieces of information that are important to their ability to function on a daily basis (Glasgow et al. 1977; Wilson 1982).

External Memory Aids

External aids to memory can take various forms, but generally they fall into the two categories of memory storage devices and memory-cuing strategies (Harris 1984). Lists and memory books are widely used by patients with brain injuries to record information that is vital to his or her daily function (e.g., the daily schedule of activities and chores to be performed) and that is then consulted at a given time. Schmitter-Edgecombe et al. (1995) supported the efficacy of memory notebook training to improve memory for everyday activities, although there was no difference in laboratory-based memory tasks, and the gains were not maintained as well at a 6-month follow-up evaluation.

With recent advances in the field of microelectronics, handheld electronic storage devices have become increasingly popular in rehabilitation settings. These devices allow for the storage of large amounts of information. Their often complicated operation requirements may obviate their use in all but the mildest cases of brain injury or disease, and the device must be consulted at the appropriate time in order to be useful. This may be a difficult task for the patient with brain injury and often requires the use of cuing strategies that remind the patient to engage in a behavior at a given time.

The application of cuing involves the use of prompts designed to remind the patient to engage in a specific behavioral sequence at a given time. To be maximally effective, the cue should be given as close as possible to the time that the behavior is required, must be active (e.g., use of an alarm clock) rather than passive, and should provide a reminder of the specific behavior that is desired (Harris 1984).

Visual-Perceptual Disorders

In addition to memory impairment, individuals with brain injuries may have diffi-
culties with visual perception (Gouvier et al. 1986). Given the importance of visual-perceptual processing to many occupational tasks and to the safe operation of an automobile (Sivak et al. 1985), the rehabilitation of deficits in this area could have important implications for the recovery of neuropsychiatric patients.

Hemispatial neglect syndrome is characterized by an inability to recognize stimuli in the contralateral visual field. One strategy that has been used extensively to treat hemispatial neglect is visual scanning training. This procedure has been designed to promote scanning to the neglected hemifield (Diller and Weinberg 1977; Gianutsos et al. 1983). The New York Medical Center program uses a light board with 20 colored lights and a target that can be moved around the board at different speeds. With this device, the patient can be systematically trained to attend to the neglected visual field (Gordon et al. 1985). Other researchers have produced similar therapeutic gains in scanning and other aspects of visual-perceptual functioning through rehabilitation strategies. (For a more complete review of this area, see Gianutsos and Matheson 1987 and Gordon et al. 1985.)

Problem Solving and Executive Functions

Patients who have sustained brain injuries often experience a breakdown in their ability to reason, to form concepts, to solve problems, to execute and terminate behavioral sequences, and to engage in other complex cognitive activities (Goldstein and Levin 1987). Deficits in these areas are among the most debilitating to the neuropsychiatric patient because they often underlie changes in the basic abilities to function interpersonally, socially, and vocationally.

Intellectual and executive functioning involve numerous processes that include motivation, abstract thinking, and concept formation, as well as the ability to plan, reason, and execute and terminate behaviors. Therefore, breakdowns in intellectual and executive functioning can occur for various reasons depending on the underlying core deficit(s) and can vary based on the area of the brain that is injured. For example, injury to the parieto-occipital area is likely to result in a problem-solving deficit secondary to difficulty with comprehension of logical-grammatical structure, whereas a frontal lobe injury may impede problem solving by disrupting the individual's ability to plan and to carry out the series of steps necessary to process the grammatical material (Luria and Tsvetkova 1990).

An apparent breakdown in the patient's ability to function intellectually also can occur secondary to deficits in other related areas of neuropsychologic functioning, such as attention, memory, and language. The type of rehabilitation strategy best suited for such a patient depends on the underlying core deficit that needs to be addressed. The goal of rehabilitation for a patient with a left parieto-occipital lesion might be to help the patient develop the skill to correctly analyze the grammatical structure of the problem. Rehabilitation efforts for a patient with frontal lobe injury might emphasize impulse control and execution of the appropriate behavioral sequence to solve the problem.

Programs designed to rehabilitate these patients have necessarily involved attempts to address these deficits in a hierarchical manner, as originally proposed by Luria (1963). One such program was developed at New York University by Ben-Yishay and associates (Ben-Yishay and Diller 1983). They developed a two-tiered approach that defines five basic deficit areas—1) arousal and attention, 2) memory, 3) impairment in underlying skill structure, 4) language and thought, and 5) feeling tone—and two domains of higher-level problem solving. This model proposes that deficits in the higher-level skills are often produced by core deficits and that the patient's behavior is likely to depend on an interaction between the two domains (Goldstein and Levin 1987).

Speech and Language

Disorders of speech and language are common, particularly when the dominant (usually left) hemisphere is injured. Because the ability to communicate is often central to the patient's personal, social, and vocational readjustment after brain injury or disease, rehabilitation efforts in this area are extremely important. In most rehabilitation settings, speech and language therapies have traditionally been the province of speech pathologists. The goal of therapy has variously been the improvement of comprehension (receptive language) and expression (expressive language), and it has been shown that patients who receive speech therapy after a stroke improve more than patients who do not (Basso et al. 1979).

It is important to consider the reason for the observed speech deficit in designing the treatment; that is, it is not sufficient simply to identify the behavioral deficit and attempt to increase the rate of production (Franzen 1991). For example, Giles et al. (1988) increased appropriate verbalizations in a patient with head injury by providing cuing to keep verbalization short and to pause in planning his speech.

Molar Behaviors

The final test of rehabilitation efforts is frequently the change in ecologically relevant molar behaviors. Examples include driving, the completion of occupational work tasks, successful social interaction, and, at a simpler level, activities of daily living. The results of standardized testing may account for most of the variance reported for molar behaviors such as driving skill (Galski et al. 1997). However, the improvement in these molar behaviors also may depend on treatment aimed directly at the production of the behaviors, even when the component cognitive skills have been optimized. Giles et al. (1997) used behavioral techniques to improve washing and dressing skills in a series of individuals with severe brain injury.

Use of Computers in Cognitive Rehabilitation

The microcomputer has great potential for use in rehabilitation settings and may offer several advantages over more conventional, therapist-based treatments (Grimm and Bleiberg 1986), including being potentially self-instructional and self-paced, requiring less direct staff time, and accurately providing direct feedback to the patient about performance. Microcomputers also facilitate research by accurately and consistently recording the large amounts of potentially useful data that are generated during the rehabilitation process.

Several cautions must be mentioned concerning the use of microcomputers in the rehabilitation process. The microcomputer is merely a tool, and its usefulness is limited by the availability of software that meets the needs of the individual patient and the skill of the therapist in implementing the program(s). As noted by Harris (1984), the danger is that cognitive rehabilitation will become centered around the software that is available through a given treatment program rather than being based on the individual needs of the patient. Microcomputers are not capable of simulating human social inter-

action and should not be used in lieu of human therapeutic contact.

Behavioral Dysfunction After Brain Injury

Relatively few follow-up studies to date have systematically investigated the efficacy of neuropsychiatric treatment programs. Much of what is known comes from studies conducted in rehabilitation settings rather than in hospitals specifically designed to treat patients with neuropsychiatric disorders.

Behavioral dysfunction associated with other neurologic disorders, such as cerebrovascular accidents and progressive dementing disorders, has not been the subject of a great deal of treatment research. The studies that have been reported have been useful in guiding the development of practical strategies for dealing with the behavioral-psychiatric consequences of brain injury. In particular, behaviorally based treatments have been heavily used. Behavioral dysfunction after brain injury can have a marked effect on the recovery process itself. The patients most needing cognitive rehabilitation services are often kept out of many treatment facilities because of their disruptive behavior (Levin et al. 1982; Lishman 1978; Weddell et al. 1980).

Levin and Grossman (1978) reported behavior problems that were present 1 month after traumatic brain injury. At 6 months after injury, those patients who had poor social and occupational recovery continued to manifest significant cognitive and behavioral disruption. Complaints of tangential thinking, fragmented speech, slowness of thought and action, depressed mood, increased anxiety, and marital and/or family conflict also were frequently noted (Levin et al. 1979). Other behavioral changes reported to have the potential to cause psychosocial disruption include increased irritability (Rosenthal 1983), social inappropriateness (Lewis et al. 1988), aggression (Mungas 1988), and expansiveness, helplessness, suspiciousness, and anxiety (Grant and Alves 1987).

Behavioral dysfunction is not limited to individuals with traumatic brain injuries. Patients with lesions in specific brain regions secondary to other pathologic conditions also can have characteristic patterns of dysfunctional behavior. For example, frontal lobe dysfunction secondary to stroke, tumor, or other disease processes is often associated with a cluster of symptoms, including social disinhibition, reduced attention, distractibility, impaired judgment, affective lability, and more pervasive mood disorder (Bond 1984; Stuss and Benson 1984). In contrast, Prigatano (1987) noted that individuals with temporal lobe dysfunction can show heightened interpersonal sensitivity, which can evolve into frank paranoid ideation.

In addition to differences between patients with different types of brain injury or disease, the variability in the severity and extent of behavioral disruption after injury within each patient group is remarkable (Eames and Wood 1985). Individuals with mild head injuries are less prone to debilitating behavioral changes but still can experience physical, cognitive, and affective changes of sufficient magnitude to affect their ability to return to preaccident activities (Dikmen et al. 1986; Levin et al. 1987).

It seems clear that adjustment after brain injury appears to be related to a multitude of neurologic and nonneurologic factors, each of which requires consideration in the choice of an appropriate course of intervention for any observed behavioral dysfunction. In addition to the extent and severity of the neurologic injury itself, some of the other factors that can contribute to the presence and type of behavioral dysfunction include the amount of time elapsed since the injury, premorbid psychiatric and psychosocial adjustment, financial resources, social supports, and personal awareness of (and reaction to) acquired deficits (Eames 1988; G. Goldstein and Ruthven 1983; Gross and Schutz 1986; Meier et al. 1987).

Given the large number of factors that influence recovery from brain injury, a multidimensional approach to the behavioral treatment of patients with brain injury is likely to result in an optimal recovery. Individuals with more severe cognitive impairments are more likely to profit from highly structured behavioral programs. Those whose neuropsychologic functioning is more intact, in contrast, may profit from interventions with a more active cognitive component that requires them to use abstract thought as well as self-evaluative and self-corrective processes.

Behavior Therapy for Patients With Brain Impairment

The domain of behavior therapy has expanded considerably in the past 20 years. (For more comprehensive and critical presentations of the recent status and direction of behavior therapies, see Haynes 1984, Hersen and Bellack 1985, and Kazdin 1979; for excellent compendia describing both assessment and treatment approaches in clinically useful terms, see Bellack and Hersen 1985b and Hersen and Bellack 1988.)

Despite a broadening scope that has included the treatment of patients with neurologic impairment, behavioral approaches remain committed to the original principles derived from experimental and social psychology. They also emphasize the empirical and objective implementation and evaluation of treatment (Bellack and Hersen 1985a).

The general assumptions about the nature of behavior disorders that form the basis of behavioral approaches include the following (Haynes 1984):

- Disordered behavior can be expressed through overt actions, thoughts, verbalizations, and physiologic reactions.
- These reactions do not necessarily vary in the same way for different individuals or for different behavior disorders.
- Changing one specific behavior may result in changes in other related behaviors.
- Environmental conditions play an important role in the initiation, maintenance, and alteration of behavior.

These assumptions have led to approaches emphasizing the objective evaluation of observable aspects of the individual and his or her interaction with the environment. The range of observable events is limited only by the clinician's ability to establish a reliable, valid quantification of the target behavior or environmental condition, ranging from a specific physiologic reaction, such as heart rate, to a self-report of the number of obsessive thoughts occurring during a 24-hour period. The goal of treatment is to alter those aspects of the environment that have become associated with the initiation or maintenance of maladaptive behaviors or to alter the patient's response to those aspects of the environment in some way.

The application of a behavioral intervention with a neuropsychiatric patient requires careful consideration of both the neuropsychologic and the environmental aspects of the presenting problem (Horton and Barrett 1988).

At present, the accumulated body of evidence remains limited regarding the specific types of behavioral interventions that are most effective in treating the various dysfunctional behaviors observed in individuals with different kinds of brain injuries. Despite this limitation, there is optimism, based on the current literature, that behavior therapy can be effective for patients with brain injuries (Horton and Miller 1985). Indeed, an increasing number of books, primarily on the rehabilitation of patients with brain injuries, describe the potential applications of behavioral approaches for persons with neurologic impairment (Edelstein and Couture 1984; G. Goldstein and Ruthven 1983; Seron 1987; Wood 1984). Such sources provide an excellent introduction to the basic models, methods, and limitations of behavioral treatments of patients with brain injuries.

Behavioral approaches can be broadly classified into at least three general models (Calhoun and Turner 1981): 1) a traditional behavioral approach, 2) a social learning approach, and 3) a cognitive-behavioral approach. The degree to which the client or patient is required to participate actively in the identification and alteration of the environmental conditions assumed to be supporting the maladaptive behavior varies across these models.

Traditional Behavioral Approach

The traditional behavioral approach emphasizes the effects of environmental events that occur after (consequences), as well as before (antecedents), a particular behavior of interest. We address these two aspects of environmental influence separately.

Interventions Aimed at the Consequences of Behavior

A consequence that increases the probability of a specific behavior occurring again under similar circumstances is termed a *reinforcer.* A behavior followed by an environmental consequence that increases the likelihood that the behavior will occur again is called a *positive reinforcer.* A behavior followed by the removal of a negative or aversive environmental condition is called a *negative reinforcer.* A behavior followed by an aversive environmental event is termed a *punishment.* The effect of punishment is to reduce the probability that the behavior will occur under similar conditions. It is useful to remember that reinforcers (positive or negative) always increase the likelihood of the behavior occurring again, whereas punishments decrease the likelihood of a behavior occurring again. When the reliable relation between a specific behavior and an environmental consequence is removed, the behavioral effect is to reduce the target behavior to a near-zero level of occurrence. This process is called *extinction.*

Interventions Aimed at the Antecedents of Behavior

Behavior is controlled or affected not only by the consequences that follow it but also by events that precede it. These events are called *antecedents.* For example, an aggressive patient may have outbursts only in the presence of the nursing staff and never in the presence of the physician. In this case, a failure to search for potential antecedents (e.g., female sex or physical size) that may be eliciting the behavior may leave half of the behavioral assessment undone and may result in difficulty decreasing the aggressive behavior. Treatment is structured to decrease the likelihood of an outburst by restructuring the events that lead to the violent behavior. Some patients are able to learn to anticipate these antecedents themselves, whereas for others, it becomes the task of the treatment staff to identify and modify the antecedents that lead to unwanted behavior. For example, if the stress of verbal communication leads to aggressive behavior in an aphasic patient, the patient may be initially trained to use an alternative form of communication, such as writing or sign language (Franzen and Lovell 1987).

Other Behavioral Approaches

Yet another class of approaches involves the use of differential reinforcement of other behaviors. In this approach, the problem behavior is not consequated—that is, the effect of the problem behavior is not addressed. Instead, another behavior that is inconsistent with the problem target behavior is reinforced. As the other behavior increases in frequency, the problem behavior decreases. Hegel and Ferguson (2000) reported the successful use of this approach in reducing aggressive behavior in a subject with brain injury. Differential reinforcement of low rates of responding also may be used to reduce undesired behaviors (Alderman and Knight 1997). Finally, noncontingent reinforcement in the form of increased attention to a subject resulted in a decrease in aggression toward others and a decrease in self-injurious behaviors (Persel et al. 1997).

Social Learning Approach

With the social learning approach, cognitive processes that mediate between environmental conditions and behavioral responses are included in explanations of the learning process. Social learning approaches take advantage of learning through modeling. Emphasis is also placed on practicing the components of social skills in role-playing situations, where the patient can receive corrective feedback.

Socially skilled behavior is generally divided into three components: 1) social perception, 2) social problem solving, and

3) social expression. Training can occur at any one of these levels. For the patient who has lost the ability to interact appropriately with conversational skills, this behavior may be modeled by staff members. (For a comprehensive review, see Bandura 1977.)

Cognitive-Behavioral Approach

The term *cognitive-behavioral approach* refers to a heterogeneous group of procedures that emphasize the individual's cognitive mediation (self-messages) in explaining behavioral responses within environmental contexts. The thoughts, beliefs, and predictions about one's own actions and their potential environmental consequences are emphasized. Treatment focuses on changing maladaptive beliefs and increasing an individual's self-control within the current social environment by changing maladaptive thoughts or beliefs. This approach is particularly useful with patients who have relatively intact language and self-evaluative abilities. Suzman et al. (1997) used cognitive-behavioral methods to improve the problem-solving skills of children with cognitive deficits following traumatic brain injury.

Assessment of Treatment Effects

Because each patient is an individual and treatment of cognitive dysfunction is still a relatively nascent endeavor, interventions often need to be specifically tailored to the individual patient. Interventions often must be applied before the period of spontaneous recovery has ended, and a method to distinguish the effects of intervention from the effects of recovery of acute physiologic disturbance is needed. The multiple baseline design is a single-subject design that addresses these issues (Franzen and Iverson 1990).

The design of multiple baselines across behaviors involves the evaluation of more than one behavior taking place at the same time. However, only one of the behaviors is targeted for intervention at a time. In this way, the nontargeted behaviors are used as control comparisons for the targeted behaviors. For example, behavior A is targeted for intervention first, and monitors on behaviors B and C are used as control comparisons. After completion of the treatment phase for behavior A, an intervention is implemented for behavior B, and monitors on behaviors A and C are used as control comparisons.

Figure 20–1 presents an example of a multiple baseline design in the treatment of an individual with brain injury and deficits in memory, attention, and visual-spatial processing. The attention skills receive treatment in the first phase, with a concomitant improvement in skill level. At the second phase, memory skills are treated, with a concomitant improvement. Finally, visual-spatial skills are treated at the third phase, and improvement is seen there. At each phase, performance in the other untreated skill areas is used as a control comparison for the treated skill areas.

In an application of the multiple baseline design to the treatment of a patient with brain injury, Franzen and Harris (1993) reported a case in which a patient had deficits in attention-based memory and in abstraction and planning as the result of a closed head injury. This patient was first seen 23 days after the closed head injury occurred. He was seen for a series of weekly appointments. At these appointments, the emotional adjustment was discussed and support was provided. Additionally, the patient received psychotherapy in the form of anger-control training and social reinforcement for increasing his daily level of activity and self-initiated social interactions, two areas identified as problems during the evaluation. Finally,

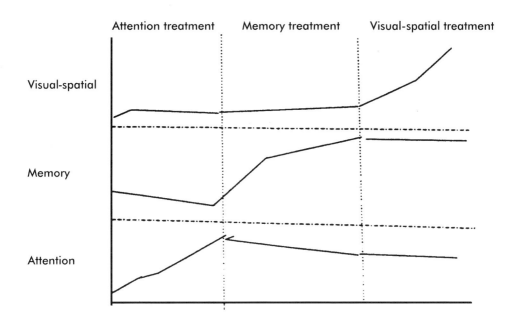

FIGURE 20–1. Multiple baseline design for the treatment of a patient with brain injury and deficits in attention, memory, and visual-spatial processing.

Attention, memory, and visual-spatial skills are each treated in sequence; improvement is seen in one area before beginning the next phase of treatment, and performance in untreated skill areas is used as a comparison for the treated areas. The vertical axis represents level of performance in each skill area (visual-spatial, memory, and attention). The passage of time is represented on the horizontal axis. The dotted vertical lines are those times at which treatment was switched from the previous focus to the current focus, such as from attention training to memory training.

cognitive-retraining exercises were implemented and taught to the patient and his family so that home practice could take place on a daily basis. The family was instructed in the methods used to record the scores from the exercises, which were then entered into a daily log.

The cognitive retraining was conducted according to a design in which multiple baselines across behaviors were used. Cognitive-retraining treatment was first aimed at improving attention and memory with a set of four exercises implemented both during outpatient appointments and at home. An assessment conducted on both of the targeted treatment areas of memory and abstraction and planning skills indicated improvement in the memory realm but not in the abstraction and

planning realm. During the second phase, treatment was aimed at improving abstraction and planning skills with a set of exercises that were again implemented during outpatient appointments and at home. Evaluations during this phase indicated improvement in abstraction and planning skills but no further improvement in memory skills. A complete neuropsychologic battery of tests was administered at the first contact and again after the termination of treatment. Additionally, short tests of relevant neuropsychologic function were administered before the initiation of treatment, at each phase change, and at the termination of treatment. The results of the standardized neuropsychologic tests were consistent with the behavioral monitoring conducted on the skill exercises, namely, improvement in attention and memory as a result of the treatment in the first phase and improvement in abstraction and planning skills as a result of the treatment in the second phase.

Conclusions

Neuropsychologic and behavioral dysfunction associated with brain injury can be varied and complex. Effective intervention requires an integrated interdisciplinary approach that focuses on the individual patient and his or her specific needs. Behaviorally based formulations can provide a valuable framework from which to understand the interaction between an individual with compromised physical, neuropsychologic, and emotional functioning, as well as the psychosocial environment in which he or she is trying to adjust.

Much work remains to define the most effective cognitive and behaviorally based treatments for various neuropsychiatric disorders. The evidence to date suggests that this area is indeed an area worthy of continued pursuit.

References

Alderman N, Knight C: The effectiveness of DRL in the management of severe behaviour disorders following brain injury. Brain Inj 11:79–101, 1997

Azouvi P, Jokic C, Attal N, et al: Carbamazepine in agitation and aggressive behaviour following severe closed-head injury. Brain Inj 13:797–804, 1999

Bandura A: Social Learning Theory. Englewood Cliffs, NJ, Prentice-Hall, 1977

Basso A, Capotani E, Vignolo L: Influence of rehabilitation on language skills in aphasic patients. Arch Neurol 36:190–196, 1979

Bellack AS, Hersen M: General considerations, in Handbook of Clinical Behavior Therapy With Adults. Edited by Hersen M, Bellack AS. New York, Plenum, 1985a, pp 3–19

Bellack AS, Hersen M: Dictionary of Behavior Therapy Techniques. New York, Pergamon, 1985b

Bellack AS, Mueser KT: Psychosocial treatment for schizophrenia. Schizophr Bull 19:317–336, 1993

Benedict RH, Harris AE, Markow T, et al: Effects of attention training on information processing in schizophrenia. Schizophr Bull 20:537–546, 1994

Ben-Yishay Y, Diller L: Rehabilitation of cognitive and perceptual deficits in people with traumatic brain damage. Int J Rehabil Res 4:208–210, 1981

Ben-Yishay Y, Diller L: Cognitive deficits, in Rehabilitation of the Head-Injured Adult. Edited by Griffith EA, Bond M, Miller J. Philadelphia, PA, FA Davis, 1983, pp 167–183

Bond M: The psychiatry of closed head injury, in Closed Head Injury: Psychosocial, Social and Family Consequences. Edited by Brooks N. New York, Oxford University Press, 1984, pp 148–178

Calhoun KS, Turner SM: Historical perspectives and current issues in behavior therapy, in Handbook of Clinical Behavior Therapy. Edited by Turner SM, Calhoun KS, Adams HE. New York, Wiley, 1981, pp 1–11

Crovitz H, Harvey M, Horn R: Problems in the acquisition of imagery mnemonics: three brain damaged cases. Cortex 15:225–234, 1979

Dikmen S, McLean A, Temkin N: Neuropsychological and psychosocial consequences of minor head injury. J Neurol Neurosurg Psychiatry 49:1227–1232, 1986

Diller L, Weinberg J: Hemi-inattention in rehabilitation: the evolution of a rational remediation program. Adv Neurol 18:63–82, 1977

Eames P: Behavior disorders after severe head injury: their nature, causes and strategies for management. J Head Trauma Rehabil 3:1–6, 1988

Eames P, Wood R: Rehabilitation after severe brain injury: a follow-up study of a behavior modification approach. J Neurol Neurosurg Psychiatry 48:613–619, 1985

Edelstein BA, Couture ET: Behavioral Assessment and Rehabilitation of the Traumatically Brain-Damaged. New York, Plenum, 1984

Flesher S: Cognitive habilitation in schizophrenia: a theoretical review and model of treatment. Neuropsychol Rev 1:223–246, 1990

Franzen MD: Behavioral assessment and treatment of brain-impaired individuals, in Progress in Behavior Modification. Edited by Hersen M, Eisler RM. Newbury Park, CA, Sage, 1991, pp 56–85

Franzen MD, Harris CV: Neuropsychological rehabilitation: application of a modified multiple baseline design. Brain Inj 7:525–534, 1993

Franzen MD, Haut MW: The psychological treatment of memory impairment: a review of empirical studies. Neuropsychol Rev 2:29–63, 1991

Franzen MD, Iverson GL: Applications of single subject design to cognitive rehabilitation, in Neuropsychology Across the Lifespan. Edited by Horton AM. New York, Springer, 1990, pp 155–174

Franzen MD, Lovell MR: Behavioral treatments of aggressive sequelae of brain injury. Psychiatr Ann 17:389–396, 1987

Galski T, Ehle HT, Williams JB: Off-road driving evaluations for persons with cerebral injury: a factor analytic study of predriver and simulator testing. Am J Occup Ther 51:352–359, 1997

Gardner H: The Shattered Mind: The Person After Brain Damage. London, Routledge & Kegan Paul, 1977

Gianutsos R, Matheson P: The rehabilitation of visual perceptual disorders attributable to brain injury, in Neuropsychological Rehabilitation. Edited by Meier MJ, Benton AL, Diller L. New York, Guilford, 1987, pp 202–241

Gianutsos R, Glosser D, Elbaum J, et al: Visual imperception in brain injured adults: multifaceted measures. Arch Phys Med Rehabil 64:456–461, 1983

Giles GM, Pussey I, Burgess P: The behavioral treatment of verbal interaction skills following severe head injury: a single case study. Brain Inj 2:75–79, 1988

Giles GM, Ridley JE, Dill A, et al: A consecutive series of adults with brain injury treated with a washing and dressing retraining program. Am J Occup Ther 51:256–266, 1997

Glasgow RE, Zeiss RA, Barrera M, et al: Case studies on remediating memory deficits in brain damaged individuals. J Clin Psychol 33:1049–1054, 1977

Glen MB: Methylphenidate for cognitive and behavioral dysfunction after traumatic brain injury. J Head Trauma Rehabil 13:87–90, 1998

Glisky EL, Schacter DL: Remediation of organic memory disorders: current status and future prospects. J Head Trauma Rehabil 4:54–63, 1986

Goldstein FC, Levin HS: Disorders of reasoning and problem solving ability, in Neuropsychological Rehabilitation. Edited by Meier MJ, Benton AL, Diller L. New York, Guilford, 1987, pp 327–354

Goldstein G, Ruthven L: Rehabilitation of the Brain-Damaged Adult. New York, Plenum, 1983

Gordon W, Hibbard M, Egelko S, et al: Perceptual remediation in patients with right brain damage: a comprehensive program. Arch Phys Med Rehabil 66:353–359, 1985

Gouvier WD, Webster JS, Blanton PD: Cognitive retraining with brain damaged patients, in The Neuropsychology Handbook: Behavioral and Clinical Perspectives. Edited by Wedding D, Horton AM, Webster J. New York, Springer, 1986, pp 278–324

Grant I, Alves W: Psychiatric and psychosocial disturbances in head injury, in Neurobehavioral Recovery From Head Injury. Edited by Levin HS, Grafman J, Eisenberg HM. New York, Oxford University Press, 1987, pp 222–246

Grimm BH, Bleiberg J: Psychological rehabilitation in traumatic brain injury, in Handbook of Clinical Neuropsychology, Vol 2. Edited by Filskov SB, Boll TJ. New York, Wiley, 1986, pp 495–560

Gross Y, Schutz LF: Intervention models in neuropsychology, in Clinical Neuropsychology of Intervention. Edited by Uzzell BP, Gross Y. Boston, MA, Martinus Highoff, 1986, pp 179–204

Gualtieri CT: Pharmacotherapy and the neurobehavioral sequelae of traumatic brain injury. Brain Inj 2:101–109, 1988

Harris JE: Methods of improving memory, in Clinical Management of Memory Problems. Edited by Wilson BA, Moffat N. Rockville, MD, Aspen, 1984, pp 46–62

Haynes SN: Behavioral assessment of adults, in Handbook of Psychological Assessment. Edited by Goldstein G, Hersen M. New York, Pergamon, 1984, pp 369–401

Hegel MT, Ferguson RJ: Differential reinforcement of other behavior (DRO) to reduce aggressive behavior following traumatic brain injury. Behav Modif 24:94–101, 2000

Hersen M, Bellack AS: Handbook of Clinical Behavior Therapy With Adults. New York, Plenum, 1985

Hersen M, Bellack AS: Dictionary of Behavioral Assessment Techniques. New York, Pergamon, 1988

Ho MR, Bennett TL: Efficacy of neuropsychological rehabilitation of mild-moderate traumatic brain injury. Arch Clin Neuropsychol 12:1–11, 1997

Holzer JC: Buspirone and brain injury (letter). J Neuropsychiatry Clin Neurosci 10:113, 1998

Horton AM, Barrett D: Neuropsychological assessment and behavior therapy: new directions in head trauma rehabilitation. J Head Trauma Rehabil 3:57–64, 1988

Horton AM, Miller WA: Neuropsychology and behavior therapy, in Progress in Behavior Modifications. Edited by Hersen M, Eisler R, Miller PM. New York, Academic Press, 1985, pp 1–55

Kazdin AE: Fictions, factions, and functions of behavior therapy. Behav Ther 10:629–654, 1979

Khouzam HR, Donnelly NJ: Remission of traumatic brain injury-induced compulsions during venlafaxine treatment. Gen Hosp Psychiatry 20:62–63, 1998

Kolata G: Brain-grafting work shows promise (letter). Science 221:1277, 1983

Kraus MF, Maki M: Effect of amantadine hydrochloride on symptoms of frontal lobe dysfunction in brain injury: case studies and review. J Neuropsychiatry Clin Neurosci 9:222–230, 1997

Levin HS, Grossman RG: Behavioral sequelae of closed head injury: a quantitative study. Arch Neurol 35:720–727, 1978

Levin HS, Grossman RG, Ross JE, et al: Long-term neuropsychological outcome of closed head injury. J Neurosurg 50:412–422, 1979

Levin HS, Benton AL, Grossman RG: Neurobehavioral Consequences of Closed Head Injury. New York, Oxford University Press, 1982

Levin HS, Mattis S, Ruff R, et al: Neurobehavioral outcome following minor head injury: a three center study. J Neurosurg 66:234–243, 1987

Lewis FD, Nelson J, Nelson C, et al: Effects of three feedback contingencies on the socially inappropriate talk of a brain-injured adult. Behavior Therapy 19:203–211, 1988

Lezak MD: Neuropsychological Assessment, 3rd Edition. New York, Oxford University Press, 1995

Liepert J, Bauder H, Miltner WHR, et al: Treatment-induced cortical reorganization after stroke in humans. Stroke 31(6):1210–1216, 2000

Lishman WA: Organic Psychiatry. St. Louis, MO, Blackwell Scientific, 1978

Luria AR: Restoration of Function After Brain Injury. New York, Macmillan, 1963

Luria AR, Tsvetkova LS: The Neuropsychological Analysis of Problem Solving. Orlando, FL, Paul Deutsch, 1990

McIntosh GC: Medical management of noncognitive sequelae of minor traumatic brain injury. Appl Neuropsychol 4:62–68, 1997

Medd J, Tate RL: Evaluation of anger management therapy programme following acquired brain injury: a preliminary study. Neuropsychological Rehabilitation 10: 185–201, 2000

Meier MJ, Strauman S, Thompson WG: Individual differences in neuropsychological recovery: an overview, in Neuropsychological Rehabilitation. Edited by Meier MJ, Benton AL, Diller L. New York, Guilford, 1987, pp 71–110

Mendez MF, Nakawatase TV, Brown CV: Involuntary laughter and inappropriate hilarity. J Neuropsychiatry Clin Neurosci 11:253–258, 1999

Moffat N: Strategies of memory therapy, in Clinical Management of Memory Problems. Edited by Wilson BA, Moffat N. Rockville, MD, Aspen, 1984, pp 63–88

Mungas D: Psychometric correlates of episodic violent behavior: a multidimensional neuropsychological approach. Br J Psychiatry 152:180–187, 1988

NIH Consensus Statement: Rehabilitation of Persons With Traumatic Brain Injury. NIH Consens Statement 16(1):1–141, October 26–28, 1998

Patten BM: The ancient art of memory. Arch Neurol 26:25–31, 1972

Persel CS, Persel CH, Ashley MJ, et al: The use of noncontingent reinforcement and contingent restrain to reduce physical aggression and self-injurious behaviour in a traumatically brain injured adult. Brain Inj 11:751–760, 1997

Posner HI, Rafal RD: Cognitive theories of attention and the rehabilitation of attentional deficits, in Neuropsychological Rehabilitation. Edited by Meier MJ, Benton AL, Diller L. New York, Guilford, 1987, pp 182–201

Prigatano GP: Personality and psychosocial consequences after brain injury, in Neuropsychological Rehabilitation. Edited by Meier MJ, Benton AL, Diller L. New York, Guilford, 1987, pp 355–378

Robertson-Tchabo EA, Hausman CP, Arenberg D: A classical mnemonic for older learners: a trip that works. Educational Gerontologist 1:215–216, 1976

Robinson RG: Neuropsychiatric consequences of stroke. Annu Rev Med 48:217–229, 1997

Rosenthal M: Behavioral sequelae, in Rehabilitation of the Head Injured Adult. Edited by Rosenthal M, Griffith ER, Bond MR, et al. Philadelphia, PA, FA Davis, 1983, pp 297–308

Schmitter-Edgecombe M, Fahy JF, Whelan JP, et al: Memory remediation after severe closed head injury: notebook training versus supportive therapy. J Consult Clin Psychol 63:484–489, 1995

Schneider WN, Drew-Cates J, Wong TM, et al: Cognitive and behavioural efficacy of amantadine in acute traumatic brain injury: an initial double-blind placebo-controlled study. Brain Inj 13:863–872, 1999

Seron X: Operant procedures and neuropsychological rehabilitation, in Neuropsychological Rehabilitation. Edited by Meier MJ, Benton AL, Diller L. New York, Guilford, 1987, pp 132–161

Sivak M, Hill C, Henson D, et al: Improved driving performance following perceptual training of persons with brain damage. Arch Phys Med Rehabil 65:163–167, 1985

Stuss DT, Benson DF: Neuropsychological studies of the frontal lobes. Psychol Bull 95:3–28, 1984

Suzman KB, Morris RD, Morris MK, et al: Cognitive remediation of problem solving deficits in children with acquired brain injury. J Behav Ther Exp Psychiatry 28:203–212, 1997

Wall P, Egger M: Mechanisms of plasticity of new connection following brain damage in adult mammalian nervous systems, in Recovery of Function: Theoretical Considerations for Brain Injury Rehabilitation. Edited by Bach-y-Rita P. Baltimore, MD, Park, 1971, pp 117–129

Weddell R, Oddy M, Jenkins D: Social adjustment after rehabilitation: a two year follow up of patients with severe head injury. Psychol Med 10:257–263, 1980

Williams SE, Ris DM, Ayyangar R, et al: Recovery in pediatric brain injury: is psychostimulant medication beneficial? J Head Trauma Rehabil 13:73–81, 1998

Wilson B: Success and failure in memory training following a cerebral vascular accident. Cortex 18:581–594, 1982

Wilson B: Identification and remediation of everyday problems in memory-impaired patients, in Neuropsychology of Alcoholism: Implications for Diagnosis and Treatment. Edited by Parsons GA, Butters N, Nathan PE. New York, Guilford, 1987, pp 322–338

Wood RL: Behavior disorders following severe brain injury: their presentation and psychological management, in Closed Head Injury: Psychological, Social and Family Consequences. Edited by Brooks N. New York, Oxford University Press, 1984, pp 195–219

Wroblewski BA, Joseph AB, Kupfer J, et al: Effectiveness of valproic acid on destructive and aggressive behaviours in patients with acquired brain injury. Brain Inj 11: 37-47, 1997.

Index

Page numbers printed in **boldface** type refer to tables or figures.

F

J

M

X

Y

Z

Reproduction of Color Figures

CHAPTER 3
Clinical Imaging in Neuropsychiatry

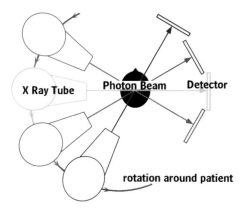

FIGURE 3–2. Schematic of conventional computed tomography X-ray tube and detector.

Note the simultaneous circular movement of both devices about the head.

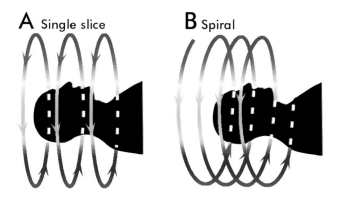

FIGURE 3–4. Schematic of computed tomography (CT) scanning path.

Panel A. Conventional CT. *Panel B.* Helical (spiral) CT. Note the continuous overlapping helical path in spiral CT.

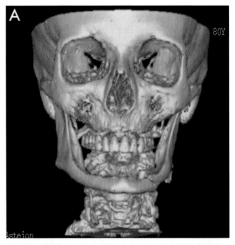

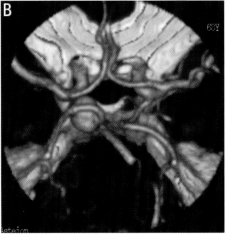

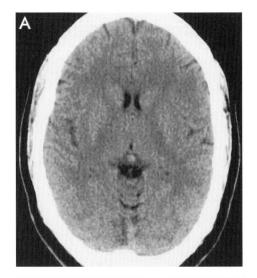

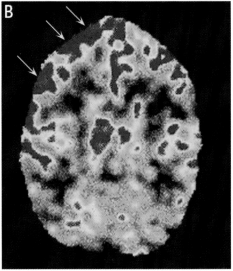

FIGURE 3–5. Three-dimensional reconstruction from helical computed tomography (CT).

Current CT scanners can acquire extremely detailed data sets in a matter of seconds. The data can be viewed as three-dimensional volume images from any desired angle. Reconstructions of bone (*Panel A*) are valuable both for diagnosis and for surgical planning. CT angiography, such as this view of an aneurysm in the circle of Willis (*Panel B*), is capable of displaying vessels from any angle. Since scanning is very rapid and noninvasive, such examinations may be performed in place of conventional angiograms.
Source. Images courtesy of Toshiba America Medical Systems, Inc.

FIGURE 3–6. Imaging of acute stroke in a 52-year-old woman who presented with left-sided weakness.

Computed tomographic (CT) images acquired 1.5 hours after onset (*Panel A*) were normal. Companion xenon-enhanced CT images (*Panel B*) showed luxury perfusion on the right (arrows), indicating that the area of the stroke had already reperfused. Magnetic resonance images acquired the next day were normal.
Source. Images courtesy of Ben Taub General Hospital, Houston, TX.

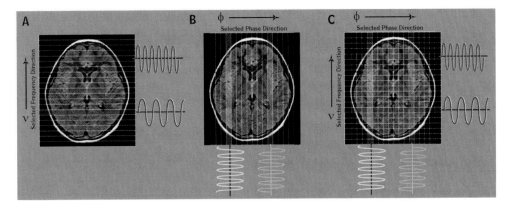

FIGURE 3–8. Origin of the imaging grid.

Panel A. Sample magnetic resonance image is overlaid with rows created by a read (frequency-encoding) gradient. *Panel B.* Sample magnetic resonance image is overlaid with columns created by a phase gradient. *Panel C.* Sample magnetic resonance image is overlaid with the grid created by the frequency and phase gradients. The computer uses the combination of frequency and phase to identify the signal from each block in the grid.

CHAPTER 4
Functional Neuroimaging in Psychiatry

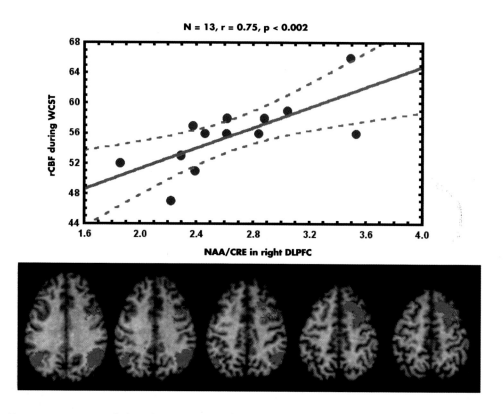

FIGURE 4–1. Correlations between metabolite ratios for the dorsolateral prefrontal cortex (DLPFC) of 13 schizophrenic patients and blood flow activation during performance of the Wisconsin Card Sorting Test (WCST).

The bottom part of the figure shows the brain locations of maximal positive correlations between blood flow activation during the WCST and the ratio of N-acetyl aspartate to creatine (NAA/CRE). The top portion shows the correlations between NAA/CRE and regional cerebral blood flow (rCBF) in the DLPFC.

Source.　　Reprinted with permission from Bertolino A, Esposito G, Callicott JH, et al.: "Specific Relationship Between Prefrontal Neuronal N-Acetylaspartate and Activation of the Working Memory Cortical Network in Schizophrenia." *American Journal of Psychiatry* 157:26–33, 2000.

CHAPTER 14
Neuropsychiatric Aspects of Alzheimer's Disease and Other Dementing Illnesses

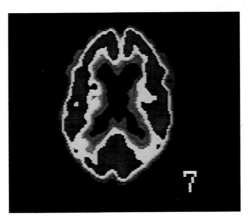

FIGURE 14–2. Transaxial single photon emission computed tomography (SPECT) of a patient with Alzheimer's disease revealing diminished cerebral perfusion in the temporoparietal regions bilaterally.

Red areas indicate normal blood flow, and yellow regions indicate diminished perfusion.

Source. Image courtesy of Dr. Ismael Mena.

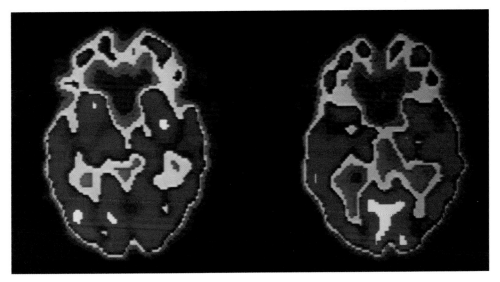

FIGURE 14–3. Transaxial single photon emission computed tomography (SPECT) of a patient with frontal lobe degeneration demonstrating decreased cerebral blood flow in the frontal lobes.

Red areas indicate normal blood flow, and yellow regions indicate diminished perfusion.

CHAPTER 15
Neuropsychiatric Aspects of Schizophrenia

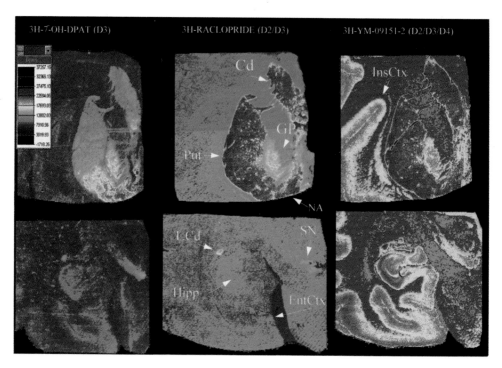

FIGURE 15–2. Binding of three different dopamine receptor ligands in human brain tissue to illustrate the localization of the dopamine type 2 (D$_2$) family receptors.

The top row includes three contiguous slices taken from a midstriatal coronal brain section; the bottom row includes three contiguous slices taken from an inferior midhippocampal coronal brain section. The left column shows binding of [^{3}H]7-OH DPAT, a ligand that labels dopamine type 3 (D$_3$) receptors, in both of these areas. D$_3$ receptors are localized chiefly in the inferior striatum nucleus accumbens (NA) and substantia nigra pars compacta (SN). The middle column shows binding of ^{3}H-raclopride, a ligand labeling D$_2$ and D$_3$ receptors. D$_2$ receptors are densely represented in the caudate nucleus (Cd) and putamen (Put) and are even apparent in the tail of the caudate nucleus (T.Cd); D$_2$ and D$_3$ receptors are intermingled in the nucleus accumbens and substantia nigra. The right column shows binding of [^{3}H]YM-09151-2, a ligand labeling D$_2$, D$_3$, and dopamine type 4 (D$_4$) receptors, in the two regions. A "mental" subtraction of the middle from the right autoradiograph suggests the D$_4$ localization to be predominantly in neocortex (InsCtx), hippocampus (Hipp), and entorhinal cortex (EntCtx). This illustration suggests that the D$_2$ receptor is predominantly localized in the caudate nucleus and putamen; the D$_2$ and D$_3$ receptors are localized in the nucleus accumbens and substantia nigra; and the D$_4$ receptor is predominant in the neocortex and in the hippocampal and parahippocampal cortices.
Source. Autoradiograph contributed by Dr. Robert Lahti.

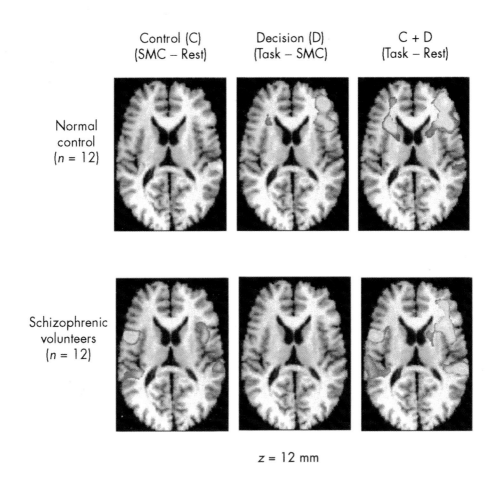

FIGURE 15–4. Regional cerebral blood flow elevations seen at an axial level 12 mm above the anterior commissure–posterior commissure (ACPC) line in healthy control (*top row*) and schizophrenic (*bottom row*) subjects, each in a sensorimotor control (SMC) (*left column*) and a decision performance (*middle column*) condition.

Control subjects merely activate the auditory cortex bilaterally (*upper left scan*) and the left motor cortex (data not shown) in the sensorimotor task, whereas the schizophrenic subjects activate those more and in more areas than control subjects (*bottom left scan*). During the decision task, the control subjects activate middle and inferior frontal cortex (*upper middle scan*) and anterior cingulate gyrus (data not shown); however the schizophrenic subjects do not recruit any additional areas or increase flow at all in their decision condition (*lower middle scan*). Overall, the schizophrenic subjects resemble the control subjects in the "task minus rest" analysis (*upper and lower right scans*), even though that activation occurred primarily in the control, not the decision, scan.

Source.   Images contributed by Dr. Henry Holcomb and Dr. Adrienne Lahti.

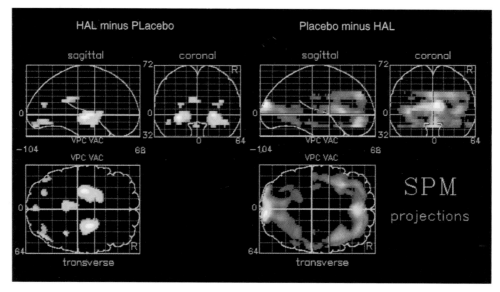

FIGURE 15-5. Projection images showing significant areas of haloperidol (HAL)–induced increases (*left*) and decreases (*right*) in regional cerebral metabolic rate for glucose (rCMRglu) from group subtraction Statistical Parametric Mapping (SPM) analyses, in within-subject comparisons.

On the left, rCMRglu increases are apparent in the caudate nucleus, putamen, and anterior thalamus; on the right, rCMRglu decreases are apparent in anterior cingulate gyrus, occipital area, and frontal cortex (middle and inferior gyri).

VAC = vertical anterior commissure line; VPC = vertical posterior commissure line.

Source. Images contributed by Dr. Henry Holcomb.

SPM, p<0.01, N=5,6 minutes

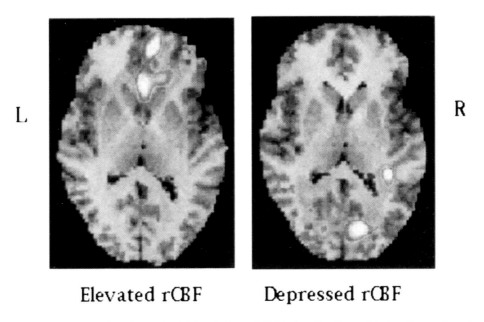

L   R

Elevated rCBF   Depressed rCBF

FIGURE 15–6. Regional cerebral blood flow (rCBF) localization of ketamine action in schizophrenic brain.

rCBF increases occurred in anterior cingulate gyrus, extending to medial frontal areas (*left scan*); rCBF decreases are apparent in hippocampus and in the lingual gyrus (*right scan*). The colored areas indicating significant flow change are plotted onto a magnetic resonance imaging template for ease of localization.

SPM = Statistical Parametric Mapping.

Source. Images contributed by Dr. Henry Holcomb and Dr. Adrienne Lahti.

CHAPTER 17
Neuropsychiatric Aspects of Anxiety Disorders

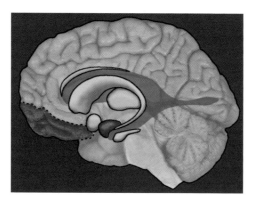

FIGURE 17–1. Neuroanatomic model of generalized anxiety disorder.

Note the increased activity in temporolimbic areas as well as in prefrontal areas.

Source. Reprinted from Stein DJ: *False Alarm!: How to Conquer the Anxiety Disorders.* Cape Town, South Africa, University of Stellenbosch, 2000. Used with permission.

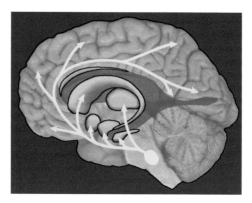

FIGURE 17–2. Serotonergic circuits project to key regions involved in the mediation of anxiety disorders: prefrontal cortex, orbitofrontal cortex, anterior cingulate, amygdala, hippocampus, basal ganglia, thalamus.

Source. Reprinted from Stein DJ: *False Alarm!: How to Conquer the Anxiety Disorders.* Cape Town, South Africa, University of Stellenbosch, 2000. Used with permission.

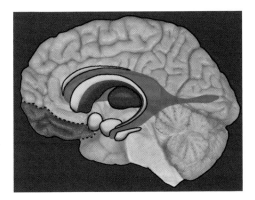

FIGURE 17–3. Neuroanatomic model of obsessive-compulsive disorder.

Note the increased activity in the ventromedial cortico-striatal-thalamic-cortical circuit.

Source. Reprinted from Stein DJ: *False Alarm!: How to Conquer the Anxiety Disorders.* Cape Town, South Africa, University of Stellenbosch, 2000. Used with permission.

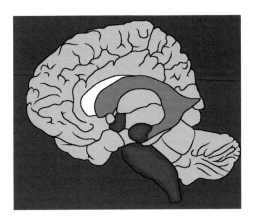

FIGURE 17–4. Neuroanatomic model of panic disorder.

Note the activation of the amygdala, which has efferents to hypothalamus and brain stem sites.

Source. Reprinted from Stein DJ: *False Alarm!: How to Conquer the Anxiety Disorders.* Cape Town, South Africa, University of Stellenbosch, 2000. Used with permission.

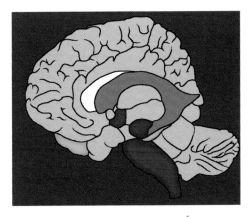

FIGURE 17–5. Neuroanatomic model of posttraumatic stress disorder.

Note the increased activity in the amygdala and its efferents (Rauch et al. 1996), decreased activity in Broca's area (Shin et al. 1997), and decreased volume of the hippocampus (Bremner et al. 1997; M.B. Stein et al. 1997).

Source. Reprinted from Stein DJ: *False Alarm!: How to Conquer the Anxiety Disorders.* Cape Town, South Africa, University of Stellenbosch, 2000. Used with permission.

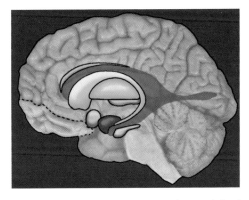

FIGURE 17–6. Neuroanatomic model of social phobia.

Note the increased temporolimbic activity, decreased basal ganglia dopaminergic activity, and perhaps some increased prefrontal activity.

Source. Reprinted from Stein DJ: *False Alarm!: How to Conquer the Anxiety Disorders.* Cape Town, South Africa, University of Stellenbosch, 2000. Used with permission.